American Academy of Orthopaedic Surgeons
American Academy of Pediatrics

2ND Edition

# ESSENTIALS
*of*
## Musculoskeletal Care

WALTER B. GREENE, MD
EDITOR

Published 2001
by the American Academy of Orthopaedic Surgeons
6300 North River Road
Rosemont, Illinois 60018

Second Edition
Copyright ©2001
by the American Academy of Orthopaedic Surgeons

The material presented in Essentials of Musculoskeletal Care, Second Edition, has been made available by the American Academy of Orthopaedic Surgeons (AAOS) for educational purposes only. This material is not intended to present the only, or necessarily best, methods or procedures for the medical situations discussed, but rather is intended to represent an approach, view, statement, or opinion of the author(s) or producer(s), which may be helpful to others who face similar situations. The recommendations in this publication do not indicate an exclusive course of treatment or serve as a standard of medical care. Variations, taking into account individual circumstances, may be appropriate.

Some drugs or medical devices demonstrated in AAOS courses or described in AAOS print or electronic publications have not been cleared by the Food and Drug Administration (FDA) or have been cleared for specific uses only. The FDA has stated that it is the responsibility of the physician to determine the FDA clearance status of each drug or device he or she wishes to use in clinical practice.

Furthermore, any statements about commercial products are solely the opinion(s) of the author(s) and do not represent an AAOS endorsement or evaluation of these products. These statements may not be used in advertising or for any commercial purpose.

ISBN 0-89203-217-0

Printed in the U.S.A.

Second printing, 2001

Library of Congress Cataloging-in-Publication Data

Essentials of musculoskeletal care / American Academy of Orthopaedic Surgeons; Walter B. Greene, editor—2nd ed.
    p. ; cm.
    Includes index.
    ISBN 0-89203-217-0
1. Pediatric orthopedics. I. Greene, Walter B. II. American Academy of Orthopaedic Surgeons.
[DNLM: 1. Musculoskeletal Diseases—diagnosis. 2. Musculoskeletal Diseases—therapy. 3. Orthopedics—methods. WE 140 E78 2000]

RD732.3.C48 E87 2000
616.7—dc21
00-067658

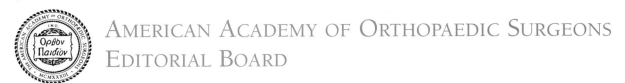
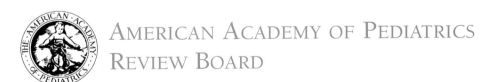

Essentials of Musculoskeletal Care *is dedicated to Robert K. Snider, MD, the editor and cultivator of the first edition and section editor of this edition, who died unexpectedly in March 2001.  Bob routinely epitomized the highest qualities of medical care, medical professionalism, and true friendship. His goodness and love of life is missed by all who knew him.*

# Contributors

William H. Anderson, Jr, MD
Department of Rehabilitation Medicine
St. Vincent Hospital and Health Center
Billings, Montana

David D. Aronsson, MD
Professor
Department of Orthopaedics and Rehabilitation
Department of Pediatrics
University of Vermont College of Medicine
Burlington, Vermont

Richard A. Balderston, MD
Philadelphia, Pennsylvania

Judith F. Baumhauer, MD
Associate Professor
Chief, Division of Foot and Ankle Surgery
Department of Orthopaedics
University of Rochester School of Medicine and Dentistry
Rochester, New York

Robert M. Bernstein, MD
Assistant Chief of Staff
Shriners Hospitals for Children—Los Angeles
Los Angeles, California

Daniel J. Berry, MD
Associate Professor of Orthopedics
Mayo Medical School
Consultant in Orthopedic Surgery, Mayo Clinic
Department of Orthopedic Surgery
Mayo Foundation
Rochester, Minnesota

Kevin P. Black, MD
Associate Professor and Vice Chairman
Department of Orthopaedics and Rehabilitation
Penn State University College of Medicine
Hershey, Pennsylvania

R. Dale Blasier, MD
Professor of Orthopaedic Surgery and Pediatrics
Division of Pediatric Orthopaedics
University of Arkansas for Medical Sciences
Little Rock, Arkansas

Darrel S. Brodke, MD
Assistant Professor
Department of Orthopedics
University of Utah Health Sciences Center
Salt Lake City, Utah

Robert D. Bronstein, MD
Associate Professor
Department of Orthopaedics
University of Rochester School of Medicine and Dentistry
Rochester, New York

Bruce R. Buhr, MD
Clinical Instructor
Section of Orthopaedics
University of Kansas Medical School—Wichita
Wichita, Kansas

Robert M. Campbell, Jr, MD
Associate Profesor
Department of Orthopaedics
University of Texas Health Science Center
San Antonio, Texas

Andrew J. Cosgarea, MD
Associate Professor
Department of Orthopaedic Surgery
Johns Hopkins University
Baltimore, Maryland

Jon R. Davids, MD
Director, Motion Analysis Laboratory
Orthopaedic Department
Shriners Hospitals for Children—Greenville
Greenville, South Carolina

Frederick R. Dietz, MD
Professor
Department of Orthopaedic Surgery
University of Iowa College of Medicine
Iowa City, Iowa

James C. Drennan, MD
Professor
Department of Orthopaedics and Rehabilitation
University of New Mexico School of Medicine
Albuquerque, New Mexico

William D. Engber, MD
Associate Professor
Department of Orthopedic Surgery
University of Wisconsin Medical School
Madison, Wisconsin

Marybeth Ezaki, MD
Associate Professor
Department of Orthopaedic Surgery
University of Texas Southwestern Medical School
Texas Scottish Rite Hospital for Children
Dallas, Texas

# CONTRIBUTORS

Jeffrey S. Fischgrund, MD
Attending Spine Surgeon
Department of Orthopaedics
William Beaumont Hospital
Royal Oak, Michigan

Keith R. Gabriel, MD
Assistant Chief of Staff
Shriners Hospitals for Children—Twin Cities
Minneapolis, Minnesota

Kevin L. Garvin, MD, FACS
Professor and Chairman
Department of Orthopaedic Surgery and Rehabilitation
University of Nebraska Medical Center
Omaha, Nebraska

Gaia Georgopoulos, MD
Associate Professor
Department of Orthopaedic Surgery
University of Colorado Health Sciences Center
Denver, Colorado

W. Lea Gorsuch, MD
Great Falls Orthopaedic Associates
Great Falls, Michigan

Merlin L. Hamer, MD
LaJolla, California

Harry N. Herkowitz, MD
Chairman
Department of Orthopaedics
William Beaumont Hospital
Royal Oak, Michigan

M. Mark Hoffer, MD
Lowman Professor
Orthopedic Hospital
Los Angeles, California

Walter W. Huurman, MD
Professor
Orthopaedic Surgery and Pediatrics
Department of Orthopaedic Surgery and Rehabilitation
University of Nebraska Medical Center
Omaha, Nebraska

Charles D. Jennings, MD
Great Falls Orthopaedic Associates
Great Falls, Michigan

Bert Jones, MD
Flathead Valley Orthopedics
Kalispell, Montana

Kosmas J. Kayes, MD
Assistant Professor, Pediatric Orthopedics
Department of Orthopaedic Surgery
Indiana University School of Medicine
Indianapolis, Indiana

Kenneth J. Koval, MD
Associate Professor
Department of Orthopaedics
New York University School of Medicine
New York, New York

Thomas H. Lee, MD
Clinical Assistant Professor
Director, Division of Foot and Ankle
Department of Orthopaedics
The Ohio State University Medical Center
Columbus, Ohio

Alan M. Levine, MD
Director, Alvin and Lois Lapidus Cancer Institute
Head, Division of Orthopedic Oncology at Sinai Hospital
Clinical Professor
Orthopaedic Surgery and Oncology
University of Maryland School of Medicine
Baltimore, Maryland

James T. Lovitt, MD
Billings, Montana

Michael D. Maloney, MD
Assistant Professor
Department of Orthopaedics
University of Rochester School of Medicine and Dentistry
Rochester, New York

Gregory S. McDowell, MD
Co-Director, Northern Rockies Regional
     Spine Injury Center
Orthopaedic Surgeons, PSC
St. Vincent Hospital and Health Center
Billings, Montana

Vincent S. Mosca, MD
Associate Professor and Chief of Pediatric Orthopedics
University of Washington School of Medicine
Director, Department of Orthopedics
Children's Hospital and Regional Medical Center
Seattle, Washington

# CONTRIBUTORS

Prasit Nimityongskul, MD
Professor and Interim Chair
Department of Orthopaedic Surgery
University of South Alabama College of Medicine
Mobile, Alabama

Brad W. Olney, MD
Clinical Professor
Section of Orthopaedics
University of Kansas Medical School—Wichita
Wichita, Kansas

Martin J. O'Malley, MD
Assistant Professor of Orthopaedic Surgery
Department of Surgery
Weill Medical College of Cornell University
Hospital for Special Surgery
New York, New York

William L. Oppenheim, MD
Professor and Head, Pediatric Orthopedics
Department of Orthopaedic Surgery
UCLA Medical Center
Los Angeles, California

Robert M. Orfaly, MD, FRCSC
Assistant Professor
Department of Orthopaedics and Rehabilitation
Oregon Health Sciences University
Portland, Oregon

John D. Osland, MD
Associate Clinical Professor
Section of Orthopaedics
University of Kansas School of Medicine—Wichita
Wichita, Kansas

Hamlet A. Peterson, MD, MS
Emeritus Professor of Orthopedic Surgery
Mayo Medical School
Division of Pediatric Orthopaedic Surgery
Mayo Clinic
Rochester, Minnesota

William A. Phillips, MD
Professor, Orthopaedics and Pediatrics
Chief, Pediatric Orthopaedics and Scoliosis
Baylor College of Medicine
Texas Children's Hospital
Houston, Texas

Michael S. Pinzur, MD
Professor
Department of Orthopaedic Surgery and Rehabilitation
Loyola University Health System
Maywood, Illinois

Peter D. Pizzutillo, MD
Director
Department of Orthopaedic Surgery
St. Christopher's Hospital for Children
Philadelphia, Pennsylvania

Charles A. Rockwood, Jr, MD
Professor and Chairman Emeritus
Department of Orthopaedics
University of Texas Health Science Center
San Antonio, Texas

Thomas L. Schmidt, MD
Chief and Professor
Pediatric Orthopaedic Surgery
The Children's Mercy Hospital
Kansas City, Missouri

Perry L. Schoenecker, MD
Chief of Staff
Shriners Hospitals for Children—St. Louis
Professor of Orthopedic Surgery
Washington University School of Medicine
Acting Chairman of Orthopedic Surgery
St. Louis Children's Hospital
St. Louis, Missouri

James F. Schwarten, MD
Orthopaedic Surgeons, PSC
Yellowstone Medical Center
Billings, Montana

Wayne Joseph Sebastianelli, MD
Associate Professor
Department of Orthopaedics and Rehabilitation
Director of Athletic Medicine
Penn State University College of Medicine
Hershey, Pennsylvania

Kit M. Song, MD
Associate Director
Department of Orthopedics
Children's Hospital and Regional Medical Center
Seattle, Washington

# CONTRIBUTORS

George Sotiropoulos, MD
Department of Child Health
University of Missouri—Columbia Hospitals and Clinics
Columbia, Missouri

L.T. Staheli, MD
Professor Emeritus
Department of Orthopedics
University of Washington School of Medicine
Seattle, Washington

J. Andy Sullivan, MD
Professor and Don H. O'Donoghue Professor and Chair
Department of Orthopaedic Surgery
Children's Hospital of Oklahoma
Oklahoma City, Oklahoma

Michael D. Sussman, MD
Former Chief of Staff
Shriners Hospitals for Children—Portland
Portland, Oregon

Peter V. Teal, MD
Billings, Montana

George H. Thompson, MD
Director, Pediatric Orthopaedics
Rainbow Babies and Children's Hospital
Department of Orthopaedics
Case Western Reserve University School of Medicine
Cleveland, Ohio

Jeffrey D. Thomson, MD
Director
Department of Orthopaedic Surgery
Connecticut Children's Medical Center
Hartford, Connecticut

Laura L. Tosi, MD
Chairman and Associate Professor
Pediatric Orthopaedic Surgery
Children's National Medical Center
Washington, DC

James P. Waddell, MD, FRCSC
A.J. Latner Professor and Chairman
Division of Orthopaedic Surgery
University of Toronto
Toronto, Ontario, Canada

Stuart L. Weinstein, MD
Ignacio V. Ponseti Chair and Professor of Orthopaedic
    Surgery
Department of Orthopaedic Surgery
University of Iowa College of Medicine
Iowa City, Iowa

# REVIEWERS

William C. Allen, MD
Professor
Department of Orthopaedic Surgery
University of Missouri School of Medicine
Columbia, Missouri

Robert D. D'Ambrosia, MD
Chair
Department of Orthopaedic Surgery
Louisiana State University School of Medicine
New Orleans, Louisiana

B. Sonny Bal, MD, MBA
Assistant Professor
Department of Orthopaedic Surgery
University of Missouri School of Medicine
Columbia, Missouri

Mark Bernhardt, MD
Clinical Associate Professor
University of Missouri—Kansas City
Dickson-Diveley Midwest Orthopaedic Clinic
St. Luke's Hospital
Kansas City, Missouri
Kansas City Orthopaedic Institute
Leawood, Kansas

Gary E. Friedlaender, MD
Wayne O. Southwick Professor and Chair
Department of Orthopaedics and Rehabilitation
Yale University School of Medicine
New Haven, Connecticut

Barry J. Gainor, MD
Professor and Vice Chairman
Department of Orthopedic Surgery
University of Missouri School of Medicine
Columbia, Missouri

James D. Heckman, MD
Editor in Chief
The Journal of Bone and Joint Surgery
Needham, Massachusetts

James A. Hill, MD
Professor
Department of Orthopaedic Surgery
Northwestern University Medical School
Chicago, Illinois

Greg A. Horton, MD
Assistant Professor
Section of Orthopaedics
University of Kansas Medical School—Kansas City
Kansas City, Kansas

Joseph P. Iannotti, MD, PhD
Chairman
Department of Orthopaedic Surgery
The Cleveland Clinic
Cleveland, Ohio

Keith Kenter, MD
Assistant Professor
Department of Orthopaedic Surgery
University of Missouri School of Medicine
Columbia, Missouri

Joe T. Minchew, MD
Assistant Professor
Department of Orthopaedics
University of North Carolina at Chapel Hill
Chapel Hill, North Carolina

William John Robb III, MD
Senior Attending
Evanston Northwestern Healthcare
Evanston, Illinois

Thomas P. Sculco, MD
Director of Orthopaedic Surgery
Hospital for Special Surgery
New York, New York

Thomas J. Selva, MD
Assistant Professor
Department of Child Health
University of Missouri—Columbia Hospitals and Clinics
Columbia, Missouri

Robert R. Slater, Jr, MD
Assistant Clinical Professor
Department of Orthopaedic Surgery
University of California School of Medicine
Davis, California

Vernon T. Tolo, MD
John C. Wilson, Jr, Professor of Orthopaedics
University of Southern California School of Medicine
Head, Division of Orthopaedic Surgery
The Children's Hospital Los Angeles
Los Angeles, California

*To my highly respected teachers during medical school and residency and my many friends and colleagues in 22 years of practice who have patiently and enthusiastically responded to my countless queries. To my wife, Debby, and our children Samuel, Aliene, and Emily, whose love and understanding have been so pivotal during this and other projects.*

# PREFACE

*Essentials of Musculoskeletal Care* is designed as a guide and easy reference for the evaluation and management of numerous and common musculoskeletal conditions. The presentation and format are based on the premise of cooperation among medical practitioners who are working to provide excellent medical care while using the limited resources of our patients and our health care system in a judicious and effective manner. The first edition of *Essentials of Musculoskeletal Care* was developed after discussion and review with many family practitioners, pediatricians, and internists. The second edition of this book relied upon the comments of many primary care practitioners in determining changes in format and the addition of topics.

The American Academy of Orthopaedic Surgeons (AAOS) is committed to excellence in medical care. Indeed, *Essentials of Musculoskeletal Care* originated from discussions by its Publications Committee, was approved and supported by its Board of Directors, and was then produced and published by the Publications Department of AAOS. Thanks also goes to the American Academy of Pediatrics (AAP) which, as an organization, recognized the value and supported the concept of this text as the first edition was being developed. Likewise for the second edition, the AAP has reviewed and approved this text as a resource for its members.

The value of this book is largely due to the contributors who were willing to share their experience and knowledge and the time needed to write these chapters. The section editors are particularly noted for their recruitment of authors, for their individual contributions to the text, and for their ongoing help in the editing process. They are George L. Lucas, MD (General Orthopaedics), Michael A. Wirth, MD (Shoulder and Elbow),

Thomas R. Johnson, MD (Elbow and Hand), Jay R. Lieberman, MD (Hip and Thigh), Kenneth E. DeHaven, MD (Knee and Lower Leg), Glenn B. Pfeffer, MD (Foot and Ankle), and Robert K. Snider, MD (Spine). We also acknowledge the assistance of the many reviewers who offered suggestions and corrections as the manuscript was being finalized.

The quality of this book is a credit to the Publications Department of AAOS. It has been a pleasure to work with them. They are a very professional and patient group who want to produce quality work that enhances reading and learning. In particular, I would like to acknowledge Lynne Shindoll who directed the development of this book, and David Stanley who directed the design, art program, and production. Their expertise, guidance, and ongoing enthusiasm were vital to the success and development of both editions.

Finally, I especially would like to acknowledge the vision and leadership of Robert K. Snider, MD. Bob was the editor of the first edition of *Essentials of Musculoskeletal Care* and significantly more than any other person was responsible for the development and success of that book. We are fortunate that Bob agreed to continue working with the second edition. Not only was he a section editor, but more importantly, he provided invaluable assistance and consultation to me as this edition was planned and prepared.

As with the first edition, we invite your observations on this second edition. It will help us and future editors plan subsequent editions. Please complete the enclosed comment card, or write to us at *Essentials of Musculoskeletal Care*, AAOS Publications Department, 6300 River Road, Rosemont, IL, 60018. You may also send e-mail comments to shindoll@aaos.org or greenew@health.missouri.edu.

*Walter B. Greene, MD*
*Editor*

# SECTION ONE
# GENERAL ORTHOPAEDICS

# SECTION TWO
# SHOULDER

# SECTION THREE
# ELBOW AND FOREARM

ESSENTIALS OF MUSCULOSKELETAL CARE | AMERICAN ACADEMY OF ORTHOPAEDIC SURGEONS

# SECTION FOUR
## HAND AND WRIST

# SECTION FIVE
## HIP AND THIGH

# SECTION SIX
## KNEE AND LOWER LEG

# PEDIATRIC ORTHOPAEDICS

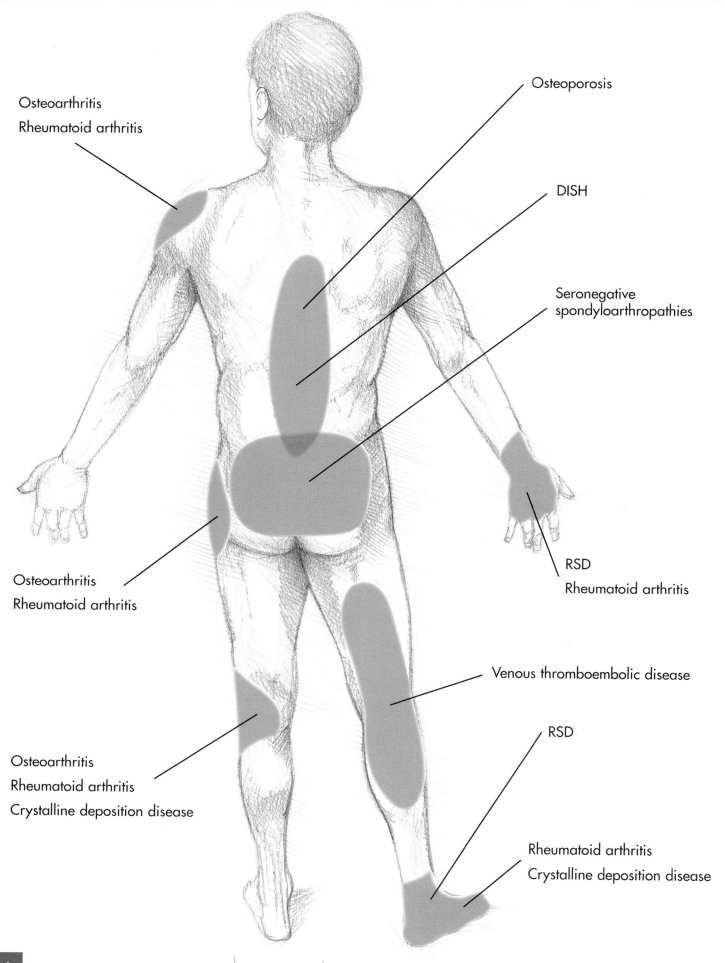

Osteoarthritis
Rheumatoid arthritis

Osteoporosis

DISH

Seronegative
spondyloarthropies

Osteoarthritis
Rheumatoid arthritis

RSD
Rheumatoid arthritis

Venous thromboembolic disease

RSD

Osteoarthritis
Rheumatoid arthritis
Crystalline deposition disease

Rheumatoid arthritis
Crystalline deposition disease

# GENERAL ORTHOPAEDICS

## Section Editor

George L. Lucas, MD
Professor and Chairman
Section of Orthopaedics
University of Kansas Medical School—Wichita
Wichita, Kansas

Bruce R. Buhr, MD
Clinical Instructor
Section of Orthopaedics
University of Kansas Medical School—
Wichita
Wichita, Kansas

Kenneth E. DeHaven, MD
Professor, Associate Chair for Clinical Affairs
Director of Athletic Medicine
Department of Orthopaedics
University of Rochester School of Medicine
and Dentistry
Rochester, New York

William D. Engber, MD
Associate Professor
Department of Orthopedic Surgery
University of Wisconsin Medical School
Madison, Wisconsin

Walter B. Greene, MD
Chairman and J. Vernon Luck, Jr,
Distinguished Professor
Department of Orthopaedic Surgery
University of Missouri School of Medicine
Columbia, Missouri

Thomas R. Johnson, MD
Orthopedic Surgeons, PSC
St. Vincent Hospital and Health Center
Billings, Montana

Kenneth J. Koval, MD
Associate Professor
Department of Orthopaedics
New York University School of Medicine
New York, New York

Jay R. Lieberman, MD
Associate Professor
Department of Orthopaedic Surgery
UCLA Medical Center
Los Angeles, California

John D. Osland, MD
Associate Clinical Professor
Section of Orthopaedics
University of Kansas School of Medicine —
Wichita
Wichita, Kansas

Michael S. Pinzur, MD
Professor
Department of Orthopaedic Surgery and
Rehabilitation
Loyola University Health System
Maywood, Illinois

Laura L. Tosi, MD
Chairman and Associate Professor
Pediatric Orthopaedic Surgery
Children's National Medical Center
Washington, DC

James P. Waddell, MD, FRCSC
A.J. Latner Professor and Chairman
Division of Orthopaedic Surgery
University of Toronto
Toronto, Ontario, Canada

# GENERAL ORTHOPAEDICS—AN OVERVIEW

Bone, cartilage, muscle, tendon, ligament, and their supporting nerve and vascular supplies are the specialized structures that make up the musculoskeletal system. In combination, these structures provide remarkable strength, movement, durability, and efficiency. Disease or injury to any of these tissues may adversely affect function and ability to perform daily activities. This section of *Essentials of Musculoskeletal Care* describes conditions that affect multiple joints and/or multiple regions, conditions that have systemic effects, and therapeutic modalities commonly used in the nonoperative treatment of musculoskeletal conditions. The purpose of this overview, as with all the others, is to highlight special conditions and to provide practical advice on diagnosis and treatment. A glossary of commonly used orthopaedic terms is provided on the inside back covers of the text.

## ARTHRITIS

The etiology of arthritis ranges from the normal degenerative process of aging to an acute infectious process. Likewise, the disability from arthritis ranges from inconsequential stiffness to severe pain and crippling dysfunction.

Osteoarthritis, the most common type of arthritis, is a noninflammatory disorder characterized by deterioration of articular cartilage and formation of new bone (sclerosis at the joint surfaces) and osteophytes (outgrowths of new bone at the joint margins). Degenerative joint disease is another term used to describe osteoarthritis and, by middle age, virtually everyone experiences some type of degenerative change in the fingers or weight-bearing joints, even though most individuals at this time are asymptomatic. Primary osteoarthritis develops without apparent cause, whereas secondary osteoarthritis can develop as a result of trauma (fracture or repetitive trauma), neuromuscular disorders that cause weakness or loss of proprioception, hemophilia, skeletal dysplasias, hemochromatosis, and other disorders that either injure or overload the articular cartilage. Stiffness and pain with activity are characteristic of osteoarthritis.

Types of inflammatory arthritides include rheumatoid arthritis, the seronegative spondyloarthropathies, crystalline deposition diseases, and septic arthritis. Of these conditions, septic arthritis is the most urgent, as it demands immediate diagnosis and an efficacious treatment plan including appropriate antibiotics and in most cases, surgical drainage and lavage. The crystalline arthropathies present with an abrupt onset of intense pain and swelling. The seronegative spondyloarthropathies are a group of disorders characterized by the following: oligoarticular peripheral joint arthritis; enthesitis; inflammatory changes in axial skeletal joints (sacroiliitis and spondylitis); extra-articular sites of inflammation; association with HLA-B27 antigen; and negative rheumatoid factor. Rheumatoid arthritis is an autoimmune disorder of unknown etiology that is characterized by a destructive synovitis, morning stiffness, and symmetrical involvement that primarily affects the joints of the hands, wrists, feet, and ankles.

## BURSITIS AND TENOSYNOVITIS

These conditions are common in adults, particularly following an injury or repetitive motion. Characteristic symptoms include pain that is worse on rising. Patients who have stiffness associated with tendinitis and bursitis usually feel better once the tendon or joint is moved. Think of it as mechanically squeezing out the edema and allowing free motion of the parts. However, with extended activity, inflammation develops and the patient notices increasing pain and the return of stiffness.

## OSTEOPOROSIS

Although bone strength and risk of fracture can be affected by diseases such as hyperparathyroidism, osteomalacia, renal osteodystrophy, and other endocrine disorders, primary osteoporosis is the most common and costly bone disease. With the population of people over age 65 years increasing, fractures and deformity related to osteoporosis have become epidemic. Preventing excessive bone loss with aging and its disabling consequences should be a concern of all physicians.

## TRAUMA

Trauma is a principal cause of musculoskeletal disorders and is more likely to affect young adults. Appropriate treatment can minimize time lost from work and, more critically, permanent impairment and predisposition to arthritis. Traumatic compartment syndrome is catastrophic if unrecognized and untreated. Appropriate splinting is necessary for all fractures, partly to reduce the likelihood of compartment syndromes, and partly to decrease soft-tissue injury and pain while the patient awaits definitive treatment. The principles used in the initial evaluation and splinting of fractures also can be helpful in the evaluation and initial management of ligament and tendon injuries.

## OTHER PAIN DISORDERS

Three conditions, considered the so-called "fuzzy areas" of arthralgias and periarticular pain, are discussed in the general section: fibromyalgia, complex regional pain syndrome, and cumulative trauma disorders also known as overuse syndromes. These processes are as difficult to treat as they are to understand, especially when issues of causation and compensation mix with issues of comfort. Like the above conditions, nonorganic behavior is often misinterpreted as a sign of nondisease, or even malingering; however, it is more likely a predictor of the patient's satisfaction with treatment outcomes than it is an indicator of psychosomatic behavior and often has a negative effect on the patient-physician relationship.

# PATIENT AGE

Trauma and conditions associated with overuse most commonly affect young adults. As adults reach their 40s, degenerative conditions that affect tendons, intervertebral disks, and joints comprise the largest source of complaints. Common presenting problems in the elderly include fractures, metastatic tumors, and arthritis.

# ABUSE

Abuse involving children, spouses, or the elderly is a complex social and medical problem. Failing to diagnose abuse (false negative) may lead to catastrophic consequences; therefore, it is essential that the appropriate social service agencies be notified if a patient's injuries are potentially from abuse. In the section on Pediatric Orthopaedics, child abuse is discussed in a separate chapter. Spouse or elder abuse may be more difficult to identify. Patients whose history is given wholly by a caregiver may feel unable to talk in their presence. In these circumstances, interview the patient and caregiver separately. A caregiver frustrated by an elderly patient's memory problems, behavior problems, alcoholism, or difficult personality may be abusing the patient regularly. Further, a financially stressed caregiver may be usurping the elderly patient's finances for his or her own benefit.

The complexity of these problems and the seriousness of the consequences demand familiarity with community resources and knowledge of the competence, compassion, and professionalism of those who will investigate the potential abuse.

# General Orthopaedics–Principles of Evaluation and Examination

Patients presenting with musculoskeletal problems usually report pain, deformity, or weakness. In evaluating pain, question the patient about the following:

## History

### Questions about the character of the pain

- Is the pain aching (joint or muscle problem), or is it sharp and associated with numbness or tingling (nerve compression)?

- Is the pain becoming worse, better, or is it relatively stable?

- Is the pain worse on movement in the morning (an inflammatory condition), or is it worse with activity (an injury or degenerative condition)?

- Is the pain waking the patient at night or preventing sleep (neoplasm or severe arthritis)?

- Does the pain radiate and, if so, what course does it take?

### Questions about any type of deformity

- When did the patient first notice the deformity? Was it associated with any injury or disease?

- Is the deformity is getting worse?

- Does the deformity affect function, including ability to work, hobbies, and/or activities of daily living?

### Questions about any type of weakness

- What is the extent of the muscle weakness? Does the patient have difficulty placing objects on shelves or climbing steps (proximal muscle weakness and a primary myopathy)?

- Does the patient have any associated sensory abnormalities (a neurologic problem), or does the patient report only weakness (a muscle disorder)?

- Has the patient had any loss of bowel or bladder function, loss of fine motor control (handwriting), or balance function (upper motor neuron involvement)?

Additional questions about the medical history, family history, and a review of systems may reveal clues that suggest the correct diagnosis. For example, weight loss may be a hint that the patient's low back pain is secondary to metastatic disease.

# PHYSICAL EXAMINATION

The principles of examining musculoskeletal problems are similar to evaluating any medical disorder. The specific techniques are detailed in subsequent sections, but the general principles used for inspection, palpation, range of motion, muscle testing, motor and sensory evaluation, and special tests are outlined below.

# INSPECTION/PALPATION

The examination starts with inspection. Ask the patient to place one finger on the one spot that hurts the most (**Figure 1**). This simple request will localize the problem and narrow the differential diagnosis. Look for swelling, ecchymosis, and muscular atrophy. Note the patient's body habitus and standing posture. Compare the affected side with the opposite extremity. This comparison is important to define subtle abnormalities and to rate the severity of the problem.

Watch the patient walk. Analyze the stance and swing phases of gait. Look for an antalgic gait, which is characterized by limited stance phase on the affected extremity. Weakness of the swing phase muscles, eg, ankle dorsiflexors (peroneal nerve dysfunction), is manifested by a drop foot gait.

The affected area should be palpated for tenderness, abnormal masses, or temperature changes (increased heat from inflammation secondary to injury, infection, or other inflammatory process).

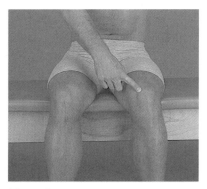

**Figure 1**
Patients can best localize a problem by identifying the one spot that hurts the most.

# RANGE OF MOTION

Measuring joint motion is important for several reasons. In acute illnesses, the degree of joint mobility is a clue to the diagnosis. For example, hip motion is restricted in children with septic arthritis of the hip or transient synovitis of the hip, but this loss of motion is much greater in patients with septic arthritis. In chronic conditions such as osteoarthritis, the degree of joint motion provides an index to the severity and progression of the disorder, as well as providing important information concerning the results of treatment.

# BASIC PRINCIPLES

Joint motion is an objective measurement that can be simply done. Therefore, the parameters for rating musculoskeletal disability, whether for governmental or other agencies, are based largely on the degree that joint motion is impaired.

Joint motion can be estimated visually; however, a goniometer enhances accuracy and is preferred at the elbow, wrist, finger, knee, ankle, and great toe. In measuring hip and shoulder motion, the overlying soft tissue does not allow the same degree of precision with a goniometer.

## ZERO STARTING POSITION

Knowing the accepted Zero Starting Position for each joint is necessary to provide consistent communication between observers. The Zero Starting Position for each joint is described in the examination chapter of each section. For most joints, the Zero Starting Position is the extended anatomic position of the extremity.

To measure joint motion, start by placing the joint in the Zero Starting Position. Place the central axis of the goniometer at the center of the joint. Align one arm of the goniometer with the proximal segment and the other end of the goniometer with the bony axis of the distal segment (**Figure 2**). The upper end of the goniometer is held in place while the joint is moved through its arc of motion. The lower arm of the goniometer is then realigned with the axis of the extremity, and the degree of joint motion is read off the goniometer.

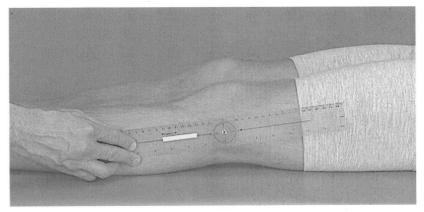

**Figure 2**
The corrected position of the goniometer in the Zero Starting Position.

## DEFINITIONS OF LIMITED MOTION

The terminology for describing limited motion is illustrated in Figure 3. The knee joint depicted in this photograph can neither be fully extended nor flexed. The restricted motion is recorded as follows: 1) the knee flexes from 30° to 90° (30° → 90°), or 2) the knee has a 30° flexion contracture with further flexion to 90° (30° FC → 90° or 30° FC W/FF 90°.

Range of motion is slightly greater in children, particularly those younger than age 10 years ge. Decreased motion occurs as adults age, but the loss of motion is relatively small in most joints. Except for motion at the distal finger joints, it is safe to say that any substantial loss of mobility should be viewed as abnormal and not attributable to aging.

Finally, motion of an injured or diseased joint is often painful. In such a situation, it is better to observe active motion first. The examiner will then

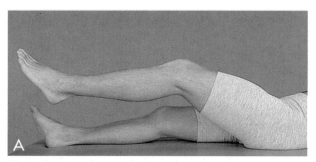 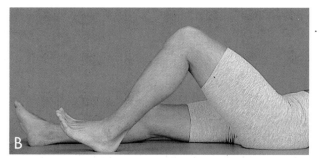

Figure 3
A, The knee flexes from 30° to 90°. B, The knee has a 30° flexion contracture with further flexion to 90°.

know how much support to provide the limb as the passive arc of motion is analyzed.

## MUSCLE TESTING

The examination techniques used in muscle testing start with placing the muscle in a shortened position and then proceed with the examiner resisting the movement. For example, when testing the biceps muscle, the patient should position the elbow in flexion and supination, and then the examiner should test resistance of the biceps by attempting to push the elbow into extension.

Manual muscle testing provides a semi-quantitative measurement of muscle strength (Table 1). The key differentiation is grade 3. For example, a patient's passive knee range of motion is normally 0 to 135°. However, if the patient can actively extend or lift the knee only to 20° of flexion, then, by definition, the quadriceps strength is less than grade 3.

## Table 1
### Grading of Manual Muscle Testing

| Numeric grade | Descriptive grade | Description |
| --- | --- | --- |
| 5 | Normal | Complete range of motion against gravity with full or normal resistance |
| 4 | Good | Complete range of motion against gravity with some resistance |
| 3 | Fair | Complete range of motion against gravity |
| 2 | Poor | Complete range of motion with gravity eliminated |
| 1 | Trace | Muscle contraction but no or very limited joint motion |
| 0 | Zero | No evidence of muscle function |

# MOTOR AND SENSORY EVALUATION

Nerve root function should be tested if the patient's presenting complaints suggest a neck or back problem. Peripheral nerve function should be tested if the disorder is localized to the extremities. In either case, the examination should be thorough and efficient. This is most readily accomplished by evaluating one muscle and one area of sensation for either a nerve root or peripheral nerve. The guidelines for assessing nerve root function are presented in the examination section of Spine.

Evaluation of peripheral nerves is outlined in Table 2. Basically, each peripheral nerve that crosses an acute injury or chronic disorder of the extremity should be evaluated. This examination can be done quickly and completely by evaluating one distal muscle group and one distal area of sensation.

## Table 2
### Evaluation of Peripheral Nerves

| Nerve | Muscle | Sensory |
|---|---|---|
| *Upper extremity* | | |
| Axillary | Deltoid–shoulder abduction | Lateral aspect arm |
| Musculocutaneous | Biceps–elbow flexion | Lateral proximal forearm |
| Median | Flexor pollicis longus–thumb flexion | Tip of thumb, volar aspect |
| Ulnar | First dorsal interosseous–abduction | Tip of little finger, volar aspect |
| Radial | Extensor pollicis longus–thumb extension | Dorsum thumb web space |
| *Lower extremity* | | |
| Obturator | Adductors–hip adduction | Medial aspect, midthigh |
| Femoral | Quadriceps–knee extension | Proximal to medial malleolus |
| Peroneal | | |
|    Deep branch | Extensor hallucis longus–great toe extension | Dorsum first web space |
|    Superficial branch | Peroneus brevis–foot eversion | Dorsum lateral foot |
| Tibial | Flexor hallucis longus–great toe flexion | Plantar aspect foot |

# SPECIAL TESTS

One basic principle to keep in mind when examining patients with joint and/or muscle pain is that stretch exacerbates pain or contracture of an injured or deformed structure. Furthermore, if a muscle/tendon crosses two joints, then both joints must be positioned to stretch the injured part. For example, if the hamstrings are injured, their involvement is elucidated by placing these structures on stretch (eg, flexing the hip to 90° and then extending the knee). Pain and/or limited knee extension typically occurs with this maneuver when a patient has an injury or contracture of the hamstring muscles.

Tests specific to individual anatomic injuries are described in the appropriate section.

Of note, as the physician becomes familiar with the musculoskeletal examination, combining different elements of inspection, palpation, range of motion, etc will make the evaluation more efficient.

# AMPUTATIONS OF THE LOWER EXTREMITY

ICD-9 Code
**997.60**
Amputation stump complication,
unspecified

## DEFINITION

Disease states, particularly diabetes and peripheral vascular disease, are the cause of approximately 75% of all lower extremity amputations in adults. In fact, these two conditions account for more than 100,000 lower extremity amputations performed yearly in the United States. Trauma accounts for 20% of lower extremity amputations in adults, and tumors for the remaining 5%.

Amputations frequently are done after extensive therapy to salvage the limb. In these situations, the patient and even the medical team may have a negative attitude concerning the procedure and subsequent rehabilitation. This attitude, however, is inappropriate because functional ambulation is restored in most amputees. Even at the transtibial (below-knee) level, almost 90% of amputees achieve a functional ambulatory capacity that approaches their preamputation level. Therefore, the physician must aggressively pursue early prosthetic limb fitting to allow patients to resume their normal daily activities.

The increased energy requirements of walking after an amputation generally are proportional to the level of amputation. Therefore, the amputation should be performed as distal as feasible for good prosthetic management. For example, an amputation performed at the hindfoot often compromises prosthetic function. In this case, performing the amputation at the next higher level (ankle disarticulation) provides better function.

## LEVELS OF AMPUTATION AND PROSTHETIC CONSIDERATIONS

### TOE(S)

Dysvascular amputees note no significant disability. Young adults with traumatic amputations may lose some propulsive function but have no significant walking difficulties. Whenever possible, isolated second toe amputation should retain the base of the proximal phalanx to prevent hallux valgus. Shoe modifications usually are not required.

### RAY RESECTION

A ray amputation includes the metatarsal and corresponding toe. A single ray resection of either the first or fifth metatarsal functions well in a standard shoe. Resection of more than one ray requires an orthotic with attached shoe filler.

### MIDFOOT

Amputation of the midfoot is done at either the transmetatarsal or tarsal-metatarsal level. The transmetatarsal procedure results in a longer lever and, therefore, better function. Prosthetic requirements are an orthotic with attached shoe filler. Patients usually do well with standard, low-counter tie shoes.

### HINDFOOT

Amputations at the talonavicular joint level do not function well. The retained talus and calcaneus frequently are pulled into equinus, and prosthetic fit is compromised.

### ANKLE DISARTICULATION

This amputation extends through the ankle (also called Syme amputation) and is considered a desirable amputation level when possible. The heel pad provides a durable end-bearing residual limb, even when the skin is insensate. The prosthesis has a foot component and extends to the proximal tibia. The gait pattern is stable and requires limited training.

### TRANSTIBIAL

This type of amputation is commonly referred to as a below-knee or BK amputation. A long posterior flap usually is better, particularly in patients with diabetes or peripheral vascular disease. Optimal length is 12 to 15 cm below the knee joint. Young adults are more likely to benefit from new developments in flexible sockets and dynamic response feet.

### KNEE DISARTICULATION

This amputation extends through the knee. New developments in prosthetic knee joints have greatly improved the walking function of patients with this type of amputation. This level of amputation also is preferred in nonambulatory patients as it maximizes sitting function and minimizes the risk of skin problems of more distal amputations.

### TRANSFEMORAL

This type of amputation is commonly referred to as an above-knee or AK amputation. Energy requirements are significantly higher with this level of amputation, and most dysvascular amputees do not have adequate cardiac function for functional ambulation. Optimal length is 8 to 12 cm above the knee joint.

### HIP DISARTICULATION

Due to the high energy requirement, even young adults with this level of amputation commonly prefer walking with crutches rather than using a prosthesis.

## PRINCIPLES OF PROSTHETIC FITTING

The soft-tissue envelope is the interface, or cushion, between the bone of the patient's residual limb ("stump") and the prosthetic socket (**Figure 1**). With disarticulation amputations at the ankle and knee levels, weight bearing is directly through the end of the residual limb. The soft-tissue envelope acts as a cushion, and the prosthetic socket simply has to prevent the prosthesis from falling off (**Figure 2**).

In through-bone amputations at the transtibial and transfemoral levels, the transected bone and soft-tissue envelope cannot accept weight-bearing forces.

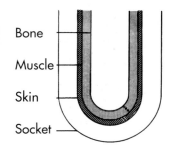

**Figure 1**
The soft-tissue envelope acts as an interface between the bone of the residual limb and the prosthetic socket. Ideally, it should be composed of a mobile nonadherent muscle mass and full-thickness skin that will tolerate the direct pressures and pistoning within the prosthetic socket.

With these amputations, the load must be distributed over the entire surface of the residual limb (**Figure 3**). Intimate fit of the prosthetic socket is crucial. If the patient gains weight, the residual limb will not be able to fit into the socket. Conversely, if the patient loses weight, he or she will "bottom out," resulting in the development of a pressure ulcer due to end-bearing pressure.

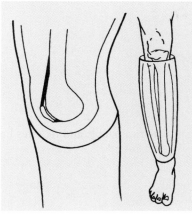 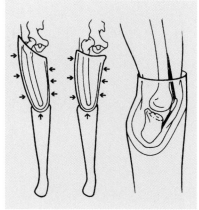

**Figure 2**
Direct load transfer is accomplished in the (left) through-knee and (right) Syme ankle disarticulation amputations.

**Figure 3**
Indirect load transfer is accomplished in above-knee amputations with either (left) a standard quadrilateral socket or (center) an adducted narrow medial-lateral socket. The below-knee amputation (right) transfers weight indirectly with the knee flexed approximately 10°.

Perfect intimate prosthetic fit is impossible; therefore, all amputees experience pistoning within the prosthetic socket. Pistoning produces shear forces. Good surgical technique produces a residual limb composed of mobile muscle and durable skin; however, if the soft-tissue envelope is thin (eg, composed of split-thickness skin graft, or adherent to bone), blisters and shearing ulcers will develop. In this situation, the prosthetist attempts to compensate by using pressure and shear-dissipating materials.

## COMPLICATIONS OF PROSTHETICS

When problems develop, a certified prosthetist should be consulted. Problems that are not related to the residual limb/prosthesis interface usually can be solved by simple measures. Revision surgery is rarely necessary.

### RESIDUAL LIMB ULCERS OR INFECTION

Most blisters, ulcers, or infections are caused by an inadequate residual limb soft-tissue envelope or poor prosthetic fit. If these problems develop, the patient should not wear the prosthesis until it can be adjusted. Oftentimes, simply modifying the socket and applying dressings with or without a hydrocolloid gel will allow the wounds to heal. Antibiotics are necessary only if the patient has signs of local or systemic infection. Revision of the amputation is not commonly indicated.

## SKIN CONDITIONS

The residual limb exists in a closed environment within the prosthetic socket. Excessive sweating or poor hygiene will lead to dermatologic eruption, so it is essential that the prosthetic socket and residual limb be kept clean and dry. Absorbent powders (other than talcum powder) or creams should be used for this purpose.

Acne can be a real nuisance for the amputee. Good hygiene and periodic treatment with oral antibiotics (usually tetracycline) usually keeps this problem in check.

Extreme swelling of the residual limb that is similar in appearance to severe venous insufficiency disease may develop if the prosthetic socket does not achieve intimate fit. Improving the fit of the socket generally prevents this problem.

## RESIDUAL LIMB PAIN

All adults perceive the continued presence of their amputated body part. This residual limb sensation is manifested by paresthesia, occasional dysesthesia, and shooting electric shocks or pains. Patient education is the only treatment necessary if symptoms are intermittent. Persistent symptoms are best controlled with antiseizure membrane-stabilizing drugs, such as gabapentin, or transcutaneous electrical nerve stimulation.

Severe, persistent phantom limb pain is unusual. Patients typically describe the pain as burning, searing, or throbbing. As in any chronic pain syndrome, treatment often requires multiple modalities. The best results are achieved when this pain is managed as a major causalgia with guidance from a specialist in pain management.

Localized stump pain may be caused by poor prosthetic socket fit or alignment. In these instances, evaluation by a prosthetist is indicated.

# CANES, CRUTCHES, AND WALKERS

Canes, crutches, and walkers (in that order) reduce weight-bearing stresses on the lower extremities and also augment balance and stability during walking. As such, these devices are helpful in the treatment of arthritic conditions and lower extremity injuries. They also improve balance and stability in elderly patients and in patients who have had a stroke, reducing the risk of a fall or fracture.

## CANES

Canes are light, easily stored, and cosmetically appealing to patients. For long-term use, a spade handle is easier on the hand than the standard crook handle. A "quad" or four-footed cane has four prongs at its base; it is more cumbersome than a single-tipped cane but provides a wider base of support and can be quite useful to patients after a stroke when they have only one functional upper extremity.

A cane should be used on the contralateral side to maximize reduction in stress on an arthritic hip.

A cane that is too long causes excessive flexion of the elbow and increases the demand on the triceps muscle, which is a major stabilizer of the upper extremity when using a cane. A cane that is too short provides inadequate support and compromises walking. The optimal length of a cane will position the elbow in 20° to 30° of flexion when the tip of the cane is placed approximately 6" in front of and 6" lateral to the little toe.

## CRUTCHES

Crutches offer more support than a cane but less than that of a walker. For short-term use, axillary wooden crutches are satisfactory and economical. Aluminum crutches are more durable but cost more and are therefore prescribed for chronic conditions. Forearm crutches only extend to the forearm and, therefore, are less bulky but require better balance and upper extremity strength. These crutches typically are used for patients with chronic conditions. Platform crutches allow forces to be transmitted through the forearm and are useful when patients have arthritic or traumatic conditions of the hand or wrist.

Crutches that are too long or that are used improperly can cause axillary artery or venous thrombosis, or a brachial plexus compression neuropathy (primarily the radial nerve). The hand piece should be positioned to provide optimal function of the triceps and latissimus dorsi muscles. Depending on the height of the patient, position the crutch tip 4" to 6" anterior and lateral to the little toe. In that position, adjust the length of the crutch to allow 2" to 2.5" clearance between the anterior axillary fold and the top of the crutch.

SECTION 1 | GENERAL ORTHOPAEDICS

Adjust the hand piece to position the elbow in 25° to 30° of flexion. As a general guideline, the length of the crutch is 77% of the patient's height. Caution the patient against wrapping towels around the axillary pad.

## WALKERS

Walkers have four points of contact and provide the greatest support and balance. Patients with balance problems more or less carry the walker while those with arthritic conditions reduce the stress on their lower extremities by transmitting more load onto the walker. The bulkiness of a walker is its major disadvantage. Some walkers fold, making storage in cars easier, but these models are more fragile. Rolling walkers require less energy to use. If balance reactions are adequate, a rolling walker may be advantageous for a patient with significant cardiopulmonary restrictions.

The same principles apply for adjusting the height of a walker (ie, the hand grip should be positioned to allow 30° flexion at the elbow when the patient is in a neutral standing position).

Gait techniques for crutches or walkers are listed in Table 1. Following injury to the lower extremity, the technique most commonly prescribed is a non–weight-bearing, swing-through gait. Walking on level ground using this method is easy to teach because it involves simply advancing both crutches, followed by a forward step with the uninjured leg. Ascending or descending steps is more difficult, but the key is to advance the crutches first when going down stairs and to advance the sound leg first when going up. A training session with a physical therapist often is helpful.

## Table 1
### Gait Patterns Used with Crutches or Walkers

| Type | Instructions |
|---|---|
| Swing-to | Advance both crutches. Lift the body to advance both feet on line with the crutches. |
| Swing-through | Advance both crutches. Lift the body to advance both feet beyond the crutches. |
| Non–weight-bearing, swing-through | Advance both crutches. Shift weight and advance the sound leg. |
| Four-point | Move one crutch forward, then advance the opposite foot, followed by the ipsilateral crutch, then the contralateral foot. (Three points of contact are always maintained.) |
| Alternating two-point | Advance one crutch and the contralateral foot at the same time. Shift weight and advance the other foot and crutch. (A progression of the four-point gait.) |

# COMPARTMENT SYNDROME

### ICD-9 Codes
355.8
    Mononeuritis of lower limb,
    unspecified (Chronic compartment
    syndrome)
958.8
    Other early complications of trau-
    ma (Acute compartment syndrome)

## SYNONYM

Volkmann ischemic contracture

## DEFINITION

A muscular compartment is defined as a group of one or more muscles and their associated nerves and vessels surrounded by fascia that is relatively unyielding. Compartment syndrome occurs when vascular perfusion of the muscle and other tissues within a compartment decreases to a level that is inadequate to sustain the viability of these tissues.

Compartment syndrome usually is acute in onset and follows trauma, especially fractures of the tibia or other long bones. Patients with severe crush injuries and/or systemic hypotension are particularly susceptible. Patients with peripheral vascular disease also are at risk, as their poor tissue perfusion leads to mild ischemia and transudation of fluid, which increases the local compartment pressure. Acute compartment syndrome also may develop after direct blows that cause only muscular injury and hemorrhage.

Chronic compartment syndrome may develop in long-distance runners, new military recruits, or others involved in a major change in activity level. In these patients, the symptoms are less acute and tend to improve with rest following exercise.

As a compartment syndrome develops, the intracompartmental tissue pressure becomes elevated, producing a secondary elevation in venous pressure that obstructs venous outflow. This causes an escalating cycle of continued increases in intracompartmental tissue pressure and a resultant decrease in arterial flow. The end result is necrosis of muscle and nerve tissues that can occur in as few as 4 to 8 hours.

Failure to recognize an acute compartment syndrome can lead to a tragic outcome with necrotic muscle that is replaced by fibrotic scar tissue, muscular contracture, and permanent dysfunction of all nerves traveling through the compartment. Prevention of this outcome requires early recognition and, in most cases, early surgical intervention.

## CLINICAL SYMPTOMS

The anterior compartment of the leg and the volar aspect of the forearm are the most commonly affected muscular compartments. Pain that is disproportionate to the injury and sensory hypoesthesia distal to the involved compartment (ie, deep peroneal nerve distribution in the foot and median nerve distribution in the hand) are characteristic early symptoms.

SECTION 1 | GENERAL ORTHOPAEDICS

# TESTS

## PHYSICAL EXAMINATION

The most important physical sign is extreme pain on stretching of the long muscles that pass through a compartment. For example, extension of the fingers will stretch the volar forearm muscles, and plantar flexion of the ankle and toes will place the anterior leg muscles on stretch. The inability to actively contract these muscles, as when making a fist or dorsiflexing the toes, is an indication of paralysis.

While passive or active stretching of muscles around fractured bones is always painful, it is usually tolerable; if it is not, the patient may have a compartment syndrome. A patient who has an extraordinary amount of pain in the leg or forearm should be examined carefully.

Examination of a patient who is wearing a cast or dressing begins by removing the cast and any padding to carefully evaluate the muscle compartments. Palpation of increased compartment pressure is subjective, but normally compartments are soft, not tight or rigid. Assess motor and sensory function of the peripheral nerves passing through the compartments, as well as passive stretch of the involved muscles.

Pulselessness indicates arterial trauma—not compartment syndrome—although a compartment syndrome may exist in combination with vascular ischemia. Pulses are typically completely normal in early compartment syndrome because, at that time, the intracompartmental pressure rarely exceeds systolic pressure levels.

## DIAGNOSTIC TESTS

When necessary, compartment pressures can be measured directly. A compartment syndrome usually is present when the diastolic pressure minus the intracompartmental pressure is less than or equal to 30 mm Hg.

# DIFFERENTIAL DIAGNOSIS

Arterial injury (pulse deficit)

Muscle contusion (local soft-tissue bleeding)

Shin-splints (exercise-induced weakness and pain)

# ADVERSE OUTCOMES OF THE DISEASE

Without immediate treatment, compartment syndrome can result in permanent loss of function. The muscles die, scar, and shorten; fingers and toes are often clawed and have little motion. The wrist is held in flexion, and sensation is impaired. Late reconstructive surgery has little chance of restoring original, normal function.

# TREATMENT

Because muscle necrosis can develop within as few as 4 to 8 hours, there is little time to delay treatment. Even a suspicion of compartment syndrome probably requires treatment, especially if intracompartmental pressure measurements support the diagnosis. Surgical fasciotomy of the compartment is essential. The wound is left open, with delayed closure or skin grafting performed after swelling subsides.

Strict instructions to patients to call at any hour, day or night, are necessary if the pain is unbearable or if they are unable to actively extend the long extensors of the fingers or toes. Patients must be able to actively extend their fingers or toes before leaving the emergency department or office so that either they or their parents/guardians know what is acceptable motion and usage.

Elevating the lower extremity on pillows placed under the calf will help reduce edema. Elevating the upper extremity with a pillow also is appropriate. Excessive elevation should be avoided because this increases hydrostatic pressure and can lower arterial pressure enough to decrease compartment perfusion.

## Adverse outcomes of treatment

There is very little negative risk in treating an acute compartment syndrome with fasciotomy, except that the scar may be unsightly. However, failure to perform a fasciotomy could be disastrous for the patient.

## Referral decisions/Red flags

Even a tentative diagnosis of compartment syndrome requires urgent evaluation so that surgical decompression by emergency fasciotomy can be considered.

# CORTICOSTEROID INJECTIONS

## GENERAL GUIDELINES

Corticosteroid injections have an accepted role in the treatment of acute and chronic inflammatory diseases. In general, these injections can decrease inflammation and improve function; but they also may occasionally cause significant adverse effects. In addition, the indications for their use in some musculoskeletal conditions are not well defined.

Many long-acting corticosteroid ester preparations enhance anti-inflammatory actions and reduce undesirable hormonal side effects. The most widely used compounds are listed in **Table 1**.

### Table 1
#### Common Injectable Corticosteroids

| Medication | Relative potency | Onset | Duration |
|---|---|---|---|
| Hydrocortisone (Cortisol) | 1 | Fast | Short |
| Prednisolone terbutate (Hydeltra) | 4 | Fast | Intermediate |
| Methylprednisolone acetate (Depo-Medrol) | 4 | Slow | Intermediate |
| Triamcinolone acetonide (Kenalog) | 5 | Moderate | Intermediate |
| Triamcinolone hexacetonide (Aristospan) | 5 | Moderate | Intermediate |
| Betamethasone (Celestone) | 25 | Fast | Long |

The choice of agent depends somewhat on the desired effect. For an acute condition that requires immediate effect (eg, carpal tunnel syndrome), a fast-acting agent would be appropriate. For chronic inflammatory conditions, a long-acting agent is preferred. Triamcinolone compounds often are used for intra-articular injections, particularly of intermediate or large joints, but because these agents are more likely to cause local tissue necrosis, other preparations often are chosen for small joint and tendon injections.

## HOW CORTICOSTEROIDS WORK

Corticosteroids suppress inflammation. They decrease collagenase and prostaglandin formation and formation of granulation tissue. They are catabolic promoters that block glucose uptake in the tissues, enhance protein breakdown, and decrease new protein synthesis in muscle, skin, bone, connective tissue, and lymphoid tissue (predominantly T cells).

SECTION 1 | GENERAL ORTHOPAEDICS

## USE OF INTRA-ARTICULAR INJECTIONS

An optimal intra-articular dose of corticosteroid is the maximum amount that can be held locally. However, it should be noted that some of the locally injected steroid is absorbed systemically and may produce transient systemic effects. Usual doses of methylprednisolone or equivalent are listed in Table 2.

### Table 2
#### Usual Doses of Methylprednisolone or Equivalent by Site

| Dose | Anatomic site |
| --- | --- |
| 5 to 10 mg | Phalangeal joints |
| 20 to 30 mg | Wrist |
| 20 to 30 mg | Elbow and ankle |
| 40 to 80 mg | Shoulder, hip, or knee |

### RHEUMATOID ARTHRITIS

Use of an intra-articular injection for active synovitis associated with rheumatoid arthritis and other inflammatory arthritides improves symptoms in the injected joint about 50% of the time and lasts from several days to several weeks. Repeated injections to suppress rheumatoid synovitis are generally effective in the knees, elbows, and interphalangeal joints. Long-term studies are limited but do not show accelerated destructive changes in the injected joints when compared with control joints.

### OSTEOARTHRITIS

Intra-articular corticosteroid injection is less effective, and its effects are of shorter duration in patients with osteoarthritis than in those with rheumatoid arthritis. The joints most often helped are the knee and the interphalangeal or metacarpophalangeal joints of the hand.

### CRYSTAL-INDUCED ARTHRITIS

Use of an intra-articular corticosteroid injection in patients with gout or pseudogout can be especially helpful for those whose comorbid conditions or allergies prohibit use of systemic medications.

### TENOSYNOVITIS AND BURSITIS

Both flexor tenosynovitis in the hand (trigger finger) and de Quervain tenosynovitis at the wrist respond well to injections of corticosteroids into the tenosynovial sheath (not the tendon). Bursitis associated with shoulder impingement often responds well to a single injection. Trochanteric bursitis usually responds well to injection (usually no more than three), and few adverse effects have been reported with multiple injections.

Injections into ligamentous structures carry the risk of spontaneous rupture of the ligament and usually are quite painful. The Achilles and patellar tendons should not be injected in the substance of the tendon. Pain in these structures usually indicates interstitial tears, which have already reduced their

SECTION 1 | GENERAL ORTHOPAEDICS

tensile strength. Lateral epicondylitis and plantar fasciitis may respond well to corticosteroid injection.

### ENTRAPMENT NEUROPATHIES

Carpal tunnel syndrome is often treated with injections into the carpal canal, but there is a substantial relapse rate and a chance of intraneural injection.

### GANGLIA

Injection of corticosteroids into ganglia is not necessary. Use a large-bore needle and make multiple punctures to decompress the ganglion. Recurrence of the ganglion is common.

## INJECTION PRINCIPLES

Prior to injecting a corticosteroid, review the following guidelines:

1. Scrub the intended injection site with a bactericidal solution. Wear sterile gloves and handle the syringes and needles with strict aseptic technique. Observe universal precautions.

2. Cleanse the top of the solution vial with an antiseptic solution.

3. Use an 18- or 20-gauge needle for easy withdrawal of solutions. Discard this needle.

4. Consider anesthetizing the injection site with ethyl chloride or a small amount of local anesthetic given with a 25- or 27-gauge needle.

5. Do not use local anesthetics that contain epinephrine when injecting the hand or foot; these can cause arterial constriction and infarction of a digit.

6. Corticosteroid and local anesthetic solutions can be mixed in the same syringe, usually in a 1:2 ratio. Injection of the site with 2 to 3 mL of a rapid-acting local anesthetic solution, advancing the same needle into the joint or tendon sheath, and injecting additional local anesthetic followed by the steroid through the same needle is less traumatic to the patient. Large joints (knee and shoulder) may need an additional 4 mL of local anesthetic.

7. Short- and long-acting local anesthetics also may be mixed in the same syringe.

8. Inject anesthetic or corticosteroid preparation with a sterile 22- to 25-gauge needle.

9. Do not inject anesthetic or corticosteroid into a nerve, a tendon, or subcutaneous fat.

10. Use multiple injections only if clear improvement has occurred. Limit the number to three injections.

11. Following the injection, have the patient rest the extremity for 24 hours and avoid the precipitating cause of the problem.

## IMPROPER USES OF INJECTIONS

Acute trauma

Injection into a tendon or nerve

Injection into an infected joint, tendon, or bursa

Multiple injections (except as above) in conditions other than
rheumatoid arthritis

## ADVERSE OUTCOMES

Adverse systemic effects include transient serum cortisol suppression and transient hyperglycemia (a particular problem in patients with diabetes). Significant effects are uncommon with doses of 25 to 50 mg of methylprednisolone. Postinjection infectious arthritis is uncommon (perhaps 1 in 13,000 injections or fewer) but potentially catastrophic.

Local side effects after injection include lipodystrophy, loss of skin pigmentation, tendon rupture, and possible accelerated joint degeneration, although recent evidence suggests this is unlikely. Up to 10% of treated patients can experience a transient flare or increased pain for 24 to 48 hours following an injection.

Nerve injection injuries can be catastrophic. Extrafascicular injection usually results in no permanent damage, but intrafascicular injection can be disastrous depending on the specific corticosteroid used. Injection of dexamethasone results in minimal damage; triamcinolone acetonide and methylprednisolone result in moderate damage. The damage has been blamed on the carrier agent, but the effect of these agents has not been distinguished from the corticosteroid.

Patients should be advised that the site of injection might be uncomfortable for a few hours after injection. Application of ice helps relieve the discomfort. Patients also should be advised that the potential beneficial effects of the steroid will not be apparent for several hours or days, although the patient typically will experience immediate but transient relief from the local anesthetic.

It is not possible to establish a safe dose of corticosteroid because of individual variability regarding sensitivity to the drug.

Olecranon and prepatellar intrabursal injections carry an increased risk for infection. These structures should be injected only when the patient's problem has not resolved with time and there is clearly no evidence of underlying infection.

Patients with diabetes mellitus are at risk for serious infection and for systemic effects of absorbed corticosteroids.

SECTION 1 | GENERAL ORTHOPAEDICS

# CRYSTALLINE DEPOSITION DISEASES

## SYNONYMS

Gout

Podagra

Calcium pyrophosphate deposition disease (CPDD)

Pseudogout

## DEFINITION

Crystalline deposition diseases are secondary to deposition of crystals in the synovium and other tissues and the subsequent inflammatory response. The arthritis is characterized by abrupt episodes of severe joint pain involving a single joint. In time, more than one joint may be involved, and joint destruction may occur.

Gout is secondary to monosodium urate crystal deposition. The disease is relatively common and increases with age and with increasing serum uric acid concentrations. The most frequent manifestation of gout is arthritis, but the uric acid crystals also may be deposited in other tissues such as bursae, tendon sheaths, skin, heart valves, and kidneys with resultant tophi, renal stones, and gouty nephropathy. Acute arthritis is the most common presentation of gout, but in some patients, nephrolithiasis is the first manifestation of the disorder.

Calcium pyrophosphate dihydrate crystals reside in cartilage and are shed into the joint, causing calcium pyrophosphate deposition disease (CPPD). How these crystals affect the joint varies widely, and CPPD can be confused with gout, osteoarthritis, rheumatoid arthritis (RA), and neuropathic (Charcot) arthropathy. Chondrocalcinosis, pseudogout, and chronic arthropathy are common manifestations of CPPD.

## CLINICAL SYMPTOMS

Acute gouty arthritis typically begins in a single joint, with symptoms first appearing at night. The pain and swelling are intense. Patients often note that the joint is so painful that even the weight of a sheet is intolerable. The overlying erythema may be confused with cellulitis or a septic joint. The metatarsophalangeal joint of the great toe (podagra) is most commonly affected, accounting for approximately 50% of the initial episodes of gouty arthritis. Other frequent sites of involvement include the ankle, tarsal joints, and the knee. Patients often also have fever and chills. As the inflammation subsides, desquamation of the skin overlying the affected joint may be noted.

Pseudogout tends to manifest itself in larger joints and is less explosive and dramatic in presentation. Approximately 50% of the episodes of pseudogout affect the knees. Other commonly involved joints include the elbows, wrists, ankles, hips, and shoulders. In the elderly, pseudogout is the most common cause of acute arthritis involving a single joint.

Tophi are soft-tissue masses resulting from urate crystal deposition that are noted several years following the onset of gout. They can develop in many locations, including the olecranon bursa, extensor surface of the forearm, Achilles tendon, or tendon sheaths in the hand. Tophi may be confused with rheumatoid nodules.

Chondrocalcinosis is calcification of articular cartilage or meniscus, usually at the periphery of the joint. The calcifications do appear on radiographs, but most patients are asymptomatic or have only mild arthritic symptoms. This disorder is more common in women and increases with age, affecting approximately half of the population over the age of 80 years.

Chronic pyrophosphate arthropathy is more common in older women. The knees, wrists, shoulders, elbows, hips, and hands are frequently affected. Symptoms include stiffness on arising and multiple joint involvement. CPPD arthropathy may be confused with RA, but patients do not have bony erosions or other features of RA, such as tenosynovitis. The symptoms also mimic osteoarthritis, but the inflammatory aspects and history of acute exacerbations help to distinguish it from osteoarthritis.

## TESTS

### PHYSICAL EXAMINATION
Document the degree of swelling, surrounding erythema, and limited motion.

### DIAGNOSTIC TESTS
For acute arthritis, joint aspiration and analysis of synovial fluid are most critical. Examination of joint fluid under polarized microscopy reveals the characteristic negatively birefringent urate crystals or weakly positive, birefringent rhomboid-shaped calcium pyrophosphate crystals. Cell counts can be quite variable in acute gouty arthritis. Because septic arthritis is a consideration, obtain a Gram stain and culture of the synovial fluid.

Radiographs are normal except for soft-tissue swelling at the onset of acute gouty arthritis, but punctate or linear calcification of articular cartilage and internal joint structures, such as menisci in the knee or the triangular fibro-cartilage in the wrist, are characteristic of pseudogout. Radiographs of established gout are characterized by subchondral bony erosions and peripheral articular spurs.

Serum uric acid levels should be checked with suspicion of gout; however, these levels may be normal during an acute episode. Plasma urate levels are variable in acute episodes, but a state of asymptomatic hyperuricemia exists prior to development of these episodes and in the intervals between them.

Some metabolic disorders, such as hyperparathyroidism, hemochromatosis, hypophosphatasia, and hypothyroidism, are associated with CPPD and should be ruled out.

## Differential Diagnosis

Cellulitis (joint not involved and motion only mildly affected by overlying skin infection)

Lyme arthritis (chronic fatigue, memory loss, history of rash, IgM or IgG antibody titer)

Neuropathic arthropathy (underlying neurologic disorder such as diabetes, insignificant pain)

Osteoarthritis (less acute, pain proportionate to activity)

Rheumatoid arthritis (younger age, multiple joint involvement, associated tenosynovitis)

Septic arthritis (severe pain, systemic signs, positive Gram stain and culture)

Trauma (history, hemarthrosis, or fracture)

## Adverse Outcomes of the Disease

Before effective control of hyperuricemia was common, development of tophi and chronic gouty arthritis was the expected course. Chronic hyperuricemia also leads to nephropathy and renal stones. End-stage arthritis may occur with CPPD, but this is infrequent.

## Treatment

Treatment of acute episodes first focuses on relieving the inflammation and then minimizing the risk of recurrence and other complications. Colchicine can be quite effective in treating acute gouty arthritis whether given orally or intravenously, but the side effects are significant. Indomethacin also can be quite effective, with an initial dose of 75 to 100 mg, followed by 50 mg every 6 hours until symptoms subside. Other NSAIDs can be used, as well. The joint also can be aspirated and injected with a corticosteroid.

Long-term treatment of gout is aimed at limiting hyperuricemia with drugs such as allopurinol and preventing recurrent acute episodes with small daily doses of colchicine or early use of indomethacin at the first sign of joint inflammation. Attention to any underlying disease in cases of secondary gout is important. Dietary discretion may help reduce the frequency of episodes.

Joint aspiration alone may relieve acute episodes of pseudogout. NSAIDs also can be effective with acute episodes of pseudogout. These medications, combined with a program of exercise, weight reduction, and canes, may be helpful in the long-term management of CPPD. Injection of intra-articular steroid may be required for a severe acute episode.

## Adverse Outcomes of Treatment

NSAIDs can interfere with drugs used concomitantly for control of hypertension and often produce gastrointestinal side effects. Complications of corticosteroid use are well known.

## Referral decisions/Red flags

Joint deformity or destruction, large tophaceous masses, or drainage of tophaceous material may require surgical attention.

# DIFFUSE IDIOPATHIC SKELETAL HYPEROSTOSIS

**ICD-9 Code**
721.6
Ankylosing vertebral hyperostosis

## SYNONYMS
Ankylosing hyperostosis
Vertebral osteophytosis

## DEFINITION
Diffuse idiopathic skeletal hyperostosis (DISH) is an idiopathic type of osteoarthritis characterized by striking osteophyte formation in the spine. Patients with DISH have confluent ossification spanning three or more intervertebral disks, most commonly in the thoracic and thoracolumbar spine. The bridging osteophytes follow the course of the anterior longitudinal ligaments and the peripheral disk margins. The disease primarily affects white men (male-to-female ratio is 2:1) who are age 60 years or older.

## CLINICAL SYMPTOMS
The principal symptom is stiffness in the spine, especially in the morning and evening. Patients often report that symptoms have been present for several months or even years. Nonradicular back pain, especially in the lumbar and thoracolumbar junction area, is relatively mild (**Figure 1**). Those with cervical spine involvement may notice dysphagia related to a large anterior cervical osteophyte located behind the esophagus. Other weight-bearing joints can be painful, but spinal pain is the most severe.

## TESTS

### PHYSICAL EXAMINATION
Examination reveals stiffness in the spine on forward flexion and on extension. Reduced hip motion or associated knee arthritis also is possible.

### DIAGNOSTIC TESTS
Radiographs of the thoracic and lumbar spine, especially the lateral view, show confluent ossification spanning the intervertebral disks of at least four contiguous vertebral bodies (three disks) (**Figure 2**). The intervertebral disk height is preserved in the fused segments. The posterior apophyseal joints and sacroiliac joints are normal as opposed to the findings characteristic of ankylosing spondylitis.

In the cervical spine, ossification of the posterior longitudinal ligament occurs and is the second most common cause of cervical myelopathy (after cervical spondylosis).

The pelvis often shows "whiskering" or shaggy hyperostotic bone at the pelvic rim. There may be hyperostotic change in the ribs, as well.

There is no human leukocyte antigen (HLA) association.

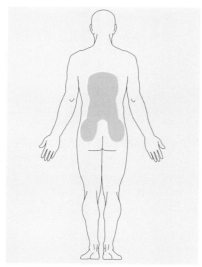

**Figure 1**
Distribution of pain in DISH.

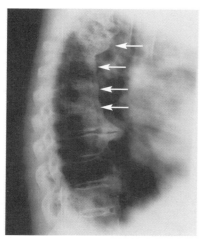

**Figure 2**
Confluent ossification anteriorly spanning multiple disk levels (arrows).

## DIFFERENTIAL DIAGNOSIS

Acromegaly (facial and phalangeal changes)

Ankylosing spondylitis (sacroiliac and apophyseal joint involvement, positive HLA-B27)

Degenerative disk disease (reduced disk height)

Paget disease (32% of patients also have DISH)

Polymyalgia rheumatica (muscle and joint pain and stiffness associated with systemic symptoms)

## ADVERSE OUTCOMES OF THE DISEASE

Spinal stiffness is common. With widespread involvement, a single mobile segment can remain, but it may become unstable and painful.

## TREATMENT

Walking and exercise programs are the most common initial treatment. Intermittent NSAIDs can help, but pain usually is mild and tolerable.

## ADVERSE OUTCOMES OF TREATMENT

Heterotopic ossification occurs five times more often following hip replacement surgery in patients with DISH. NSAIDs can cause gastric, renal, or hepatic complications.

## REFERRAL DECISIONS/RED FLAGS

Symptoms of neurogenic claudication, myelopathy, or dysphagia indicate the need for further evaluation.

SECTION 1 | GENERAL ORTHOPAEDICS

# FALLS AND MUSCULOSKELETAL INJURIES IN THE ELDERLY PATIENT

## DEFINITION

The elderly are the fastest growing segment of our population. Fall prevention is a critical wellness issue in this age group because nearly one third of all elderly people fall each year. Of these, 50% fall repeatedly. One percent of falls result in a hip fracture. Falls also constitute 40% of nursing home admissions.

Intrinsic factors causing falls are those associated with the aging body, as follows:

- visual changes (often due to diseases such as glaucoma, macular degeneration, diabetic retinopathy, and improper use of corrective lenses);

- hearing problems and/or vestibular dysfunction;

- neurologic conditions (such as Parkinson disease, weakness from stroke, transient ischemic attacks);

- cardiovascular problems (arrhythmia, hypertension, hypotension, peripheral vascular disease);

- dementia;

- musculoskeletal conditions (arthritis, stiffness, osteoporosis);

- systemic illness (leading to metabolic defects or malignancy causing pathologic fractures).

Extrinsic factors causing falls are related to the environment and include obstacles or design flaws in the home, poor supervision, weather conditions, and improper footwear. The elderly often do not have adequate assistance to help with their daily routine; as a result, they may be forced to engage in risky behavior, such as climbing to reach objects in the kitchen or closet. Bathing also poses numerous hazards, most notably a slippery wet floor. Obstacles such as furniture or rugs can contribute to falls, particularly at night. Cracks in sidewalks and ice contribute to outdoor falls. Assistance in and out of the home can decrease these risks. Attention to layout in the home, including clearing obstructed pathways and installing handrails and traction pads in the bathroom, can decrease the risk of falls.

Many elderly patients present in poor nutritional condition and/or are weakened and confused as a result of multiple drug use (polypharmacy). The use of sedatives specifically in the elderly is associated with an increased risk of falls and injury. Communicating with elderly patients can be difficult because of poor hearing, poor eyesight, or confusion. Despite the frustrations in communication, it is important to treat elderly patients with dignity and respect.

## CLINICAL SYMPTOMS

The most common fractures involve the hip, wrist, shoulder, and spine. Specific information about these different fractures is detailed in individual chapters.

Hip fracture is a common injury in the elderly, with significant morbidity and mortality, and should be suspected when a fall results in the inability to walk. Surgical treatment is optimal for nearly all hip fractures. Mortality has been shown to increase significantly with an operative delay of more than 3 calendar days following injury. Following surgery, early mobilization is ideal.

Wrist fractures most often follow a fall on an outstretched hand. Presenting symptoms include pain, swelling, and obvious deformity. Many wrist fractures can be treated by closed reduction and splinting or casting for approximately 6 weeks.

Proximal humerus fractures typically occur following low-energy trauma such as a simple fall. Patients report shoulder pain that becomes worse with motion. Treatment typically is immobilization in a sling or shoulder immobilizer; early motion is encouraged. Occasionally, surgical treatment with open reduction and internal fixation or prosthetic replacement is necessary. While the patients are usually pain-free following fracture union, they are often left with functional limitations.

Vertebral compression fractures are nearly synonymous with osteoporosis. These fractures typically occur in the low thoracic and/or upper lumbar region, often after minimal trauma. Though pain and deformity occasionally occur, neurologic injury is rare. Vertebral compression fractures are usually treated by a short period of rest and pain medication, followed by early mobilization and short-term bracing.

## TESTS

Clinical and diagnostic tests depend on the specific conditions.

## ADVERSE OUTCOMES OF THE DISEASE

Elderly patients are susceptible to many medical complications following fracture. Ability to manage without assistance and/or to ambulate may deteriorate despite optimal fracture care and may result in loss of independence.

Osteoporosis affects fracture management. Surgical fixation is more difficult because of the difficulties in obtaining stable fixation in weak bone.

## TREATMENT

While all intrinsic causes are a natural part of aging, many can be prevented or mitigated by appropriate medical intervention. Pharmacologic treatment of osteoporosis has been shown to prevent or delay decrease in bone density. Medical management of chronic conditions such as diabetes can improve vision. Proper nutrition and exercise throughout life can decrease the incidence of cardiovascular disease. Medications, particularly antihypertensives and sedatives, must be closely monitored to prevent orthostatic hypotension, syncope, and oversedation.

SECTION 1 | GENERAL ORTHOPAEDICS

The goal of fracture treatment is to restore preinjury level of function. Therefore, treatment must be tailored to the patient and the specific injury. The patient's ability to actively participate and comply with a rehabilitation program factors into the treatment decision. Evaluate polypharmacy, vision, balance, and associated medical conditions. Ask a friend or family member to remove throw rugs or other objects that may cause the patient to trip. Also advise the removal of obstacles from hallways or frequently traveled pathways. Prescribe single-vision glasses (without bifocals) for ambulation to the bathroom at night. Emphasize the importance of handrails for the toilet and bathtub and nonslip mats in the bathtub.

The medical condition of elderly patients also impacts on fracture management. Because cardiovascular and pulmonary disease are so common in this population, the risks associated with surgery and general anesthesia are greater. These risks must be considered when deciding on treatment options.

## ADVERSE OUTCOMES OF TREATMENT

Medications must be continuously monitored in elderly patients to avoid polypharmacy, oversedation, and adverse drug interactions. Postoperative complications are common; therefore, frequent, careful monitoring of cerebrovascular, cardiovascular, neurologic, and hematologic function is mandatory.

## REFERRAL DECISIONS/RED FLAGS

Pain with walking may signal a hip problem that requires evaluation. If initial radiographs are inconclusive, then a second series or adjunctive studies such as a bone scan or MRI may be indicated.

# Fibromyalgia Syndrome

ICD-9 Code
729.1
Myalgia and myositis, unspecified

## Definition

Fibromyalgia syndrome (FMS) is a chronic condition characterized by generalized pain, fatigue, and tender areas in the soft tissues. The joints, however, are spared. Women between the ages of 20 and 60 years are at greatest risk. The cause is unknown, and a cure is not available.

## Clinical symptoms

In 1990, the American College of Rheumatology established the following criteria for the diagnosis of fibromyalgia:

- Widespread pain that has been present for 3 months.

- Pain is considered widespread when all of the following are present: pain in the left side of the body, pain in the right side of the body, pain above the waist, and pain below the waist. In addition, axial skeletal pain must be present (neck, anterior chest, or thoracic or low back). By definition, shoulder and buttock pain is considered as pain for each involved side. Low back pain is considered pain below the waist.

- Pain and tenderness at 11 or more of 18 trigger point sites on digital palpation with an approximate force of 4 kg. For a tender point to be considered positive, the patient must state that the palpation was "painful" in contrast to "tender" (**Figure 1**).

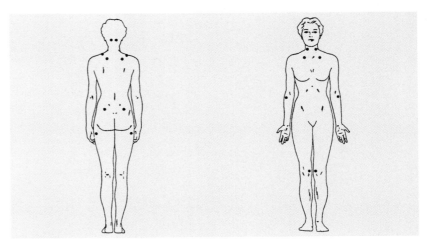

**Figure 1**
Posterior and anterior trigger points.

*Reproduced with permission from the Arthritis Foundation, Atlanta, GA.*

SECTION 1 | GENERAL ORTHOPAEDICS

## POSTERIOR TRIGGER POINT SITES

Occiput: Bilateral, at the occipital muscle insertions

Supraspinatus: Bilateral, at origins, above the scapular spine near the medial border

Trapezius: Bilateral, at the midpoint of the upper border

Gluteal: Bilateral, in upper outer quadrants of buttocks in anterior fold of muscle

Greater trochanter: Bilateral, posterior to the trochanteric prominence

## ANTERIOR TRIGGER POINT SITES

Low cervical: Bilateral, at the anterior aspects of the intertransverse spaces at C5-7

Second rib: Bilateral, at the second costochondral junctions, just lateral to the junctions on upper surfaces

Lateral epicondyle: Bilateral, 2 cm distal to the epicondyles

Knee: Bilateral, at the medial fat pad proximal to the joint line

A wide variety of symptoms can accompany FMS. Sleep disturbances and stiffness often are present. Short-term memory loss may be reported. Fatigue, which is worse in the morning and late in the day, is a common complaint. Mood changes include depression and anxiety and often develop concurrently with multiple somatic complaints, such as migraine and tension headaches, substernal chest pain, bursitis and tendinitis, cystitis, irritable bowel syndrome, urinary frequency, and paresthesias in the hands and feet.

## TESTS

### PHYSICAL EXAMINATION

Examination reveals tenderness to palpation over several of the 18 tender point sites. Sufficient pressure should be applied so that the patient's skin blanches under the examiner's fingers. These tender points are limited to the soft tissues (muscle, tendon, ligament, or bursa); examination of the joints is normal.

### DIAGNOSTIC TESTS

No radiographs or laboratory tests are diagnostic of FMS.

## DIFFERENTIAL DIAGNOSIS

AIDS (blood test)

Bursitis or tendinitis (usually single joint or extremity)

Complex regional pain syndrome (usually a single extremity)

Hypothyroidism (abnormal thyroid function tests)

Lyme disease (serology test)

Multiple sclerosis (abnormal MRI of the brain)

Polymyalgia rheumatica (elevated erythrocyte sedimentation rate)

Polymyositis (skin rash)

Rheumatoid arthritis (positive rheumatoid factor)

Systemic lupus erythematosus (antinuclear antibodies, elevated erythrocyte sedimentation rate)

Tenosynovitis (single focus, associated with tendon motion)

## ADVERSE OUTCOMES OF THE DISEASE

The chronic pain associated with FMS can result in depression, anxiety, and inactivity. The multiple tests ordered and the multiple clinicians consulted to make the correct diagnosis can be expensive.

## TREATMENT

Patients should be advised that FMS is not a life-threatening or progressive disease. No cure is available, but symptom relief is possible. The optimal treatment program is multifaceted. Tricyclic antidepressants and NSAIDs can be helpful in controlling the pain. Amitriptyline in doses of 10 to 50 mg or cyclobenzaprine in doses of 10 to 40 mg, taken at bedtime, can be useful. Fluoxetine, taken in the morning, is useful to reduce a severe depression. Short-term or intermittent NSAIDs may help diminish pain, but corticosteroids and narcotic analgesics are contraindicated. The non-narcotic analgesic tramadol taken in divided doses of 50 to 400 mg per day has been shown to help the pain in FMS. Topical agents such as capsaicin cream applied to the tender point areas may be beneficial.

Patients should be instructed in a stretching program to increase flexibility. Exercise programs for FMS should begin slowly and increase gradually to build endurance while minimizing pain. In addition, initiation of an aerobic exercise program to increase cardiac fitness is recommended. Referral to a dietitian for weight loss supervision often is indicated. Many patients will benefit from participation in FMS support groups, which are a useful source of information and encouragement. Many larger medical centers have established FMS clinics, which use a multidisciplinary approach in the treatment of these patients.

## ADVERSE OUTCOMES OF TREATMENT

Patients can become dependent on narcotics and tranquilizers. Medications also have side effects, including drowsiness, dry mouth, change in appetite, and constipation. Tachyphylaxis (decreased response) can develop with long-term use of amitriptyline and/or cyclobenzaprine.

## REFERRAL DECISIONS/RED FLAGS

Severe symptoms that interfere with patients' ability to work or the presence of serious psychiatric problems indicates the need for evaluation at an FMS treatment center.

# FRACTURE PRINCIPLES

## DEFINITION

A fracture is a disruption in the continuity of bone that occurs as a result of a direct blow to the bone or an indirect force applied to the limb. Most fractures result in gross interruption of the bone matrix. Fractures, however, may occur at a microscopic level, as seen in stress fractures.

## CLINICAL SYMPTOMS

The classic symptoms of acute fractures are swelling, pain that is aggravated by movement, deformity, and decreased function. Nondisplaced fractures may not exhibit any obvious deformity. Stress fractures often present with the indolent onset of mild swelling and tenderness and pain with weight bearing. Table 1 lists the defining characteristics of specific types of fractures.

## TESTS

### PHYSICAL EXAMINATION

Examination reveals localized tenderness, swelling, and often deformity. A complete examination should include an evaluation of the surrounding skin integrity, stability of the adjacent joints, and function of the nerves and vessels distal to the site of injury. *Any laceration or abrasion of the skin should be considered an open fracture.* All suspected open fractures require further evaluation for exploration and debridement.

### DIAGNOSTIC TESTS

Radiographs usually identify an acute fracture. With stress fractures and some nondisplaced fractures, the injury may not be visible on radiographs until bone resorbs from the fracture ends (1 to 4 weeks). Carpal navicular fractures often are missed for this reason. Tomography, CT, and MRI usually are not indicated in the initial assessment of fractures unless the diagnosis cannot be confirmed with routine radiographs.

## DIFFERENTIAL DIAGNOSIS

Dislocation (marked deformity, disruption of normal joint alignment on radiographs)

Infection (no history of trauma, fever, elevated erythrocyte sedimentation rate)

Sprain (normal radiographs)

Tumor (gradual onset, bone destruction evident on radiographs)

## ADVERSE OUTCOMES OF THE DISEASE

Any fracture can exhibit delayed union (slower healing than normal), nonunion (failure to heal by bone), or malunion (healing with unacceptable

## Table 1
## Fracture Classification

| Location in the bone | Description |
| --- | --- |
| Epiphyseal | The end of the bone, forming part of the adjacent joint |
| Metaphyseal | The flared portion of the bone at the ends of the shaft |
| Diaphyseal | The shaft of a long bone |

| Orientation/Extent of the fracture line(s) | Description |
| --- | --- |
| Transverse | A fracture that is perpendicular to the shaft of the bone |
| Oblique | An angulated fracture line |
| Spiral | A multiplanar and complex fracture line |
| Comminuted | More than two fracture fragments |
| Segmental | A completely separate segment of bone bordered by fracture lines |
| Intra-articular | The fracture line crosses the articular cartilage and enters the joint |
| Torus | A buckle fracture of one cortex, often seen in children |
| Compression | Impaction of bone, such as in the vertebrae or proximal tibia |
| Greenstick | An incomplete fracture with angular deformity, seen in children |
| Pathologic | A fracture through bone weakened by disease or tumor |

| Amount of displacement of the fracture fragments | Description |
| --- | --- |
| Nondisplaced | A fracture in which the fragments are in anatomic alignment |
| Displaced | A fracture in which the fragments are no longer in their usual alignment |
| Angulated | A fracture in which the fragments are malaligned |
| Bayonetted | A fracture in which the distal fragment longitudinally overlaps the proximal fragment |
| Distracted | A fracture in which the distal fragment is separated from the proximal fragment by a gap |

| Integrity of the skin and soft-tissue envelope around the fracture | Description |
| --- | --- |
| Closed | The skin over and near the fracture is intact |
| Open | The skin over and near the fracture is lacerated or abraded by the injury |

deformity). Limb function can be adversely affected by nearby joint contractures, stiffness, limb shortening, or malalignment to such a degree that the patient cannot easily compensate using the nearby joints. Osteomyelitis may develop if the fracture is open. In severe fractures, nerve and/or vascular damage may jeopardize the viability or usefulness of the extremity. A compartment syndrome can develop if there is excessive swelling. This complication requires early recognition and emergency treatment. Complex regional pain syndrome can develop but is rare.

## TREATMENT

Treatment is guided by the four Rs: Recognition, Reduction, Retention of reduction while achieving union, and Rehabilitation. The key to recognition is awareness of the subtle injuries that may occur at different anatomic locations. Reduction is not necessary with nondisplaced or minimally displaced injuries. For fractures with significant displacement, however, reduction will be required. Some fractures can be manipulated to an acceptable position by closed techniques, whereas others require open reduction and internal fixation. Retention of reduction may involve a splint, circular cast, or internal fixation device. Rehabilitation is extremely important. Even nondisplaced fractures treated by splinting result in muscle atrophy and adjacent joint stiffness. Many patients can be treated by a gradual increase in activities and simple instructions in range-of-motion and strengthening exercises. Table 2 lists factors that influence fracture healing.

## ADVERSE OUTCOMES OF TREATMENT

Malunion, nonunion, stiffness, arthritis, or vascular or nerve injury is possible. One of the most devastating problems is unrecognized compartment syndrome from the injury or from a cast that is too tight.

### Table 2
**Factors That Influence Fracture Healing**

---

**Factors that increase fracture stability, facilitate treatment, and offer a good prognosis**

Skeletal immaturity—thick periosteum, faster rate of healing, potential for remodeling

Single bone fractures in forearm (radius or ulna) or lower leg (tibia or fibula)

Nondisplaced pelvic fractures

Transverse fractures—tend to be stable when reduced

Presence of adjacent bone for support (eg, finger buddy taped to adjacent finger)

Thoracic spine fractures

---

**Factors that decrease fracture stability and render fracture more difficult to treat**

Skeletal maturity—thin periosteum and poor potential for remodeling

Both-bone fractures of forearm or lower leg

Comminuted, displaced pelvic fractures

Oblique fractures

Marked displacement (indicates severe soft-tissue stripping)

Unstable cervical and lumbar spine fractures

Comminuted and segmental fractures

Fractures involving a joint

## Referral decisions/Red flags

Patients with open fractures, unstable fractures, or irreducible fractures, or those with suspected compartment syndrome, or nerve, vascular, or muscle damage need further evaluation. Most patients who have displaced fractures require further evaluation, as even fractures that appear innocuous may be associated with poor outcomes.

# IMAGING PRINCIPLES AND TECHNIQUES

Imaging studies are expensive, time consuming, and may be painful for the patient. The simplest studies should be ordered and interpreted before more specialized studies are considered. MRI, CT, and other specialized studies are rarely needed in the initial evaluation.

## RADIOGRAPHY

Plain radiographs are the mainstay of bone and joint imaging. Radiographic examination of a long bone for fracture should meet the following criteria:

- Any radiograph of a long bone should include the joints above and below to avoid missing a dislocation associated with a fracture.

- Images should be obtained in at least two planes perpendicular to each other (ie, AP and lateral). Radiographs of a joint may be confusing if the extremity is in a nonstandard position (Table 1).

## Table 1
### Standard Radiographic Views

| Region | Views | Special considerations |
|---|---|---|
| Hand | PA and lateral | |
| Wrist | PA and lateral | |
| Elbow/Forearm | AP and lateral | Comparison views may be helpful (opposite elbow) |
| Shoulder | AP of shoulder, AP of glenohumeral joint, axillary | Transscapular lateral view if unable to obtain axillary view |
| Cervical spine | AP and lateral | Include from C1 through C7 in the lateral view; swimmer's view may help visualize C7 |
| Thoracic | AP and lateral | Swimmer's view may help visualize C7-T5 |
| Lumbar spine | AP and lateral | Spot lateral of L5 if not seen well on standard lateral; try to see from T12-sacrum |
| Pelvis | AP | |
| Hip | AP and groin lateral or true lateral | |
| Knee | Weight-bearing AP in full extension and 30° flexion in patients older than 40 years; otherwise, standard AP, lateral, and bilateral/axial (Merchant) views | |
| Ankle | AP, lateral, and mortise | |
| Foot | Weight-bearing AP and lateral, supine oblique | |

## INDICATIONS

Deformity of a bone or joint, inability to use the extremity or a joint, or unexplained pain in a bone or joint indicates the need for radiographic examination. Children and women of child-bearing age should be protected with lead shields whenever possible.

# MAGNETIC RESONANCE IMAGING

Magnetic resonance imaging (MRI) offers the advantage of seeing soft-tissue detail and often identifies the extent of tumors. MRI is an excellent technique for imaging the spine, joints, and soft tissues. Combining MRI with contrast material distinguishes between scar and avascular tissues.

## INDICATIONS

MRI often is very valuable in preoperative planning, especially in certain soft-tissue conditions, tumors, or chronic osteomyelitis; however, the underlying diagnosis usually can be made by less expensive means. MRI also is valuable in situations of diagnostic dilemma. Patients whose conditions are associated with issues of liability, such as personal injury or workers' compensation claims, can require MRI to determine the anatomic extent of injury or disease for purposes of claim settlement. Claustrophobia precludes MRI in some patients.

# COMPUTED TOMOGRAPHY

Computed tomography (CT) offers axial visualization of bone, muscle, and fat tissues. Bone visualization is usually excellent, and soft-tissue structures less so.

## INDICATIONS

CT is helpful in preoperative planning for bony procedures to help localize lesions and appreciate the scope of bony changes. Complex or extensive fracture patterns, especially those with joint involvement, also are best visualized with CT. This imaging technique often is used with myelography in patients who have degenerative spine disease.

# ARTHROGRAPHY

Arthrography is an invasive but less expensive technique than CT or MRI in which contrast material is injected into the joint to evaluate the joint capsule and articular surface integrity. At times, arthrography is combined with CT or MRI. Arthrography is associated with a risk of infection and allergic reaction to the contrast material.

## INDICATIONS

Rotator cuff tears, interosseous ligament tears at the wrist, and meniscal tears are conditions well evaluated by arthrography; however, MRI often provides superior imaging of these conditions.

## BONE SCAN

Bone scan, or scintigraphy, is a radioisotope technique that shows blood flow and metabolic activity in the bone, thereby indicating bone formation or destruction.

### INDICATIONS

A bone scan is useful for identifying infection, tumor, and fractures.

# LYME DISEASE

## DEFINITION

Lyme disease is a multisystem illness with acute and chronic manifestations caused by the spirochete *Borrellia burgdorferi* that is borne by the deer tick *Ixodes dammini*. Lyme disease is named after a town in Connecticut where, in 1975, several children developed a mysterious arthritis of unknown cause that was subsequently found to be caused by this spirochete. Lyme disease is the most prevalent vector-borne illness in the United States, with nearly 50,000 cases reported since 1982. The incidence is highest in the Northeast (Maryland to northern Massachusetts), the upper Midwest (Wisconsin and Minnesota), and the far West (northern California and Oregon). Lyme disease has been reported in 48 states, as well as in Asia and Europe.

## CLINICAL SYMPTOMS

Patients with Lyme disease initially have variable constitutional and flulike symptoms. In adults, these symptoms are commonly accompanied by a distinctive skin lesion (erythema migrans) originating and expanding from the site of the tick bite. A subacute or intermediate stage of Lyme disease can follow the acute episode and is characterized by arthralgia and arthritis in up to 80% of untreated patients. The knee is most commonly affected. Multiple joint involvement is rare. Cardiovascular involvement occurs in 4% to 8% of patients at this stage, and neurologic symptoms develop in 15% of patients. Half of these neurologic complications are either Bell palsy or other types of cranial nerve paralysis. Dermatologic and ocular symptoms also may occur in the intermediate phase. The chronic stage of Lyme disease often does not appear for several months or even years after the initial episode and is characterized by chronic arthritis and recurrent arthralgias. Other symptoms include chronic fatigue, polyradiculopathy, and encephalopathy with loss of memory and inability to concentrate.

## TESTS

### PHYSICAL EXAMINATION

Patients with arthralgia should be examined for synovitis and restricted joint motion.

### DIAGNOSTIC TESTS

Lyme disease is a clinical diagnosis, but serologic testing for *Borrellia* titer is important, particularly in the later stages of the disease.

## DIFFERENTIAL DIAGNOSIS

Acute rheumatic fever

Idiopathic Bell palsy (physical examination)

Meningitis (lumbar puncture)

Multiple sclerosis (abnormal MRI of the brain)

Peripheral neuritis (specific nerve involvement)

Reiter syndrome (iritis, urethritis)

## ADVERSE OUTCOMES OF THE DISEASE

Lyme disease can be complicated by arthritis in major weight-bearing joints, facial paralysis, chronic fatigue, concentration defects, cardiac conduction block, and peripheral neuritis.

## TREATMENT

When diagnosed early, Lyme disease is effectively treated with antibiotics. Doxycycline 100 mg twice a day for 10 to 30 days or amoxicillin 500 mg three times a day for 10 to 30 days has been shown to be effective. For children younger than age 8 years, amoxicillin 20 mg/kg in divided doses is indicated.

Clinical trials are presently under way to test vaccines that will prevent the development of Lyme disease. One recombinant vaccine, LYMErix, has been approved by the FDA. Although studies have shown that three doses provided protective efficacy of more than 80%, several questions remain regarding its safety in children and its duration of protection. Therefore, at this time prevention is still the best course of action. People in high-risk areas should avoid or minimize walking in the woods. Those living in heavily wooded areas should wear long-sleeved shirts tucked into trousers with the trouser legs tucked into socks. Most importantly, the skin and clothing should be checked for ticks. If the tick is removed within 24 to 36 hours, the risk of Lyme disease is minimal. Tick removal is best done by carefully teasing with fine tweezers. Heat and chemicals should not be used on the tick as these can cause the tick to burst or regurgitate and expel fluid onto the skin.

## ADVERSE OUTCOMES OF TREATMENT

Allergic reactions or adverse drug interactions to antibiotics can occur.

## REFERRAL DECISIONS/RED FLAGS

Patients with suspected Lyme disease may require evaluation by an infectious disease specialist.

# Nonorganic Symptoms and Signs

ICD-9 Code

ICD-9 lists psychophysiologic disorders according to body system.

## Synonyms

Psychosomatic illness

Functional overlay

## Definition

Patient responses or symptoms that do not fit known patterns of illnesses or injury are considered nonorganic. These findings are not considered malingering; rather, they often are the way that some patients communicate their perception of the seriousness of their problem or their perception that they are not receiving the care they think they need. True malingering is rare and typically is a manifestation of bizarre social behavior.

Nonorganic findings should not be construed as indicating lack of concomitant disease because significant underlying pathology can be present. Nonorganic findings occur three to four times more often in situations where workers' compensation and litigation are issues than in situations where they are not.

## Clinical symptoms

Pain or symptoms that appear to "travel" from one side or area of the body to another in a nonanatomic fashion and global pain are characteristic. Nonsegmental numbness (ie, does not fit a nerve root or peripheral nerve pattern) also occurs.

## Tests

### Physical examination

Exaggerated responses: Light touch causes a jerk or withdrawal. Other findings include grimacing, groaning, and grabbing the affected extremity during examination when there is no obvious trauma or medical problem.

Axial loading (low back pain): With the patient standing, place both hands on the head and push down, asking if it causes pain. Low back pain elicited in this position is a nonorganic finding; however, neck pain may be a legitimate finding.

Axial rotation (spine): With the patient's hands on the iliac crests, grasp and rotate the pelvis, asking the patient if this causes back pain. This maneuver should not elicit back pain, since the motion occurs at the hips, not in the back. Because this test may be positive in 20% of patients, it is not as sensitive in identifying nonorganic behavior as are exaggerated responses and axial loading.

Flip sign: This sign is elicited with the patient seated leaning slightly forward with his or her hands on the edge of the examination table. While asking if the patient has knee problems, lift the foot and extend the knee. This maneuver increases tension on the sciatic nerve, and patients with lower lumbar herniated disks or other similar conditions will involuntarily "flip" back against the wall, reporting back and leg pain. A negative flip sign in the presence of supine straight leg raising test that produces leg and back pain at less than 45° of leg elevation is a significant nonorganic finding, as these maneuvers are the same test.

Distraction: A provocative test (such as palpation) may be negative when the patient is distracted with conversation, but positive when attention is drawn to the test or body part.

Giving way: During muscle testing, a nonorganic finding is a lack of sustained effort. Typically, the patient "gives way" or "lets go" in a ratchety, uneven pattern. Another variant is the patient who gives a poor effort on muscle testing and then, with coaxing, may intermittently contract the muscle, then let go.

Stocking or nonanatomic numbness: Some patients report hypoesthesia that affects the extremity in a circumferential (stocking glove) distribution or covers nonanatomic patterns. Patients with diabetes mellitus or multiple sclerosis may develop sensory abnormalities in a stocking glove or nonsegmental pattern.

Pain diagram: On a diagram of the body, ask the patient to draw representations of symptoms, using dashes, slashes, Xs, etc. Bizarre drawings do not indicate malingering or mental disease. Many people have perceptual disorders that blunt the scientific validity of these drawings, but they often yield insight into how pain is perceived by patients, and what areas of the body they feel are related in their current problem (**Figure 1**).

The kneeling bench test of Burns: This is another test of exaggerated response. Ask a patient who reports back pain to kneel on a stool. Hold the patient's ankles to ensure confidence and ask the patient to bend forward and touch the floor. Patients who are exaggerating symptoms will bend forward a few degrees and then grab their back, saying they cannot bend. Note that these patients are already bending forward significantly.

A thorough neurologic examination is required to give the above tests perspective and to rule out concomitant disease.

## DIAGNOSTIC TESTS
None

## DIFFERENTIAL DIAGNOSIS

Acute injury (withdrawal from a painful examination maneuver may be an appropriate response)

Diabetes mellitus (stocking-type peripheral neuropathy)

Multiple sclerosis (bizarre sensory patterns that are not segmental)

Stroke or other central lesions with altered sensory appreciation

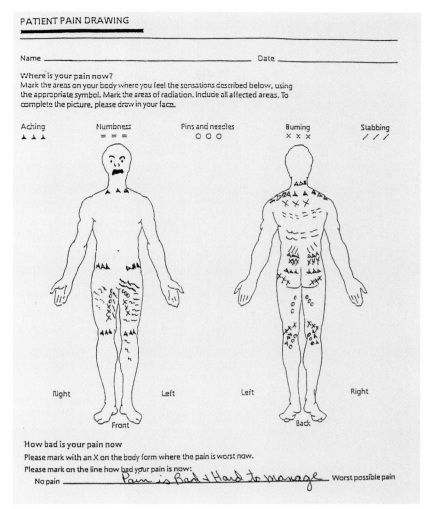

**PATIENT PAIN DRAWING**

Name _____ Date _____

Where is your pain now?
Mark the areas on your body where you feel the sensations described below, using the appropriate symbol. Mark the areas of radiation. Include all affected areas. To complete the picture, please draw in your face.

| Aching | Numbness | Pins and needles | Burning | Stabbing |
|---|---|---|---|---|
| ▲ ▲ ▲ | = = = | O O O | x x x | / / / |

Right     Left          Left     Right
Front                          Back

How bad is your pain now
Please mark with an X on the body form where the pain is worst now.
Please mark on the line how bad your pain is now:
No pain _____ *Pain is Bad + Hard to manage* _____ Worst possible pain

**Figure 1**
Pain diagram for patient with nonorganic physical findings.

## TREATMENT

Rule out serious disorders that may be masked by these symptoms and discuss the absence of specific disorders with the patient. Because patients with this condition often are indirectly indicating that they are not getting the support or help they need, discuss psychological and social support interventions and inquire about contributing factors such as occupational stress and marital difficulties.

## ADVERSE OUTCOMES OF TREATMENT

Failure to identify an associated serious condition is possible.

## REFERRAL DECISIONS/RED FLAGS

True diminished pinprick, diminished light touch with or without areflexia, clonus, or spasticity usually indicates neurologic involvement.

# Nonsteroidal Anti-Inflammatory Drugs

## Definition

Nonsteroidal anti-inflammatory drugs (NSAIDs) are a group of drugs used to treat inflammatory conditions such as arthritis, bursitis, and tendinitis. Aspirin is a nonsteroidal anti-inflammatory drug, but the term NSAID usually is reserved for the newer aspirin-like agents that were developed to decrease the severity of gastritis associated with long-term use of aspirin.

Inflammation is an essential, normal protective mechanism associated with injury to the musculoskeletal system, but in addition to trauma, inflammation may be triggered by infection, allergy, or an autoimmune response, as in rheumatoid arthritis. The inflammatory response is mediated by chemicals, such as prostaglandins, which are released from mast cells, granulocytes, and basophils. NSAIDs block prostaglandin by interfering with the action of the enzyme cyclooxygenase (COX). Corticosteroids also block the formation of prostaglandins but do so at a different step in the production chain.

In addition to their anti-inflammatory properties, all NSAIDs exhibit analgesic and antipyretic activity. These drugs also decrease platelet adhesiveness and may inhibit the production of prothrombin.

NSAIDs vary in chemical structure, cost, frequency of side effects, and duration of action (**Table 1**). Effective use of these drugs often requires some experimentation because patients may respond to certain NSAIDs but not to others, and an initial good response may wane with time. Switching to another class of NSAIDs as opposed to switching within the class is likely to be more effective, and for this reason, Table 1 is organized by group.

Two isoforms of COX have been identified. COX-1 is expressed in many tissues, but COX-2 is an enzyme that primarily mediates the inflammatory response. Most NSAIDs inhibit COX-1 and COX-2 production, thereby affecting gastric mucosa, renal blood flow, and platelet aggregation as well as inflammation. Recently developed COX-2 inhibitors selectively affect COX-2 enzymes and, therefore, are much less likely to cause gastric ulcers and bleeding. Renal and hepatic complications have been reported in patients taking COX-2 inhibitors. COX-2 inhibitors should not be used in patients who are at greater risk and need reduced platelet aggregation to reduce the risk of cardiac events.

## Side effects

NSAIDs cause similar side effects, but in varying degrees. Minor dyspepsia is common, even with COX-2 drugs. Gastric ulcers and bleeding are less common but more serious. In patients older than 65 years, approximately 30% of hospitalizations and deaths from gastrointestinal hemorrhage are secondary to NSAID treatment.

## Table 1
### Types of NSAIDs

| Drug | Strength | Trade name | Typical dosage |
|---|---|---|---|
| *Salicylates* | | | |
| Aspirin | 300, 325, 600, 650 | Several | 325 mg qid |
| Choline magnesium trisalicylate | 500, 750, 1000 | Trilisate | 1,500 mg bid |
| Salsalate | 500, 750 | Disalcid | 1,000 mg tid, 1,500 mg bid |
| Diflunisal | 500 | Dolobid | 250 mg bid or tid, 500 mg bid |
| *Propionic acids* | | | |
| Naproxen sodium | 220 | Aleve | 220 mg bid |
| | 375, 500 | Naprelan 375, 500 | 750-1000 mg/day |
| | 275, DS 550 | Anaprox | 275 mg bid or tid 550 mg bid |
| Naproxen | 250, 375, 500 | Naprosyn | 250, 375, or 500 mg bid |
| Naproxen EC | 375, 500 | EC Naprosyn | 375 or 500 mg/day |
| Flurbiprofen | 50, 100 | Ansaid | 100 mg bid |
| Oxaprozin | 600 | Daypro | 600-1,200 mg/day |
| Ibuprofen | 400, 600, 800 | Motrin | 400-800 mg bid or tid |
| Ibuprofen (OTC) | 200 | Motrin IB, Advil, Rufin, Nuprin | 200-400 mg bid or tid |
| Ketoprofen | 25, 50, 75 | Orudis | 50 mg qid, 75 mg tid |
| Ketoprofen extended release | 100, 150, 200 | Oruvail | 200 mg/day |
| Ketorolac tromethamine | 10 | Toradol Oral | 10 mg qid; 5 days max of oral and IM combined |
| *Indolacetic acids and related compounds* | | | |
| Sulindac | 150, 200 | Clinoril | 150-200 mg bid |
| Indomethacin | 25, 50 | Indocin | 25-50 mg tid |
| Indomethacin sustained release | 75 | Indocin SR | 75 mg/day |
| Etodolac | 200-500 | Lodine | 200-400 mg tid, 500 mg |

Reversible hepatotoxicity is observed in 10% to 15% of patients with long-term usage. Nephrotoxicity is less common but can develop early in treatment and results from loss of the vasodilatory effects of renal prostaglandins. Fluid retention can increase blood pressure in susceptible patients. The inhibition of prostaglandin synthesis also can be responsible for hives and acute episodes of asthma in some patients.

### CHOICE OF THERAPEUTIC AGENTS

Because of decreased side effects, an NSAID usually is selected to initiate treatment of an arthritic condition. If the problem is likely to be of several weeks' or months' duration, one of the second- or third-generation medications typically is chosen. Cost, side effects, the dosage schedule, and physician familiarity are all factors to consider. Once or twice daily dosage schedules are optimal for patients with poor compliance. Although long-term use in patients with rheumatoid arthritis or osteoarthritis is standard practice, short-term use for most other conditions is encouraged. For osteoarthritis that has a minimal inflammatory component, the use of acetaminophen for primary management with intermittent use of NSAIDs for breakthrough pain can help reduce gastric complications.

In general, all NSAIDs should be taken with food to decrease gastric irritation. Oral hypoglycemic agents or warfarin sodium may be unfavorably potentiated by some NSAIDs in some patients. Full-dose aspirin or other NSAIDs should not be taken at the same time as another NSAID; however, low-dose aspirin often is used with other NSAID medications in patients with cardiac disease. NSAIDs should be used with caution in patients with hypertension; indomethacin is particularly hazardous in elderly patients.

Patients who are at risk for gastric complications can choose from the following alternatives, in addition to those described previously:

- A nonacetylated NSAID such as salsalate (Disalcid) appears to cause less mucosal injury.

- NSAIDs that are nonacidic (such as nabumetone)

- Prodrugs (drugs that must undergo biotransformation to an active metabolite) are reported to decrease gastric injury.

- NSAIDs of the pyranocarboxylic acid class, such as etodolac (Lodine), are appropriate in high-risk patients.

- COX-2 inhibitors should cause the lowest incidence of gastritis but are more expensive.

# OSTEOARTHRITIS

## ICD-9 Codes

715.0
  Osteoarthrosis, generalized
715.1
  Osteoarthrosis, localized, primary
715.2
  Osteoarthrosis, localized, secondary
715.3
  Osteoarthrosis, localized, not specified whether primary or secondary
716.1
  Traumatic arthropathy

## SYNONYMS

Osteoarthrosis

Degenerative joint disease

Wear and tear arthritis

## DEFINITION

Osteoarthritis (OA), or perhaps more appropriately osteoarthrosis, is a progressive, currently irreversible condition involving loss of articular cartilage that leads to pain and sometimes deformity, principally in the weight-bearing joints of the lower extremities and the spine. It is the most common type of arthritis and is most often associated with age, obesity, and previous trauma or other disorders that change the mechanics of the joint.

## CLINICAL SYMPTOMS

The common symptoms are stiffness, pain, and deformity. Even when there is a joint effusion, patients more commonly report stiffness rather than swelling. Until the later stages of the disease, the pain of OA usually is relieved by rest. Osteophytes (spurs) may physically block joint motion in advanced disease.

## TESTS

### PHYSICAL EXAMINATION

Osteophytes are often palpable at the joint margins in the knee, ankle, elbow, hand, and foot. An effusion sometimes is present but is typically mild. Range of motion is decreased. The loss of motion usually is mild unless the disease is severe. Genu varum (bowleg) or genu valgum (knock-knee) are common findings. With OA of the hip, the patient often walks "toes out" with the limb externally rotated and tilts or lurches to the affected side with each step.

### DIAGNOSTIC TESTS

Radiographs of the affected joint usually demonstrate loss of joint space, sclerosis, subchondral cysts, and/or osteophytosis or spurs at the joint margin.

## DIFFERENTIAL DIAGNOSIS

Charcot joint (primarily foot and ankle, diabetic neuropathy)

Chondrocalcinosis (crystals in joint aspirate)

Degenerative changes secondary to inflammatory arthritis (positive rheumatoid factor)

Epiphyseal dysplasia (short stature)

Hemochromatosis (abnormal liver function studies)

Hemophilia (bleeding tendency)

## ADVERSE OUTCOMES OF THE DISEASE

Pain, deformity, loss of joint motion, loss of limb function, and joint instability are possible.

## TREATMENT

Continued reassurance, patient education, and protection from overuse are critical. Simply telephoning patients periodically can often help them cope with this irreversible disorder. Gentle, regular joint exercises help maintain function and manage pain. Water exercise, bicycling, and non–weight-bearing exercises can help to reduce symptoms and preserve muscle support in the affected joints. Isometric exercises help improve strength if patients are unable to tolerate exercises involving joint motion.

Weight loss is important, especially for the joints of the lower extremity, not only to reduce symptoms but also to improve the survival of joint implants, placed when symptoms are intolerable.

Pain management with acetaminophen, propoxyphene, or salicylates and NSAIDs often is helpful. Many elderly patients are better able to cope with symptoms if they can manage their pain. Simple medications may allow them to postpone or avoid surgery and its associated risks.

Intra-articular corticosteroids often relieve symptoms, but the duration of relief may be short (1 to 2 weeks) in the lower extremities, the shoulder, or the elbow. In the hand, intra-articular steroids may relieve symptoms for months. No more than two injections should be given in any weight-bearing joint. Viscosupplement injections are useful for OA at the knee (see Alternative Therapies for Osteoarthritis, pp 53-54).

Surgery, typically joint replacement or arthrodesis, is appropriate when patients have pain at rest, pain at night, or unacceptable loss of joint function. Hip and knee replacement surgery is especially effective in reducing pain and increasing function.

## ADVERSE OUTCOMES OF TREATMENT

Salicylates and NSAIDs often help but can cause renal, hepatic, or gastric problems. In addition, NSAIDs may inhibit joint repair by interfering with prostaglandin synthesis. This is currently only a theoretic consideration.

Removal of prosthetic implants due to infection or loosening is possible. Patients who have an earlier, preemptive procedure, such as an arthroscopic joint debridement or osteotomy, may ultimately require a second operation (ie, joint replacement).

## REFERRAL DECISIONS/RED FLAGS

Patients who have pain at rest, pain at night, or unacceptable loss of joint function need further evaluation.

# ALTERNATIVE THERAPIES FOR OSTEOARTHRITIS

Osteoarthritis (OA) is the most common form of arthritis and a leading cause of disability in adults. NSAIDs are commonly used to alleviate the symptoms of OA, but these medications can have significant side effects. For that reason, alternative medications and therapies often are actively sought by patients and frequently publicized in the lay press and in other venues. Furthermore, patients frequently inquire about these new treatments. This chapter reviews four alternative therapies that may be of benefit in the treatment of OA. It is important to advise patients that the indications, benefits, and long-term efficacy of these treatments are still relatively unknown.

## GLUCOSAMINE AND CHONDROITIN SULFATE

Articular cartilage is composed of chondrocytes, water, collagen, and proteoglycans. Glycosaminoglycans are an important component of proteoglycans. In OA, there is a breakdown of the proteoglycans, resulting in increased water permeability and resultant deterioration of cartilage. Glucosamine is a hexosamine sugar and a building block for glycosaminoglycans. Chondroitin sulfate is a glycosaminoglycan that is found in proteoglycans.

Glucosamine and chondroitin are currently extracted from animal products and sold as over-the-counter dietary supplements. The usual dosages for glucosamine and chondroitin sulfate are 1,500 mg/day and 1,200 mg/day, respectively, for at least 6 weeks. These compounds also are sold in combination, but taking the combination does not appear to be beneficial. The absorption of chondroitin sulfate through the gastrointestinal tract has been reported to be inconsistent, and some authors recommend initial treatment with glucosamine. Only mild side effects such as dyspepsia have been reported, but there are theoretical concerns that glucosamine might increase blood glucose levels in patients with diabetes and that chondroitin sulfate might increase clotting time in patients taking anticoagulants.

Theoretically, these compounds can be ingested and absorbed into the blood stream to cross into the joint to promote analgesia and healing of cartilage. In vitro and animal studies have shown that both compounds demonstrate anti-inflammatory activities and favorably affect cartilage metabolism. Clinical studies have reported that both are considered safe and effective in treating OA. However, a recent review and rigorously conducted meta-analysis of randomized controlled trials of these supplements raised serious concerns of publication bias and design flaws in previous studies that had reported both analgesic and disease-modifying benefits of glucosamine and chondroitin sulfate.

At the time of the publication of this book, the National Institutes of Health has initiated a double-blinded, randomized controlled trial of glucosamine and chondroitin sulfate in patients with OA of the knee. Until the results of

SECTION 1 | GENERAL ORTHOPAEDICS

that study are known, patients should be advised that these compounds appear to be safe and may be effective in treating OA, but that there is no definitive proof of their benefits.

## S-ADENOSYL-L-METHIONINE (SAM)

S-adenosyl-L-methionine (SAM) is available as an over-the-counter dietary supplement used to treat OA and depression. SAM is synthesized in the body from the essential amino acid methionine. Theoretically, by forming sulfur compounds, SAM can augment cartilage formation. In some clinical studies, SAM has been as effective as NSAIDs and has fewer side effects. The usual dosage is 200 to 400 mg three times a day. Although SAM may be an alternative pain medication, more evidence is needed to prove whether this medication promotes cartilage repair.

## VISCOSUPPLEMENTS

Hyaluronic acid is a large glycosaminoglycan produced by chondrocytes and type B synoviocytes. It is a key biochemical for synovial viscoelasticity, boundary lubrication, and joint motion. Patients with OA have a diminished concentration of hyaluronic acid. Due to poor gastrointestinal absorption, hyaluronic acid must be injected into the joint. Theoretic mechanisms by which hyaluronic acid may be therapeutic include: 1) providing additional lubrication of the synovial membrane; 2) controlling permeability of the synovial membrane, thus diminishing joint effusions; and 3) directly blocking inflammation by scavenging free radicals. Several clinical trials have shown pain relief, but it is not known whether the use of viscosupplements will delay progression of OA.

Currently, the FDA approves viscosupplementation for OA of the knee only. Two preparations are available. One is produced from rooster combs and the other is manufactured through bacterial cultures. Injection schedules are either three over 15 days or weekly injections for 5 weeks. This therapy is relatively expensive. Local reactions are self-limiting and consist of increased joint pain with swelling, erythema, and itching. Systemic effects are uncommon but have included muscle cramps, especially the calf, and hemorrhoid formation.

# OSTEOMYELITIS

## SYNONYM

Bone infection

## DEFINITION

Bone, like any other tissue, is susceptible to invasion by microorganisms. Osteomyelitis usually is caused by pyogenic organisms, but other sources such as tuberculosis, syphilis, and viral or fungal elements also are causative of osteomyelitis. The infecting agent creates an inflammatory response that progresses to an abscess that then destroys bone. The organism usually reaches the bone by hematogenous spread but can also infect the bone by direct spread of a soft-tissue infection or by a penetrating wound, eg, an open fracture. *Staphylococcus aureus* is the most common causative organism, with hemolytic streptococci next.

## CLINICAL SYMPTOMS

Unrelenting pain is the first symptom. The patient may report a history of an injury, which can delay the diagnosis. Fever develops early, followed by other symptoms, including localized tenderness, particularly over the metaphyseal area of the bone, generalized aches and pains, and a flushed appearance. In a neonate or infant, diagnosis is more difficult, and the bone infection may accompany other infectious causes such as meningitis, septicemia, or pneumonia.

## TESTS

### PHYSICAL EXAMINATION

Patients, including neonates, will not use the limb and often hold it in a protective manner. Motion is possible but painful. Gentle attempts at motion can be used to help differentiate osteomyelitis from a septic joint, as motion is extremely painful in an infected joint. Focal bone tenderness leads to the diagnosis and also to the site for possible aspiration. More established lesions will demonstrate swelling, erythema, and increased localized warmth. These findings typically are less dramatic with chronic osteomyelitis or osteomyelitis caused by nonpyogenic organisms. However, the latter may be associated with soft-tissue ulceration or draining sinuses.

### DIAGNOSTIC TESTS

Obtain a white blood cell count, erythrocyte sedimentation rate, AP and lateral radiographs of the affected area, blood culture, and aspiration of the suspected site for culture. Early radiographs will be negative or will show only soft-tissue swelling but should be obtained to rule out other conditions. A bone scan usually is not necessary in the acute situation but indicates osteomyelitis very early. MRI also is usually not necessary but can provide early diagnosis in complicated cases.

The most important diagnostic step is aspiration of the suspected site, which provides material for culture and identification of the organism. Even a tiny drop of pus may be adequate for culture and Gram stain.

## DIFFERENTIAL DIAGNOSIS

Septic arthritis (extremely painful joint motion)

Trauma (deformity, open wound)

Tumor (Ewing sarcoma, eosinophilic granuloma)

## ADVERSE OUTCOMES OF THE DISEASE

In the preantibiotic era, osteomyelitis often resulted in death—quickly in the case of hematogenous disease and more slowly in chronic disease. Delay in treatment can still lead to death or serious compromise of growth and function of the extremity. Pathologic fracture or progression of the acute illness to the chronic stages with persistent drainage, repeated episodes of pain and fever, and soft-tissue destruction are avoided by early, aggressive treatment.

## TREATMENT

After diagnostic aspiration has been attempted, parenteral antibiotic treatment with bactericidal drugs should be initiated. Do not wait for culture results but consider that *Staphylococcus aureus* or *Streptococcus* are the likely causative organisms and use appropriate intravenous antibiotics against these organisms. Negative results on aspiration do not exclude the diagnosis.

If a dramatic decrease in temperature and diminished pain and tenderness do not occur within 24 to 36 hours, surgical decompression is indicated. Different antibiotic regimens and surgical treatments are indicated for non-pyogenic cases or for chronic conditions.

## ADVERSE OUTCOMES OF TREATMENT

Damage to the physis or adjacent joint by needle aspiration, bone biopsy, or open surgery is possible. Serious allergic reaction to penicillin or other antibiotics also is possible.

## REFERRAL DECISIONS/RED FLAGS

Most patients with acute osteomyelitis should be hospitalized. Aspiration or surgical decompression may require specialty consultation. Infectious disease consultation may be helpful when dealing with unusual organisms.

# OSTEOPOROSIS

ICD-9 Code
733.00
Osteoporosis, unspecified

## DEFINITION

Osteoporosis is a disease characterized by low bone mass leading to microarchitectural deterioration. As a result, there is increased fragility of the bone and an increased risk of fracture. Other adverse outcomes include deformity, pain, loss of independence, and premature death, particularly following hip fracture. Although osteoporosis has long been considered an inevitable consequence of aging, the natural history can be altered by diet and treatment strategies.

Osteoporosis is defined as primary (type I or II) or secondary. Type I osteoporosis, frequently called postmenopausal osteoporosis, is six times more common in women than in men. Estrogen deficiency in women and testosterone deficiency in men lead to trabecular bone loss. These patients commonly present with vertebral compression fractures or fractures of the distal radius. Type II osteoporosis, previously called senile osteoporosis, is twice as common in women than in men. It affects most individuals over the age of 70 years. Altered calcium metabolism and intrinsic problems in bone formation lead to a decrease in formation of new bone. Hip and pelvic fractures are common in this group. In secondary osteoporosis, an identifiable agent or disease process causes loss of bone.

## CLINICAL SYMPTOMS

Osteoporosis frequently is not recognized until a patient seeks medical attention for back pain, fracture, loss of height, or spinal deformity. Table 1 summarizes risk factors for osteoporotic fractures.

Secondary osteoporosis is seen commonly in patients taking long-term steroid therapy. It is also seen in a wide range of disorders such as hormone abnormalities (hyperthyroidism, hyperparathyroidism), neoplastic disorders (multiple myeloma), metabolic abnormalities (osteomalacia), and connective tissue diseases (osteogenesis imperfecta). It is a serious problem for patients who require prolonged immobilization.

## TESTS

### PHYSICAL EXAMINATION

The physical examination is normal in the early stages. In advanced disease, findings may include tenderness to palpation over an area of fracture, spinal deformity, loss of height (often more than 2"), lax abdominal musculature with a protuberant abdomen, hypermobility, and exaggerated thoracic kyphosis (dowager hump) (Figure 1).

Athletes, particularly those participating in endurance activities, gymnastics, skating, and dance, are prone to developing low bone density and subsequent stress or overt fractures because of poor diet and overtraining. It is

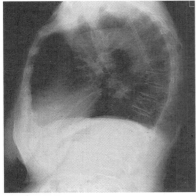

**Figure 1**
Kyphosis secondary to osteoporosis and vertebral collapse.

imperative to thoroughly question female athletes about their menstrual history and all athletes about their diet and exercise habits.

## DIAGNOSTIC TESTS

Diagnostic tests are performed to identify the presence and severity of the disease, measure response to therapeutic interventions, and rule out secondary causes of osteoporosis.

Because there is no specific measurement for bone strength, bone mineral density (BMD) is used as a surrogate. This quick, painless test helps estimate bone strength and predict future fracture risk. Dual energy x-ray absorptiometry (DXA or DEXA) is currently the gold standard for bone density measurement. It is fast, reproducible, and involves very low radiation exposure. DEXA currently is the best test for monitoring the results of osteoporosis treatment. However, for reasons of cost, speed, and availability, quantitative ultrasound frequently is used as a screening tool.

Because osteoporosis typically is a "silent" disease, the decision to test should be based on a patient's risk profile. The National Osteoporosis Foundation recommends BMD testing for the following individuals:

- All postmenopausal women under age 65 who have one or more additional major risk factors for osteoporosis besides menopause;

- All women ages 65 or older, regardless of risk factors;

- Postmenopausal women who present with fractures (to confirm diagnosis and determine disease severity);

- Women who are considering therapy for osteoporosis (perimenopausal or postmenopausal) if BMD testing would facilitate the decision;

- Women who have been on hormone replacement therapy for prolonged periods.

Tests to rule out secondary causes of osteoporosis include complete blood cell count, erythrocyte sedimentation rate, serum protein level, and immunoelectrophoresis to rule out a bone marrow disorder. Thyroid function tests and parathyroid hormone level tests are performed to rule out hyperthyroidism or hyperparathyroidism. Cushing disease and diabetes are ruled out by history. Tests for serum levels of calcium, phosphorus, alkaline phosphatase, and 25-hydroxyvitamin D (along with parathyroid hormone levels) rule out osteomalacia. Other studies include renal and liver function tests and a 24-hour urine calcium test.

## DIFFERENTIAL DIAGNOSIS

Disuse osteopenia (prolonged immobilization or bed rest)

Osteomalacia (deformity, renal osteodystrophy)

Poor imaging technique on radiographs (overpenetration)

Primary osteoporosis (type I or type II)

Secondary osteoporosis

## ADVERSE OUTCOMES OF DISEASE

Adverse outcomes of osteoporosis include fracture, deformity, chronic pain, social withdrawal, loss of independence, and death, particularly following hip fracture.

## TREATMENT

### PREVENTION

Women should be encouraged to maximize bone formation during youth (peak bone mass) and minimize bone loss during adulthood. Recommendations for the general population include an adequate intake of calcium and vitamin D, regular weight-bearing exercise, and avoidance of tobacco use and alcohol abuse.

Older patients should be educated about the importance of maintaining their body weight and reducing their risk factors for falls by walking for exercise, avoiding long-acting benzodiazepams, minimizing caffeine intake, and treating impaired visual function (**Table 1**).

---

**Table 1**
**Risk Factors for Osteoporotic Fracture**

| Nonmodifiable | Potentially modifiable |
|---|---|
| **Personal history of fracture as an adult\*** | **Current cigarette smoking\*** |
| **History of fracture in a first-degree relative\*** | **Low body weight (< 127 lb)\*** |
| Caucasian or Asian race (recent data suggest that African- and Hispanic Americans are at a significant risk, as well) | Estrogen deficiency<br>  Early menopause (< age 45) or bilateral ovariectomy<br>  Prolonged premenopausal amenorrhea (> 1 year) |
| Advanced age | Low calcium intake (lifelong) |
| Female gender | Use of certain medications such as corticosteroids and anticonvulsants |
| Dementia | Alcoholism |
| Poor health/Fragility\*\* | Impaired eyesight despite adequate correction |
| | Recurrent falls |
| | Inadequate physical activity |
| | Poor health/Fragility\*\* |

\*These items in boldface are major factors in determining the risk of hip fracture, independent of bone density.
\*\*Note that poor health and fragility may or may not be modifiable and thus occur under both headings.
*Adapted from National Osteoporosis Foundation: Physician's Guide to the Prevention and Treatment of Osteoporosis. Washington, DC, National Osteoporosis Foundation, 1998.*

---

Standards for the optimal type and duration of exercise have not been established. The ideal exercise program includes impact-loading exercise (such as walking), strength training, and balance training (such as tai chi).

Recommendations for calcium intake are listed in **Table 2**. Most Americans consume far less calcium than what is recommended, particularly in their elder years. Calcium supplements are frequently required.

## Table 2
### Dietary Reference Intake Values for Calcium by Life-Stage Group

| Life-stage group* | Adequate intake (mg/day) | Pregnancy | Adequate intake (mg/day) |
|---|---|---|---|
| 0 to 6 months | 210 | ≤ 18 years | 1,300 |
| 6 to 12 months | 270 | 19 through 50 years | 1,000 |
| 1 through 3 years | 500 | | |
| 4 through 8 years | 800 | Lactation | Adequate intake (mg/day) |
| 9 through 13 years | 1,300 | ≤ 18 years | 1,300 |
| 14 through 18 years | 1,300 | 19 through 50 years | 1,000 |
| 19 through 30 years | 1,000 | | |
| 31 through 50 years | 1,000 | | |
| 51 through 70 years | 1,200 | | |
| > 70 years | 1,200 | | |

*All groups except Pregnancy and Lactation are both males and females

Adapted from National Osteoporosis Foundation: Physician's Guide to the Prevention and Treatment of Osteoporosis. Washington, DC, National Osteoporosis Foundation, 1998.

Vitamin D is essential for intestinal absorption of calcium, and requirements increase with age because skin production of this vitamin decreases even with adequate sun exposure. Current recommendations for vitamin D intake are 400 IU/day in young adults and 800 to 1,200 IU/day in the elderly.

### INTERVENTION

In the best circumstances, treatment of osteoporosis is initiated before a fracture occurs. Physicians should encourage all patients to follow prevention strategies listed above. The National Osteoporosis Foundation recommends pharmacologic intervention for osteoporosis in white women whose BMD scores are 2 standard deviations below those of a "young normal" adult in the absence of risk factors and in women whose BMD scores are 1.5 standard deviations below those of a "young normal" adult if other risk factors are present. The Foundation also notes that white women over age 70 with multiple risk factors (especially those with previous nonhip, nonspine fractures) are at high enough risk of fracture to initiate treatment without BMD testing.

Current medications approved by the FDA for osteoporosis treatment are all antiresorptive agents and include calcium and vitamin D, hormone replacement therapy, alendronate, calcitonin, and raloxifene (a selective estrogen receptor, frequently termed SERM). Bone stimulation agents are still considered experimental.

### ADVERSE OUTCOMES OF TREATMENT

Hormone replacement therapy may be associated with an increased risk of breast cancer and deep vein thrombosis. Side effects can include vaginal bleeding, breast tenderness, mood disturbances, and gallbladder disease. Alendronate has a somewhat difficult dosing schedule, and a significant proportion of patients report upper gastrointestinal disturbance. Calcitonin has fewer side effects but is less effective than either hormone replacement therapy or alendronate. Long-term data on raloxifene are not available, but it has been shown to increase the risk of deep vein thrombosis at the same rate as estrogen. It also causes hot flashes and does not treat menopausal symptoms.

## REFERRAL DECISIONS/RED FLAGS

Osteoporosis and fragility fractures are not inevitable in any age group. All appropriate patients should be referred for BMD testing and offered treatment.

Many physicians may feel uncomfortable evaluating bone density studies, ruling out secondary causes of osteoporosis, or initiating pharmacologic treatment. Referral to an osteoporosis specialist may be appropriate.

# OVERUSE SYNDROMES

## SYNONYMS

Cumulative trauma disorder
Occupational arm pain
Occupational stress syndrome
Repetitive strain injury
Work-related pain disorder
Writer's cramp

## DEFINITION

Overuse injuries are caused or aggravated by repetitive motion or sustained exertion of a particular body part, resulting in microtrauma to a musculo-tendinous unit. Overuse syndrome is an umbrella term that encompasses specific conditions such as carpal tunnel syndrome, tennis elbow, wrist flexor and extensor tendinitis (de Quervain disease), Achilles and posterior tibial tendinitis, patellar tendinitis, stress fractures of the lower extremity, shin-splints, exertional compartment syndromes, epicondylitis, and flexor tendinitis, as well as generalized myofascial pain. While more attention has been focused on overuse syndromes in the upper extremity, some conditions such as stress fractures and exertional compartment syndromes, are actually more common in the lower extremity.

Overuse syndromes reflect an interplay of physical, psychosocial, and sociopolitical factors. While the exact cause of overuse syndromes remains controversial, contributing factors may include repetitive tasks, forceful exertions, exposure to vibration or cold temperatures, awkward postures in the workplace, the ergonomic environment, lack of job satisfaction, psychological makeup, boredom, the state's workers' compensation laws, and the social environment.

## CLINICAL SYMPTOMS

Unfortunately, a precise definition of overuse syndromes is lacking, and there is no agreement concerning the diagnostic criteria. Likewise, whether certain jobs or occupations cause overuse syndromes remains controversial. The many synonyms listed above illustrate the confusion that surrounds these conditions. Overuse syndromes develop over time—from a few weeks to years. Frequently, the onset is insidious, and patients may not report their problems early on in anticipation that the condition will improve.

Typical complaints include pain, fatigue, numbness, or any combination of the above. While patients often have difficulty localizing their pain, they may have specific complaints related to carpal tunnel syndrome, lateral elbow epicondylitis, or flexor tenosynovitis in the palm, associated with vague and nonanatomic discomfort elsewhere in the arm. Patients with overuse syndromes may report numbness in a nonanatomic or nondermatomal distribution. Patients also may report a sensation of swelling in the extremity, although it is not generally apparent on examination.

Certain individuals are at risk for overuse syndromes, principally those with exposure to physical stresses (eg, repetition, force, awkward postures, temperature extremes, and vibration) and those with psychosocial stresses (eg, fast work pace, inflexibility in the workplace, monotonous demanding tasks, and depression). At least 25% of adult athletes also experience overuse injuries. Certain jobs and occupations appear to predispose workers to overuse syndromes. Professional dancers, musicians, grocery store checkers, computer keyboard operators, and dental hygienists are particularly susceptible. Women with serious psychosocial problems, such as a history of physical and sexual abuse, are at increased risk for unexplained musculoskeletal pain. Individuals who are poorly educated or who work in mundane, low-paying jobs also are at risk. Note, too, that highly skilled individuals who believe that they are overworked, underpaid, overstressed, and unappreciated also are at higher risk.

## TESTS

### PHYSICAL EXAMINATION

Patients should be asked specific job-related questions, including questions about job satisfaction, working conditions, the relationship with the supervisor and coworkers, exposure to repetitive and forceful exertions, vibration, cold temperature, and job harassment. Identifying the type of industry and specific job also is important, as the incidence of claims for overuse syndromes is higher for certain industries and jobs, such as meat packers, assembly line workers, grocery store checkers, and clerical workers.

Many of the conditions listed in the differential diagnosis may be present concomitantly.

### DIAGNOSTIC TESTS

Radiographs are indicated if there is a clear history of trauma, but they are often normal. A bone scan may be necessary to identify a stress fracture. Likewise, nerve conduction velocity studies can be ordered to rule out carpal tunnel syndrome or ulnar nerve entrapment at the elbow, but results of these studies usually are normal. Exertional compartment syndrome can be confirmed by measuring compartment pressure after exercise.

## DIFFERENTIAL DIAGNOSIS

Angina with referred arm pain (abnormal electrocardiogram)

Claudication (decreased peripheral pulses)

Deep vein thrombosis (abnormal venogram)

Fibromyalgia (11 of 18 tender points in four body quadrants)

Herniated cervical or lumbar disk (abnormal spine radiographs, myelogram, and MRI)

## ADVERSE OUTCOMES OF THE DISEASE

With these disorders, patients often lose time from work and experience psychological changes. They may even change occupations or simply never return to work.

## TREATMENT

A satisfactory outcome for the patient depends on the cooperative efforts of the employer, the insurance carrier, and a physician-directed health care team that might include physical and occupational therapists, occupational health nurses, and vocational rehabilitation counselors. A case manager, such as an occupational health nurse, can be invaluable in coordinating the efforts of these groups to return the patient to work.

Initial treatment should include ice and rest of the affected part, along with a progressive exercise program of subsymptomatic stresses to strengthen the extremity. At the workplace, modify tasks and work schedules, and consider job change if the symptoms persist.

NSAIDs may reduce the musculoskeletal pain associated with these conditions. Narcotics should be avoided because of the possibility of addiction. Antidepressants can be a useful adjunct if depression is a significant part of the clinical picture.

Although surgery may be indicated, it is seldom urgent. The results of surgery are less predictable in these patients. Better results are obtained when the overuse has caused a specific, clearly identifiable syndrome such as carpal tunnel syndrome. Lack of job satisfaction and depression are also important predictors of recovery. Poor prognosis is associated with both long-standing disability (longer than 6 months) and litigation.

## ADVERSE OUTCOMES OF TREATMENT

Drug dependence from narcotics or antidepressants is possible. If the patient has had multiple, ill-advised surgeries, persistently tender scars may be left.

## REFERRAL DECISIONS/RED FLAGS

Once a diagnosis of overuse syndrome is suspected, treatment by a team of health care professionals may be the best way to manage these difficult problems.

# Reflex Sympathetic Dystrophy and Complex Regional Pain Syndromes

### ICD-9 Codes

337.21
Reflex sympathetic dystrophy of the upper limb
337.22
Reflex sympathetic dystrophy of the lower limb

## Synonyms

RSD

Causalgia

Sympathetically maintained pain (SMP)

Shoulder-hand syndrome

Sudeck atrophy

Pain dysfunction syndrome

## Definition

Complex regional pain syndrome (CRPS) is a spectrum of conditions that have in common dysfunction and pain that is out of proportion to what would be expected from the original injury. The cause is not understood. The terminology was developed in 1993 by a consensus group of the American Pain Society in an attempt to correct the confusion over the terms reflex sympathetic dystrophy (RSD) and causalgia. Two types of CRPS are recognized: type I (RSD syndrome) is characterized by pain that extends beyond the area supplied by a peripheral nerve and is out of proportion to the inciting event; type II (causalgia) is similar to type I in all aspects but follows a nerve injury. The pain associated with either type of CRPS can be influenced by a dysfunction of the sympathetic nervous system (eg, sympathetically maintained pain [SMP]). If the sympathetic nervous system is not contributing to the pain, the condition is referred to as sympathetically independent pain (SIP). Both types of CRPS can have SMP and SIP operating simultaneously.

Fracture of the distal radius is the most common injury that precipitates type I CRPS (RSD). Although RSD is most often associated with the upper extremity, it also can develop in the knee, foot, and ankle. Up to 30% of patients have no apparent injury, indicating the innocuous nature of the events that precipitate RSD. Patients between the ages of 30 and 50 years are most at risk, with women three times more likely to be affected. Smokers also are at increased risk. Although patients with RSD often have significant anxiety and depression, even to the point of suicide, there is no evidence that predisposing psychological factors are causative.

## Clinical symptoms

The clinical presentation can vary, but RSD typically occurs in three stages. Stage 1, which can last up to 3 months, is characterized by severe pain that is out of proportion to the injury. This pain often is described as burning, throbbing, or cutting and can be triggered by an innocuous stimulus (allodynia). Not uncommonly, following a normally painful stimulus, the perception of pain is delayed and is felt well beyond the normal nerve distribution (hyperpathia). Autonomic nervous system dysfunction in this state is manifested by swelling in the affected extremity, increased sweating, a change in skin color from red to cyanotic, temperature changes, an increased amount of hair growth, and excessive nail growth. Stage 2 occurs after 3 or 4 months and is marked by loss of skin lines, which causes the skin to look pale and waxy, joint stiffness, brittle nails, muscle spasms, and persistent pain. Stage 3 occurs with loss of muscle and skin, permanent joint contractures, and loss of motion, and the persistent pain becomes severe (**Figure 1**).

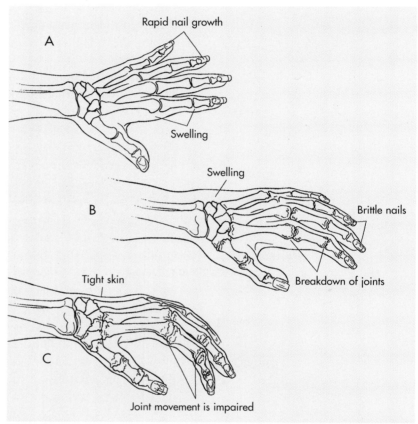

**Figure 1**
Clinical presentations of RSD. A, Early RSD stage 1. B, Middle RSD stage 2. C, Late RSD stage 3.

## TESTS

### PHYSICAL EXAMINATION
Inspect for swelling, color changes in the skin, and abnormal hair and nail growth. Palpate for changes in skin temperature and altered sweat patterns. Measure joint motion and document swelling by measuring the circumference of the extremity and comparing it with that of the contralateral side.

### DIAGNOSTIC TESTS
In late stage 1 through stage 3, plain radiographs should be ordered, as they may show spotty areas of osteopenia or demineralization in the bones of the affected extremity. Three-phase bone scans, especially the third phase, may

show increased uptake in the extremity and correlate with RSD. Other tests, such as quantitative pain questionnaires, cold stress tests with laser Doppler fluximetry, and endurance testing, can be ordered but are probably best done at a pain center. The bone scan findings usually correlate with the patchy osteopenia seen on the radiograph.

## DIFFERENTIAL DIAGNOSIS

Neuropathic pain disorders (carpal tunnel syndrome, tarsal tunnel syndrome, cubital tunnel syndrome, Morton neuroma)

## ADVERSE OUTCOMES OF THE DISEASE

Chronic, possibly debilitating pain, joint contractures and stiffness, and skin and muscle atrophy can develop. More serious consequences include loss of function in the affected extremity. Psychiatric problems, including depression, anxiety, and even the potential to commit suicide, also have been noted.

## TREATMENT

Early recognition and prompt treatment appear to decrease the severity of the symptoms, although the cure may be incomplete. Eighty percent of patients with type I CRPS (RSD) will improve dramatically if diagnosis is established and treatment initiated within 1 year of injury. If left untreated for more than a year, more than half the patients will have significant disability. Variables indicating a poor prognosis include delay in diagnosis of more than 6 months, history of smoking, and female gender. Remember to look for the remedial lesion, such as the median nerve compression associated with a distal radial fracture.

Use of sympathetic anesthetic blocks can be therapeutic as well as diagnostic. If an anesthetic block provides relief, a series of three to six blocks over a 2- to 3-week period is indicated. Note that a single block does not distinguish the placebo effect (in which up to one third of patients report temporary improvement following an injection of normal saline) from true pain relief. A positive response to the block indicates that the pain is at least partially sympathetically mediated. Sympathetically mediated pain often is easier to treat and has a better prognosis.

Immediately after each block, range-of-motion exercises and a graduated stress-loading program are begun, usually under the direction of a physical or occupational therapist. For example, when RSD affects the hand, a typical home stress-loading program includes performing routine chores, such as scrubbing a 3-foot-square area of kitchen floor (of tile or wood) for 20 minutes three times a day and bearing as much weight through the wrist and hand as tolerated. The home program also includes lifting and carrying household objects, such as a 25-lb suitcase three times a day, and generally using the affected hand as often as is practical.

Oral steroids and NSAIDs can decrease pain, but they do not alter the course of the disease. In stage 1, narcotic analgesics may be required for pain control; however, use of narcotics requires special caution as these can result

SECTION 1 | GENERAL ORTHOPAEDICS

in drug dependency. Tricyclic antidepressants (amitriptyline) in doses of 25 to 50 mg taken at night allow patients to sleep and can offer partial pain relief during the day. Other medications that can help the nerve pain include gabapentin and phenytoin.

A transcutaneous electrical nerve stimulation (TENS) unit applied to the extremity, under the supervision of a physical therapist, is a useful adjunct for pain control and can decrease the need for stronger narcotic pain medications. Biofeedback also can be tried. With biofeedback, patients are taught to control the autonomic functions of the body that regulate sweating, skin temperature, and blood flow. Acupuncture and injections of corticosteroid and local anesthetic into trigger points also can provide transient relief. Psychological counseling may help the patient deal with the pain.

## ADVERSE OUTCOMES OF TREATMENT

Side effects from cervical sympathetic blocks include hoarseness, weakness or numbness in the arm, pneumothorax, and possible seizure from vertebral artery injection. Use of narcotics can lead to addiction, and excessive use of NSAIDs can result in gastric, hepatic, and renal symptoms. Fractures also can occur from too vigorous manipulations.

## REFERRAL DECISIONS/RED FLAGS

Excessively severe pain and swelling associated with any type of injury to an extremity indicate the need for further evaluation at a center where a multidisciplinary team is available to treat this difficult problem. Also, patients with severe, unexplainable pain following even a trivial injury may need further evaluation.

# REHABILITATION PRINCIPLES AND THERAPEUTIC MODALITIES

## DEFINITION

Rehabilitation is the key to maximal recovery following injury and should be recognized as an integral part of treatment. The goal is a return to optimal function as quickly as possible. For many injuries, rehabilitation does not require complicated equipment, extensive therapy sessions, or detailed knowledge of physiatry or physiotherapy. For these patients, a physician who understands the basic principles can usually outline and monitor an effective program. Other patients with complex conditions such as paraplegia, chronic arthritis, amputations, or multisystem trauma are best rehabilitated through the coordinated efforts and expertise of a multidisciplinary health care team.

## TREATMENT

The principle to restoring full function is regaining range of motion (ROM), strength, and coordination. A standard treatment plan begins with restoring ROM. Stretching and gentle isometric strengthening exercises also are initiated. As the ROM improves, endurance strengthening exercises with light resistance and higher repetitions are added. As strength returns, coordination and functional activities, such as sport- or work-related activities, are added to progressively more advanced strengthening and ROM exercises. Table 1 lists basic types of rehabilitation exercises and therapeutic modalities.

Modalities that decrease swelling and pain are useful adjuncts. Because these modalities frequently produce comforting sensations, their psychological effect may be difficult to separate from their physiologic benefit.

## ADVERSE OUTCOMES OF TREATMENT

Overaggressive therapy can cause tendinitis, tendon rupture, fracture, surgical wound dehiscence, or failure of the surgical treatment. Modalities can cause skin irritation, burns, frostbite, or electrical shock.

## REFERRAL DECISIONS/RED FLAGS

Complex problems, lack of treatment progression, or requirement for special equipment indicate referral to a physical therapist. Patients who are not able to do therapy on their own also will benefit from referral. When ordering therapy, the physician should specify the type, duration, and frequency of treatments.

## Table 1
### Basic Types of Rehabilitation Exercises and Therapeutic Modalities

| Exercise/Modality | Directions |
| --- | --- |
| Stretching | Performed slowly and maintained for 20 to 30 seconds without bouncing. |
| Active ROM | The patient performs the stretch or movement. |
| Passive ROM | The therapist or outside force is used to stretch or move the joint. |
| Strengthening | Performed at a slow, controlled rate through safe parameters of the patient's ROM. |
| Cryotherapy | Used to decrease swelling, inflammation, and pain. Avoid areas of compromised circulation or patients with cold sensitivities (ie, Raynaud syndrome). |
| Thermotherapy | Increases blood flow, promotes healing and muscular relaxation. It should not be used in acute or subacute injuries, as there is risk of increased hemorrhage or swelling. |
| Ultrasound | Commonly used for chronic inflammation and increasing ROM in joints. Do not use in areas of acute hemorrhage, tumor, active infection, or open epiphysis. |
| Phonophoresis | Type of ultrasound used to deliver topical medications. Same indications as for ultrasound. |
| Electrical stimulation | Commonly used for decreasing pain and edema, regaining strength, and preventing atrophy. Do not use over abraded skin or scars. |
| Iontophoresis | Uses topical medication with electrical stimulation for chronic inflammatory conditions. More effective on superficial areas and often tried before injections. |

# RHEUMATOID ARTHRITIS

ICD-9 Code
714.0
    Rheumatoid arthritis

## DEFINITION

Rheumatoid arthritis (RA) is a systemic autoimmune disorder characterized by an inflammatory synovitis that can erode and ultimately destroy the articular cartilage. The etiology is unknown, but most likely an unknown agent activates an immune response in synovial tissue.

RA more commonly affects women, and the prevalence increases with age with peak onset in the late 40s and early 50s. The arthritis typically is symmetrical and most often involves the joints of the hands, wrist, feet, and ankles.

## CLINICAL SYMPTOMS

By definition, symptoms of RA must be of at least 6 weeks' duration. Pain, morning stiffness, swelling, and systemic symptoms are common. The 1987 revised criteria of the American College of Rheumatology require at least four of the following seven criteria to be satisfied before a diagnosis can be established.

- Morning stiffness that is periarticular and lasts at least an hour

- Arthritis (synovitis with periarticular soft-tissue swelling) of three or more joints for at least 6 weeks

- Arthritis of hand joints (wrist, metacarpophalangeal, or proximal interphalangeal) for at least 6 weeks

- Symmetrical arthritis for at least 6 weeks

- Rheumatoid nodules (subcutaneous nodules over extensor surfaces or bony prominences)

- Positive serum rheumatoid factor

- Radiographic changes

Extra-articular symptoms include generalized malaise, fatigue, tenosynovitis (particularly of the hands and feet) that may be complicated by carpal tunnel syndrome or other tenosynovitis manifestations, vasculitis manifested by palpable purpura, dry eyes secondary to keratoconjunctivitis sicca, pulmonary nodules, and inflammatory pericarditis.

The hypertrophic synovium stretches the ligaments and joint capsules. As a result, these supporting structures become less effective. Erosion of the articular cartilage in combination with the ligamentous changes results in deformity and contractures such as ulnar drifting and subluxation of the metacarpophalangeal joints of the hand and hallux valgus and claw toe deformities in the foot. With progression of the disease, pain and deformity increase.

Patients with severe RA typically have multiple affected joints in the upper and lower extremities. Joints of the cervical spine may be involved as well.

SECTION 1 | GENERAL ORTHOPAEDICS

Neck pain and stiffness occur, and with atlantoaxial subluxation, cervical myelopathy may develop.

## TESTS

### PHYSICAL EXAMINATION

Joint contractures, joint effusions, deformity (genu valgum or knock-knee), and painful motion are common. Swelling of the proximal interphalangeal joints and stiffness in the hands usually occurs early. An associated carpal tunnel syndrome, manifested by severe, neuritic-type pain and a positive Phalen test, may appear acutely.

Most joints show increased warmth and synovial bogginess. Joint aspirations often produce less fluid than expected because much of the enlargement comes from synovial hypertrophy.

Rheumatoid nodules often appear, especially along the extensor aspect of the arm.

### DIAGNOSTIC TESTS

Rheumatoid factors (mostly IgM antibodies against the Fc portion of IgG) are elevated in 75% to 90% of patients. This test, however, is not specific for RA, because rheumatoid factors also are elevated in chronic inflammatory conditions that cause sustained elevation of IgG. The erythrocyte sedimentation rate usually is elevated.

Radiographs often show periarticular osteopenia and bony erosion at the joint margin (correlates with insertion site of synovium). Lateral flexion and extension views of the neck may demonstrate C1-2 instability secondary to erosion of the ligaments that hold the odontoid in place. These findings are important if the patient is anticipating any surgery that involves intubation or manipulation of the neck, as it could lead to quadriparesis or death.

## DIFFERENTIAL DIAGNOSIS

Hepatitis (abnormal liver function tests)

Lyme disease (serology, rash, anemia)

Seronegative arthropathies (HLA tests, abnormal radiographs, urethritis)

Systemic lupus erythematosus (antinuclear antibodies, peripheral blood smear)

## ADVERSE OUTCOMES OF THE DISEASE

Joint contractures, pain, loss of function, loss of ambulation, and multisystem disorders leading to death are possible. Osteoporosis is common, in part related to the disease, inactivity, and steroid use.

## TREATMENT

Describing complete medical treatment for this condition is beyond the scope of this text. Commonly, salicylates, NSAIDs, splinting, and oral and intra-articular corticosteroids are used to treat the polyarthralgias and pain. Disease-modifying agents, such as hydroxychloroquine, methotrexate, and gold are used at earlier stages of the disease. Corticosteroid injections into selected joints and the carpal tunnel may relieve acute synovitis and carpal tunnel syndrome. Splints can help manage acute episodes of pain associated with synovitis as well as positioning joints to minimize progressive deformity. Custom shoes are helpful with severe foot deformities. Physical therapy in the form of range-of-motion, strengthening, and other modalities is important. Selective surgical intervention by synovectomy or tenosynovectomy may prevent tendon rupture and progression of joint deformity. End-stage arthritis requires total joint arthroplasty or arthrodesis.

## ADVERSE OUTCOMES OF TREATMENT

Infection secondary to injection or surgery; gastric, hepatic, or renal complications associated with NSAID use; and osteonecrosis of bone or osteoporosis associated with steroid use are possible. Skin rash and other side effects of various medications also can develop.

## REFERRAL DECISIONS/RED FLAGS

Patients whose symptoms persist for more than 3 months, or who have uncontrollable joint pain at rest, or who have deformity need further evaluation. Patients with foot deformities not responsive to custom shoes also need additional evaluation, as do those in whom extra-articular manifestations develop.

# SEPTIC ARTHRITIS

ICD-9 Code
711.0
    Pyogenic arthritis

## DEFINITION

Septic arthritis usually occurs as a result of inoculation of bacteria into a joint. The inoculation can occur as a hematogenous event, by direct penetration of a joint, or by spread from an adjacent focus of infection. Septic arthritis has a wide variety of presentations depending on the age and general health of the patient, virulence of the infecting organism, and circumstances of the inoculation, eg, tissue necrosis with a penetrating injury.

Septic arthritis occurs most commonly in children as a result of hematogenous spread of bacteria. When hematogenous septic arthritis occurs in adults, there is often an associated arthritic condition such as rheumatoid arthritis or an underlying medical condition that affects the immune system. Gonoccocal infections also may cause septic arthritis.

## CLINICAL SYMPTOMS

An infant or child with septic arthritis often appears seriously and acutely ill, with a high fever, tachycardia, irritability, and pain with any motion of the limb. Children who previously have been walking may now refuse to walk. Older patients with sepsis secondary to a total joint arthroplasty might have only a vague sense of discomfort in the joint and a variable history of pain on weight bearing or motion. Between these two extremes, symptoms of discomfort, limited joint motion, swelling, or deformity vary widely depending on the type of organism. The onset of symptoms with fungal or mycobacterial infections is quite indolent compared with that of pyogenic bacteria.

## TESTS

### PHYSICAL EXAMINATION

Examination of a patient with a suspected septic arthritis should include a generalized examination to identify a source of the infection, such as a furuncle or abscessed tooth, or site of penetrating wound near the joint. Note swelling and the position of the joint. With septic arthritis, the patient holds the joint in a position of comfort, such as flexion of the hip or knee. Passive motion of the joint causes severe pain. Palpate the joint for increased warmth and effusion. With a chronic infection, hypertrophy of the synovium will be present.

### DIAGNOSTIC TESTS

A white blood cell count (WBC), erythrocyte sedimentation rate (ESR), screening AP and lateral radiographs, blood culture, and aspiration of joint fluid for analysis, Gram stain, and culture are standard. The WBC may be normal or elevated, and the ESR is frequently but not always elevated. The radiographs usually are normal or show only soft-tissue swelling but are useful in ruling out other pathologic conditions. Blood cultures are important because this study may identify the causative organism when joint fluid cultures are negative. Analysis of the synovial fluid typically shows a WBC of >50,000/mm³, and often the WBC is >100,000/mm³. However, the WBC of the joint fluid typically is less elevated in gonococcal arthritis. Culture of joint fluid mandates special considerations when *Haemophilus influenzae* or *Neisseria gonorrheoae* is considered.

With chronic infections, cultures should include study for acid-fast and fungal organisms, as well as pyogenic bacteria. A negative culture does not necessarily exclude septic arthritis, particularly in chronic cases that may be caused by organisms of low virulence or that are fastidious in their growth.

## DIFFERENTIAL DIAGNOSIS

Acute rheumatic fever (migratory arthralgia, carditis, increased antistreptolysin titer, group A streptococcal infection)

Juvenile rheumatoid arthritis (morning stiffness, usually mild joint swelling)

Lyme disease (indolent onset, erythema migrans, cardiac and neurologic manifestations)

Osteoarthritis (evident on radiographs)

Rheumatoid arthritis (morning stiffness, symmetric involvement, positive rheumatoid factor, elevated erythrocyte sedimentation rate)

Transient synovitis of the hip (pediatric disorder, limited hip motion, afebrile)

## ADVERSE OUTCOMES OF THE DISEASE

The most serious associated outcomes clearly are generalized sepsis or death. In infants and children, joint destruction or physeal damage is possible. In older patients, less dramatic loss of joint function usually occurs, but chronic infection may never be eradicated. In these situations, arthrodesis of the joint or even amputation of the extremity may be necessary.

## TREATMENT

Antibiotics also must be started immediately, beginning with broad-spectrum coverage based on age-related factors until culture and sensitivity results are known (**Table 1**). Surgical decompression and drainage by arthroscopic or open arthrotomy should be considered at presentation with either severe involvement or involvement of the hip (to prevent osteonecrosis). Surgical drainage also should be considered in patients who do not demonstrate a clinical response to antibiotic therapy in 24 to 48 hours.

SECTION 1 | GENERAL ORTHOPAEDICS

## Table 1
### Likely Infecting Organism and Early Antibiotic Treatment of Septic Arthritis

| Age | Likely organism | Initial antibiotic regimen |
| --- | --- | --- |
| Neonate | S aureus, group B Streptococcus | Oxacillin plus gentamicin<br>Enteric gram-negative bacterium |
| Child < 5 years | S aureus, group A Streptococcus, Streptococcus pneumoniae, H influenzae | Second-generation cephalosporin |
| Child 5 years to adolescence | S aureus | Oxacillin |
| Adolescence to adults | N gonorrhoeae, S aureus | Ceftriaxone (third-generation cephalosporin) |
| Older adults | S aureus | Gram-negative bacterium<br>Oxacillin or cefazolin, aminoglycoside |

## ADVERSE OUTCOMES OF TREATMENT

Allergic reactions or adverse drug interactions related to antibiotics can occur. Strict aseptic technique must be followed in aspiration of joints to avoid additional contamination or joint injury.

## REFERRAL DECISIONS/RED FLAGS

Acute septic arthritis requires emergent antibiotic treatment and consideration of surgical drainage. Patients with chronic septic arthritis may require evaluation by an infectious disease specialist.

# SERONEGATIVE SPONDYLOARTHROPATHIES

## SYNONYMS

Ankylosing spondylitis

Reiter disease

Arthritis of inflammatory bowel disease

Psoriatic arthritis

## DEFINITION

The seronegative spondyloarthropathies are a group of arthritides that have common clinical and genetic features. The genetic factor is an association with the HLA-B27 antigen. The associated clinical features include involvement of the spine and sacroiliac joints, oligoarticular peripheral joint arthritis, enthesitis (inflammation at sites of tendon and ligament insertion into bone), and unique eye, skin, and intestinal manifestations. The seronegative spondyloarthropathies are not associated with rheumatoid factor or antinuclear antibodies.

### ANKYLOSING SPONDYLITIS

Ankylosing spondylitis affects 1 in every 2,000 persons. In the past, ankylosing spondylitis was thought to primarily affect men, but studies now indicate a more equivalent gender ratio, but with milder disease in women. Ankylosing spondylitis particularly involves the sacroiliac joints and the spine. Involvement of peripheral joints correlates with the severity of the disease but typically is less than that observed in the other seronegative spondyloarthropathies. The association with the HLA-B27 antigen is high, particularly in white patients who have an HLA-B27 positive rate of approximately 95%. Uveitis, carditis, or enthesitis may occur.

### REITER DISEASE

Reiter disease is a seronegative arthritis that develops after urethritis, cervicitis, or dysentery. It is considered to be a reactive arthritis that is typically an asymmetric oligoarthritis of the lower extremities that starts 2 to 8 weeks after an infection. Other musculoskeletal manifestations include enthesitis of the Achilles tendon or plantar fascia, dactylitis ("sausage digit" with swelling of an entire toe or finger), and sacroiliitis. Conjunctivitis commonly develops. Other associated lesions include iritis and cutaneous manifestations such as balanitis circinata and keratoderma blennorrhagica. Chronic, recurrent episodes of arthritis are most common, but some patients have no recurrence of joint problems while others have unremitting arthritis.

### PSORIATIC ARTHRITIS

Psoriatic arthritis affects approximately 5% to 10% of patients who have psoriasis. The gender ratio is approximately equal. Skin disease usually, but not always, precedes joint symptoms. Patients with joint problems have a high association of nail disorders, including pitting, ridging, and oncolysis. Iritis may develop.

### ARTHRITIS ASSOCIATED WITH INFLAMMATORY BOWEL DISEASE

Arthritis associated with inflammatory bowel disease occurs in patients with ulcerative colitis or Crohn disease. The incidence is 10% to 20% and is more common in patients with Crohn disease. In those who develop arthritis, the HLA-B27 incidence is 50% to 70%. Sacroiliitis, spondylitis, and arthritis of the knee and ankle are common. The peripheral arthritis usually parallels the course of the bowel disease, but the severity of the spondylitis bears no relation to the activity of the bowel disorder.

## CLINICAL SYMPTOMS

Back pain may be the presenting complaint, particularly in young men with ankylosing spondylitis. Stiffness may be worse in the morning, with patients needing up to 30 minutes to "warm up" on arising. Enthesitis is common, particularly at the Achilles tendon insertion and origin of the plantar fascia (heel pain). Extraskeletal manifestations such as iritis, conjunctivitis, and urethritis may occur.

## TESTS

### PHYSICAL EXAMINATION

With spondylitis, limited spinal motion is common. Measure a 15-cm span in the midline distally from the posterior iliac spine (dimples of Venus) to the upper lumbar region. Then have the patient flex (lean forward) as much as possible. The distance between the two points should increase by 5 to 7 cm (See Physical Examination—Spine). With spondylitis, spinal motion is limited, and the skin distraction on forward flexion is decreased. The FABER maneuver (flexion, abduction, and external rotation of the hip) will place stress across the sacroiliac joint, and patients with sacroiliitis will have increased pain. Examine the patient for enthesitis, swelling and restricted motion, particularly of the lower extremity joints, and abnormalities of the digits and nails.

### DIAGNOSTIC TESTS

Although HLA-B27 antigen is positive in many of these patients, this relatively expensive test usually is not needed to make the diagnosis. A detailed history and examination are more important. In patients with sacroiliitis, radiographs demonstrating narrowing of the sacroiliac joints can be helpful (**Figures 1, 2**). With spondylitis, early radiographic findings in the spine include squaring of the superior and anterior margins of the vertebral bodies thought to be caused by enthesitis at the attachment of the annulus fibrosus (ligament surrounding the disk) into the vertebral body. Later findings include ossification of the anterior longitudinal ligament of the spine and autofusion of the facet joints leading to the classic "poker spine," which may be fused along the entire length of the spine.

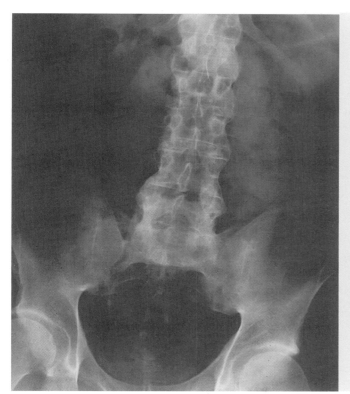

**Figure 1**
AP radiograph of the pelvis demonstrating advanced sacroiliitis.

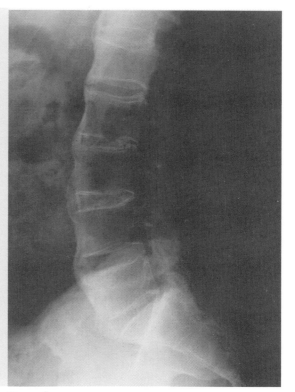

**Figure 2**
Lateral radiograph of the lumbar spine demonstrating bridging syndesmophytes.

## DIFFERENTIAL DIAGNOSIS

Degenerative disk disease (no associated symptoms, normal skin distraction on flexion of the spine)

Localized Achilles tendinitis or plantar fasciitis (no associated symptoms)

Rheumatoid arthritis (positive rheumatoid factor, peripheral joint involvement)

## ADVERSE OUTCOMES OF THE DISEASE

Severe spinal deformity may occur in ankylosing spondylitis. End-stage arthritis may affect the peripheral joints. Uveitis with visual impairment may occur. Occasionally carditis may cause aortic insufficiency in patients with ankylosing spondylitis.

## TREATMENT

NSAIDs, particularly indomethacin, are effective in controlling symptoms in many patients. Tetracycline is appropriate for suspected *Chlamydia* infections associated with Reiter disease. Topical treatment of psoriatic skin lesions is important. Methotrexate has been used with success for both skin and joint lesions in psoriatic arthritis. Methotrexate also may be useful for severe Reiter disease. Regular exercise is important, particularly for patients with ankylosing spondylitis. Surgery (total joint replacement) can provide relief of end-stage arthritic pain. An occasional patient may require a spinal osteotomy for correction of deformity associated with ankylosing spondylitis.

## ADVERSE OUTCOMES OF TREATMENT

Postoperative infection and/or loosening of total joint implants following surgery is possible, while heterotopic ossification can complicate total hip arthroplasty. NSAIDs can cause gastric, renal, or hepatic complications.

## REFERRAL DECISIONS/RED FLAGS

Patients with kyphosis, pain at rest, or pain at night in a weight-bearing joint need further evaluation. Accompanying problems with the eyes, skin, or pulmonary system may require additional attention.

# SPLINTING PRINCIPLES

Splinting of fractures, dislocations, or tendon ruptures often is required as part of initial emergency management. A well-applied splint reduces pain, bleeding, and swelling by immobilizing the injured part. Splinting also helps prevent a number of problems:

- Further damage of muscles, nerves (including the spinal cord), and blood vessels by the sharp ends of fractured bones

- Laceration of the skin by sharp fracture ends

- Constriction of vascular structures by malaligned bone ends

- Further contamination of an open wound

## GENERAL PRINCIPLES OF SPLINTING

1. Remove clothing from the area of any suspected fracture or dislocation to inspect the extremity for open wounds, deformity, swelling, and ecchymosis.

2. Note and record the pulse and capillary refill and neurologic status distal to the site of injury.

3. Cover all wounds with a dry, sterile dressing before applying a splint. If further evaluation is necessary, notify the receiving physician of all open wounds.

4. Ensure that the splint immobilizes the joints above and below the suspected fracture.

5. With injuries in and around the joint, ensure that the splint immobilizes the bones above and below the injured joint.

6. Pad all rigid splints to prevent local pressure.

7. During application of the splint, use your hands to minimize movement of the limb and to support the injury site until the splint has set and the limb is completely immobilized.

8. Align a limb severely deformed with constant gentle manual traction so that it can be incorporated into a splint.

9. If you encounter resistance to limb alignment when you apply traction, splint the limb in the position of deformity.

10. When in doubt, splint.

## MATERIALS

Although prefabricated plastic, fabric, or metal splints are available, they generally are unsatisfactory except for very brief periods of emergency treatment. If a splint is expected to be effective and to remain in place for more than a few hours, custom application of a well-padded plaster or fiberglass splint is preferred. Because plaster is cheaper, more readily available, more versatile, and can be more easily molded to the extremity, it is usually preferred. Caution: Many-layered "homemade" splints or thick commercial plaster splints can generate enough heat to burn the patient. See Table 1 for the materials needed for splinting. Store these materials in a dry cabinet or closet.

## Table 1
### Splinting Materials

| Thumb/finger | Arm | Short leg splint |
|---|---|---|
| 1 to 2 rolls 4" cast padding (adults) or 3" cast padding (children) | 2 or 3 rolls 4" cast padding (adults) or 3" cast padding (children) | 2 rolls of 4" to 5" wide cast padding |
| 4" × 15" splints, six thicknesses (adults) or 3" roll folded into splint of appropriate length (children) | 5" × 30" splints six thicknesses (adults) or 4" roll folded to necessary length (children) | 12 to 14 thicknesses of 5" × 30" or 5" × 45" plaster strips |
| | | One 3" to 4" wide roll of plaster |
| 2" or 3" elastic bandage | 3" or 4" elastic bandage | One roll of 4" wide elastic bandage |
| Tepid water (≈24°C) | Tepid water (≈24°C) | One bucket of tepid water |
| Nonsterile gloves | Nonsterile gloves | Nonsterile gloves |

| Wrist and forearm | | Long leg splint |
|---|---|---|
| 2 rolls 4" cast padding (adults) or 3" cast padding (children) | | 3 to 4 rolls of 6" wide cast padding |
| 5" × 30" splints, six thicknesses (adults) for "sugar tong" or 4" × 15" six thicknesses splints (children) for simple dorsal or volar splint | | 3 to 4 rolls of 5" or 6" wide plaster or 5" × 45" plaster splints |
| 2" or 3" elastic bandage | | One roll each of 4" and 6" wide elastic bandages |
| Tepid water (≈24°C) | | One bucket of tepid water |
| Nonsterile gloves | | Nonsterile gloves |

## SPLINTING THE UPPER EXTREMITY

### FRACTURES OR INJURIES OF THE HAND OR WRIST

1. Position the patient supine or sitting and have an assistant hold the patient's thumb and/or index fingers.

2. Loosely wrap cast padding from the palm to the elbow, making sure that there are three layers of padding at any bony prominence.

3. Place a 4" × 15" preassembled splint in the palm and carry it up the volar aspect of the forearm to just below the elbow (**Figure 1**). If the injury involves the thumb, wrap it separately with 2" or 3" of cast padding.

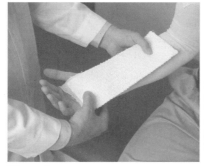

**Figure 1**
Begin in the palm and extend up the volar surface of the forearm to below the elbow.

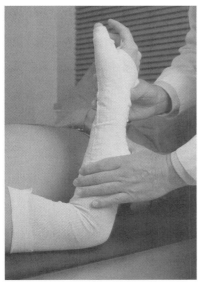

**Figure 2**
Apply the splint along the volar aspect of the thumb, extending across the wrist to the proximal forearm.

4. Place the splint on the volar or radial aspect and fold the plaster around the thumb, extending across the wrist to the proximal forearm. Leave the dorsal or ulnar side open for swelling (**Figure 2**).

5. Wrap the cast padding loosely over the plaster, then wrap an elastic bandage loosely over the cast padding as you mold the splint.

6. Trim the palmar portion of the splint back to the distal palmar flexion crease, proximal to the metacarpophalangeal (MP) joint.

### FRACTURES OR INJURIES OF THE FOREARM AND ELBOW

1. With the patient sitting or supine, have an assistant support the patient's hand with the elbow flexed to 90°. If sitting, the patient should lean slightly to the affected side so that the elbow falls away from the body.

2. Loosely wrap cast padding from the palm to above the elbow, taking care to avoid creating a constriction in the antecubital fossa. Make sure that there are three layers of padding at any bony prominence, such as the wrist and elbow.

3. Begin the splint in the palm, carry it up the forearm to the elbow, around the posterior elbow, then distally on the extensor aspect of the forearm to the dorsum of the hand (sugar tong) (**Figure 3**). Use multiple 4" × 15" preassembled splints, or a 5" × 30" preassembled splint if that size is appropriate.

4. Wrap cast padding loosely over the plaster, then wrap an elastic bandage loosely over the cast padding as you mold the splint.

5. Trim the palmar portion of the splint back to the distal palmar flexion crease, proximal to the MP joint.

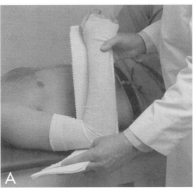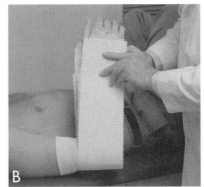

**Figure 3**
Splinting the elbow and forearm. A, Begin in the palm and extend proximally around the posterior elbow. B, Complete the splint distally on the extensor aspect of the forearm to the dorsum of the hand.

### FRACTURES OR INJURIES ABOVE THE ELBOW

1. With the patient sitting, have an assistant support the patient's hand with the elbow flexed to 90°. The patient should lean slightly to the affected side so that the elbow falls away from the body.

2. With an elbow injury, loosely wrap cast padding from the palm to the upper arm. Begin the splint below the axilla, carry it under the elbow, then up the lateral aspect of the arm (**Figure 4**).

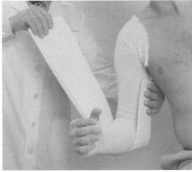

**Figure 4**
Begin the splint below the axilla, extending it under the elbow, then up the lateral aspect of the arm.

3. For unstable humeral fractures, continue the splint over the top of the shoulder, cover the plaster with a layer of cast padding, and then loosely wrap the entire arm with an elastic bandage (elephant ear splint) (**Figure 5**).

4. For lower humeral fractures or elbow injuries, end the splint below the lateral shoulder, cover the plaster with a layer of cast padding, and then loosely wrap the entire arm with an elastic bandage (coaptation splint). Provide the patient with a strap sling that loops around the wrist, then around the neck, and back to the wrist (**Figure 6**). The sling should be long enough to allow the elbow to be maintained at 90°.

5. Ensure that the sling has padding at the neck and wrist; these straps do not slide at night and can be adjusted for different arm lengths.

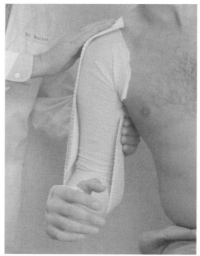

**Figure 5**
For lower humeral or elbow fractures, end the splint below the lateral shoulder.

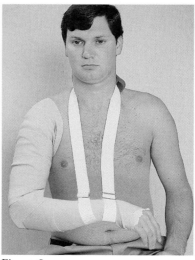

**Figure 6**
Proper positioning of a sling to maintain the elbow at 90°.

## PATIENT INSTRUCTIONS

Patients should be advised to protect the splint for 24 hours, until the plaster cures and hardens (fiberglass splints harden faster than plaster splints). A splinted arm should not be placed on any plastic covered surfaces (including pillows) until the plaster has cooled. Patients also should be reminded to watch for changes in skin color (circulation), sensation, and motion in the hand.

## SPLINTING THE LOWER EXTREMITY

### LONG LEG SPLINT

1. For unstable fractures of the leg or ankle, a long leg splint with the knee flexed 30° and the ankle 90° should be used.

2. With the patient supine, move his or her buttocks to the edge of the table, allowing the entire leg to hang suspended with an assistant holding the patient's forefoot. Ask the patient to allow the heel to sink so that the foot will be maintained at 90° during splinting.

3. Use either a stirrup-type splint or a long posterior splint. For a stirrup splint, have an assistant hold the patient's forefoot as you wrap the leg with three layers of 6" cast padding. Place extra padding over the kneecap and lateral knee (fibular head).

4. Begin the 5" × 45" plaster splint (10 to 12 thicknesses) on the lateral aspect of the thigh, extend it down the lateral aspect of the leg, under the heel, and then back up the medial side (**Figure 7**).

5. Start a second splint medially, and extend it beneath the foot and up the lateral side.

6. Apply a layer of cast padding over the plaster, and wrap a 5" or 6" elastic bandage over the padding as you mold the splint.

7. Ensure that the knee is positioned in 25° to 30° of flexion and the foot is positioned at 90° to the tibia (**Figure 8**).

Avoid folds in the plaster over the area of the peroneal nerve below the lateral knee (fibular head) or around the ankle. Preassembled foam padded splints are convenient, but use them with caution as they may develop folds or ridges in critical areas.

Use tepid or cool—never hot—water when applying the splint. The heat generated by the reaction of the plaster, if coupled with the use of hot water, can seriously burn the skin. For the same reason, place the leg on a cloth (not plastic) pillow and leave it uncovered for about 10 minutes following application to allow better convection of the heat.

Hold the splint in place with a loosely applied elastic bandage or bias-cut stockinet, rolled on with almost no tension. As the splint hardens, maintain the ankle at 90°. Mold or support the splint with the flat of the hand—only while it hardens—to avoid causing dents. Dents not only make the splint uncomfortable, but can cause cast sores or peroneal nerve palsy and foot drop.

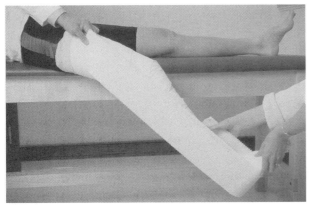

**Figure 7**
Begin the splint on the lateral aspect of the thigh, extending it down the lateral aspect of the leg, under the heel, and then back up the medial side.

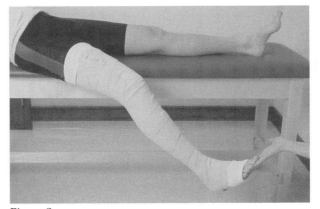

**Figure 8**
Maintain the knee in 25° to 30° of bend, maintaining the ankle at 90°.

## SHORT LEG SPLINT

1. With the patient sitting, have an assistant hold the forefoot to maintain the ankle at 90°, wrap the foot, ankle, and leg loosely with three thicknesses of cast padding.

2. Use either 5" × 45" cast padding or fashion a splint with 4" or 5" rolls folded to length.

3. Begin the splint laterally, three fingerbreadths below the knee flexion crease, and extend it down and wrap it under the heel and then up the medial side of the leg (**Figure 9**).

4. Apply the splint like a stirrup, extending material under the foot, covering the heel and arch.

5. Place a single layer of cast padding over the splint, and loosely wrap a 4" elastic bandage to secure the splint as you mold it to the extremity.

6. Maintain the ankle at 90° as the splint hardens (**Figure 10**).

An additional splint may be placed posteriorly if needed. Leave the plaster open in front and/or back for swelling, so the patient can unwrap the elastic bandage and spread the splint if needed.

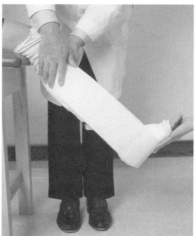

**Figure 9**
Begin the splint laterally, three finger-breadths below the knee flexion crease, and extend it down and wrap it under the heel and then up the medial side of the leg.

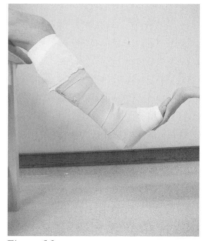

**Figure 10**
Maintain the angle of the ankle at 90° as the splint hardens.

## PATIENT INSTRUCTIONS

Patients should be advised to keep their injured leg elevated to the level of their heart as much as possible. Sitting in a reclining chair with a pillow beneath the leg is useful for this. In addition, ice bags should be kept on the injured leg as much as possible for the next 2 to 3 days to reduce pain and minimize swelling.

If the pain becomes a lot worse, the foot begins to feel numb or like it is "going to sleep," or the patient cannot move his or her toes up and down, the splint should be loosened by unwrapping the elastic bandage and tearing the padding down the front of the leg. If the leg does not feel better in 20 to 30 minutes, the patient should be advised to call the doctor because problems with circulation to the leg may be developing, which can have serious consequences.

The splint must be kept dry. Patients should be advised to place a plastic bag or commercially available cast cover over their leg, prop their leg on the side of the tub, and fill the tub around them, keeping the splinted leg out of the water. They should not shower.

Patients should be advised to contact the physician if they notice any places where the splint feels as though it is chafing or digging into the skin. Patients also should be reminded to watch for changes in skin color (circulation), sensation, and motion in the foot.

## ADVERSE OUTCOMES OF TREATMENT

Compartment syndrome, burns, and pressure sores can occur in splints of both the upper and lower extremities. Plantar flexion contractures of the ankle can develop if the ankle is splinted for prolonged periods with the ankle plantar flexed beyond the neutral position.

# SPORTS MEDICINE PRINCIPLES

## DEFINITION

The term "sports medicine" means different things to different people. A general definition is the application of professional training to the understanding, prevention, care, and rehabilitation of sports-related problems. This necessarily makes sports medicine a multidisciplinary field that encompasses other disciplines, such as physical therapy, athletic training, and exercise physiology. Thus, all areas of general and specialized primary care and internal medicine, as well as all surgical specialties, have legitimate roles in the management of sports-related problems. Orthopaedic surgeons represent the surgical specialty most frequently involved because of the large number of musculoskeletal injuries associated with sports and fitness participation.

Anyone who applies his or her area of expertise to sports-related problems is involved in sports medicine, although only a relative few serve as team physicians. Being a team physician involves coordination of preparticipation physical evaluations; determining readiness for participation; ensuring medical coverage of high-risk practices and competitions; arranging regular visits to the training room to evaluate and monitor problems; arranging appropriate referrals; communicating with parents, coaches, and administrators; and ensuring that adequate records are kept.

The fact that these patients are athletes on teams does not change their status as patients, and physicians providing their care must keep the best interests of the athlete-patient in mind, regardless of the relationship with the team.

## GENERAL ISSUES OF IMPORTANCE IN SPORTS MEDICINE

- Know and appreciate the importance of sports and/or fitness participation to athlete-patients. Communicate your understanding and commitment to helping them return as effectively and safely as possible.

- Competitive athletes and serious fitness participants need a prompt diagnosis and treatment plan; they also need to know the prognosis. If they are part of a team, all concerned must understand these issues and the anticipated lost playing time as soon as possible so appropriate team planning can be initiated. Parents need to know this information for their peace of mind.

- Communication plays a critical role. Prompt, authoritative, and efficient communication among parents, coaches, trainers, and involved colleagues is essential. Telephone calls can be notoriously inefficient. An immediately available sports injury report form with multiple copies can be a big help.

- Personal coverage of competitions is optimal for team physicians but is not always feasible. When not physically present, a team physician needs to be available for timely communication with coaches, trainers, parents, or athletes.

- Provide a team approach to the care of the athlete. Coordinated involvement of all concerned with the athlete and the team (athletes, parents, coaches, trainers, colleagues, and therapists) optimizes outcomes.

- Recognize public interest in the status of injured athletes. Treating physicians frequently are approached by the media for information about prominent athletes who are injured. It is important to protect physician-patient confidentiality. A practical, successful approach is to prepare a brief factual statement that includes no details that should remain confidential. This statement can be released upon request, with the proviso that any additional information has to come from the team or the athlete.

- Many more nonoperative illnesses and injuries are encountered than operative. Nonoperative treatment does not mean no treatment. Aggressive nonoperative treatment is the mainstay of sports medicine.

- Sports-oriented physical therapy plays a critical role by understanding the extent of recovery required to return safely and effectively to competitive sports. While many of these needs apply to virtually all sports and fitness activities, many are sport specific, and some are also position specific. Traditional physical therapy rarely provides adequate or timely rehabilitation for an in-season or preseason competitive athlete.

## CLINICAL SYMPTOMS

Symptoms are exactly the same for athletes as for nonathletes in situations of sprains/strains, tendinitis, or fractures. Certain injuries are somewhat specific to athletics, such as turf toe or myositis ossificans. Shoulder and elbow tendinitis in baseball players and tennis players is another example.

## TESTS

Physical examination and appropriate radiographs are needed, as indicated for the specific situation.

## TREATMENT

Sports-oriented rehabilitation includes four phases: initial, functional, sport-specific, and graduated return to play. It is essential that the injured structures be protected to the extent necessary and that the injury not be aggravated. The principles of rest, ice, compression, and elevation (RICE) should be followed. Pain control modalities and electrical stimulation also can be helpful. Joint range of motion; muscle flexibility, strengthening, and endurance; and apparatus-based functional and aerobic activities are initiated as tolerated. It is not possible to make injuries heal faster, but the healing process should not be impaired. Athletes and serious fitness participants can maintain their aerobic fitness by doing other activities that do not aggravate or jeopardize the injury.

Functional rehabilitation begins when the healing status is appropriate, and when joint motion, muscle flexibility, strength, and endurance are adequate. The program should be disciplined, independent, and emphasize normal form. A gradual running program is initiated for lower extremity problems. It should begin with straight line running, progressing from jogging to half-speed to three-quarter speed to sprinting as tolerated. Agility drills are then added starting at half-speed intensity, progressing to three-quarter speed and to full speed as tolerated. Jumping activities are added last.

For upper extremity and spine injuries, individual programs that apply general and sport-specific principles should be used. Once a general functional program has been successfully completed, sport-specific and position-specific drills can be initiated.

Graduated return to play should include transition to increasing partial practice and then to full practice as tolerated. A helpful guideline is to require at least two full practices without restriction and without problems before returning to full competition. This helps the athlete, coaches, and family to know that the athlete is truly ready to return to competition effectively and safely.

# Sprains and Strains

## Definition

Sprains and strains are both injuries, but they differ in the tissue that is affected. Sprains involve the supporting structures of a joint and, therefore, a sprain is a stretching or tearing of a ligament or joint capsule. Strains involve muscles, or more precisely the muscle-tendon unit. A strain is a stretching or partial tear of a muscle. A complete tear of a muscle or tendon typically is described as a rupture.

Sprains may occur in patients of any age, but they are much more common in older adolescents, young adults, and middle-aged adults. In children the physis is the weak link, and similar forces or injuries result in a fracture of the growth plate. In older adults, the bone again is the weak link and similar injuries cause a fracture.

Strains likewise may occur in patients of any age but are more common in middle-aged and older adults. With aging, the collagen in a muscle-tendon unit changes. As a result, muscles have decreased elasticity and are more susceptible to injury.

## Clinical symptoms

Sprains usually are a result of sudden trauma, such as a fall causing an inversion stress to the ankle resulting in tearing of the lateral ligaments of the ankle. Patients often report a pop or snap at the time of the acute event, followed by pain, swelling, stiffness, and difficulty bearing weight. Ecchymosis can appear within 24 to 48 hours.

Strains and muscle ruptures commonly result from a sudden stretch on a muscle that is actively contracting. For example, a strain or rupture of the quadriceps muscle commonly occurs when a person falls and lands with the knee flexed and the quadriceps contracting to absorb the energy of the fall. Severe strains also are associated with a snap or tearing sensation; however, pain and swelling with a mild strain may not be noted on the day of injury.

## Tests

### Physical examination

Swelling, tenderness, and ecchymosis at the site of the torn ligament or capsule usually are seen early and persist until healing is well underway in joints that are superficial. Swelling, tenderness, and ecchymosis are not as well defined with muscle injuries or with sprains of joints that are deep and covered by muscles.

Palpate the injured area for the site of maximal tenderness. This leads to or narrows the diagnostic possibilities. Gently place the injured structure on stretch. This increases the pain and provides additional information concerning what structure has been injured. For example, for a patient who has tenderness over the medial aspect of the proximal tibia after a fall, gently stress the knee into valgus. If the pain is increased with a valgus stress and the radiographs are negative for a fracture, then the patient has a sprain of the medial collateral ligament of the knee. Likewise, the diagnostic test for a patient who reports acute pain in the posterior thigh while running is to position the limb so that the hamstring muscles are put on stretch (flex the hip to 90° and then extend the knee).

With a sprain, the degree of injury and stability of the joint should be assessed. This assessment is not always precise, particularly if the patient has marked swelling and tenderness. Some ligamentous injuries require unique clinical maneuvers to determine injury and instability. When possible, however, classifying sprains provides useful information concerning the degree of disability and requirements for treatment (Table 1). For example, a grade I sprain is a partial tear of the ligament.

## Table 1
### Classification of Sprains

| Grade | Degree of injury | Treatment principles |
|---|---|---|
| I | Partial tear but no instability, or opening of the joint on stress maneuvers | Symptomatic treatment only |
| II | Partial tear with some instability indicated by partial opening of joint on stress maneuvers | Immobilization to protect injured part, but full healing expected |
| III | Complete tear with complete opening joint on stress | Immobilization or possibly repair |

With a muscle injury, it is important to distinguish a strain from a complete rupture. The latter sometimes require operative repair. If a patient can move the joint, that is suggestive evidence of a strain. For example, a patient with a strain of the quadriceps muscle can hold the knee extended, but with a complete rupture of the quadriceps tendon, the patient is unable to straighten the knee. Pain and resultant inhibition of muscle contraction sometimes makes this clinical test imprecise.

### DIAGNOSTIC TESTS

Radiographs are helpful only in the negative sense. Thus, they should be obtained only if a fracture is suspected. The Ottawa guidelines are useful in patients with suspected foot or ankle sprain. These guidelines delineate that radiographs of the ankle are necessary only if there is pain near the malleoli or if either of the following findings are present: inability to bear weight (four steps) both immediately and in the emergency department; or bony tenderness at the posterior edge or tip of the malleoli. Similarly, radiographs of the foot are necessary only if there is midfoot pain and either of the following conditions: inability to bear weight (four steps) both immediately and in the emergency department; or bony tenderness at the navicular or the base of the fifth metatarsal.

## DIFFERENTIAL DIAGNOSIS

Fracture (evident on radiographs)

## ADVERSE OUTCOMES OF THE DISEASE

The tissue damaged as a result of a sprain might not heal, resulting in a chronic condition, such as chronic ankle instability. Prolonged weakness, tightness, and tenderness can follow a muscle strain or tear. Complex regional pain syndrome (CRPS) can develop after a seemingly minor strain or sprain. Compartment syndrome occasionally occurs.

## TREATMENT

Rest, ice, compression, and elevation (RICE) are the mainstays of treatment. Heat can be helpful later, but ice should be used initially. NSAIDs are useful for the first few days. Grade I sprains need immobilization only for comfort. Grade II and III sprains should be protected. Most grade III sprains can be treated nonoperatively, but certain injuries require surgical repair.

## ADVERSE OUTCOMES OF TREATMENT

Overemphasis on treatment in the suggestible patient can lead to chronic impairment and disability, particularly in workers' compensation situations.

## REFERRAL DECISIONS/RED FLAGS

Patients with grade III sprains, severe grade II sprains, or complete muscle-tendon ruptures require further evaluation. Patients whose symptoms are out of proportion to their injury and findings can be at risk for chronic conditions or CRPS, and a second opinion should be sought early. Equivocal radiographs should be repeated in these cases.

# TUMORS OF BONE

## ICD-9 Code
**238.0**
Neoplasm of uncertain behavior of other and unspecified sites and tissues, bone and articular cartilage

## SYNONYMS
Malignancy
Neoplasm
Bone lesion
Bone cancer

## DEFINITION

Bone tumors are classified as either benign or malignant. Benign tumors of bone are relatively common, but primary malignant tumors of bone are rare. Bone, however, is a common site for metastasis, and any malignant lesion of bone in a patient older than age 40 years must be considered as a possible skeletal metastasis.

Bone tumors also are classified by their tissue of origin: benign and malignant tumors can develop from cartilage, bone, fibrous tissue, and marrow elements.

Age is an important factor in predicting the type of bone tumor. Gender, history of trauma, and site are of limited or no diagnostic benefit (**Table 1**).

## Table 1
### Bone Tumors and Tumor-like Conditions by Age

| 1 year to 5 years | 6 to 18 years | 19 to 40 years | 40 + years |
|---|---|---|---|
| Osteomyelitis | Simple bone cyst | Ewing sarcoma | Metastases |
| Metastatic neuroblastoma | Aneurysmal bone cyst | Giant cell tumor | Multiple myeloma |
| Leukemia | Nonossifying fibroma | Osteosarcoma | Chondrosarcoma |
| Eosinophilic granuloma | Ewing sarcoma | | Fibrosarcoma |
| Simple bone cyst | Osteomyelitis | | Malignant fibrous histiocytoma |
| | Osteosarcoma | | Chordoma |
| | Enchondroma | | |
| | Chondroblastoma | | |
| | Chondromyxoidfibroma | | |
| | Osteoblastoma | | |
| | Fibrous dysplasia | | |
| | Osteofibrous dysplasia | | |

# CLINICAL SYMPTOMS

Pain is the usual presenting complaint. Malignant tumors are associated with a constant, deep aching pain that does not go away with rest and is present at night. However, certain benign tumors also cause night pain. This is particularly true of osteoid osteoma, but it also occurs with benign tumors that are relatively large and have weakened the bone. A sudden increase in pain following trivial trauma that was preceded by a history of mild, dull, aching pain suggests a pathologic fracture.

The presence of a mass also may be the presenting complaint. If the mass is painless, it is most likely benign. Bony tumors may press on adjacent nerves and cause radicular symptoms. The size and locations of some tumors interfere with joint and muscle function.

Ask about fever, malaise, weakness, weight loss, and other constitutional symptoms that are more common with malignant tumors, particularly Ewing sarcoma, primary tumors of bone that have metastasized, and secondary skeletal metastasis.

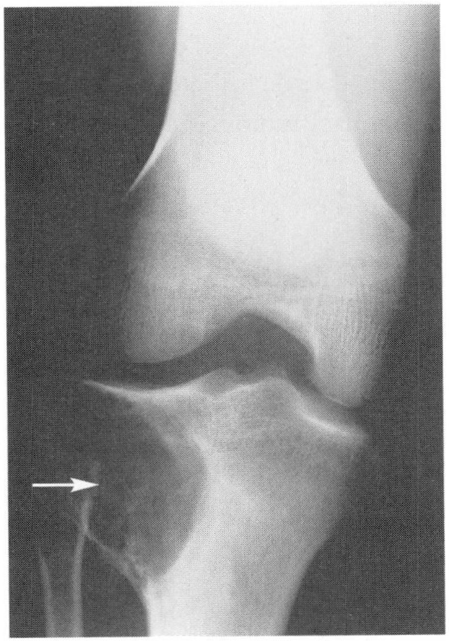

# TESTS

## PHYSICAL EXAMINATION

Physical examination should focus on identifying masses, sites of tenderness, reduced range of motion, a limp, and regional adenopathy. In patients older than age 40 years, careful examination of other systems, particularly the lungs, breasts, prostate, kidneys, and thyroid, should be done to rule out a metastatic carcinoma.

## DIAGNOSTIC TESTS

AP, lateral, and oblique radiographs usually identify the location of the lesion. Associated findings can include the following; the characteristics of the borders of the lesion (well circumscribed or not well delineated); periosteal elevation and reactive bone formation adjacent to the lesion; the presence of calcification within the lesion; and whether the lesion is eccentric or central, lytic, or blastic. These factors help to distinguish the lesion and, most importantly, whether the mass is benign or malignant (**Figure 1**).

The goal in staging a bone neoplasm is to determine the extent of the disease before performing a biopsy and initiating definitive treatment. CT is excellent for demonstrating bony changes and degree of calcification within the lesion and, therefore, is often better for benign bony lesions (**Figure 2**). MRI is better for malignant tumors because of its superiority in defining extension of the lesion through the medullary canal and into the surrounding muscle compartments. Bone scans are helpful in identifying the presence or absence of other skeletal lesions. If a malignant tumor is suspected, a chest radiograph, bone scan, and usually CT of the chest also should be obtained.

Routine laboratory tests are of limited value in the diagnosis of many bone tumors, but with certain tumors they can help to narrow the differential diagnosis. With suspected malignant tumors, laboratory studies can provide baseline values for patients who need chemotherapy. The following laboratory

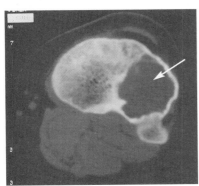

**Figure 1**
Lytic tumor destroying bone of proximal lateral tibia.

*Reproduced with permission from Kasser JR (ed): Orthopaedic Knowledge Update 5. Rosemont, IL, American Academy of Orthopaedic Surgeons, 1996, pp 133–148.*

**Figure 2**
CT scan of tumor shown in Figure 1.

*Reproduced with permission from Kasser JR (ed): Orthopaedic Knowledge Update 5. Rosemont, IL, American Academy of Orthopaedic Surgeons, 1996, pp 133–148.*

SECTION 1 | GENERAL ORTHOPAEDICS

studies usually are obtained: CBC with differential, erythrocyte sedimentation rate, serum electrolytes, blood urea nitrogen, creatinine, calcium, phosphorus, and alkaline phosphatase. Tests for patients age 40 years and older include the following additional studies: urinalysis, urine and serum protein electrophoresis, and prostate specific antigen (PSA) for men.

A biopsy is performed to determine if the lesion is benign or malignant, to determine the cell type of lesion, and to determine the grade of the lesion. The biopsy should be performed by a surgeon who has the training to perform the definitive surgical procedure.

## DIFFERENTIAL DIAGNOSIS (PARTIAL LIST)

### BENIGN CARTILAGINOUS

Chondroblastoma (age 8 to skeletal maturity, rare, located in epiphysis)

Chondromyxoid fibroma (adolescents, eccentric, metaphyseal, tibia)

Enchondroma (young adults, phalanges and metacarpals, speckled calcification)

Osteochondroma (children and teenagers, cartilaginous cap on bony stalk)

### BENIGN BONY

Osteoid osteoma (children and teenagers, night pain relieved by NSAIDs, small size)

Osteoblastoma (children, young adults, rare, spine)

### BENIGN MARROW ELEMENTS

Eosinophilic granuloma (young children, "hole in a bone")

### BENIGN FIBROUS TISSUE

Nonossifying fibroma (children and teenagers, eccentric metaphyseal location)

Fibrous dysplasia (ages 6 years to maturity, diaphyseal, bone deformity, limb shortening)

### BENIGN WITH TISSUE OF UNCERTAIN ORIGIN

Aneurysmal bone cyst (children and teenagers, metaphyseal, expansile)

Giant cell tumor (young adults, epiphysis and metaphysis, eccentric and lytic)

Simple bone cyst (children and teenagers, metaphyseal, lytic)

### MALIGNANT CARTILAGINOUS, BONY, AND FIBROUS TISSUE ORIGIN

Chondrosarcoma (age over 40 years, central metaphyseal location, calcification)

Fibrosarcoma/malignant fibrous histiocytoma (older adults, metaphyseal, lytic)

Osteosarcoma (second decade, metaphyseal, long bones, mixed blastic and lytic areas)

Secondary osteosarcoma (originates in Paget disease or irradiated bone)

### MALIGNANT TUMORS OF MARROW ORIGIN

Ewing sarcoma (second decade, may simulate osteomyelitis, lytic)

Leukemia (in young children may present as bone lesion in limbs or spine)

Multiple myeloma or plasmacytoma (age over 40 years, spine and pelvis, lytic)

## ADVERSE OUTCOMES OF THE DISEASE

Pathologic fracture (minimal trauma, poor healing), disability, and even death are possible.

## TREATMENT

Observation is appropriate for benign bone tumors that are causing minimal symptoms, that are not likely to enlarge, and for which the diagnosis is clear on radiographs. Other benign bony tumors should be excised. Malignant lesions usually require surgery, often in conjunction with chemotherapy and radiation therapy.

## ADVERSE OUTCOMES OF TREATMENT

Disability, disfigurement, pathologic fracture, infection, failure of implant, nerve and vascular deficits, and death are possible and depend on the size and growth potential of the tumor.

## REFERRAL DECISIONS/RED FLAGS

Suspicious bone or soft-tissue masses, unusual pain or night pain, constitutional symptoms in association with bone pain or lytic or blastic changes of bone, soft-tissue calcification, or periosteal reaction on radiography all require further evaluation.

# Tumors of Soft Tissue

## ICD-9 Code

238.1
Neoplasm of uncertain behavior of other and unspecified sites and tissues, connective and other soft tissue

## DEFINITION

Soft-tissue tumors of the extremities can be classified as benign or malignant. Benign soft-tissue tumors are much more common than malignant tumors (ratio of more than 100:1). Some benign lesions, such as ganglia, popliteal cysts, and epidermoid cysts, although classified as tumors, are not neoplastic but result from degenerative changes. Compared to bony tumors, malignant soft-tissue tumors cannot be clearly distinguished from benign lesions. However, sarcomas arising in the soft tissue of the extremities are more likely with lesions that are at least 5 cm in diameter, fixed to the surrounding tissues, and deep to the fascia. Pain, however, is not a defining characteristic of malignant soft-tissue somatic tumors. For example, a lipoma can occur anywhere on the extremity or even on the trunk. All soft-tissue masses should be considered as neoplasms because failure to do so can have serious consequences. Although most musculoskeletal tumors are benign, the possibility of malignancy always should be considered.

## CLINICAL SYMPTOMS

Most soft-tissue tumors are asymptomatic, except for the presence of an enlarging mass. A much smaller mass will be discovered earlier in the hand or foot than around the pelvis or shoulder. Mild pain and tenderness may be present.

## TESTS

### PHYSICAL EXAMINATION

Inspect the limb for swelling and adherence of the surrounding structures. Palpate the lesion to determine size, discreetness, and texture. Benign lesions tend to be more discreet with well-defined margins, while malignant lesions can be less well defined. A lipoma has a rubbery consistency, while a fibroma is firm. Auscultation can yield the sound of a bruit or the to-and-fro murmur of an arteriovenous fistula. Cystic lesions may transilluminate, which distinguishes them from solid tumors.

### DIAGNOSTIC TESTS

Routine laboratory studies are nonspecific. If a malignant lesion is possible, obtain a baseline CBC with differential, erythrocyte sedimentation rate, routine blood chemistries, and radiographs of the involved area. MRI is the best imaging study to define the extent and characteristics of a soft-tissue malignancy; however, a fine-needle or open biopsy is necessary to make a definitive diagnosis of most lesions.

# DIFFERENTIAL DIAGNOSIS (PARTIAL LIST)

## BENIGN TUMORS

Angiomyoma (middle-aged adults, lower limbs, small, subcutaneous)

Ganglia (children, teenagers, and young adults, degenerative lesions arising from joint capsule or tendon sheath, may transilluminate)

Giant cell tumor of tendon sheath (middle-aged adults, hand and foot, close proximity to the tendon sheath)

Hemangioma and vascular malformations (children and adolescents)

Lipoma (adults, most common soft-tissue tumor, lobular nature, rubbery consistency)

## MALIGNANT TUMORS

Fibrosarcoma (young and middle-aged adults, subfascial)

Liposarcoma (young, middle-, and older-aged adults, subfascial)

Malignant fibrous histiocytoma (middle- and older-aged adults, often deep but may be superficial to fascia)

Rhabdomyosarcoma (children and teenagers, subfascial)

Synovial cell sarcoma (teenagers and young adults, small focal calcification)

## ADVERSE OUTCOMES OF THE DISEASE

Continued growth, discomfort, and impaired function due to location of the mass or patient concerns about the identification of the mass may necessitate removal. Malignant soft-tissue tumors have a variable prognosis depending on several factors, but loss of limb or even death can be the end result.

## TREATMENT

If the diagnosis is reasonably certain, many benign soft-tissue tumors can be observed for signs of growth, change in character, or interference with function. Patients, however, are often uncomfortable with this approach and prefer biopsy and, if indicated, surgical excision. For malignant lesions, surgical excision, in conjunction with chemotherapy, radiation, or immunotherapy, is indicated, with a variable response depending on the patient's age, tumor type, duration, and location.

## ADVERSE OUTCOMES OF TREATMENT

Aside from injury to adjacent nerves or other structures and a cutaneous scar, few adverse effects are associated with excision of a small, benign tumor. Disfigurement, disability, loss of more vital neurovascular structures, and extensive scarring may be the consequence of the much more extensive surgery required for malignant lesions.

## REFERRAL DECISIONS/RED FLAGS

All but the smallest, clearly benign lesions in nonthreatened locations require further evaluation.

SECTION 1 | GENERAL ORTHOPAEDICS

# VENOUS THROMBOSIS

| ICD-9 Code |
| --- |
| 451.1 |
| Phlebitis and thrombophlebitis, of deep vessels of lower extremities |

## DEFINITION

Deep venous thrombosis (DVT) is characterized by hypercoagulation, obstruction of venous outflow, and/or endothelial trauma that precipitates venous clot formation. Proximal propagation of clots can lead to pulmonary embolism and even death. Major musculoskeletal procedures (eg, total hip arthroplasty, total knee arthroplasty, hip fracture surgery), multiple trauma, and spinal cord injuries increase the likelihood of DVT and subsequent pulmonary embolism. Other risk factors include previous thrombosis; immobilization; stroke; congestive heart failure; malignancy; deficiencies in antithrombin III, protein C, or proteins S; myeloproliferative diseases, estrogen use; inflammatory bowel disease; diabetes; obesity; and age older than 40 to 50 years.

## CLINICAL SYMPTOMS

Many patients with venous thrombosis are asymptomatic, but some report pain or swelling in the calf or thigh. Patients with pulmonary embolism often report dyspnea, pleuritic or substernal chest pain, and hemoptysis.

## TESTS

### PHYSICAL EXAMINATION

Clinical signs of venous thrombosis often are nonspecific. Swelling, whether painful or not, is common. However, pulmonary embolism can occur without any prior warning. Patients with superficial saphenous vein thrombophlebitis have a tender, warm, ropy vein, which may be serious if it extends into the common femoral vein. A positive Homans sign is calf pain with forced ankle dorsiflexion.

The clinical signs of pulmonary embolism include dyspnea, hemoptysis, tachycardia, pleural rub, tachypnea, and sometimes circulatory collapse.

### DIAGNOSTIC TESTS

If patients report swelling and pain, duplex ultrasound is highly accurate in diagnosing proximal clot formation. However, the role of a duplex scan in screening for asymptomatic thrombi remains controversial. Venography remains the gold standard to confirm DVT but is an invasive procedure that may cause pain, allergic reactions to contrast medium, or, rarely, a DVT.

## DIFFERENTIAL DIAGNOSIS

Ruptured popliteal (Baker) cyst (no history of prior trauma or surgery)

Cellulitis (erythema, superficial tenderness)

Contusion of calf muscles (direct blow, subsequent ecchymosis and tenderness)

Lymphedema (nontender, diffuse swelling)

Strain of the calf or thigh muscles (history of injury, pain with stretch of the involved muscle)

## ADVERSE OUTCOMES OF THE DISEASE
Both distal and proximal clots can lead to pulmonary embolism and/or death. Symptomatic proximal leg vein thromboses may have silent pulmonary emboli in as many as 50% of patients. Other possible problems include post-thrombotic syndrome with venous stasis ulceration, chronic edema, venous claudication, and recurrent thromboses.

## TREATMENT
Most patients who die of a pulmonary embolism do so within 30 minutes of the acute event, which is too soon for therapeutic anticoagulation to be effective. Consequently, prophylaxis is needed to reduce the incidence of thromboembolism or prevent proximal propagation of the clots. There is no universally accepted regimen (agent or duration) for prophylaxis in orthopaedic surgical conditions. The effect of early hospital discharge on the duration of prophylaxis and the impact on the prevalence of symptomatic thromboembolism following discharge are unclear. Effective prophylaxis can be obtained with both pharmacologic and mechanical methods. There is general agreement that patients undergoing total hip or knee arthroplasty and multiple-trauma patients require DVT prophylaxis. There is, however, disagreement concerning the preferred approach.

The ultimate goal of prophylaxis is to prevent a symptomatic pulmonary embolism or chronic venous insufficiency. Warfarin may be given the night following surgery, although some physicians prefer to give a low dose before surgery. The dose of warfarin is adjusted to keep the international normalized ratio (INR) between 1.8 and 2.5. Warfarin prophylaxis usually continues for 2 to 3 weeks. The prophylaxis regimen used with low-molecular-weight heparin depends on the particular drug being prescribed. In general, these drugs have a very short half-life, and they should not be administered immediately after surgery. Monitoring of INR or partial thromboplastin time (PTT) is not necessary. The recommended duration of prophylaxis is approximately 10 to 14 days. Compared with warfarin, low-molecular-weight heparin is effective in reducing the overall asymptomatic DVT rates, but there has been no difference compared with warfarin noted in the prevalence of symptomatic pulmonary embolism.

The duration of prophylaxis remains controversial. The use of in-hospital prophylaxis with a screening study at discharge is not recommended at this time. When using standard unfractionated (adjusted-dose) heparin, give the first subcutaneous injection of 5,000 USP units 1 to 2 hours preoperatively or within 12 hours after the procedure. Subsequent doses are given every 8 to 12 hours and are adjusted to achieve an activated PTT of 1.5 to 2.0 times more than the upper limit of normal. The blood sample for the measurement of the activated PTT is obtained 4 to 6 hours after the morning dose of heparin.

## 1

Although this regimen provides effective prophylaxis, it is associated with higher bleeding rates than other modalities.

Pneumatic compression boots or plantar arch compression devices reduce the overall risk of DVT and should be applied during and after surgery. The advantage to using these devices is that they do not require laboratory monitoring, and there is no risk of bleeding. However, patient compliance can be a problem, and the efficacy of these devices in limiting proximal clot formation in patients undergoing total hip arthroplasty requires further study. These devices can serve as an adjunct to pharmacologic prophylaxis.

Effective prophylaxis after total hip arthroplasty includes warfarin, low-molecular-weight heparin, and adjusted-dose heparin. Effective prophylaxis after total knee arthroplasty includes low-molecular-weight heparin, warfarin, pneumatic compression boots, and plantar compression devices. Low-molecular-weight heparin also provides effective prophylaxis for most multiple-trauma patients.

The purpose of treatment of a pulmonary embolism or proximal or popliteal thrombus is to reduce the likelihood of recurrence or propagation of the thrombus. When a patient is diagnosed with a proximal venous thrombosis or a pulmonary embolism, start IV heparin with a bolus dose of 5,000 USP units. Follow this with a continuous infusion beginning at 30,000 USP units per day (which is adequate for most patients) to maintain a PTT between 1.5 and 2.0 times normal while starting warfarin therapy. Stop the heparin when the INR has been maintained between 2.0 and 3.0 for 2 consecutive days. Continue warfarin therapy for at least 3 months.

Intravenous heparin is currently the mainstay for early therapy of acute pulmonary embolism or proximal thrombus. However, low-molecular-weight heparin has been demonstrated to be effective in treating acute thromboembolic disease in clinical trials. These agents eventually may be the treatment of choice for acute thromboembolic disease as hospital stays and costs can be reduced.

Contraindications of long-term warfarin therapy include pregnancy, liver insufficiency, severe liver disease, noncompliance, severe alcoholism, uncontrolled hypertension, active major hemorrhage, and inability to return for monitoring.

## ADVERSE OUTCOMES OF TREATMENT

Bleeding has been associated with all anticoagulants. Thrombocytopenia occurs with standard heparin but occurs infrequently with low-molecular-weight heparin. However, bleeding risks are low, and it is important that high-risk patients receive prophylaxis despite these potential problems. Skin necrosis can develop with warfarin but is uncommon.

## REFERRAL DECISIONS/RED FLAGS

None

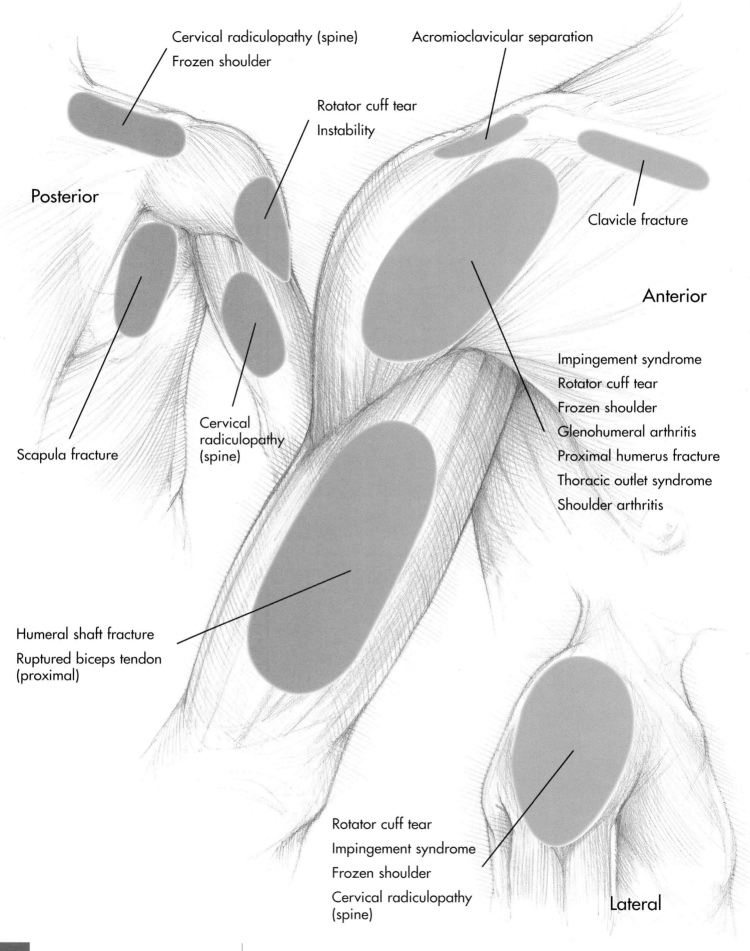

Cervical radiculopathy (spine)

Frozen shoulder

Acromioclavicular separation

Rotator cuff tear

Instability

Posterior

Clavicle fracture

Anterior

Scapula fracture

Cervical radiculopathy (spine)

Impingement syndrome

Rotator cuff tear

Frozen shoulder

Glenohumeral arthritis

Proximal humerus fracture

Thoracic outlet syndrome

Shoulder arthritis

Humeral shaft fracture

Ruptured biceps tendon (proximal)

Rotator cuff tear

Impingement syndrome

Frozen shoulder

Cervical radiculopathy (spine)

Lateral

# SHOULDER

**Section Editor**
Michael A. Wirth, MD
Associate Professor
Department of Orthopaedics
University of Texas Health Science Center
Chief, Shoulder Service
Audie Murphy Veterans Hospital
San Antonio, Texas

Robert M. Orfaly, MD, FRCSC
Assistant Professor
Department of Orthopaedics and Rehabilitation
Oregon Health Sciences University
Portland, Oregon

Charles A. Rockwood, Jr, MD
Professor and Chairman Emeritus
Department of Orthopaedics
University of Texas Health Science Center
San Antonio, Texas

# Shoulder—An Overview

This section of *Essentials of Musculoskeletal Care* focuses on the common conditions affecting the shoulder girdle in adults. These include acute injuries (fractures, dislocations, and acute tendon ruptures), chronic or repetitive injuries (impingement syndrome and most rotator cuff tears and biceps tendon ruptures), and degenerative, inflammatory, or idiopathic conditions (glenohumeral and acromioclavicular arthritis, frozen shoulder). While there have been many technological advances in diagnostic aids, most shoulder disorders can be diagnosed from a careful history, physical examination, and plain radiographs.

A concise differential diagnosis often is achieved by evaluating the patient's chief complaint in the context of its chronicity and the patient's age. The chief complaint is usually related to pain or instability. Symptoms of decreased motion, power, or function can accompany complaints of pain or instability, but they are rarely the chief complaint.

## Pain

Patients with acute symptoms (less than 2 weeks' duration) usually have an injury, such as a fracture or a dislocation, or a rotator cuff tear. Common physical findings include local tenderness, deformity, swelling, and ecchymosis. Determining the mechanism and magnitude of the injury and the anatomic location of symptoms helps in making the diagnosis. For example, a football player who has severe pain and deformity at the superior aspect of the shoulder after falling directly on that shoulder most likely has an acromioclavicular (AC) joint separation.

Similarly, for patients with chronic shoulder pain, knowledge of the activities related to the onset of symptoms and the location and character of symptoms often leads to the correct diagnosis. Pain localized to the top of the shoulder suggests AC joint arthritis or chronic separation. This pain often is exacerbated by cross-body adduction in the horizontal plane. Pain from subacromial bursitis, frozen shoulder, and rotator cuff pathology is typically referred to the lateral deltoid region and may radiate to the lateral aspect of the upper arm. Overhead activities most commonly exacerbate this pain. In contrast, shoulder pain arising from cervical nerve root irritation usually follows a dermatomal distribution, is associated with numbness and/or tingling, and is often relieved by placing the forearm on top of the head. Degenerative arthritis of the glenohumeral joint can cause pain along the anterior and posterior joint lines. Both rotator cuff tears and arthritis can cause night pain, which makes sleeping on the affected side difficult.

# INSTABILITY

Instability can be classified by the frequency of symptomatic episodes, as well as the direction and degree of instability. Acute injuries may be a first-time dislocation or a recurrent episode. The instability episode may be partial (subluxation) with spontaneous reduction or may be complete (dislocation). The instability can be anterior, posterior, inferior, or multidirectional. Most traumatic dislocations are anterior. Multidirectional instability should be considered in patients who present with recurrent episodes of subluxations or dislocations and no history of significant trauma.

# RANGE OF MOTION, MUSCLE STRENGTH, AND FUNCTION

In assessing motion, it is important to determine if there is a discrepancy between active and passive motion. While some loss of passive range can occur secondary to disuse, patients with rotator cuff tears primarily lose active elevation and external rotation. Equal losses of active and passive range of motion can be secondary to soft-tissue contracture, as in frozen shoulder, or the result of joint incongruity from trauma or arthritis.

Muscle strength should be assessed and compared with the opposite shoulder. Tears of the rotator cuff and neurologic injury can produce weakness. Pain inhibition can affect the accuracy of muscle testing.

Functional status relates to a patient's ability to perform his or her normal activities. The level of functional disability depends on the specific type and intensity of activities the patient normally performs. Motivation and ability to adapt to impairment also play a significant role.

# PATIENT AGE

## YOUNGER PATIENTS

Patients younger than 30 years of age most commonly present with traumatic injuries or instability such as glenohumeral dislocations and AC joint separations. Impingement syndrome and rotator cuff tears rarely occur in this age group.

## MIDDLE-AGED PATIENTS

Impingement syndrome and rotator cuff tears are common in this group. These must be distinguished from frozen shoulder, which produces a global loss of passive and active range of motion. Glenohumeral dislocations are much less common and must be treated with a high index of suspicion for a concomitant rotator cuff tear (50% of patients over 40 years of age will have an acute tear).

## OLDER PATIENTS

Patients older than 50 years of age are likely to have rotator cuff tears or degenerative arthritis. Acute pain following a fall in an elderly patient is most commonly a fracture of the proximal humerus.

# RADIOGRAPHS

The standard trauma series starts with two good quality radiographs of the shoulder taken 90° from one another. This ideally consists of an anteroposterior (AP) view of the shoulder and an axillary lateral view. These views are sufficient to reveal most fractures and dislocations. Several techniques of obtaining axillary views have been described to minimize patient discomfort in the acute trauma setting. The transscapular lateral view occasionally can serve as a substitute but is much more prone to misinterpretation.

# PHYSICAL EXAMINATION
# SHOULDER

## Inspection/Palpation

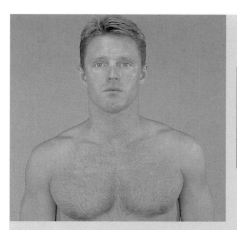

### Anterior view

Look for abnormal contours and bony prominences. An AC separation produces a "step-off" deformity with prominence of the distal clavicle. An anterior shoulder dislocation produces a prominent acromion and anterior fullness of the deltoid, and the arm typically is held in slight abduction and external rotation. By contrast, with a posterior dislocation, the coracoid and anterior acromion are prominent, there is posterior fullness, and the arm is held in adduction and internal rotation.

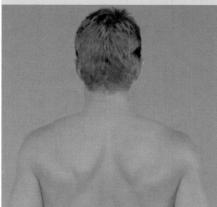

### Posterior view

Note symmetry of shoulder heights and contours (dominant shoulder often rests slightly lower than the opposite shoulder). Look for muscle atrophy, particularly of the trapezius, deltoid, and supraspinatus/infraspinatus muscles. Diminished posterior contour from neck to shoulder indicates atrophy of the trapezius. Loss of lateral shoulder contour occurs at the deltoid, and a prominent suprascapular ridge can be seen with atrophy of the supraspinatus/infraspinatus muscles.

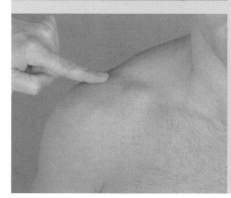

### AC joint

Palpate the end of the clavicle and the acromion for tenderness or spurs. Tenderness usually is most pronounced at the posterior joint interval and is exaggerated when the patient adducts the arm toward the opposite shoulder.

# Inspection/Palpation

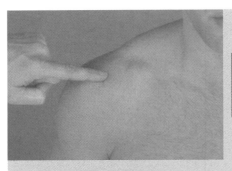

### Subacromial bursa

Palpate the anterolateral portion of the acromion, moving down toward the deltoid until you feel the acromiohumeral sulcus. Tenderness in this area usually is related to subacromial bursitis or a rotator cuff tear (supraspinatus tendon).

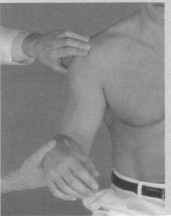

### Long head biceps tendon

Palpate over the humeral head in the region of the bicipital groove. With tendinitis, there is tenderness and swelling and the area of tenderness should move with the humeral head as the shoulder is rotated.

# Range of Motion

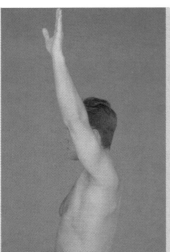

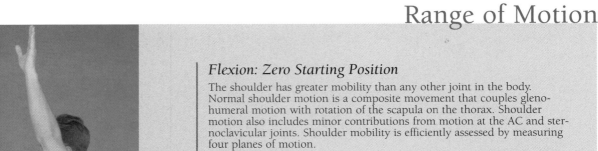

### Flexion: Zero Starting Position

The shoulder has greater mobility than any other joint in the body. Normal shoulder motion is a composite movement that couples glenohumeral motion with rotation of the scapula on the thorax. Shoulder motion also includes minor contributions from motion at the AC and sternoclavicular joints. Shoulder mobility is efficiently assessed by measuring four planes of motion.

The Zero Starting Position is with the arm at the side of the body. Flexion, sometimes called elevation, is the maximum upward motion of the arm. Slight external rotation and abduction are required to reach maximum elevation. These accessory motions are permitted because maximal elevation correlates better with functional impairment. Ask the patient to raise the arm in the most comfortable plane, and then measure active and passive motion in reference to the trunk. Normal shoulder flexion is 160° to 180°.

# Range of Motion

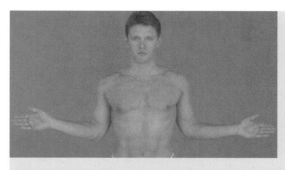

### External rotation, arm at the side

The Zero Starting Position is with the arm held comfortably against the thorax, the elbow flexed to 90°, and the forearm parallel to the sagittal plane of the body. Measure external rotation by evaluating the maximum outward rotation of the arm. Restricted rotation in this position is often observed in patients with degenerative arthritis of the shoulder.

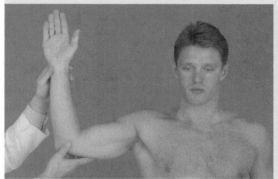

### External rotation, arm abducted 90°

The Zero Starting Position is with the arm abducted 90° and aligned with the plane of the scapula, the elbow flexed 90°, and the forearm parallel to the floor. Measure external rotation in this position by evaluating how many degrees the forearm moves away from the floor. Limited external rotation in this position is seen in some athletes who emphasize strengthening exercises without including an appropriate stretching program and in patients who have had reconstructive surgery of the shoulder.

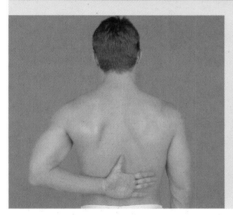

### Internal rotation

Internal rotation is defined as the highest midline spinous process that is reached by the hitchhiking thumb. Assess internal rotation of the shoulder by evaluating the patient's posterior reach. This maneuver is simple and easy to reproduce, but represents a composite motion that also depends on shoulder extension as well as elbow, wrist and thumb motion. Internal rotation may be severely limited in patients with adhesive capsulitis or degenerative arthritis. In these patients, internal rotation may be limited to the sacrum, gluteal region, or greater trochanter. In young adults, internal rotation typically extends beyond the interior tip of the scapula (approximately T7 level).

# Muscle Testing

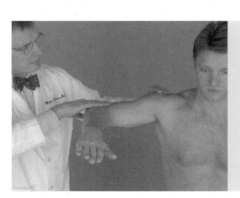

### Deltoid

Place the arm in 90° of abduction. Push down on the arm as the patient resists this pressure. This position also activates the supraspinatus and, to some degree, the other rotator cuff muscles. The anterior deltoid is isolated by moving the arm forward. The posterior deltoid is isolated by moving the arm backward and then doing the muscle test.

# Muscle Testing

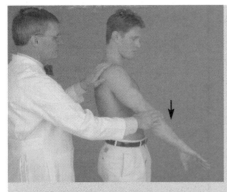

### Supraspinatus

Place the arm in 90° of abduction, 30° of forward flexion, and internal rotation (the "thumbs down" position). Push down on the arm as the patient resists this pressure.

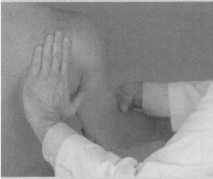

### Infraspinatus and teres minor

Apply resistance with the arm at the side and externally rotated 30° to test strength in the infraspinatus and teres minor.

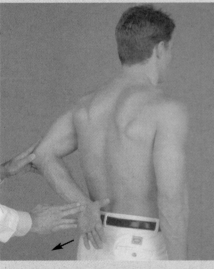

### Subscapularis

Test subscapularis strength and possible tendon rupture by asking the patient to place a hand behind the back and then lift it away from the back against resistance (lift-off test).

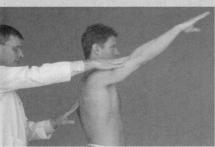

### Serratus anterior

Test serratus anterior strength by asking the patient to elevate the arm as you depress the arm with one hand and palpate the scapula with the other. With normal strength of the serratus anterior, the scapula remains in position on the chest wall. Winging and prominence of the vertebral border occurs with a weak serratus anterior muscle. Stretch or avulsion injuries of the long thoracic nerve with resultant paralysis of the serratus anterior also causes winging of the scapula and fatigue with overhead activities.

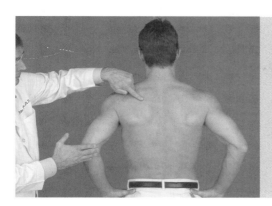

### Rhomboid

Test rhomboid function by asking the patient to place both hands on the side of the iliac crest as you push the patient's arm forward with your hand and palpate the vertebral border of the scapula with the other hand. An intact rhomboid maintains the scapula against the chest wall.

# Special Tests

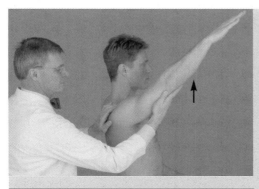

### Neer impingement sign

With the patient seated, depress the scapula with one hand while elevating the arm with the other. This maneuver compresses the greater tuberosity against the anterior acromion and elicits discomfort in patients who have a rotator cuff tear or impingement syndrome.

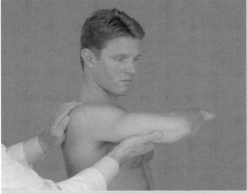

### Hawkins impingement sign

This test reinforces a positive Neer impingement sign. Elevate the patient's shoulder to 90°, flex the elbow to 90°, and place the forearm in neutral rotation. Support the arm and then internally rotate the humerus. Pain elicited with this test is indicative of rotator cuff tear or impingement syndrome.

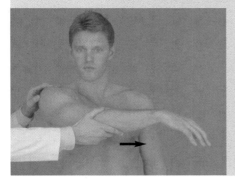

### Cross-body adduction

Elevate the shoulder to 90° and then adduct the arm across the body in the horizontal plane. Pain over the AC joint suggests arthritis of this joint.

# Special Tests

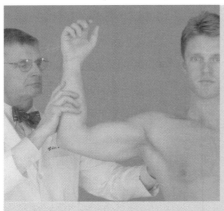

### Apprehension sign

Place the arm in 90° of abduction and then maximal external rotation. Patients with anterior instability may report apprehension and a sense of impending dislocation. A report of pain without apprehension is less specific.

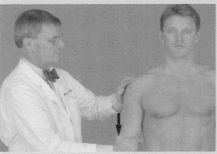

### Sulcus sign

Apply traction in an inferior direction with the arm relaxed at the patient's side. In patients with inferior shoulder laxity, this maneuver causes inferior subluxation of the humeral head and a widening of the sulcus between the humerus and acromion.

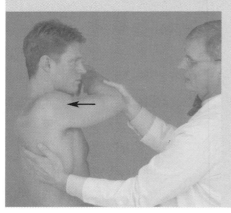

### Jerk test

Place the arm in 90° of flexion and maximum internal rotation with the elbow flexed 90°. Adduct the arm across the body in the horizontal plane while pushing the humerus in a posterior direction. The test is positive if a posterior subluxation or dislocation occurs. If this maneuver cause a dislocation, the humeral head can be felt to clunk back into the joint as the arm is then abducted.

# ACROMIOCLAVICULAR INJURIES

ICD-9 Code

831.04
Closed dislocation acromioclavicular joint

## SYNONYMS

Shoulder separation

Acromioclavicular separation

## DEFINITION

Acromioclavicular (AC) injuries commonly result from a fall onto the tip of the shoulder. A common example is a patient who falls off a bicycle. When the acromion is driven into the ground, variable degrees of ligamentous disruption occur.

These injuries can be classified into one of six types based on the severity of injury and the degree of clavicular separation (**Figure 1**). In type I injuries, the AC joint ligaments are partially or completely disrupted, but the strong coracoclavicular (CC) ligaments are intact. As a result, there is no superior separation of the clavicle from the acromion. In type II injuries, the AC ligaments are torn and, in addition, the CC ligaments are partially disrupted. As a result, there is partial separation of the clavicle from the acromion. This superior separation may not be apparent unless the joint is stressed. In type III injuries, the CC ligaments are completely disrupted, and there is complete

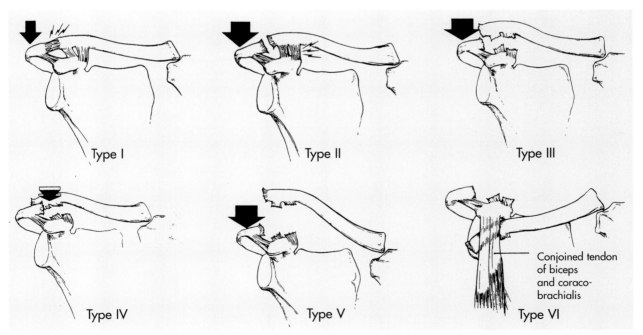

**Figure 1**
Classification of AC separations.

*(Adapted with permission from Rockwood CA Jr: Subluxation and dislocations about the shoulder, in Rockwood CA Jr, Green DP (eds): Rockwood and Green's Fractures in Adults, ed 3. Philadelphia, PA, JB Lippincott, 1988, pp 722-985.*

separation of clavicle from the acromion. Types IV through VI are uncommon. In these injuries, the periosteum of the clavicle and/or the deltoid and trapezius muscle are also torn, causing wide displacement.

## CLINICAL SYMPTOMS

Patients report pain over the AC joint and pain on lifting the arm. With type III and higher injuries, there is an obvious and cosmetically displeasing deformity.

## TESTS

### PHYSICAL EXAMINATION

Patients support the arm in an adducted position, and any motion, especially abduction, causes pain. Tenderness to palpation can be elicited over the AC joint. The distal end of the clavicle may be prominent and slightly superior to the acromion in type II injuries, and there is an obvious deformity in types III and higher. Elevating the arm or depressing the clavicle will temporarily reduce the AC joint, except in types IV and VI injuries, in which there is soft-tissue and bony interposition, respectively.

### DIAGNOSTIC TESTS

AP radiographs of both shoulders will confirm type II or higher AC separations. A weighted radiographic view in which a 10-lb weight is strapped to each wrist can aid in diagnosis by increasing the separation in the injured shoulder.

Type I injuries are sprains; therefore, patients have pain and tenderness, but radiographs are normal.

Type II injuries display some AC joint widening on radiographs. However, the distance between the clavicle and coracoid remains normal.

Type III injuries show complete displacement of the clavicle above the superior border of the acromion with a 30% to 100% increase in the coracoclavicular interspace.

Type IV injuries may show superior displacement of the clavicle on AP radiographs, but an axillary lateral view will clearly show the predominant posterior displacement.

Type V injuries show the coracoclavicular interspace to be increased over 100% of that seen in the opposite shoulder without the application of weights.

Type VI injuries are rare and show the distal end of the clavicle to lie either in the subacromial or subcoracoid space.

## DIFFERENTIAL DIAGNOSIS

Fracture of the acromion (evident on radiographs)

Fracture of the end of the clavicle (evident on radiographs)

Rotator cuff tear (most tenderness over the subacromial space, not the AC joint; no visible deformity or radiographic findings)

## ADVERSE OUTCOMES OF THE DISEASE

Cosmetic deformity, weakness on lifting the arm, chronic shoulder pain, and numbness in the arm are possible. Arthritis of the AC joint may eventually develop.

## TREATMENT

Nonoperative treatment of type I and II injuries consists of wearing a sling for a few days until the pain subsides. Ice is helpful for the first 48 hours, and analgesics can be used to control severe pain. Patients can resume everyday activities as pain allows, with a full return to normal activities and sports within 4 weeks. Treatment of type III injuries is controversial. Many type III injuries can be treated nonoperatively with good functional results. However, operative repair may be considered in a young manual laborer who does heavy overhead work. Type IV, V, and VI injuries require evaluation for operative repair.

## ADVERSE OUTCOMES OF TREATMENT

Following prolonged immobilization in a sling, stiffness can develop; use of a sling or tape can also cause skin breakdown. AC arthritis can be a late sequela of any grade of injury, regardless of treatment.

## REFERRAL DECISIONS/RED FLAGS

Patients with types IV, V, or VI injuries and laborers with type III injuries may be candidates for early operative repair. Injuries that remain painful warrant further evaluation.

# ARTHRITIS OF THE SHOULDER

## ICD-9 Codes
714.0
  Rheumatoid arthritis
715.11
  Primary osteoarthritis, shoulder
715.21
  Secondary osteoarthritis, shoulder
  (rotator cuff arthropathy)
716.11
  Traumatic arthropathy, shoulder
716.91
  Arthropathy, unspecified, shoulder

## SYNONYMS
Glenohumeral arthritis

## DEFINITION
Arthritis of the shoulder is characterized by destruction of joint cartilage with loss of joint space (**Figure 1**). As in other joints, glenohumeral arthritis generally affects patients over age 50 years and occurs as a result of many conditions. Common etiologies include osteoarthritis, rheumatoid arthritis, and posttraumatic arthritis. Less common causes include osteonecrosis, infection, seronegative spondyloarthropathies, and rotator cuff tear arthropathy (a type of arthritis that results from large, long-standing rotator cuff tears).

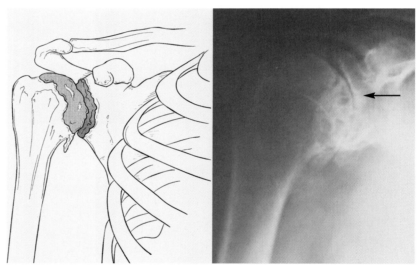

**Figure 1**
Osteoarthritis of the shoulder.

## CLINICAL SYMPTOMS
Patients can report diffuse or deep-seated pain but most often localize the worst pain to the posterior aspect of the shoulder. Initially, the pain is aggravated by any strenuous activity. As the disease progresses, any movement of the shoulder causes pain, and rest and night pain become prominent complaints.

Along with pain, range of motion is progressively limited. As a result, activities of daily living, such as dressing, combing the hair, and reaching overhead, are increasingly difficult.

Osteoarthritis typically involves a single joint in an older patient, whereas multiple and symmetrical joint involvement and a positive rheumatoid factor suggest rheumatoid arthritis. Generally, there is no apparent relationship between the development of osteoarthritis in the shoulder and the patient's previous level of physical activity. A history of previous fracture or dislocation suggests posttraumatic arthritis or osteonecrosis. Superior migration of the humeral head can develop in association with long-standing rotator cuff tears, which results in eccentric loading of the glenoid and can lead to rotator cuff tear arthropathy (**Figure 2**).

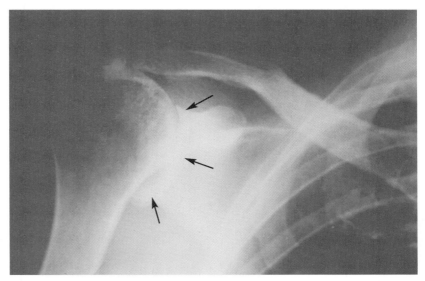

**Figure 2**
Rotator cuff tear arthropathy (arrows show loss of space).

## TESTS

### PHYSICAL EXAMINATION

Examination can reveal generalized atrophy of the muscles about the shoulder. Swelling within the shoulder joint is not common and is difficult to detect. Palpation elicits tenderness over the front and back of the shoulder. Bone-on-bone crepitus is commonly present with rotation or flexion of the shoulder. Range of motion is usually decreased. Patients with concomitant rotator cuff tears often have less active than passive range of motion.

### DIAGNOSTIC TESTS

AP and axillary views of the shoulder are indicated. The axillary view most reliably demonstrates the joint space narrowing that is indicative of cartilage destruction. Other radiographic findings that support a diagnosis of osteoarthritis include flattening of the humeral head, an inferior osteophyte, and posterior erosion of the glenoid. Rheumatoid arthritis is suggested by the presence of periarticular erosions, osteopenia, and central wear of the glenoid. Superior migration of the humeral head suggests a large rotator cuff deficiency.

## DIFFERENTIAL DIAGNOSIS

Adhesive capsulitis (normal radiographs)

Charcot joint (gross destruction of the joint without trauma and relatively little pain)

Fracture of the humerus (history of trauma, evident on radiographs)

Herniated cervical disk (unilateral or bilateral radicular pain, positive Spurling test)

Infection (acute onset, systemic symptoms, elevated WBC)

Rotator cuff tear (normal radiographs, pain mostly with overhead use)

Tumor of the shoulder girdle (variable presentation, radiographic lesion)

## ADVERSE OUTCOME OF THE DISEASE

Chronic shoulder pain and loss of strength and motion can develop. Severe losses of strength and motion can be difficult to recover, even with joint replacement surgery. Addiction to narcotic pain medication is also a possibility.

## TREATMENT

Nonoperative treatment is recommended initially, including use of NSAIDs and application of heat and/or ice to relieve symptoms, and gentle stretching exercises to preserve motion. A trial of glucosamine and/or chondroitin sulfate can be considered but their efficacy needs further investigation. Activity modifications are beneficial in reducing pain. Corticosteroid injections rarely provide relief, except in some cases of inflammatory (eg, rheumatoid) arthritis.

For advanced arthritis, total shoulder replacement or hemiarthroplasty offers a very satisfactory solution, even in younger patients (30 to 50 years of age) who do not use their shoulders for strenuous activities. Manual laborers may be better served by glenohumeral arthrodesis because the heavy demands placed on their shoulders often lead to early loosening of the prosthetic components.

## ADVERSE OUTCOMES OF TREATMENT

NSAIDs can cause gastric, renal, and hepatic complications. Corticosteroid injection has a small but possible risk of causing an infection in the joint that may preclude or compromise later joint replacement. Patients who undergo shoulder replacement surgery may also experience perioperative complications.

## REFERRAL DECISIONS/RED FLAGS

Patients with intolerable shoulder pain and/or a progressive loss of motion who do not respond to at least 3 months of nonoperative treatment need further evaluation.

# Burners and Other Brachial Plexus Injuries

## Synonyms

Stingers

Brachial plexopathy

## Definition

Brachial plexus injuries include a broad array of neurologic dysfunction ranging from momentary paresthesias to completely flail extremities. The mechanism of injury is equally diverse, from high-energy motor vehicle crashes, falls from a height, and gunshot wounds, to lower-energy injuries such as most athletic injuries.

Burners or stingers (transient brachial plexopathy) are transient injuries to the upper trunk of the brachial plexus involving the C5 and C6 nerve roots. The most common mechanism of injury is a traction force when the shoulder is forcefully depressed and the head and neck are tilted toward the opposite side or by compression of the upper plexus between a shoulder pad and the scapula. These injuries are relatively common among college and professional athletes in contact sports, especially football.

Brachial plexus injuries involving axonal disruption can be further categorized as occurring proximal to the dorsal root ganglion in the spinal foramen (preganglionic) or anywhere distal to the ganglion (postganglionic). This distinction is important because operative repair is impossible, and the prognosis for recovery is poor for preganglionic root avulsions.

## Clinical symptoms

The symptoms of a brachial plexus injury depend on the position of the plexus when it is injured. The mechanism of injury to the upper and middle trunks (C5, C6, and C7, respectively) usually involves a direct blow to the top of the shoulder accompanied by tilt of the head in the opposite direction, causing traction on the plexus with the arm adducted at the side. Lower trunk injuries (C8, T1) occur when these nerves are stretched with the arm abducted, as when grabbing onto a ledge when falling from a height. Injuries involving the entire plexus result from extreme traction from a major trauma.

A typical presentation is a football player injured by a direct blow to the head, neck, or shoulder. The classic symptom is sharp, burning shoulder pain that radiates down the arm. Weakness is also common, and the patient often is seen holding the arm on the affected side, which often is limply hanging at the side. Burners usually last seconds to minutes, though some lasting several weeks have been reported.

# TESTS

## PHYSICAL EXAMINATION

A detailed neurologic examination is the cornerstone of an accurate diagnosis. At a minimum, sensation to light touch, motor power, and deep tendon reflexes should be tested. Deficits should be mapped out by nerve root and peripheral nerve distribution. The neurologic examination also should include evaluation of the lower extremities because spasticity or weakness in the ipsilateral leg suggests a concomitant spinal cord injury.

Injuries to C8 and T1 are more likely to be preganglionic, which is confirmed by the presence of an ipsilateral ptosis, myosis, anhydrosis, and enophthalmos (Horner syndrome). Because the dorsal scapular nerve and the long thoracic nerve arise from the C5 and C5-7 nerve roots, respectively, intact function of the rhomboids and serratus anterior muscles in upper plexus injuries indicates that the injury is distal to these nerves and hence is postganglionic.

Examination of the neck (with cervical spine precautions if indicated) and shoulder, as well as a general examination, is indicated to rule out associated injuries such as cervical spine fractures or disk herniations, clavicle, scapular or humeral fractures, or scapulothoracic dissociation.

As with other plexus injuries, the sideline evaluation of a burner should include the cervical spine and a neurologic examination of the extremities. Bilateral upper extremity burners or radicular symptoms into the legs should be treated as a spinal cord injury until proven otherwise.

## DIAGNOSTIC TESTS

Plain radiographs should be obtained if injury to the cervical spine or shoulder girdle is suspected. Recurrent episodes of burners or prolonged symptoms should be investigated with cervical spine radiographs, including flexion and extension lateral views, to rule out instability, congenital anomaly, or cervical stenosis (assessed by the relative width of the cervical body and the spinal canal). An MRI is helpful in patients with abnormal plain radiographs or when symptoms persist.

# DIFFERENTIAL DIAGNOSIS

Cervical spine fracture or instability (evident on radiographs)

Peripheral nerve injury (isolated weakness or sensory deficit confined to a specific nerve distribution)

Transient quadriplegia (neurapraxia of the cervical spinal cord producing bilateral paresthesias and weakness)

# ADVERSE OUTCOMES OF THE DISEASE

Burners, by definition, resolve spontaneously, though recurrent episodes may suggest cervical stenosis and an associated increased risk for catastrophic spinal cord injury. Depending on the location and severity of a brachial plexus injury, persistent pain, sensory loss, paresthesias, and weakness or paralysis are possible.

## TREATMENT

Complete resolution of pain and neurologic symptoms, as well as a normal neurologic examination and full range of cervical spine motion, are required before an athlete with a burner is allowed to return to play. Athletes with prolonged or bilateral symptoms or recurrent episodes should not return to play without further evaluation.

Treatment options for more severe brachial plexus injuries vary, including nonoperative measures and a variety of operative repair and reconstruction procedures. Nonoperative management is aimed at strengthening and stretching exercises and splinting to maintain passive range of motion of the joints affected by muscle paralysis or weakness, protection of anesthetic areas of skin, and pain relief. Referral to a pain clinic is often helpful in this regard.

## ADVERSE OUTCOMES OF TREATMENT

The effectiveness of therapy, splinting, and pain control must be monitored frequently. While operative techniques are continuously evolving, the prognosis for severe brachial plexus injuries, especially root avulsions, remains guarded.

## REFERRAL DECISIONS/RED FLAGS

Any injury that is persistent, recurrent, bilateral, or associated with other concomitant injuries requires further evaluation. Cervical spine precautions should be followed if a cervical injury is suspected.

# FROZEN SHOULDER

## SYNONYMS

Adhesive capsulitis

Stiff shoulder

## DEFINITION

Adhesive capsulitis of the shoulder, commonly called frozen shoulder, is defined as an idiopathic loss of both active and passive motion. It is considered distinct from posttraumatic shoulder stiffness, a condition that is related to a significant shoulder injury or operative procedure (**Figure 1**).

Frozen shoulder most commonly affects patients between ages 40 and 60 years, with no clear predisposition based on gender, arm dominance, or occupation. Diabetes mellitus, especially type I, is the most common risk factor. Patients with diabetes tend to be more refractory to treatment, and 40% to 50% will have bilateral involvement. Other conditions related to frozen shoulder include hypothyroidism, Dupuytren disease, cervical disk herniation, Parkinson disease, cerebral hemorrhage, and tumors.

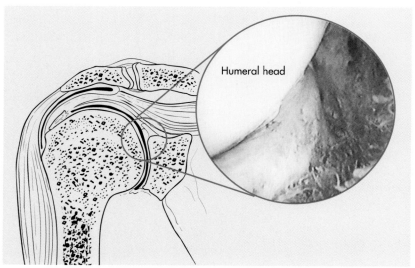

**Figure 1**

Contracted soft tissue about the glenohumeral joint in frozen shoulder. The arthroscopic view reveals that the capsule is snug against the humeral head.

*The arthroscopic view is reproduced with permission from Harryman DT II: Shoulders: Frozen and stiff, in Heckman JD (ed): Instructional Course Lectures 42. Rosemont, IL, American Academy of Orthopaedic Surgeons, 1993, pp 247-257.*

## CLINICAL SYMPTOMS

Patients typically progress from an early "freezing" phase of pain and progressive loss of motion to a "thawing" phase of decreasing discomfort associated with a slow but steady improvement in range of motion. The process typically takes 6 months to 2 years or more to resolve, with most patients experiencing minimal long-term pain or functional deficit, though some motion loss remains.

## TESTS

### PHYSICAL EXAMINATION

Examination reveals significant reduction in both active and passive range of motion, at least 50%, when compared with the opposite normal shoulder. Motion is painful, especially at the extremes. Pain and tenderness are common at the deltoid insertion. Diffuse tenderness about the shoulder also can be present.

### DIAGNOSTIC TESTS

AP and axillary radiographs of the shoulder are indicated to ensure that smooth, concentric joint surfaces with an intact cartilage space are present and to rule out other pathology such as osteophytes, loose bodies, calcium deposits, or tumors. Other studies, such as arthrography, CT, or MRI are rarely indicated if plain radiographs are normal.

## DIFFERENTIAL DIAGNOSIS

Chronic posterior shoulder dislocation (evident on axillary radiographs)

Impingement syndrome (motion preserved and pain primarily with elevation)

Osteoarthritis (evident on radiographs)

Posttraumatic shoulder stiffness (history of clear and significant preceding trauma)

Rotator cuff tear (normal passive range of motion)

Tumor (rare, but evident on shoulder or ipsilateral chest radiograph)

## ADVERSE OUTCOMES OF THE DISEASE

Residual pain and/or stiffness can persist for years in some patients.

## TREATMENT

NSAIDs, non-narcotic analgesics, and moist heat are indicated, followed by a gentle stretching program. Intra-articular injection of corticosteroid also can be considered. The patient should be instructed in a home stretching program that is to be done within a comfortable range that does not cause significant pain (see Shoulder Rehabilitation). Ideally, the stretching program should be performed three to four times per day. Advise patients that, on average, a recovery period of 1 to 2 years is to be expected before motion is fully restored and pain completely relieved.

## ADVERSE OUTCOMES OF TREATMENT

Therapy that is too aggressive can aggravate symptoms and/or cause a fracture of the humerus.

## REFERRAL DECISIONS/RED FLAGS

Patients who fail to show significant improvement in pain and motion after 3 months of consistent rehabilitation need further evaluation.

# FRACTURE OF THE CLAVICLE

810.00
Fracture of clavicle, closed,
unspecified part

## SYNONYM

Collar bone fracture

## DEFINITION

Clavicle fractures are the most common bony injury. The most common location of injury is the middle third of the clavicle (**Figure 1**). Approximately 80% occur in this location, 15% occur in the lateral one third, and 5% involve the medial end.

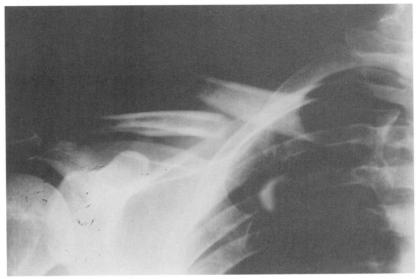

**Figure 1**
Fracture of the middle third of the clavicle.

## CLINICAL SYMPTOMS

Patients typically report a history of significant injury, such as falling on the shoulder or being struck over the clavicle with a heavy object. Patients cannot lift their arm because of pain at the fracture site.

## TESTS

### PHYSICAL EXAMINATION

Examination typically reveals an obvious deformity, or "bump," at the fracture site. Gentle pressure over the fracture site will elicit pain, and a grinding sensation can be felt when the patient attempts to raise the arm. The skin can appear tented over a fracture fragment, but the fragment rarely penetrates through the skin to create an open fracture. Assess neurologic function distal to the fracture, including the axillary, musculocutaneous, median, ulnar, and radial nerves. Check the radial pulse and capillary refill.

## DIAGNOSTIC TESTS

An AP radiograph of the clavicle will confirm most clavicle fractures (**Figure 1**). Fractures or dislocations at the medial end of the clavicle are uncommon and are often difficult to see on plain radiographs, so if there is an index of suspicion, CT should be ordered.

## DIFFERENTIAL DIAGNOSIS

Acromioclavicular separation (deformity near the tip of the shoulder)

Sternoclavicular dislocation (deformity at the sternoclavicular junction)

## ADVERSE OUTCOMES OF THE DISEASE

Nonunion is rare, occurring in only 1% to 4% of patients. Some degree of malunion is common, and a visible lump can occur, even when the fracture is well approximated. This lump can be of cosmetic concern to some patients but has little functional significance. Neurovascular complications can occur on an early or delayed basis.

## TREATMENT

Most clavicle fractures can be treated nonoperatively with either a simple arm sling or a figure-of-8 clavicle strap. Support for 3 to 4 weeks is adequate for a child younger than age 12 years, whereas 4 to 6 weeks is usually required for an adult. After 2 to 3 weeks, the patient is encouraged to begin gentle shoulder exercises, as pain allows.

## ADVERSE OUTCOMES OF TREATMENT

Pressure over the nerves and vessels in the armpit from a tight clavicle strap can cause numbness and paresthesias in the arm. Malunion may produce an unsightly bump. Nonunion is rare.

## REFERRAL DECISIONS/RED FLAGS

Painful nonunion after 4 months of treatment indicates the need for further evaluation. Patients with widely displaced lateral or midshaft clavicle fractures have a greater risk of nonunion and should be evaluated for internal fixation.

# FRACTURE OF THE HUMERAL SHAFT

**ICD-9 Code**
812.21
Fracture of shaft of humerus, closed

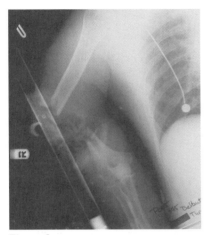

**Figure 1**
Humeral shaft fracture.

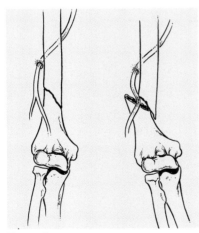

**Figure 2**
Entrapment of the radial nerve at the fracture site.

## DEFINITION

Fractures of the humeral shaft often result from a direct blow to the arm, such as occurs in a motor vehicle accident, or from a fall on the outstretched arm (**Figure 1**). These fractures can also occur as a result of sports activities involving a vigorous throwing motion, but these instances are rare. Most of these fractures can be treated nonoperatively with a rate of union of nearly 100%.

## CLINICAL SYMPTOMS

Severe pain, swelling, and deformity are characteristic of a displaced fracture of the humerus. With gentle palpation and movement of the arm, it is often possible to detect motion at the fracture site. Radial nerve injuries are associated with this fracture. If the radial nerve has been injured, patients are unable to extend the wrist or fingers and may have loss of sensation over the back of the hand (**Figure 2**).

## TESTS

### PHYSICAL EXAMINATION

Examination reveals marked swelling and contusion. Look for puncture wounds in the skin near the fracture site, as these indicate an open (compound) fracture. Assess neurologic function distal to the fracture including the median, radial, and ulnar nerves. Check the radial pulse and record the color and temperature of the hand. The shoulder and elbow should be evaluated for pain, tenderness, and swelling or deformity because concomitant injury proximal or distal to the shaft fracture can be easily missed in the acute setting.

### DIAGNOSTIC TESTS

AP and lateral radiographs confirm the diagnosis. These views should include both the shoulder and elbow joints, as well.

## DIFFERENTIAL DIAGNOSIS

Fracture of the proximal humerus (evident on AP and lateral radiographs)

Fracture of the distal humerus (evident on radiographs)

Ruptured biceps tendon (swelling localized to biceps muscle)

## ADVERSE OUTCOMES OF THE DISEASE

Radial nerve injury, indicated by weakness in the wrist or finger extensors and numbness in the first dorsal web space, is possible. Injury to the brachial plexus or vascular system can also occur. Healing of the fracture with angulation is common but results in little functional impairment, unless it is severe.

SECTION 2 | SHOULDER

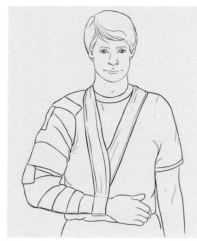

**Figure 3**
Coaptation splint.

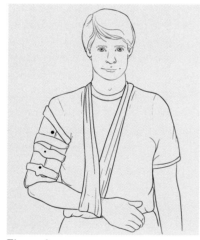

**Figure 4**
Humeral fracture brace.

Nonunion is possible but uncommon. Persistent stiffness in the shoulder and elbow can be a problem.

## TREATMENT

Most humeral shaft fractures can be treated nonoperatively. Fractures with minimal shortening (2 cm or less) can be treated with a U-shaped coaptation splint for 2 weeks (**Figure 3**), followed by a humeral fracture brace (**Figure 4**). A coaptation splint is applied as follows: place 12 thicknesses of plaster or a commercially available prepackaged splint in a U-shaped fashion from the axilla around the elbow and extend it to the top of the shoulder. Use a collar and cuff made from stockinette to support the forearm and wrist. (See Splinting Principles, pp 81-87.) Instruct the patient to exercise the fingers, wrist, and elbow at least three times a day. Allow the patient to flex the elbow as tolerated, and to extend the elbow to full extension, as pain allows. The coaptation splint may need to be reapplied during these first 2 weeks. After 2 weeks, the patient is fitted with a humeral fracture brace, which is worn for at least the next 6 weeks or until there is radiographic evidence of healing. During this time, continue to encourage range of motion exercises for the shoulder, elbow, wrist, and hand.

Radial nerve injuries associated with fractures of the humerus should be observed. Within 6 months, 95% of patients will regain nerve function. During this period of observation, the patient should be fitted with a wrist splint and receive instruction in stretching exercises to avoid flexion contractures of the wrist and fingers. Electromyography is indicated after 3 to 4 months if radial nerve function does not return.

## ADVERSE OUTCOMES OF TREATMENT

Radial nerve injury occurring after manipulation, stiffness of the shoulder and elbow, and discomfort and/or skin irritation from the splint are possible. The patient may need to sleep sitting in a chair to maintain fracture alignment.

## REFERRAL DECISIONS/RED FLAGS

Patients who have one of the following conditions need further evaluation: associated vascular injury; a nerve injury that develops after manipulation; an open fracture; a segmental fracture; a "floating elbow" in which the radius and ulna are fractured along with the humerus; nonunion following 3 months of treatment; an associated head injury, seizure disorder, or multiple injuries; a pathologic fracture; or skin breakdown under the fracture brace.

# FRACTURE OF THE PROXIMAL HUMERUS

ICD-9 Code

812.00
  Fracture of humerus, upper end,
  closed

## SYNONYMS

Humeral head fracture

Surgical neck fracture

## DEFINITION

Fractures of the proximal humerus commonly occur in elderly patients with osteoporosis, especially women. Most of these fractures are minimally displaced and can be treated with a sling and early motion.

These fractures are generally classified according to which parts of the proximal humerus are fractured and the amount of displacement. The four parts are 1) the greater tuberosity (the bony prominence that provides attachment for the supraspinatus, infraspinatus, and teres minor muscles), 2) the lesser tuberosity (attachment site for subscapularis), and 3) the humeral head and 4) shaft (**Figure 1**). The most common two-part fracture occurs at the surgical neck (region just distal to the tuberosities). Other two-part fractures include fracture at the anatomic neck, isolated fracture of the greater tuberosity, and isolated fractures of the lesser tuberosity. Three-part fractures involve the humeral head, the shaft, and one of the tuberosities. Four-part fractures involve all four components of the proximal humerus. Three- and four-part fractures are severe injuries that are fortunately uncommon.

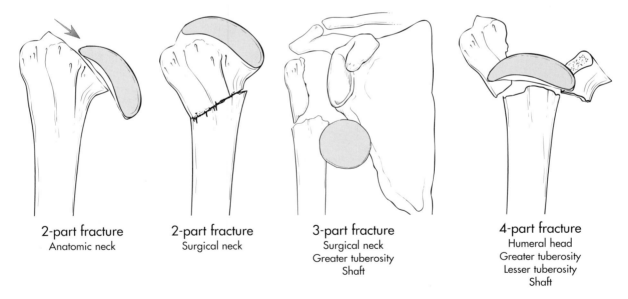

| 2-part fracture | 2-part fracture | 3-part fracture | 4-part fracture |
| Anatomic neck | Surgical neck | Surgical neck<br>Greater tuberosity<br>Shaft | Humeral head<br>Greater tuberosity<br>Lesser tuberosity<br>Shaft |

**Figure 1**

Fracture patterns for displaced fractures of the proximal humerus (Neer classification).

*Adapted with permission from Neer CS II: Displaced proximal humeral fractures: I. Classification and evaluation. J Bone Joint Surg Am 1970;52:1077-1089.*

## CLINICAL SYMPTOMS

Patients typically have severe pain, swelling, and bruising around the upper arm and shoulder following an injury, such as a fall. The pain is worse with even the slightest movement of the arm. If the patient reports a loss of feeling in the arm, a nerve injury is more likely. If the forearm and hand appear pale, the axillary artery may have been injured.

## TESTS

### PHYSICAL EXAMINATION

Examination reveals swelling and discoloration around the shoulder and upper arm. Assess neurologic function distal to the fracture, including the axillary, musculocutaneous, median, radial, and ulnar nerves. Check the radial pulse and capillary refill as well.

### DIAGNOSTIC TESTS

A trauma series of plain radiographs of the shoulder should include a true AP and an axillary lateral view (**Figure 2**). Several techniques are available to obtain an axillary view on a patient with a painful shoulder. If the axillary view is impossible to obtain, a transscapular lateral (or scapular 'Y') view should be obtained. Great care must be taken in interpreting the AP and the scapular 'Y' views, as errors are easier to make (**Figure 3**). The most common error is misdiagnosis of an associated shoulder dislocation because of inadequate radiographs. AP views alone are insufficient to document an associated shoulder dislocation.

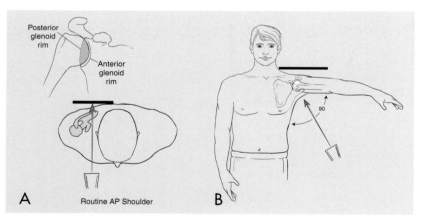

**Figure 2**
Plain radiographs of the shoulder should be obtained in these views: routine AP (lateral) (A), and axillary lateral (B).

*Adapted with permission from Rockwood CA, Szalay EA, Curtis RJ, et al: X-ray evaluation of shoulder problems, in Rockwood CA, Matsen FA III (eds): The Shoulder. Philadelphia, PA, WB Saunders, 1990.*

## DIFFERENTIAL DIAGNOSIS

Acromioclavicular (AC) separation (pain localized to the AC joint)

Rotator cuff tear (weakness with elevation and external rotation, normal radiographs)

Rupture of the long head of the biceps tendon (asymmetrical bulge of arm musculature with biceps contraction)

Shoulder dislocation (evident on AP and lateral radiographs of the gleno-humeral joint)

## ADVERSE OUTCOMES OF THE DISEASE

Chronic pain, along with loss of motion, and nerve and vascular injury are possible. Nonunion is also a possibility. Patients may also have posttraumatic arthritis and/or osteonecrosis of the humeral head.

## TREATMENT

Patients with minimally displaced (less than 1 cm) fractures can be treated safely with a sling and, after the first week, can often begin an exercise program consisting of pendulum and circumduction exercises. Isometric exercises of the deltoid and rotator cuff also are encouraged within the first 2 weeks following the injury. Beginning these exercises prior to bony union is important because disabling stiffness is very common, especially in the elderly. After 3 weeks, the sling can be worn part time, or it can be removed if pain is minimal.

Two-part fractures in which the greater tuberosity is separated more than 1 cm require operative repair to restore normal function of the rotator cuff muscles. If the patient has a two-part fracture in which the lesser tuberosity is fractured, an associated posterior dislocation is also quite possible. Displaced two-part fractures through the humeral neck and displaced three- and four-part fractures require consideration for operative treatment. Displaced four-part fractures disrupt the blood supply to the humeral head and in most cases require prosthetic replacement of the proximal humerus rather than internal fixation of the fracture.

## ADVERSE OUTCOMES OF TREATMENT

Nonunion and malunion are both possible. Missed shoulder dislocation is also a possibility, especially if insufficient radiographs are obtained. Patients often report persistent stiffness in the shoulder.

## REFERRAL DECISIONS/RED FLAGS

Patients with displaced two-part and all three- and four-part fractures need further evaluation. In addition, patients with associated neurovascular symptoms require further evaluation as soon as possible.

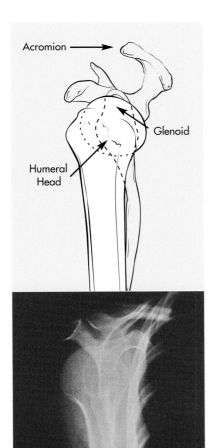

**Figure 3**
Illustration and radiograph showing lateral scapula view of the shoulder.

*Radiograph reproduced with permission from Frymoyer JW (ed): Orthopaedic Knowledge Update 4. Rosemont, IL, American Academy of Orthopaedic Surgeons, 1993, p 286.*

Labels on illustration: Acromion, Glenoid, Humeral Head

SECTION 2 | SHOULDER

# FRACTURE OF THE SCAPULA

ICD-9 Code
811.00
    Fracture of scapula, unspecified
    part, closed

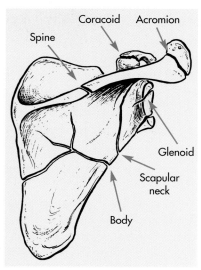

**Figure 1**
Fracture patterns in the scapula.

*Reproduced with permission from Zuckerman JD, Koval KJ, Cuomo F: Fractures of the scapula, in Heckman JD (ed): Instructional Course Lectures 42. Rosemont, IL, American Academy of Orthopaedic Surgeons, 1993, pp 271-281.*

## SYNONYMS

Glenoid fracture

Fracture of the acromion

Fracture of the shoulder blade

Fracture of the coracoid process

## DEFINITION

Scapular fractures typically result from high-energy trauma such as motorcycle accidents or falls from a significant height. These fractures can involve the body of the scapula, the glenoid, the acromion, and/or the coracoid process (**Figure 1**). Ninety percent of patients with scapula fractures have associated injuries, including rib fractures, which are the most common; pneumothorax; pulmonary contusion; and head, spinal cord and brachial plexus injuries. Because of the common association with life-threatening injuries, the diagnosis is easily missed on initial examination.

## CLINICAL SYMPTOMS

Pain and tenderness about the back of the shoulder are the most common complaints. The patient typically holds the arm securely at the side, and any attempts to actively move the extremity result in pain.

## TESTS

### PHYSICAL EXAMINATION

Skin abrasions, swelling, and ecchymosis over the back of the shoulder are common. Tenderness to gentle palpation over the back of the shoulder or acromion suggests a possible scapula fracture.

### DIAGNOSTIC TESTS

Radiographic visualization of scapular fractures can be difficult. An AP view of the shoulder and a chest radiograph should be obtained. If the patient is cleared to sit upright, a transscapular lateral radiograph can be helpful in the diagnosis of a displaced scapular body fracture (**Figure 2**). The axillary view is more useful in revealing acromial and coracoid fractures. Poorly visualized fractures and any fracture involving the glenoid should be further evaluated with CT.

## DIFFERENTIAL DIAGNOSIS

Acromioclavicular (AC) separation (maximum tenderness over the AC joint)

Fracture of the proximal humerus (radiograph needed to confirm diagnosis)

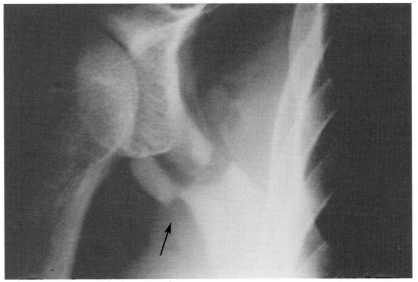

**Figure 2**
Fracture of the body of the scapula.

Fracture of the rib (evident on plain radiographs of the chest)

Os acromiale (nontender, no history of trauma, incidental finding on radiographs)

Shoulder dislocation (deformity of the anterior and lateral shoulder, evident on radiographs)

## ADVERSE OUTCOMES OF THE DISEASE

Persistent loss of motion and chronic pain are possible. Malunion is common but usually asymptomatic. Complications such as suprascapular nerve injury or impingement syndrome are rare.

## TREATMENT

Nonoperative treatment using a sling is adequate for most patients, followed by early range of motion as tolerated, usually within 1 week of injury. Patients with scapular body fractures should be considered for hospital admission because of the risk of pulmonary contusion.

## ADVERSE OUTCOMES OF TREATMENT

Prolonged immobilization can result in shoulder stiffness.

## REFERRAL DECISIONS/RED FLAGS

Patients with displaced fractures of the glenoid articular surface (greater than 2 mm), fractures of the neck of the scapula with severe angular deformity (greater than 30°), and fractures of the acromion process with impingement syndrome need further evaluation.

# IMPINGEMENT SYNDROME

**ICD-9 Code**
726.10
  Rotator cuff syndrome NOS

## SYNONYMS

Rotator cuff tendinitis
Shoulder bursitis

## DEFINITION

Four muscles come together to form the rotator cuff that covers the anterior, superior, and posterior aspects of the humeral head. As these muscles assist in elevation of the arm, the rotator cuff, primarily the supraspinatus tendon, is pulled repetitively under the coracoacromial arch (**Figure 1**). The coracoacromial arch includes the coracoid process, the coracoacromial ligament, the acromion, and the acromioclavicular joint capsule.

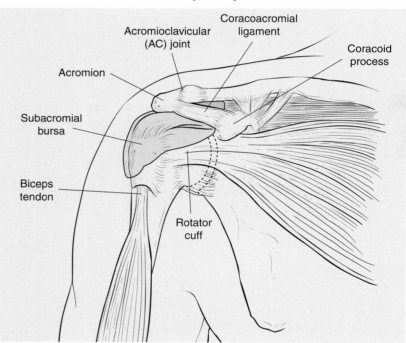

**Figure 1**
Anatomy of the front of the shoulder.

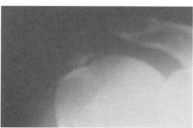

**Figure 2**
Radiograph showing calcific tendinitis in a person with impingement syndrome.

Inflammation of the subacromial bursa and underlying rotator cuff tendons is a common cause of shoulder pain in middle-aged patients. Rotator cuff pathology presents a continuum from edema and hemorrhage to chronic inflammation and fibrosis to microscopic tendon fiber failure progressing to full-thickness rotator cuff tears. The etiology is likely a combination of factors, including loss of microvascular blood supply to the tendon and repeated mechanical insult as the tendon passes under the coracoacromial arch (**Figure 2**).

# CLINICAL SYMPTOMS

Gradual onset of anterior and lateral shoulder pain exacerbated by overhead activity is characteristic. Night pain and difficulty sleeping on the affected side are also common. Atrophy of the muscles about the top and back of the shoulder may be apparent if the patient has had symptoms for several months.

# TESTS

## PHYSICAL EXAMINATION

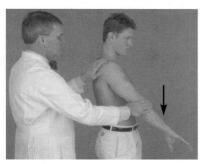

**Figure 3**
Testing the strength of the supraspinatus.

Palpation over the greater tuberosity and subacromial bursa commonly elicits tenderness and crepitus with shoulder motion. Pain will be elicited by having the patient slowly lower the abducted arm against downward resistance. Patients with impingement generally have positive Neer and Hawkins signs (see Physical Examination–Shoulder). After completing these tests, 10 mL of 1% plain local anesthetic can be injected into the subacromial space (see Subacromial Bursa Injection), followed by impingement testing. Complete pain relief supports a diagnosis of impingement syndrome.

To demonstrate weakness of the supraspinatus tendon, position the arm in 90° elevation and internal rotation (thumb turned down). Ask the patient to resist while pushing the arm down (**Figure 3**). Compare the result with that of the opposite shoulder. If the patient initially demonstrates weakness but is strong following subacromial injection, pain inhibition from inflammation and fibrosis rather than a full-thickness rotator cuff tear is the likely cause of the weakness. Muscle atrophy about the top and back of the shoulder usually indicates a rotator cuff tear (**Figure 4**).

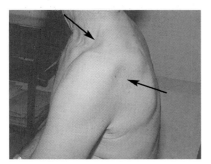

**Figure 4**
Visible muscle atrophy.

## DIAGNOSTIC TESTS

AP and axillary radiographs of the shoulder are usually normal. Narrowing of the space between the head of the humerus and the under surface of the acromion (normally greater than 7 mm) suggests a long-standing rotator cuff tear.

# DIFFERENTIAL DIAGNOSIS

Acromioclavicular (AC) arthritis (tenderness over the AC joint)

Frozen shoulder (active and passive motion loss)

Glenohumeral arthritis (pain with any motion, evident on radiographs)

Herniated cervical disk (associated neck stiffness, deltoid weakness with absent biceps reflex, possible sensory loss)

Rotator cuff tear (weakness of the supraspinatus that does not improve following subacromial injection of local anesthetic)

Suprascapular nerve entrapment (atrophy of the supraspinatus and infraspinatus muscles, negative impingement sign)

# ADVERSE OUTCOMES OF THE DISEASE

Pain can be persistent or recurrent. Rotator cuff tendinitis can progress to a full-thickness tear.

## TREATMENT

Rest from the offending activity and NSAIDs can relieve an acute exacerbation of pain. The patient should begin a stretching program (see Shoulder Rehabilitation, pp 153-156) with emphasis on posterior capsule stretching. If a home therapy program performed three to four times a day for 6 weeks does not result in any improvement, a subacromial corticosteroid injection can be considered, followed by continued stretching. Steroid injections should not be repeated if the previous injection did not produce significant and sustained (more than 2 months) relief.

A rotator cuff strengthening program should be added to the stretching program once the shoulder is supple and pain is improved.

## ADVERSE OUTCOMES OF TREATMENT

NSAIDs may cause gastric, renal, or hepatic complications. Tearing of the rotator cuff and rupture of the long head of the biceps tendon can occur after repeated corticosteroid injections. The latter is more likely with more than three injections.

## REFERRAL DECISIONS/RED FLAGS

Significant weakness of the rotator cuff or failure of 2 to 3 months of rehabilitation (with or without subacromial steroid injection) are indications for further evaluation and operative consideration.

# PROCEDURE

## SUBACROMIAL BURSA INJECTION

### MATERIALS

Sterile gloves

Bactericidal skin prep solution

1% lidocaine solution without epinephrine

2 mL of 40 mg/mL of a betamethasone or similar steroid

10-mL syringe with a 22-gauge, 1¼" needle

3-mL syringe with a 25-gauge, ¾" needle

Adhesive bandage

### STEP 1

Wear protective gloves at all times during this procedure and use sterile technique.

### STEP 2

Seat the patient with the arm hanging down to distract the subacromial space. The injection site can be anterior or anterolateral (Figure 1).

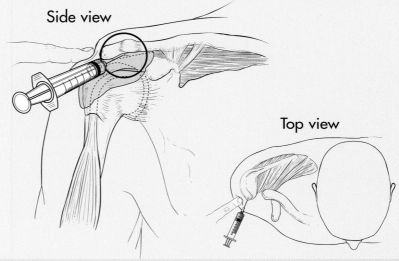

Side view

Top view

**Figure 1**
Location for needle insertion.

### STEP 3

Palpate the acromion both anteriorly and laterally until the anterolateral corner is located.

### STEP 4

Cleanse this area with a bactericidal solution.

### STEP 5

With an index finger on the lateral acromion, insert the 25-gauge needle about 1 cm below the palpating finger and raise a wheal with the local anesthetic.

### STEP 6

Insert the syringe with the 22-gauge needle. Angle the needle superiorly approximately 20° to 30° to access the subacromial space. Most use 8 to 10 mL of the 1% lidocaine solution. If there is a resistance while attempting to inject the solution, partially withdraw the needle and reinsert. If the needle is in the proper place, there is little resistance to injection. If you feel the needle hit bone, redirect it superiorly if the bony obstruction is thought to be the humerus, or inferiorly if the bone is thought to be the acromion.

## Step 7

Detach the syringe from the needle hub, leaving the needle in the correct location. Attach the second syringe with 2 mL of corticosteroid preparation and inject it into the subacromial space. The syringe can again be exchanged and local anesthetic injected as the needle is withdrawn to avoid steroid deposition subcutaneously. This reduces the risk of depigmentation in dark-skinned patients or fat atrophy.

## Step 8

Dress the puncture wound with a sterile adhesive bandage.

## Adverse outcomes

Temporarily increased pain is possible and, although rare, infection can occur. Subcutaneous atrophy and depigmentation also may occur.

## Aftercare/Patient instructions

One third of patients will experience a temporary increase in pain for 24 to 48 hours from the corticosteroid injection. Advise the patient to apply ice bags to the shoulder and take an NSAID or acetaminophen if increased pain occurs the night following the injection. Instruct the patient to resume usual activities as soon as tolerated, but no later than 24 to 48 hours after the injection.

# ROTATOR CUFF TEAR

**ICD-9 Codes**
726.10
    Rotator cuff syndrome NOS
727.61
    Nontraumatic complete rupture of
    rotator cuff
840.4
    Rotator cuff sprain

## SYNONYMS

Rotator cuff rupture
Rotator cuff tendinitis
Musculotendinous cuff rupture

## DEFINITION

The rotator cuff is composed of four muscles: the supraspinatus, the infraspinatus, the subscapularis, and the teres minor (**Figure 1**). These muscles form a cover around the head of the humerus and function to rotate the arm and stabilize the humeral head against the glenoid.

While rotator cuff tears can occur with acute injury, most are the result of age-related degeneration, chronic mechanical impingement, and altered blood supply to the tendons. Tears generally originate in the supraspinatus tendon and can progress posteriorly and anteriorly. Full-thickness tears are uncommon in individuals younger than age 40 years, but are present in 25% of individuals over age 60 years. Most older people with rotator cuff tears are asymptomatic or have only mild, nondisabling symptoms.

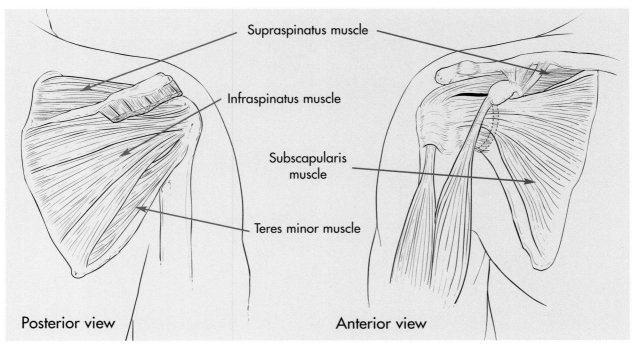

Supraspinatus muscle

Infraspinatus muscle

Subscapularis muscle

Teres minor muscle

Posterior view

Anterior view

**Figure 1**
Muscles of the rotator cuff.

*Posterior view adapted with permission from Rockwood CA, Matsen FA (eds): The Shoulder. Philadelphia, PA, WB Saunders, 1990.*

## CLINICAL SYMPTOMS

Patients often report recurrent shoulder pain for several months and a specific injury that triggered the onset of the pain. Night pain and difficulty sleeping on the affected side are characteristic. Weakness, catching, and grating are common symptoms, especially when lifting the arm overhead.

## TESTS

### PHYSICAL EXAMINATION

The back of the shoulder may appear sunken, indicating atrophy of the supraspinatus and infraspinatus muscles following a long-standing cuff tear. Passive range of motion is near normal, but active range of motion can be limited. With large tears, the patient can only shrug or "hike" the shoulder when asked to lift the arm (**Figure 2**) and cannot hold the arm elevated when it is lifted parallel to the floor. Some patients, however, maintain remarkably good active motion despite large cuff tears. As the patient lifts the arm, a grating sensation about the tip of the shoulder can be felt. Tenderness to palpation over the greater tuberosity is usually present as well.

### DIAGNOSTIC TESTS

With large, long-standing tears, AP radiographs may reveal a high-riding humerus relative to the glenoid. A 30° caudal tilt view will often show a spur projecting down from the inferior surface of the acromion (**Figure 3**).

If the diagnosis is equivocal or if operative treatment is being considered, MRI has become the imaging study of choice as it can provide additional information on the status of the muscle and on the size of full-thickness and some partial-thickness tears.

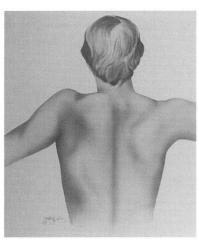

**Figure 2**
Atrophy of the supraspinatus and infraspinatus muscles and shoulder shrug with attempted abduction.

*Reproduced with permission from Rockwood CA Jr: Subluxations and dislocations about the shoulder, in Rockwood CA Jr, Green DP (eds): Rockwood and Green's Fractures in Adults, ed 2. Philadelphia, PA, JB Lippincott, 1984, pp 722-805.*

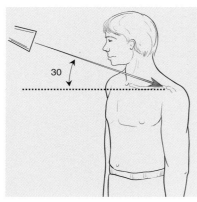

**Figure 3A**
Proper angle for a radiograph of the rotator cuff.

*Adapted with permission from Rockwood CA, Matsen FA (eds): The Shoulder. Philadelphia, PA, WB Saunders, 1990.*

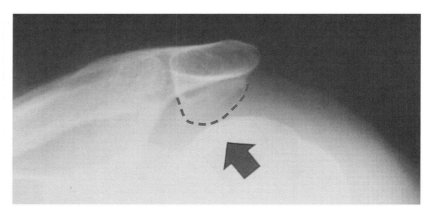

**Figure 3B**
Radiograph showing a bone spur of the inferior acromion.

## DIFFERENTIAL DIAGNOSIS

Acromioclavicular joint arthritis (localized pain and tenderness and preserved motion)

Cervical spondylosis (neck stiffness, absent biceps reflex, sensory changes)

Frozen shoulder (restricted active and passive motion)

Glenohumeral joint arthritis (evidence of arthritis on radiographs)

Impingement syndrome/cuff tendinitis (similar pain, but preserved active motion)

Pancoast tumor (venous distention, pulmonary changes, or bony metastases)

Thoracic outlet syndrome (ulnar nerve paresthesias, worse with "military brace" position)

## ADVERSE OUTCOMES OF THE DISEASE

Loss of shoulder motion, especially the ability to lift the arm overhead, chronic pain, and/or weakness in the affected arm are possible. Long-standing large tears can sometimes lead to joint degeneration.

## TREATMENT

Nonoperative treatment includes NSAIDs, physical therapy with stretching and strengthening exercises (see Shoulder Rehabilitation, pp 153-156), and avoiding overhead activities. Corticosteroid injections should be used judiciously. The steroid injection may decrease inflammation of an associated subacromial bursitis and provide short-term pain relief, but the steroid injection also weakens the tendon. Repeated injections can ultimately accelerate propagation of the rotator cuff tear. Therefore, patients should never receive more than three subacromial injections.

Only patients with significant symptoms and failed rehabilitation should be considered candidates for surgery. The exception to the rule is the patient younger than age 60 years who has an acute traumatic cuff tear. In this uncommon scenario, rotator cuff repair is best done within 6 weeks of injury.

## ADVERSE OUTCOMES OF TREATMENT

NSAIDs can cause gastric, renal, or hepatic complications. Corticosteroid injections can result in a transient increase in pain because of the injection itself and degeneration of cuff tissue. Repair of large rotator cuff tears has a high incidence of failure, though the debridement alone may relieve persistent pain.

## REFERRAL DECISIONS/RED FLAGS

Failure of 6 weeks of nonoperative treatment is indication for further evaluation.

# RUPTURE OF THE BICEPS TENDON

## DEFINITION

Rupture of the biceps tendon usually involves the proximal long head of the biceps (**Figure 1**). Most often, ruptures occur in older adults who have a long history of shoulder pain secondary to an impingement syndrome. The tendon of the long head of the biceps, by its position in the intertubercular groove, has an active role in depressing the humeral head. This position, however, also predisposes the tendon to attritional changes, and the tendon ultimately ruptures, often as a result of a trivial event.

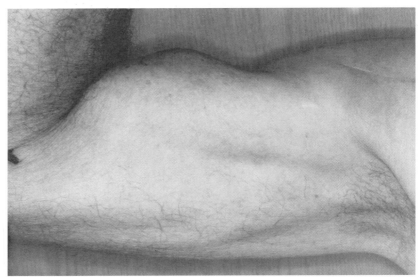

**Figure 1**
Rupture of the proximal biceps tendon.

Rupture of the proximal biceps tendon is uncommon in young adults but may occur in athletic individuals involved in weight lifting or throwing sports. Rupture of the distal biceps tendon also may occur but is rare.

## CLINICAL SYMPTOMS

Sudden pain in the upper arm, often accompanied by an audible snap, is often reported. Subsequently, patients notice a bulge in the lower arm. Pain in the acute stage is often mild.

## TESTS

### PHYSICAL EXAMINATION

Examination reveals a bulge in the lower arm, which results from the muscle belly of the biceps retracting into the lower arm after the long head ruptures.

A defect can also be palpated proximally. Acutely, ecchymosis can be seen tracking down the middle and lower arm.

The bulge can be accentuated by having the patient contract the biceps against resistance with the elbow flexed or by doing the Ludington test (the patient puts his or her hands behind the head and flexes the biceps muscle) (**Figure 2**). Gentle pressure over the bicipital groove of the humerus with the arm in 10° of internal rotation will elicit pain (**Figure 3**).

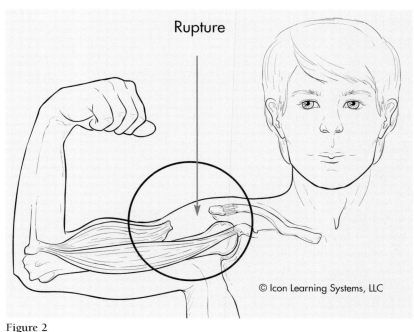

**Figure 2**
Rupture made more obvious by attempted contraction.

*Adapted with permission from Netter FH: The CIBA Collection of Medical Illustrations. Summit, NJ, CIBA-GEIGY, 1987.*

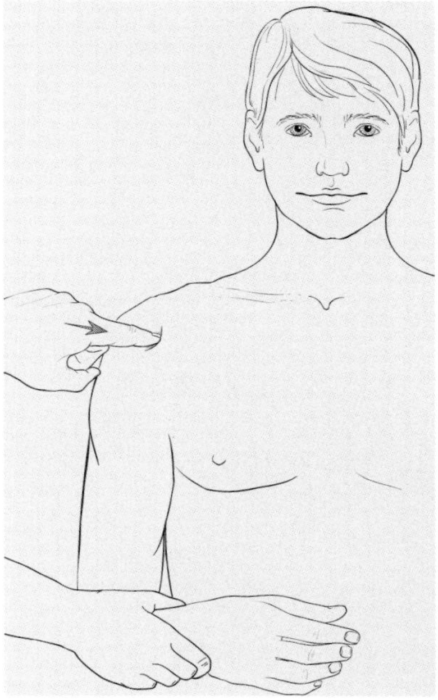

**Figure 3**
Palpation of the bicipital groove.

## DIAGNOSTIC TESTS

AP and axillary radiographs of the shoulder are useful to rule out a fracture but are not helpful in confirming a diagnosis of a ruptured biceps tendon. For patients with a previous history of disabling shoulder pain, a shoulder arthrogram or MRI should be considered to rule out a rotator cuff tear.

## DIFFERENTIAL DIAGNOSIS

Dislocated biceps tendon (tenderness over the bicipital groove, but no distal muscle bulge)

Distal biceps rupture (pain and ecchymosis distally with high-riding muscle belly, often missed until late)

Glenohumeral arthritis (pain in the joint exacerbated with motion, evident on radiographs)

Impingement syndrome (can coexist with biceps tendon rupture)

Rotator cuff tear (often coexists with biceps tendon rupture)

Rupture of the pectoralis major muscle (abnormal muscle contour apparent in anterior axillary fold)

## ADVERSE OUTCOMES OF THE DISEASE

Patients can lose approximately 10% of elbow flexion and forearm supination strength (the motion required to use a manual screwdriver). Cosmetic deformity of the arm in the form of a bulge in the lower arm can also be of concern to the patient.

## TREATMENT

Nonoperative treatment is effective for most patients, resulting in little loss of function and acceptable cosmetic deformity. Most patients regain full range of motion and normal elbow flexion strength with an exercise program consisting of range of motion and strengthening, as pain allows. Patients with persistent shoulder pain and young athletes need evaluation for a concomitant rotator cuff tear.

In young athletes and in adults younger than age 40 years who work as heavy laborers and need the extra strength for lifting, repair of the biceps tendon should be considered. Ruptures of the distal biceps are more disabling because all continuity of the biceps muscle has been lost. These injuries should be repaired acutely.

## ADVERSE OUTCOMES OF TREATMENT

Functional improvement from surgery is often modest, and postoperative stiffness is a potential concern. Bodybuilders may trade a distal muscle bulge for a surgical scar with little subjective cosmetic improvement.

## REFERRAL DECISIONS/RED FLAGS

Young patients who are heavy laborers and older patients with a concomitant rotator cuff tear and persistent symptoms need further evaluation.

# SHOULDER INSTABILITY

ICD-9 Codes
718.81
    Instability of shoulder joint NOS
831.00
    Closed dislocation shoulder,
    unspecified

## SYNONYMS

Dislocation
Subluxation
Multidirectional instability
Recurrent dislocation

## DEFINITION

With its shallow glenoid and loose capsule, the shoulder joint has great mobility. As a corollary, instability is also most common at the shoulder. Patients with shoulder instability have recurrent episodes of subluxation (humeral head partially slips out of the socket) and/or dislocation. Instability can be anterior, posterior, inferior, or multidirectional. Anterior and multidirectional account for most cases (**Figure 1**). Anterior instability can be categorized by the acronym TUBS—Traumatic, Unidirectional, Bankart lesion present (a tear of the anterior glenoid labrum) (**Figure 2**), Surgery is often required.

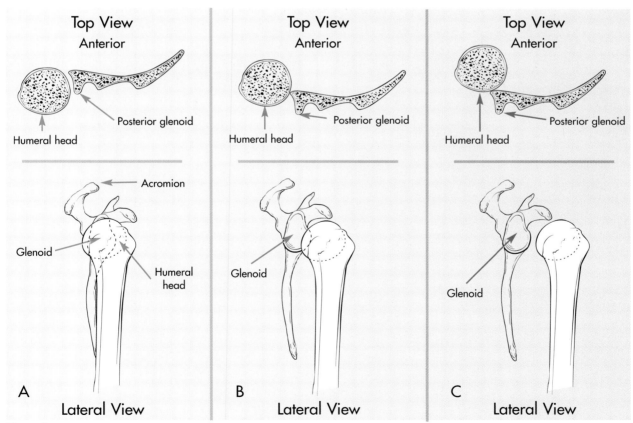

**Figure 1**
A, Humeral head reduced. B, Humeral head subluxated anteriorly. C, Humeral head dislocated anteriorly.

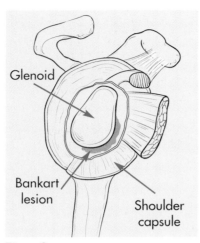

**Figure 2**
Detachment of the labrum—Bankart lesion.

*Adapted with permission from Matsen F III (ed): Practical Evaluation and Management of the Shoulder. Philadelphia, PA, WB Saunders, 1994, p 103.*

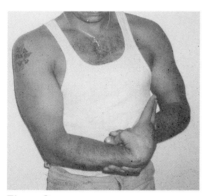

**Figure 3**
Patient who has generalized laxity.

*Reproduced with permission from Bigliani LU (ed): The Unstable Shoulder. Rosemont, IL, American Academy of Orthopaedic Surgeons, 1996.*

Multidirectional instability can be categorized by the acronym AMBRI—Atraumatic, Multidirectional, Bilateral signs of laxity, Rehabilitation as the preferred treatment, and Inferior capsular shift as the indicated procedure if surgery becomes necessary. Posterior dislocations result from a posteriorly directed force when the arm is in adduction and internal rotation. This uncommon injury is associated with seizures or electric shock injuries.

## CLINICAL SYMPTOMS

Patients with anterior instability typically describe the sensation of the shoulder slipping out of joint when the arm is abducted and externally rotated. The initial anterior shoulder dislocation is associated with significant trauma from a fall or forceful throwing motion, but with recurrent dislocations, the patient may experience instability by simply positioning the arm overhead. With multidirectional instability, symptoms may be vague but tend to be activity-related. Ask the patient whether he or she can voluntarily dislocate the shoulder, as this is an important clue.

## TESTS

### PHYSICAL EXAMINATION

With an acute dislocation, any movement of the shoulder is associated with considerable pain. With an anterior dislocation, the patient supports the arm in a neutral position. Patients with a posterior dislocation hold the arm in adduction and internal rotation, external rotation is impossible. Neurovascular function, particularly that of the axillary nerve, should be carefully assessed before and after reduction.

Assessment of a patient believed to have recurrent instability should include the apprehension test for anterior instability, the sulcus sign test for inferior laxity, and the jerk test for posterior instability (see Physical Examination–Shoulder). The patient should also be assessed for generalized ligamentous laxity. Ask the patient to touch the thumb against the volar (flexor) surface of the forearm (**Figure 3**). Bend the fingers back at the knuckle to determine how far they extend past neutral with the finger and hand in a straight line. Patients with ligamentous laxity are more likely to have multidirectional instability, but other types of instability are still possible.

### DIAGNOSTIC TESTS

AP and axillary radiographs of the shoulder should be obtained. The axillary view may show a bony defect at the anterior edge of the glenoid rim (**Figure 4**). A compression fracture of the posterior humeral head (a Hill-Sachs lesion) is created when the head is pressed against the anterior edge of the glenoid. A Hill-Sachs lesion is clear evidence of an anterior dislocation. Patients older than age 40 years with a history of traumatic dislocation are also prone to tear the rotator cuff at the time of dislocation. A shoulder arthrogram or MRI may be indicated in these cases.

Posterior dislocation of the shoulder is easily missed if only an AP radiograph is obtained. If an axillary view cannot be obtained, request a transscapular lateral view.

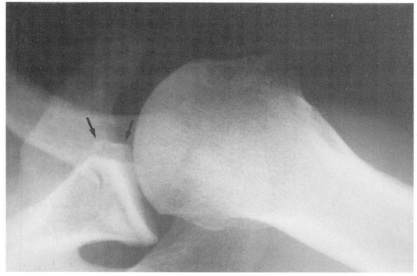

**Figure 4**
Axillary view showing erosion (arrows) of the glenoid rim associated with anterior glenohumeral instability.

*Reproduced with permission from Bigliani LU (ed): The Unstable Shoulder. Rosemont, IL, American Academy of Orthopaedic Surgeons, 1996.*

## DIFFERENTIAL DIAGNOSIS

Glenohumeral arthritis (confirm with radiographs)

Impingement syndrome (pain but not apprehension of instability)

Rotator cuff tear (pain and weakness without apprehension)

## ADVERSE OUTCOMES OF THE DISEASE

Axillary nerve injury (deltoid dysfunction and numbness over lateral arm) is not uncommon but usually resolves. The risk of recurrent instability is greater in younger patients and in those with multiple episodes.

## TREATMENT

Most acute shoulder dislocations can be reduced in the emergency department. While there are several ways to reduce a shoulder, only two are described here (see Reduction of Anterior Shoulder Dislocation, pp 151-152). Patients with a first-time dislocation can be treated with a physical therapy program that emphasizes strengthening the rotator cuff muscles, especially the subscapularis muscle (see Shoulder Rehabilitation, pp 153-156).

Patients with atraumatic or voluntary instability (AMBRI) should be treated nonoperatively with the shoulder exercise program described above. Educating patients to avoid voluntarily dislocating the shoulder and to avoid positions of known instability is an important part of the treatment plan.

## ADVERSE OUTCOMES OF TREATMENT

Axillary nerve injury, osteoarthritis of the glenohumeral joint, and/or persistent dislocation are possible. Failure to recognize a posterior dislocation can also occur.

## REFERRAL DECISIONS/RED FLAGS

Failure to reduce an acute dislocation by closed manipulation, recurrent dislocations (two or more) despite a 3-month trial of shoulder rehabilitation exercises, and patients with multidirectional instability whose symptoms are intolerable and who do not respond to a rehabilitation program also can benefit from further evaluation.

# Procedure
## Reduction of Anterior Shoulder Dislocation

Prior to reduction, a neurovascular examination should be performed. Assess function of the axillary, musculocutaneous, median, radial, and ulnar nerves with emphasis on evaluating the axillary nerve through voluntary isometric contraction of the deltoid and sensation over the lateral deltoid region. Obtain AP and axillary radiographs to document the dislocation and rule out any fractures that may displace during the reduction maneuver. Reducing a first-time dislocation is most safely done in the emergency department with a resuscitation cart available.

Establish an intravenous line, ensure that naloxone is available, and initiate pulse oximetry and cardiac monitoring if narcotics are used for anesthesia. Apply oxygen by mask or nasal cannula throughout the procedure. Fentanyl in a dose of 100 µg is given IV over 1 minute, and then repeated every 3 to 5 minutes until adequate sedation is achieved. The usual total dose of fentanyl is 3 µg/kg. Patients with recurrent dislocations may not require any anesthesia.

### First technique

#### Step 1

Place the patient prone on a stretcher with the dislocated arm hanging off the cart. Secure the patient to the stretcher with a sheet.

#### Step 2

Either have an assistant sit on the floor and provide downward traction, or attach 10 to 15 lb of weight to the patient's arm (**Figure 1**). The weights should not touch the floor.

#### Step 3

For reduction of the left shoulder, place your left thumb on the patient's acromion and the fingers of your left hand over the front of the humeral head.

#### Step 4

As the muscles relax, gently push the humeral head caudally until it reduces.

### Second technique

#### Step 1

Place the patient supine on the stretcher with a sheet folded into a band 4" to 5" wide around the patient's chest (**Figure 2**). Stand next to the patient on the same side as the injured shoulder, at or below the patient's waist.

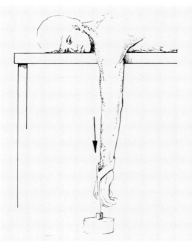

**Figure 1**
Stimson technique (gravity assisted reduction with patient lying on stomach).

*Figure 2 is reproduced with permission from Rockwood CA Jr: Subluxations and dislocations about the shoulder, in Rockwood CA Jr, Green DP (eds): Rockwood and Green's Fractures in Adults, ed 2. Philadelphia, PA, JB Lippincott, 1984, pp 722-805.*

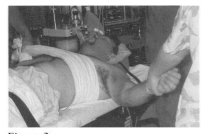

**Figure 2**
Second technique for shoulder reduction.

## STEP 2

Position the patient's elbow in 90° of flexion to relax the biceps muscle. An assistant applies traction to the sheet that is wrapped around the patient's thorax while you apply a steady traction to the arm.

## STEP 3

Reduction may be aided if you gently rotate the arm while the longitudinal traction is applied. You usually can feel and see the shoulder reduce. Occasionally, especially in large patients, the reduction may be subtle, and you may neither feel nor see it.

## ADVERSE OUTCOMES

Axillary nerve palsy can develop with reduction. Be sure to test axillary nerve function (motor and sensory) before and after the reduction. Inability to reduce the shoulder without general anesthesia is also possible. Fentanyl overdose is treated with naloxone. Initially, give 0.2 to 0.4 mg IV, and if there is no response, administer repeated doses of up to 4 to 5 mg; doses as high as 15 to 20 mg may be administered with resistant opioids, such as fentanyl. Patients older than age 40 with a first-time dislocation should be examined for a possible rotator cuff tear.

## AFTERCARE/PATIENT INSTRUCTIONS

Obtain postreduction AP and axillary radiographs to confirm the reduction. Immobilize the arm in a sling, but have the patient remove the sling and extend the elbow several times daily to prevent elbow stiffness. Begin isometric exercises for the rotator cuff. Have the patient externally rotate the arm to 0° with the hand pointing straight ahead, and flex the shoulder to 90° with the humerus parallel with the floor, at least 10 times each day for 2 weeks.

Begin strengthening exercises for the subscapularis and infraspinatus muscles at 2 to 3 weeks in the older patient and at 6 weeks in the younger patient.

Increase shoulder external rotation to 30° or 40° and shoulder flexion to 140°. This occurs at 6 weeks in patients younger than age 30 years and at 3 weeks in patients older than age 30 years.

Begin vigorous shoulder motion at 6 weeks in patients older than age 30 years, but delay this step to 3 months for patients younger than age 30 years.

The propensity for shoulder stiffness in patients older than age 30 years is an advantage in regaining stability; however, these patients are more likely to suffer a rotator cuff tear at the time of the dislocation.

In the athlete, allow return to sports activities once near full flexion and rotation of the arm and normal strength of the cuff have been regained.

# SHOULDER REHABILITATION

The rehabilitation program for most patients consists of two basic phases: stretching exercises to restore range of motion and strengthening exercises to improve muscle power. Attempting to strengthen a stiff shoulder is likely to cause or increase pain; therefore, stretching exercises alone should be prescribed until the patient has a near-normal range of motion. Strengthening exercises should then be added as appropriate for the condition. These exercises are done with the elbow maintained fairly close to the side because resistance work with the arm horizontal and overhead is more likely to exacerbate symptoms.

Once the patient has achieved the prescribed goals of stretching and strengthening with the rehabilitation routine described below, a period of sport- or work-specific training should begin. Performing the actions normally required with gradually increasing intensity and duration provides the necessary conditioning for a successful return to normal work or competitive sport.

The focus of rehabilitation should be on having the patient understand and commit to a home exercise program. The principal role of physical therapy is to instruct patients on exact techniques for a home exercise program, including alternate methods as necessary to minimize pain with exercise.

Pain control modalities also can be helpful. Forcing stretching or strengthening to the point of pain is always deleterious and should be avoided. Progress is achieved by performing the exercises frequently (two to four times a day, 7 days a week) and making small gains.

## STRETCHING EXERCISES

Before performing stretching exercises, the patient should apply moist heat by using a moist-heat heating pad, taking a hot shower, or soaking in a hot tub to help "loosen up" the shoulder. If prescribed, NSAIDs can be taken 20 to 30 minutes prior to stretching for added benefit.

The most gentle way to begin stretching is with pendulum exercises. The patient leans forward and relaxes the muscles of the involved arm so it will hang freely. The arm is then gently moved in up/down, side-to-side, and circular motions (**Figure 1**).

Passive stretching is accomplished with stick and pulley exercises. The involved arm does not do any active work but is passively pushed or pulled in the specific directions (**Figure 2**). The shoulder should be stretched to the point of feeling a pull on the muscles without pain and then held for 5 seconds. The stretch is released and after a moment of relaxation is repeated. Normally, five repetitions of each stretch are performed.

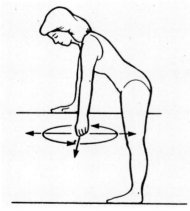

**Figure 1**
Pendulum exercise.

*Reproduced with permission from Shoulder Service, Department of Orthopaedics, The University of Texas Health Science Center at San Antonio, San Antonio, TX.*

SECTION 2 | SHOULDER

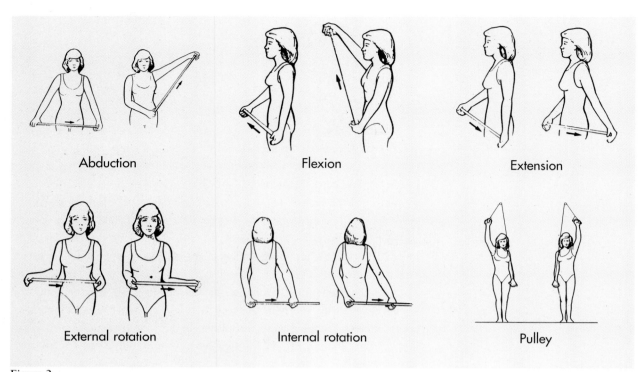

**Figure 2**
Stick and pulley exercises.

*Reproduced with permission from Shoulder Service, Department of Orthopaedics, The University of Texas Health Science Center at San Antonio, San Antonio, TX.*

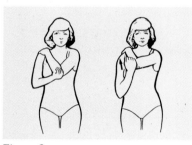

**Figure 3**
Posterior capsule stretch.

*Reproduced with permission from Shoulder Service, Department of Orthopaedics, The University of Texas Health Science Center at San Antonio, San Antonio, TX.*

The capsule and muscles of the posterior shoulder can become quite tight, especially in impingement syndrome and rotator cuff tears. Stretching the posterior capsule involves gently pulling the elbow of the involved arm across the chest as far as possible and holding it for 5 seconds (**Figure 3**). This stretch also should be done in sets of five repetitions.

## STRENGTHENING EXERCISES

Exercises to strengthen the deltoid and rotator cuff muscles can be done most easily using commercially available rubber bands, which come in different thicknesses, to provide progressive resistance. The same exercises can also be performed with pulleys or light free weights. Each motion is performed and held at the indicated endpoint for 5 seconds and repeated five times (**Figure 4**). It usually takes 2 to 3 weeks to progress from one band to the next. However, the patient should be advised not to progress to the next band if he or she still has difficulty using the current band or if pain develops when trying the new one. The patient should also be instructed to continue stretching exercises during this stage so that the hard-won gains in range of motion are not lost.

Strengthening the scapular stabilizers, as well as the rotator cuff and deltoid muscles, is important as strong, coordinated function of all shoulder muscle groups helps stabilize the glenohumeral joint (**Figure 5**). The shoulder shrug strengthens the trapezius muscle by lifting a weight off the ground

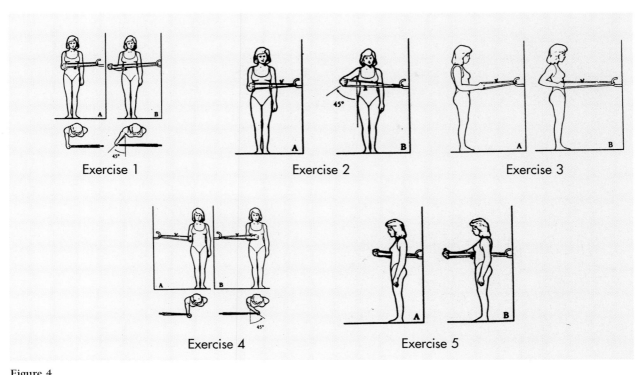

**Figure 4**
Rubber band exercises.

*Reproduced with permission from Shoulder Service, Department of Orthopaedics, The University of Texas Health Science Center at San Antonio, San Antonio, TX.*

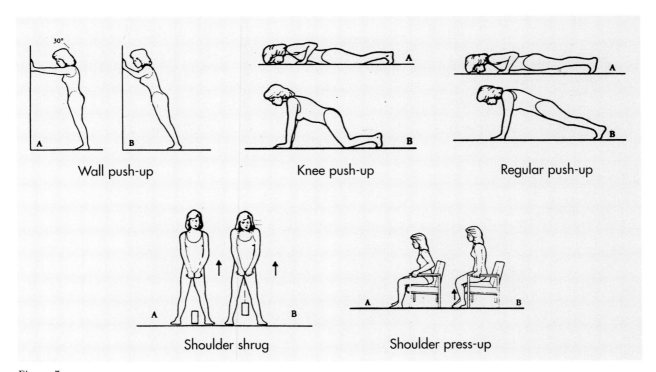

**Figure 5**
Exercises to strengthen the scapular stabilizers.

*Reproduced with permission from Shoulder Service, Department of Orthopaedics, The University of Texas Health Science Center at San Antonio, San Antonio, TX.*

as the shoulders are shrugged without bending the elbows. Most patients will start with about 5 lb and increase by 2 to 5 lb every 2 to 3 weeks. The serratus anterior and rhomboid muscles are conditioned with push-up exercises. Depending on their level of fitness, patients can start with wall push-ups, knee push-ups, or regular push-ups and then gradually progress. As with the other exercises described, each push-up should be held for 5 seconds, with a set of five repeated two to four times per day. Finally, the latissimus dorsi is strengthened with press-up exercises. These are performed by pushing up out of an armchair and holding the position just short of full elbow extension. The legs should be used to assist to the extent required to perform the exercise without pain.

# THORACIC OUTLET SYNDROME

ICD-9 Code
353.0
    Brachial plexus lesions

## DEFINITION

Thoracic outlet syndrome (TOS) is compression of the brachial plexus and/or subclavian vessels as they exit the narrow space between the superior shoulder girdle and the first rib (**Figure 1**). These structures can be affected individually or in combinations. Women between the ages of 20 and 50 years are most commonly affected.

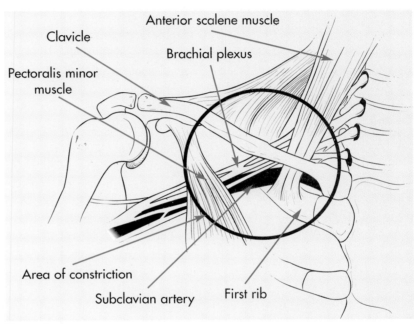

**Figure 1**
Anatomy of the thoracic outlet.

*Adapted with permission from Rockwood CA Jr: Subluxation and dislocations about the shoulder, in Rockwood CA Jr, Green DP (eds): Rockwood and Green's Fractures in Adults, ed 3. Philadelphia, PA, JB Lippincott, 1988, pp 722-985.*

The etiology of TOS may be secondary to congenital anomalies such as a cervical rib or abnormally long transverse process of C7, or an anomalous fibromuscular band in the thoracic outlet. Posttraumatic fibrosis of the scalene muscles also is a possibility.

## CLINICAL SYMPTOMS

Symptoms are often vague and variable. Compression of the brachial plexus accounts for most presenting symptoms and can mimic distal nerve entrapment, especially of the ulnar nerve with small and ring finger paresthesias. Aching pain and paresthesias can extend from the neck into the shoulder, arm, medial forearm, and the fingers. Symptoms from vascular compression include intermittent swelling and discoloration of the arm. The aching fatigue and weakness are worse when the arm is in an overhead position. Psychological disturbances such as depression are seen with TOS, but whether they contribute to the causation or are the result of a chronically painful condition is unclear.

## TESTS

### PHYSICAL EXAMINATION

Inspect for swelling or discoloration of the arm and palpate the supraclavicular fossa to rule out a mass lesion. Auscultation over this area may reveal the presence of a bruit, especially while doing the provocative maneuvers described below. Compare distal pulses with those on the opposite side. Assess sensory and motor function of the axillary, musculocutaneous, medial antebrachial cutaneous, median, radial, and, most important, ulnar nerve.

Several clinical tests have been described to diagnose TOS. Perhaps the simplest and most reproducible provocative maneuver is the elevated arm stress test (EAST) (**Figure 2**). With both shoulders abducted at least 90° and braced somewhat posteriorly, ask the patient to open and close his or her fists at a moderate speed for 3 minutes. Reproduction of neurologic and/or vascular symptoms is a positive test. A sense of fatigue without neurologic or vascular symptoms is considered a negative or inconclusive test.

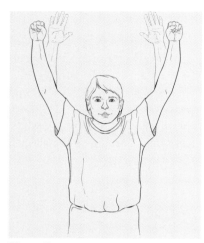

**Figure 2**
Elevated arm stress test (EAST).

### DIAGNOSTIC TESTS

No laboratory studies currently exist to confirm the diagnosis. AP and lateral radiographs of the cervical spine identify cervical ribs or overly long C7 transverse processes. PA and lateral views of the chest help rule out an apical lung tumor or infection. MRI of the cervical spine may be needed if the patient has signs and symptoms of a cervical disk rupture or a cervical spondylosis. AP and axillary radiographs of the shoulder are indicated if the patient has shoulder symptoms. Somatosensory evoked potentials, nerve conduction velocity studies, and ultrasound are not reliable in confirming the diagnosis but can be useful in ruling out alternative diagnoses (eg, ulnar nerve entrapment).

## DIFFERENTIAL DIAGNOSIS

Brachial plexus neuritis (sudden onset, severe pain, proximal muscle weakness)

Carpal tunnel syndrome (numbness on the radial side of the hand, positive Phalen test)

Herniated cervical disk (neck pain and stiffness with unilateral or bilateral pain and neurologic findings in a radicular pattern)

Impingement syndrome (localized shoulder pain with positive impingement signs)

Pancoast tumor (venous congestion, lesion on apical lordotic chest radiograph)

Ulnar nerve entrapment (Tinel sign at elbow, abnormal nerve conduction velocity studies, no symptoms above the elbow)

## ADVERSE OUTCOMES OF THE DISEASE

Weakness and loss of coordination of the upper extremity, chronic headaches, and the inability to work with the arm overhead are possible. Ulcerations on the arm and hand and the Raynaud phenomenon are rare. Serious problems such as venous thrombosis and aneurysm of the subclavian artery are uncommon but can develop.

## TREATMENT

Most patients can be treated nonoperatively with 3 months of physical therapy that emphasizes muscle strengthening and postural education exercises (Figure 3). Strenuous activities, such as carrying heavy objects, should be avoided, as should placing straps over the affected shoulder, including bras, purses, and seat belts. Activities that aggravate symptoms, such as prolonged overhead activities, strenuous aerobic exercises, and sleeping on the affected shoulder, should be discouraged as well.

---

**The following exercises are designed to stretch the soft-tissue structures that may be compressing the neurovascular bundle. Do the exercises two times daily, 10 repetitions each.**

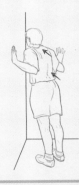

**1. Corner stretch**
Stand in a corner with your hands at shoulder height. Lean into corner until you feel a gentle stretch. Hold for 5 seconds.

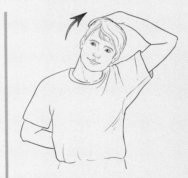

**2. Neck stretches**
Put your left hand on your head with your right hand behind your back. Pull your head towards your left shoulder until you feel a gentle stretch. Hold for 5 seconds. Switch hand positions and repeat the exercise in the opposite direction.

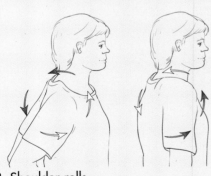

**3. Shoulder rolls**
Shrug your shoulders up, back, and then down in a circular motion.

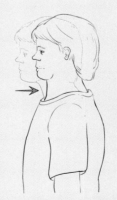

**4. Neck retraction**
Pull your head straight back, keeping your jaw level. Hold for 5 seconds.

*If any of these exercises causes an increase in your symptoms, discontinue exercises and consult your physician.*

**Figure 3**
Thoracic outlet syndrome exercise protocol.

*Adapted with permission from Visual Health Information, Tacoma, WA.*

Maintaining proper posture is important. The patient should be taught to stand up straight with the shoulders back, not slumped forward. The use of NSAIDs, muscle relaxants, and transcutaneous electrical nerve stimulation (TENS) units can help decrease the severity of the symptoms. Weight reduction, when indicated, should be encouraged as well. A multidisciplinary approach, including physical therapists, occupational therapists, and physiatrists, may be beneficial.

Because the success rate from surgery is variable and the complication rate is significant, every effort should be made to treat these patients nonoperatively.

## ADVERSE OUTCOMES OF TREATMENT

The following conditions can develop following or as a result of treatment: complex regional pain syndrome, intercostal neuroma, frozen shoulder, brachial plexus injury, or pneumothorax.

## REFERRAL DECISIONS/RED FLAGS

Vascular compromise with swelling and/or ulceration necessitates early consultation. Similarly, patients with TOS and a cervical rib or extra-long transverse process need early specialty evaluation when these findings are associated with loss of sensation, muscle atrophy, and weakness. Finally, failure of a well-supervised exercise program in a patient with disabling symptoms is an indication for further evaluation.

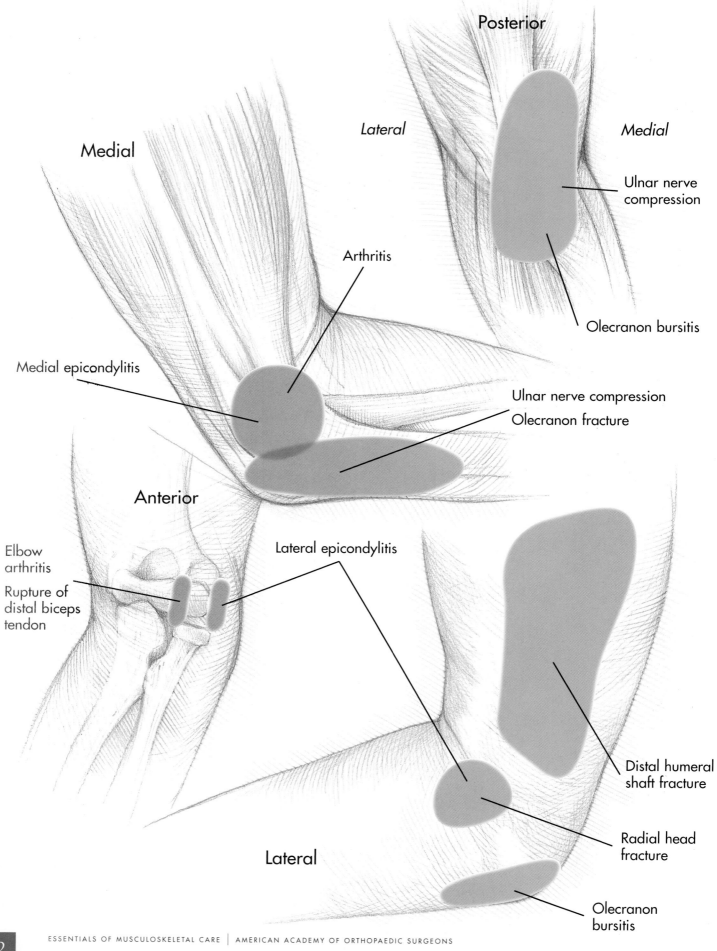

Medial

Posterior

Lateral

Medial

Ulnar nerve compression

Olecranon bursitis

Arthritis

Medial epicondylitis

Ulnar nerve compression

Olecranon fracture

Anterior

Elbow arthritis

Rupture of distal biceps tendon

Lateral epicondylitis

Distal humeral shaft fracture

Radial head fracture

Lateral

Olecranon bursitis

# ELBOW AND FOREARM

Section Editor
Thomas R. Johnson, MD
Orthopedic Surgeons, PSC
St. Vincent Hospital and Health Center
Billings, Montana

Section Editor
Michael A. Wirth, MD
Associate Professor
Department of Orthopaedics
University of Texas Health Science Center
Chief, Shoulder Service
Audie Murphy Veterans Hospital
San Antonio, Texas

Robert M. Orfaly, MD, FRCSC
Assistant Professor
Department of Orthopaedics and Rehabilitation
Oregon Health Sciences University
Portland, Oregon

# ELBOW AND FOREARM—AN OVERVIEW

This section of *Essentials of Musculoskeletal Care* focuses on the more common and important conditions encountered in the elbow and forearm. Making a correct diagnosis of a condition in the elbow or forearm begins with clearly defining the nature of the patient's chief complaint and the anatomic location. The chief complaint usually is related to pain or stiffness or both. Unlike the shoulder, the elbow has considerable articular congruency, and elbow instability is a much less common problem than with the shoulder.

The elbow joint comprises three distinct articulations: ulnohumeral, radiocapitellar, and proximal radioulnar. The proximal radioulnar joint is linked to the distal radioulnar joint at the wrist to achieve forearm pronation and supination.

Basic radiographic assessment consists of an AP view of the extended elbow and a lateral view with the elbow flexed 90° with the forearm supinated. Oblique views can be helpful in identifying subtle fractures and when the elbow cannot be extended enough to obtain an AP view.

## ACUTE PAIN

Acute pain and swelling after an injury can be caused by a fracture, dislocation, or tendon rupture. The location of the pain, tenderness, deformity, and ecchymosis are important physical findings. Pain with elbow flexion/extension suggests involvement of the ulnohumeral articulation, whereas pain with forearm pronation/supination should direct attention to the radiocapitellar and proximal radioulnar joints.

Radiographs will confirm a fracture or dislocation, although some radial head or other articular surface fractures can be easily missed. When radiographs are normal, a tendon rupture, such as of the distal biceps, is possible.

Acute pain in the absence of trauma most commonly is associated with swelling over the tip of the elbow, indicating an acute olecranon bursitis. Intra-articular conditions include septic arthritis (especially in intravenous drug abusers), rheumatoid arthritis, or other inflammatory conditions, such as crystalline deposition diseases (gout, pseudogout).

## CHRONIC PAIN

Most elbow and forearm complaints are chronic in nature (greater than 2 weeks' duration) and represent overuse injuries from work or sport. Localization of the pain and tenderness, as well as identifying the movement or position that provokes pain, is important.

Pain and tenderness localized to the lateral epicondyle and the "common extensor origin" of forearm muscles extending from it are referred to as lateral epicondylitis (tennis elbow). The pain of lateral epicondylitis is exacerbated by forearm supination and wrist extension against resistance. When the pain and tenderness is localized about 5 cm distal to the lateral epicondyle, entrapment of the posterior interosseous branch of the radial nerve (radial tunnel syndrome) might be present. Because this nerve compression syndrome typically produces pain without distal motor or sensory deficits, distinguishing it from tennis elbow sometimes can be difficult.

Posterior elbow pain usually is associated with chronic olecranon bursitis. Overhead-throwing athletes can develop painful spurs on the posteromedial olecranon secondary to repetitive valgus strain on the elbow during the throwing motion.

Pain over the medial aspect of the elbow is probably the result of one of two conditions: ulnar nerve entrapment or medial epicondylitis (golfer's elbow). Ulnar nerve entrapment is associated with localized pain at the elbow accompanied by numbness and tingling in the little finger and ulnar half of the ring finger that is exacerbated by tapping over the nerve in the ulnar groove. Patients with medial epicondylitis have pain and tenderness over and just lateral and distal to the medial epicondyle. This pain is increased with wrist flexion or forearm pronation against resistance.

Anterior elbow pain occurring acutely and associated with tenderness, ecchymosis, and change in the contour of the biceps muscle indicates a distal biceps tendon rupture. This rupture typically occurs in middle-aged men who also report weak supination (screwdriver motion) following a sudden jerking movement or heavy lifting.

Elbow arthritis can be posttraumatic arthritis, inflammatory (rheumatoid) arthritis, or osteoarthritis. The pain can be diffuse or localized, based on the area of greatest involvement. For example, lateral elbow pain that is exacerbated by forearm rotation is likely caused by arthritis in the radiocapitellar articulation. These symptoms are often the initial presentation of rheumatoid arthritis involving the elbow or of posttraumatic arthritis after a radial head fracture. Loose bodies often develop in arthritic elbows and can produce catching or locking.

## STIFFNESS

The normal elbow has range of motion from 0° (arm out straight) to 140° to 150° of flexion. Normal pronation and supination are 80° each way. The elbow has a particular predisposition to develop stiffness with arthritis, trauma, or immobilization; however, mild loss of motion causes no significant disability because most daily activities are performed in an arc of motion from 30° to 130° of flexion and 50° each of pronation and supination.

# PHYSICAL EXAMINATION
# ELBOW AND FOREARM

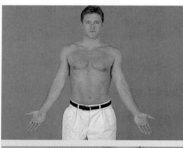

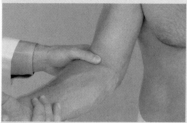

### Anterior view

Inspect the elbow for swelling and ecchymosis. Measure the "carrying angle" (ie, the angle made by the axis of the humerus and the forearm) with the elbow extended and the forearm supinated (top). Note that the normal carrying angle is a cubitus valgus of 5° to 8°. Cubitus varus usually results from a malunion of a supracondylar humerus fracture.

The biceps tendon can be easily palpated in the middle of the antecubital fossa, especially when the patient flexes the elbow against resistance (bottom). Absence of this normally palpable tendon with associated tenderness and ecchymosis indicates a complete biceps tendon rupture. A partial rupture also can occur. The brachial artery is deep and medial to the biceps tendon. The median nerve is medial to the brachial artery.

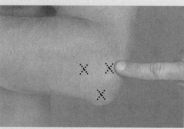

### Lateral view

Check for an effusion by inspecting and palpating the area in the center of a triangle bounded by the lateral epicondyle of the humerus, the tip of the olecranon, and the radial head. Confirm the position of the radial head by feeling it move with forearm pronation/supination.

Palpate the area over the radial head to check for pain and crepitus. These findings, along with limited forearm rotation, suggest a radial head fracture. Tenderness to palpation just distal to the lateral epicondyle indicates lateral epicondylitis (tennis elbow). Tenderness 5 cm distal to the lateral epicondyle that is localized deep to the extensor muscles suggests entrapment of the posterior interosseous branch of the radial nerve.

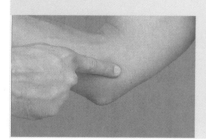

### Medial elbow

Pain and tenderness immediately distal to the medial epicondyle suggest medial epicondylitis. The ulnar nerve passes in the ulnar groove just posterior to the medial epicondyle. Palpation and light percussion in this area can produce local pain and paresthesias in the forearm and ulnar two fingers in association with ulnar nerve entrapment.

# Inspection/Palpation

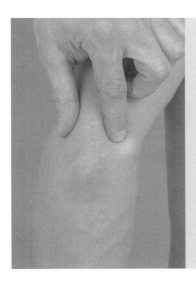

### Posterior view

Inspect the area over the olecranon for focal swelling and palpate for tenderness to confirm the presence of olecranon bursitis. An olecranon fracture produces a broader area of swelling with ecchymosis and a possible skin abrasion at the point of impact. Palpate just above the olecranon (as shown in figure) to identify elbow effusion.

# Range of Motion

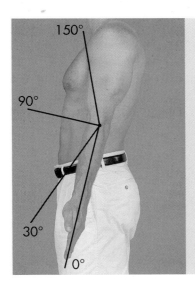

150°

90°

30°

0°

### Flexion/extension: Zero Starting Position

Use the Zero Starting Position (ie, with the extremity straight) to measure elbow flexion/extension. Young children commonly extend the elbow by 10° to 15°, but adults show minimal, if any, elbow extension. Normal elbow flexion is 135° to 145°. Mild flexion contractures are of little functional consequence, as most activities of daily living are accomplished in an arc of elbow flexion from 30° to 130°.

Limited motion may be expressed in the following ways: 1) the elbow flexes from 30° to 90°; 2) the elbow has a flexion contracture of 30° with further flexion to 90°.

# Range of Motion

## Forearm rotation

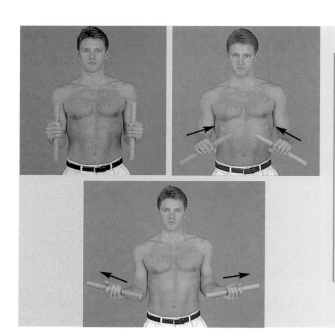

Forearm rotation (pronation/supination) is a composite motion occurring at the proximal and distal radioulnar joints, as well as the radiohumeral joint. Measure forearm rotation by stabilizing the arm against the chest wall and flexing the elbow to 90°. The Zero Starting Position is with the extended thumb aligned with the humerus (left). Palpate the radial and ulnar styloid as the forearm is rotated to estimate pronation and supination. Ask the patient to grasp a pencil or similar object to facilitate visual estimation of forearm rotation.

Pronation is the position in which the palm is turned down (right). Supination the position in which the palm is turned up (bottom). Normal pronation and supination is 70° to 85°. Many activities of daily living are accomplished in an arc of motion between 50° pronation to 50° supination. A very restricted arc of forearm rotation may be of limited consequence if shoulder mobility is normal and if the forearm is ankylosed in a neutral position.

# Muscle Testing

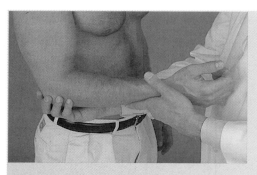

## Resisted supination

Test the strength of the forearm supinators, the most powerful of which is the biceps muscle, by grasping the patient's distal forearm and resisting the patient's maximum effort to turn the palm up. Weakness will be evident with rupture or tendinitis of the biceps tendon, subluxation of the biceps tendon at the shoulder, a lesion of the musculocutaneous nerve, or a lesion involving the C5 and C6 nerve roots. Patients with lateral epicondylitis also may experience pain with this maneuver.

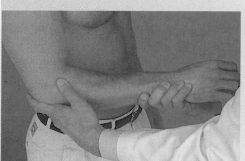

## Resisted pronation

Test the strength of the forearm pronators, the most powerful of which is the pronator teres muscle, by grasping the patient's distal forearm and resisting the patient's maximum effort to turn the palm down. Weakness will be evident with rupture of the pronator origin from the medial epicondyle, fracture of the medial elbow, or lesions involving the median nerve or the C6 and C7 nerve roots. Patients with medial epicondylitis also may experience pain with this maneuver.

# Muscle Testing

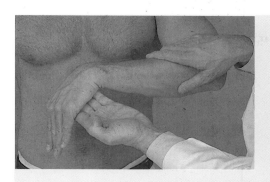

## Resisted wrist flexion

Test the strength of the wrist flexors by positioning the wrist in flexion and the fingers in extension (eliminates wrist flexion activity by the finger flexors). Ask the patient to keep the wrist flexed while you push the wrist into extension. Weakness will be evident with rupture of the muscle origin, fracture of the medial elbow, tendinitis of the medial elbow, or lesions involving the ulnar nerve (C8 and T1 nerve roots) or median nerve (C6 and C7 nerve roots).

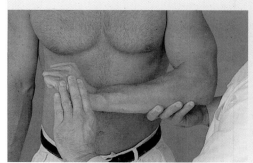

## Resisted wrist extension

Test the strength of the wrist extensors, the most powerful of which are the extensor carpi ulnaris and extensor carpi radialis brevis muscles, by positioning the wrist in extension and the fingers in flexion (eliminates wrist extension activity by the finger extensors). Ask the patient to hold the wrist in extension as you push the wrist into flexion. Weakness will be evident with rupture of the extensor origin, fracture of the lateral elbow, epicondylitis, or lesions involving the radial nerve or C6 to C8 nerve roots.

# ARTHRITIS OF THE ELBOW

SECTION 3 | ELBOW AND FOREARM

## ICD-9 Codes

714.12
  Rheumatoid arthritis of the elbow
715.12.1
  Osteoarthritis, primary, of the elbow
715.22
  Osteoarthritis, secondary, of the elbow
716.12
  Traumatic arthritis of the elbow

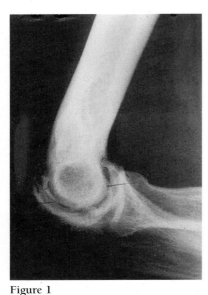

**Figure 1**
Lateral radiograph of an arthritic elbow.

*Reproduced with permission from Norberg FB, Savoie FH III, Field LD: Arthroscopic treatment of arthritis of the elbow, in Price CT (ed): Instructional Course Lectures 49. Rosemont, IL, American Academy of Orthopaedic Surgeons, 2000, p 248.*

## DEFINITION

Arthritis of the elbow can be the result of rheumatoid arthritis, trauma, or osteoarthritis. Rheumatoid arthritis (RA) is the most common cause of elbow joint destruction and nearly always develops in patients with multiple joint involvement. Concomitant wrist and hand involvement occurs in 90% and shoulder involvement in 80% of patients with RA. Similar to other joints, an active synovitis of the elbow causes periarticular erosions and symmetric joint narrowing. Further progression causes gross destruction of the bone and soft-tissue constraints. The end result is a grossly unstable elbow (**Figure 1**).

Posttraumatic arthritis results from primary injury to the articular cartilage at the time of trauma, as well as fracture malunion. The end result is incongruity of the articular cartilage and progressive arthritis. Because posttraumatic arthritis often presents as an isolated joint impairment in an otherwise young and active patient, treatment options and the patient's expectations are often quite different from those of patients with RA.

Because the elbow is not a weight-bearing joint, osteoarthritis (OA) is not nearly as common in the elbow as it is in the hip, knee, or even the shoulder. Elbow OA most often is seen in manual laborers and overhead-throwing athletes, suggesting repetitive overuse as an underlying cause. Repetitive overuse of the elbow also commonly causes intra-articular loose bodies that can act as gravel and promote joint degeneration.

## CLINICAL SYMPTOMS

RA of the elbow causes pain and swelling, as it does in other joints. In the early stages, the pain can be primarily localized to the lateral side of the joint and exacerbated by forearm rotation. Advanced disease causes diffuse pain and often gross instability that makes even light household tasks impossible.

The primary complaint with posttraumatic arthritis can be pain or stiffness, depending on the type of injury. With malunion of a radial head fracture, the pain can be isolated to the lateral side of the joint and also exacerbated by forearm rotation.

OA is characterized by pain and restricted motion. Intra-articular loose bodies are associated with symptoms of catching and locking. Posterior osteophytes typically cause limited extension and pain on terminal extension. Less commonly, anterior osteophytes can cause pain and limited flexion. Pain during midrange motion and at rest are symptoms of late disease. Osteophytes on the medial side of the elbow can cause ulnar nerve irritation.

## TESTS

### PHYSICAL EXAMINATION

Inspection of the rheumatoid elbow demonstrates joint swelling, best seen laterally, and occasionally rheumatoid nodules over the olecranon and extensor surface of the forearm. Tenderness may occur primarily over the radial head or may be diffuse. Range of motion and varus/valgus stability also should be assessed.

Elbows with posttraumatic arthritis or OA typically do not have an effusion. The joint lines should be palpated for tenderness, and range of motion measured. Impingement pain from posterior and anterior osteophytes can be elicited by gently "jogging" the joint in full extension and flexion, respectively.

### DIAGNOSTIC TESTS

AP and lateral radiographs of the elbow usually are sufficient for diagnosis. RA produces the typical picture of osteopenia, symmetric joint narrowing, and periarticular erosions, or may show gross joint destruction. Malunion, nonunion, and joint space narrowing are possible findings in posttraumatic arthritis. Radiographs of OA reveal osteophytes and narrowing of the joint space. Loose bodies may be multiple and present in the anterior and posterior portion of the elbow.

## DIFFERENTIAL DIAGNOSIS

Fracture of the distal humerus (evident on radiographs)

Fracture of the radial head (evident on radiographs)

Osteochondritis dissecans of the elbow (typically affects adolescent boys, capitellum usually involved, seen with repetitive overuse, and may produce loose bodies)

Septic arthritis of the elbow (fever, redness, swelling)

## ADVERSE OUTCOME OF THE DISEASE

Progressive pain and stiffness are common to all arthritic conditions. Rheumatoid arthritis can lead to an unstable, essentially flail elbow.

## TREATMENT

Mild limitation of elbow motion does not interfere with daily activities and is well tolerated. Because the elbow is not a weight-bearing joint, modification of job or sports activities can be very helpful.

Medical management of RA should be optimized. Intra-articular corticosteroid injection and gentle physiotherapy may be of benefit. Static and hinged splints can be helpful for some patients. Synovectomy with or without radial head excision can provide pain relief in early stages of RA that are resistant to nonoperative management. Total elbow arthroplasty is the best option for patients with RA who have advanced joint destruction.

Nonoperative measures for posttraumatic and osteoarthritic elbows are limited to analgesics and gentle stretching to preserve motion. Arthroscopic debridement and removal of loose bodies can be quite helpful. Unless the patient is elderly, total elbow replacement generally is not considered beneficial because of concern for prosthesis loosening and breakage.

## ADVERSE OUTCOMES OF TREATMENT

Patients with RA require regular monitoring for side effects from NSAIDs and disease-modifying agents. Nerve injury and infection are possible with surgery. Joint replacements can loosen or fracture with time.

## REFERRAL DECISIONS/RED FLAGS

Patients with persistent pain or significant loss of motion require further evaluation.

# DISLOCATION OF THE ELBOW

ICD-9 Code
832.0
    Dislocation of elbow, unspecified

## DEFINITION

The elbow is the most common joint to dislocate during childhood and is second only to the shoulder and finger in adults. Typically, a dislocated elbow is the result of a fall on an outstretched hand. More than 80% of elbow dislocations are posterior unless associated with an olecranon fracture (**Figure 1**). A dislocation can be complete or perched (subluxation, with the trochlea resting "perched" on top of the coronoid process). The medial collateral ligament usually is disrupted and other soft-tissue restraints commonly are injured, as well. Concomitant fractures of the radial head (adults) or medial epicondyle (children) may be present. Neurovascular structures, such as the brachial artery, median nerve, and ulnar nerve, may be injured, as well.

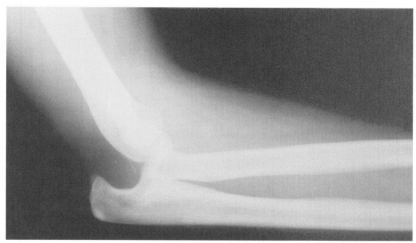

**Figure 1**
Posterior dislocation of the elbow.

*Reproduced with permission from Crosby LA, Lewallen DG (eds): Emergency Care and Transportation of the Sick and Injured, ed 6 revised. Rosemont, IL, American Academy of Orthopaedic Surgeons, 1997, p 544.*

## CLINICAL SYMPTOMS

Extreme pain, swelling, and inability to bend the elbow after a fall on the outstretched hand are characteristic of a dislocated elbow.

## TESTS

### PHYSICAL EXAMINATION

Note areas of abnormal prominence and tenderness. The most important part of the examination is the neurovascular evaluation. Check the radial pulse and capillary refill. Assess motor and sensory function of the median, radial, and ulnar nerves.

### DIAGNOSTIC TESTS

AP and lateral radiographs of the elbow are adequate to make a diagnosis. Look carefully for associated fractures and bony fragments incarcerated in the joint, as these may cause widening of the joint space.

### DIFFERENTIAL DIAGNOSIS

Fracture-dislocation of the elbow (same deformity, evident on radiographs)

Fracture of the distal humerus (evident on radiographs)

Fracture of the olecranon process of the ulna (evident on radiographs)

Hemarthrosis (positive fat pad sign)

Occult fractures (positive fat pad sign)

Synovitis (normal radiographs, no deformity or ecchymosis)

### ADVERSE OUTCOMES OF THE DISEASE

Persistent loss of motion is common, especially in extension. Although most simple dislocations (that is, without fractures) are stable after reduction, persistent or recurrent instability is possible and should be specifically addressed rather than treated with prolonged immobilization. Heterotopic bone formation and the development of arthritis of the elbow joint also are possible.

### TREATMENT

Reduction of an elbow dislocation should be performed as soon as possible after the injury. The reduction usually can be accomplished in the emergency department with the patient under conscious sedation. The sedation can be supplemented by aspirating the hemarthrosis and injecting 10 mL of 1% lidocaine into the joint from a lateral approach (**Figure 2**). If muscle spasm or marked swelling precludes reduction with the patient under conscious sedation, then general anesthesia may be required.

Flexing the elbow tenses the triceps attachment to the olecranon and makes the reduction more difficult. The reduction should be performed by holding the elbow relatively extended (flexed about 45°) and applying slow, steady, downward traction on the forearm in line with the long axis of the humerus. The reduction usually is easily felt ( a "clunk") and, once achieved, is most stable with the elbow flexed and forearm pronated. The stability of the reduction should be tested by slowly extending the elbow until the beginning of some subluxation is felt. The arm should be splinted in its stable range but avoiding more than 100° of flexion, which can contribute to vascular compromise as swelling develops.

After completing the reduction, the neurovascular examination must be repeated. After applying the splint, obtain AP, lateral, and oblique radiographs to confirm the reduction. Failure to obtain a perfectly concentric reduction suggests the possibility of a bony or cartilaginous intra-articular loose body or extensive soft-tissue injury, either of which may require operative treatment.

Motion should begin 5 to 7 days later and gradually progress during the next 3 to 4 weeks. A brace that blocks terminal extension may be required

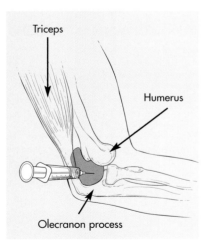

**Figure 2**
Site of aspiration of hemarthrosis and injection of local anesthetic.

during this time if some instability persists. NSAIDs can be useful during this period and may decrease the incidence of heterotopic bone formation.

## ADVERSE OUTCOMES OF TREATMENT

Fracture and neurovascular injury are possible during the reduction maneuver. Subsequent vascular problems can result from compressive bandages or splinting in more than 100° of elbow flexion. Failure to identify and address persistent instability can lead to a difficult situation of chronic instability. Prolonged immobilization leads to elbow contracture and pain and at the same time may not correct the underlying instability.

## REFERRAL DECISIONS/RED FLAGS

Patients with associated neurovascular or bony injury require further evaluation, although a gentle reduction can be attempted to avoid lengthy delays. Incomplete reduction, as shown on radiographs, should never be accepted. Patients with persistent instability or greater than a 45° flexion contracture 3 weeks after injury also require further evaluation.

# EPICONDYLITIS AND RADIAL TUNNEL SYNDROME

ICD-9 Codes
384.3
    Posterior interosseous nerve syndrome
726.31
    Medial epicondylitis
726.32
    Lateral epicondylitis

## SYNONYMS

Lateral epicondylitis

Tennis elbow

Lateral tendinosis of the elbow

Medial epicondylitis

Golfer's elbow

Medial tendinosis of the elbow

## DEFINITION

Lateral epicondylitis and tennis elbow are the most commonly used terms to describe a condition that produces pain and tenderness at the site of origin of the extensor carpi radialis brevis muscle (lateral epicondyle of the humerus). Although the term epicondylitis is commonly used, the pathology and point of maximal pain are in the tendon substance just distal to the epicondyle (**Figure 1**). The term elbow tendinitis also is inaccurate because it implies an inflammatory origin. In fact, the histologic pattern of lateral epicondylitis is one of tissue degeneration with fibroblast and microvascular hyperplasia and the absence of inflammation. The term lateral tendinosis of the elbow is probably the most accurate but rarely is used.

Compression of the posterior interosseous nerve (radial tunnel syndrome) is another cause of lateral elbow pain and is commonly misdiagnosed as lateral epicondylitis. The posterior interosseous nerve has no sensory distribution but innervates the thumb and finger extensors and the extensor carpi ulnaris. The posterior interosseous nerve is most commonly compressed by fibrous bands between the two heads of the supinator muscle in a region termed the radial tunnel.

Medial epicondylitis, or golfer's elbow, is similar to lateral epicondylitis in etiology and pathology and occurs in the common tendinous origin of the flexor/pronator muscles just distal to the medial epicondyle. Both radial tunnel syndrome and medial epicondylitis are much less commonly encountered than lateral epicondylitis.

## CLINICAL SYMPTOMS

The typical patient with lateral epicondylitis is between 35 and 50 years of age who reports the gradual onset of pain in the lateral elbow and forearm during activities involving wrist extension, such as lifting, turning a screwdriver, or hitting a backhand in tennis. With time, the pain can become severe and occur at rest. Less commonly, the patient may relate the onset of symptoms to

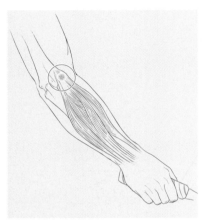

**Figure 1**
Location of pain in lateral epicondylitis.

an acute event, such as a direct blow to the elbow or a sudden maximal muscle contraction.

Patients with radial tunnel syndrome present with similar symptoms but with pain that is 4 to 5 cm more distal than lateral epicondylitis. Because the posterior interosseous nerve contains only motor fibers, there is no numbness or tingling. Obvious muscular weakness is rarely encountered until late in the disease process.

Medial epicondylitis typically occurs with active wrist flexion and forearm pronation, such as takes place with a golf swing, baseball pitching, or the pull-through strokes of swimming.

## TESTS

### PHYSICAL EXAMINATION

The most consistent finding in lateral epicondylitis is localized tenderness over the common extensor origin 1 cm distal to the lateral epicondyle (**Figure** 2). During the examination, it is best to have the patient's elbow flexed to 90° and the forearm supinated. Tapping lightly on the lateral epicondyle may be painful. Pain in the region also can be produced with resisted extension of the wrist when the elbow is in extension. Ask the patient to lift a stool or chair with the palm up (using the wrist flexors) and then the palm down (using the wrist extensors) to help differentiate lateral epicondylitis from other painful elbow conditions. Patients with lateral epicondylitis will have pain when lifting with the palm down.

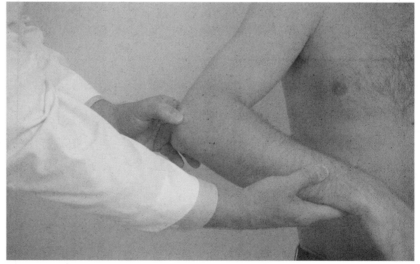

**Figure 2**
Palpating the point of maximum tenderness.

The area of tenderness with posterior interosseous nerve compression is directly over the radial tunnel, which lies 4 to 5 cm distal and slightly anterior to the lateral epicondyle. With radial tunnel syndrome, pain in the proximal forearm may be noted by extending the long finger against resistance (middle finger test).

With medial epicondylitis, the area of tenderness is just distal to the medial epicondyle, and the pain is exacerbated by pronating the forearm and flexing the wrist against resistance. These patients also may have pain when lifting a chair with the palm up.

## DIAGNOSTIC TESTS

AP and lateral radiographs of the elbow are necessary to rule out arthritis or osteochondral loose bodies. Rarely, an area of calcification may be seen at the attachment of the extensor muscles to the lateral epicondyle of the humerus.

## DIFFERENTIAL DIAGNOSIS

Cubital tunnel syndrome (compression of the ulnar nerve, paresthesias in little and ring fingers)

Fracture of the radial head (pain and tenderness over the radial head that is exacerbated by passive pronation and supination)

Osteoarthritis of the radiocapitellar portion of the elbow joint (similar examination to radial head fracture but without a history of acute trauma)

Osteochondral loose body (medial or lateral joint line pain, symptoms of locking)

Synovitis of the elbow (swelling, palpable fluid)

Triceps tendinitis (tenderness above the olecranon)

## ADVERSE OUTCOMES OF THE DISEASE

Persistent pain is the most common problem. Weakness or poor endurance with motions that involve forceful wrist extension or forearm supination, such as heavy or repetitive lifting, also is common.

## TREATMENT

Modifying or eliminating the activities that cause symptoms is the most important step in treatment, such as changing to a lighter weight tennis racquet or overwrapping the handle to make it slightly larger. For severe and long-standing cases, this activity modification may have to be permanent. NSAIDs can be helpful during acute exacerbations. Use of a commercial tennis elbow strap worn just below the elbow during heavy-lifting activities is helpful, as well. Application of heat or ice (whichever works best) may relieve pain and inflammation. Once the pain has decreased, gentle stretching and forearm-strengthening exercises can be initiated.

If symptoms persist, corticosteroid injection into the area of maximum tenderness may be helpful with lateral epicondylitis or medial epicondylitis (see Tennis Elbow Injection, pp 180-181). Advise patients that they might experience an increase in pain for 1 to 2 days after the injection. No more than three injections should be given. If the pain recurs and the symptoms are severe, surgery should be considered.

Decompression of the radial tunnel is indicated for patients with radial tunnel syndrome who have significant discomfort.

## ADVERSE OUTCOMES OF TREATMENT

NSAIDs can cause gastric, renal, or hepatic complications. Although surgery always carries a small risk of complications, such as wound infection or nerve injury, the most common adverse outcome is incomplete pain relief despite adequate surgical release. Return to a workplace that was related to the onset of symptoms can be difficult to achieve.

## REFERRAL DECISIONS/RED FLAGS

Failure of nonoperative management indicates the need for further evaluation.

# PROCEDURE

## TENNIS ELBOW INJECTION

### MATERIALS

Sterile gloves

Bactericidal skin preparation solution

5-mL syringe with a 25-gauge, 1¼" needle

3 to 4 mL of a 1% lidocaine solution without epinephrine

2-mL syringe

2 mL of a corticosteroid preparation

Adhesive bandage

The classic tender spot in lateral epicondylitis of the elbow (tennis elbow) is just distal to the lateral epicondyle of the humerus with the elbow in 90° of flexion.

### STEP 1

Wear protective gloves at all times during this procedure and use sterile technique.

### STEP 2

Place the patient's arm against the chest or abdomen, with the elbow flexed at least 90° and the forearm fully pronated.

### STEP 3

Prep the skin with a bactericidal solution.

### STEP 4

Palpate just distal to the lateral epicondyle and locate the patient's point of maximal tenderness. At this point, insert the 25-gauge needle, make a subcutaneous skin wheal with the local anesthetic, and advance through the tendon of the extensor carpi radialis brevis muscle to inject the remaining 2 to 3 mL of local anesthetic (**Figure 1**).

### STEP 5

Exchange syringes on the needle and inject the corticosteroid preparation.

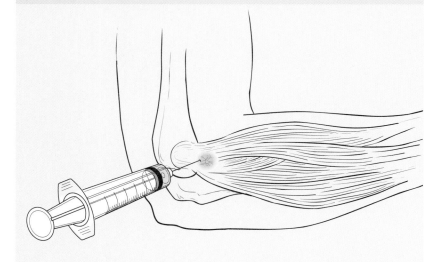

**Figure 1**
Location for needle insertion.

## STEP 6

Dress the puncture wound with a sterile adhesive bandage.

## ADVERSE OUTCOMES

Subcutaneous infiltration of the corticosteroid preparation can cause subcutaneous fat atrophy, leading to a waxy appearing depression in the skin, and can cause depigmentation in dark-skinned patients. Although rare, infection is possible. Between 25% and 33% of patients will experience a "flare" characterized by increased pain at the injection site.

## AFTERCARE/PATIENT INSTRUCTION

Advise the patient that pain may increase for 24 to 48 hours after the injection. Pain often improves with the application of ice. Acetaminophen or an NSAID also is beneficial.

# FRACTURE OF THE DISTAL HUMERUS

## ICD-9 Code

812.40
    Fracture of the distal humerus,
    unspecified

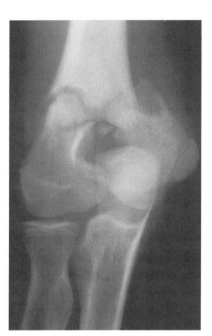

**Figure 1**
Radiograph of displaced supracondylar fracture.

*Reproduced with permission from Beaty JH, Kasser JR: Fractures about the elbow, in Jackson DW (ed): Instructional Course Lectures 44. Rosemont, IL, American Academy of Orthopaedic Surgeons, 1995, pp 199–215.*

## FRACTURE PATTERNS

Supracondylar fracture
Transcondylar fracture
Intercondylar fracture
T condylar fracture
Lateral/medial condylar fracture

## DEFINITION

Fractures of the distal humerus are relatively uncommon, accounting for only 2% of fractures in adults (**Figure 1**). Because these fractures are often comminuted and intra-articular, the potential morbidity is high. Classification schemes used for these fractures can be quite complex, but the most important factors to consider in deciding the best course for initial treatment are whether the fracture is displaced (**Figure 2**), whether the fracture involves the joint surface, and whether the skin and neurovascular structures are involved.

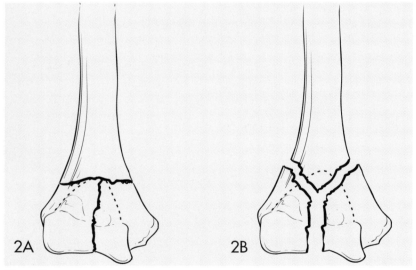

**Figure 2**
A, Nondisplaced T condylar fracture of the distal humerus. B, Displaced intercondylar fracture of the distal humerus.

*Part B is adapted from Mehne DK, Jupiter JB: Fractures of the distal humerus, in Browner BD, Jupiter JB, Levine AM, et al (eds): Skeletal Trauma: Fractures, Dislocations, Ligamentous Injuries. Philadelphia, PA, WB Saunders, 1992, pp 1146–1176.*

## CLINICAL SYMPTOMS

Marked swelling, ecchymosis, deformity, and pain around the elbow after an injury are common. Patients report increased pain with attempted flexion of the elbow.

## TESTS

### PHYSICAL EXAMINATION

Swelling and deformity usually are clearly visible with any displaced fracture. Inspect the skin around the site to identify any open wounds. Palpation around the joint may reveal an effusion, and crepitus may be felt with gentle flexion. Palpate the radial pulse and check capillary refill. Assess median, radial, and ulnar function. All peripheral nerves crossing the fracture may be injured, but ulnar nerve dysfunction is most common. Brachial artery occlusion is less common but requires early diagnosis and treatment to avoid devastating complications. Check the wrist and shoulder on the affected side for associated injuries.

### DIAGNOSTIC TESTS

AP and lateral radiographs of the elbow, with other radiographs as clinically indicated, should be adequate in most patients. Without radiographic evidence of fracture, look carefully for a fat pad sign, which indicates bleeding into the joint, often from an occult fracture (**Figure 3**).

## DIFFERENTIAL DIAGNOSIS

Elbow dislocation (evident on radiographs)

Olecranon fracture (evident on radiographs)

Radial head fracture (evident on radiographs)

Rupture of the distal biceps tendon (tenderness, weakness on supination, ecchymosis)

## ADVERSE OUTCOMES OF THE DISEASE

Unfortunately, some degree of residual pain and stiffness is common. Other complications include deformity with malunion, nonunion, and ulnar neuropathy. Vascular injury can lead to ischemia in the forearm and hand or to compartment syndrome of the forearm muscle compartments (see Compartment Syndrome, pp 17-19). Prompt treatment is required to salvage a functional arm.

## TREATMENT

The goal of treatment is to achieve and maintain a stable reduction that permits early motion. Stable, nondisplaced fractures can be treated with splinting for 10 days. Nearly all displaced fractures require open reduction and internal fixation. Other techniques, such as hinged external fixation or primary total elbow replacement, might be considered under circumstances such as severe osteoporosis and/or fracture comminution.

## ADVERSE OUTCOMES OF TREATMENT

Pain and stiffness can persist after treatment. Deformity, nonunion, and ulnar neuropathy can develop, as can symptoms related to the prominent implants used for internal fixation.

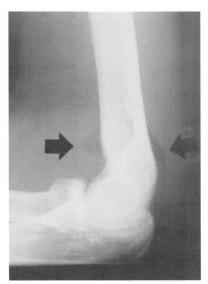

**Figure 3**
Anterior and posterior fat pad signs.

SECTION 3 | ELBOW AND FOREARM

## Referral decisions/Red flags

Patients with displaced fractures of the distal humerus need further evaluation to determine whether surgical stabilization of the fracture is necessary. Likewise, patients with associated neurovascular injury need further evaluation.

Patients treated with nonoperative management require close follow-up for complications such as fracture displacement and joint stiffness. Delayed vascular compromise can occur because of progressive swelling and/or tight splinting. Failure to regain motion is also an indication for referral.

# FRACTURE OF THE OLECRANON

## DEFINITION

The olecranon is the portion of the ulna that constitutes the bony prominence of the posterior elbow. Because of its subcutaneous position, the olecranon is easily fractured as a result of a direct blow to the elbow or a fall on an outstretched arm with the elbow flexed. As with other fractures, an important consideration is whether the fracture is displaced or nondisplaced. Most olecranon fractures are displaced and can be further classified as two-part fractures with either transverse or oblique fracture lines, comminuted fractures, or fracture-dislocations (**Figure 1**).

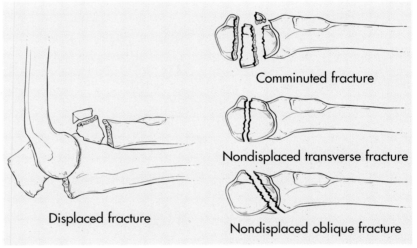

Comminuted fracture

Nondisplaced transverse fracture

Displaced fracture

Nondisplaced oblique fracture

**Figure 1**
Types of olecranon fractures.

*Adapted with permission from Jupiter JB, Mehne DK: Trauma to the adult elbow and fractures of the distal humerus, in Browner BD, Jupiter JB, Levine AM, et al (eds): Skeletal Trauma: Fractures, Dislocations, Ligamentous Injuries. Philadelphia, PA, WB Saunders, 1992, vol 2, pp 1125–1175.*

## CLINICAL SYMPTOMS

A history of trauma followed by marked swelling and ecchymosis is typical. When the patient has an associated dislocation, the elbow will appear deformed as well. Because of the close proximity of the ulnar nerve, the trauma itself or the resultant swelling can contuse the nerve and cause numbness in the little and ring fingers.

## TESTS

### PHYSICAL EXAMINATION

Examination usually reveals marked swelling of the entire elbow joint. Superficial abrasions at the site of impact are common and must be distinguished from deep wounds, which would make the injury an "open" fracture. Gentle palpation may reveal a defect if the fracture is displaced. Flexion of the elbow produces pain and is met with resistance. Median, radial, and ulnar nerve function should be assessed; of these, ulnar nerve injury is most common. Radial and ulnar pulses and capillary refill should be assessed, but significant vascular injury is uncommon with this fracture.

## DIAGNOSTIC TESTS

AP and lateral radiographs usually are adequate to confirm the diagnosis.

## DIFFERENTIAL DIAGNOSIS

Dislocation of the elbow (more grotesque deformity, evident on radiographs)

Fracture of the coronoid process of the olecranon (nearly always associated with an elbow dislocation)

Fracture of the distal humerus (more proximal area of pain, evident on radiographs)

Fracture of the radial head (lateral elbow pain increases with forearm rotation, fracture can be difficult to see on radiographs)

## ADVERSE OUTCOMES OF THE DISEASE

Loss of motion and/or stability in the elbow is possible. Because the triceps inserts on the tip of the olecranon, active elbow extension can be lost with displaced fractures. Arthritis of the elbow may develop.

## TREATMENT

Nondisplaced fractures of the olecranon can be treated with a posterior splint. To avoid excessive pull on the triceps and possible loss of reduction, position the elbow in approximately 45° of flexion. Follow-up radiographs should be obtained 7 to 10 days after the injury to ensure that the fracture has not become displaced. To maintain hand strength and flexibility, instruct patients to squeeze a rubber ball or commercially available hand exerciser for 5 minutes at least twice each day.

Most displaced fractures are best treated surgically. Occasionally, a displaced fracture in a debilitated elderly patient who is a poor risk for surgery can be treated with a sling and early range of motion, as pain allows.

## ADVERSE OUTCOMES OF TREATMENT

Elbow stiffness and loss of motion can develop despite treatment. Nonunion or displacement of the fracture also is possible. After operative treatment, irritation from the implants used to fix the fracture commonly occurs, necessitating a second procedure for implant removal.

## REFERRAL DECISIONS/RED FLAGS

Patients with displaced fractures or open fractures need further evaluation for possible operative treatment.

# FRACTURE OF THE RADIAL HEAD

ICD-9 Codes
813.05
    Fracture radial head
813.06
    Fracture radial neck

## DEFINITION

Fractures of the radial head and neck result from falls on the outstretched hand. The most commonly used classification system (modified Mason classification) separates these fractures into three types (**Figure 1**). Type I is a nondisplaced or minimally displaced fracture. Type II includes radial head fractures that are displaced more than 2 mm at the articular surface or angulated neck fractures that produce articular incongruity or a mechanical block. Type III fractures are severely comminuted fractures of the radial head and neck.

## CLINICAL SYMPTOMS

Following a fall on the outstretched arm, pain and swelling develop over the lateral aspect of the elbow. Loss of elbow motion may be related to pain inhibition and joint effusion, but a mechanical block to full forearm pronation and supination will be present in type II and III injuries. Radial head fractures also can be present in the context of an elbow dislocation.

## TESTS

### PHYSICAL EXAMINATION

Tenderness to palpation is localized to the lateral aspect of the joint, and a joint effusion can often be palpated. Passive forearm rotation is limited and may be associated with palpable crepitus. Elbow flexion and extension also may be limited by pain.

Tenderness over the forearm and/or wrist can signify a more extensive soft-tissue injury involving the radioulnar interosseous membrane and the distal radioulnar joint. Presence of this type of injury makes treatment more difficult.

### DIAGNOSTIC TESTS

Type I fractures may be difficult to visualize radiographically but should be suspected based on positive clinical findings. Type II and III fractures are usually obvious on AP and lateral radiographs.

## DIFFERENTIAL DIAGNOSIS

Elbow dislocation (clinical deformity and diffuse pain)

Hemarthrosis of the elbow (present with radial head fracture or with other bony or soft-tissue injury)

Olecranon fracture (pain and tenderness over the posterior tip of the elbow)

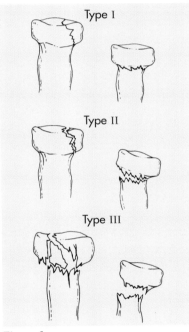

**Type I**

**Type II**

**Type III**

**Figure 1**
Classification of radial head fractures.

*Adapted with permission from Jupiter JB, Mehne DK: Trauma to the adult elbow and fractures of the distal humerus, in Browner BD, Jupiter JB, Levine AM, et al (eds): Skeletal Trauma: Fractures, Dislocations, Ligamentous Injuries. Philadelphia, PA, WB Saunders, 1992, vol 2, pp 1125–1175.*

SECTION 3 | ELBOW AND FOREARM

Supracondylar fracture of the humerus (location of pain, tenderness, and deformity)

## ADVERSE OUTCOMES OF THE DISEASE

Loss of motion, especially the last 10° to 15° of extension, is common, even with type I injuries. Posttraumatic arthritis of the radiocapitellar joint also may develop.

## TREATMENT

Type I fractures should be treated with a sling or splint for comfort and early active motion as soon as pain allows. Because early motion is the key to a successful outcome, aspiration of the associated elbow hemarthrosis should be considered.

Aspiration with local anesthetic injection is useful diagnostically in type II fractures to determine whether a mechanical block to forearm rotation is present. When the fracture involves displacement of less than 30% of the head and no block is present, treatment should consist of early range of motion, as in type I fractures. Otherwise, open reduction and internal fixation is preferred.

Type III fractures usually are best treated by early excision of the bone fragments. If the patient has associated injuries of the medial collateral ligament or interosseous membrane, other treatment considerations are required.

## ADVERSE OUTCOMES OF TREATMENT

Loss of motion, instability, and wrist pain caused by proximal radial migration after radial head excision can all occur.

## REFERRAL DECISIONS/RED FLAGS

Type II fractures that block rotation or involve more than 30% of the head, type III fractures, and any fracture associated with elbow dislocation or instability should be referred for surgical consideration. Failure of nonoperative treatment, manifested by persistent pain or limited motion, also indicates the need for further evaluation.

# OLECRANON BURSITIS

ICD-9 Code

726.33
Olecranon bursitis

## DEFINITION

Because of its superficial location on the extensor side of the elbow, the olecranon bursa is easily irritated and inflamed (**Figure 1**). Olecranon bursitis may be secondary to trauma, inflammation, or infection. Falls or direct blows may cause an acute inflammatory bursitis. Prolonged irritation from excessive leaning on the elbow results in chronic inflammation. The latter is associated with certain occupations and avocations. Olecranon bursitis also may develop in patients with chronic lung disease who lean on their elbows to aid breathing. Infection of the olecranon bursa (septic bursitis) may occur primarily or develop as a secondary complication of an aseptic bursitis.

## CLINICAL SYMPTOMS

The swelling associated with bursitis develops either gradually (chronic) or suddenly (infection or trauma). Pain is variable but can be intense and can limit motion after an acute injury or when infection is present. Severe swelling of the bursa may occur such that patients report difficulty putting on long-sleeved shirts. As the mass recedes, patients may feel firm "lumps" that are tender when the elbow is bumped. These lumps or nodules are scar tissue left as the fluid recedes.

Olecranon bursitis also occurs in patients with gout or rheumatoid arthritis. Gouty tophi (masses of monosodium urate crystals) can form in the olecranon bursa as well as along the ulnar border of the forearm, in the synovium of the elbow joint, and in numerous distant locations. Tophi are found only in patients with fairly advanced gout. As with gout, rheumatoid nodules can appear in several subcutaneous locations, such as over the olecranon and the ulnar border of the forearm. With time, these nodules can spontaneously shrink or disappear.

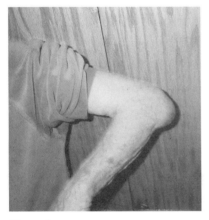

**Figure 1**
Swollen olecranon bursa.

*Adapted with permission from Jupiter JB, Mehne DK: Trauma to the adult elbow and fractures of the distal humerus, in Browner BD, Jupiter JB, Levine AM, et al (eds): Skeletal Trauma: Fractures, Dislocations, Ligamentous Injuries. Philadelphia, PA, WB Saunders, 1992, vol 2, pp 1125–1175.*

## TESTS

### PHYSICAL EXAMINATION

Examination can reveal a large mass, up to 6 cm in diameter, over the tip of the elbow. The skin might be abraded or even lacerated if related to trauma. Redness and heat are not uncommon with acute bursitis and could indicate infection. Exquisite tenderness usually results from an infectious or traumatic origin. Chronic, recurrent swelling usually is less tender. The dimensions of the bursa should be measured periodically to monitor progress.

### DIAGNOSTIC TESTS

When the mass is large and symptomatic, aspiration can be both diagnostic and therapeutic (see Olecranon Bursa Aspiration, pp 191-192). After an acute injury, bloody fluid can be found. Any fluid that is cloudy or has a foul odor should be cultured. When the origin is traumatic, radiographs should be obtained to rule out a fracture of the olecranon process of the ulna.

## DIFFERENTIAL DIAGNOSIS

Fracture of the olecranon process of the ulna (evident on radiographs)

Gout (elevated serum uric acid)

Rheumatoid arthritis (multiple joint involvement, positive results on serologic tests)

Synovial cyst of the elbow joint (synovial fluid positive for crystals, lateral or medial location)

## ADVERSE OUTCOMES OF THE DISEASE

Infection, chronic recurrence or drainage, and swelling or limited motion can develop.

## TREATMENT

If it is small and mildly symptomatic, the bursitis should be left alone or treated symptomatically with activity modifications and possibly NSAIDs. Patients with more symptomatic bursitis should undergo aspiration of the bursa, followed by Gram stain and culture of any suspicious fluid. If there is no indication of septic bursitis, a compression bandage consisting of a circularly shaped piece of foam, 8 cm in diameter, and an elastic wrap should be applied. Reassess the patient in 2 to 7 days. If cultures are negative and fluid has reaccumulated in the bursa, repeat the aspiration and, if the fluid does not look infected, inject 1 mL of a corticosteroid preparation into the sac. The bursal sac may have to be aspirated two or more times. If the patient's elbow is at risk for repeated trauma, then recommend an elbow protector to prevent further trauma.

Septic olecranon bursitis requires aspiration for culture, antibiotic coverage for penicillin-resistant *Staphylococcus aureus*, and decompression by either surgical drainage or daily aspiration. Oral antibiotics may be administered if the septic bursitis is treated early and the patient is not immunocompromised. Hospitalization with intravenous antibiotics and surgical drainage and irrigation is indicated if the patient does not respond to oral antibiotics or if the patient has a more serious infection.

Excision of chronically inflamed aseptic bursitis is not commonly necessary and should be avoided because a chronically draining or infected sinus can develop.

## ADVERSE OUTCOMES OF TREATMENT

Infection, chronic drainage, or recurrence are possible.

## REFERRAL DECISIONS/RED FLAGS

Recurrence of fluid despite repeated (three or more) aspirations or septic bursitis needs further evaluation.

# PROCEDURE

## OLECRANON BURSA ASPIRATION

### MATERIALS

Sterile gloves

Bactericidal skin preparation solution

2 - 1-mL syringes

27-gauge, ¾" needle

1 mL of 1% lidocaine without epinephrine

10-mL syringe

18-gauge needle

1 mL of a 40 mg/mL cortico-steroid preparation (optional)

Adhesive bandage

The olecranon bursa lies on the extensor aspect of the elbow, over the olecranon process of the ulna. The ulnar nerve lies adjacent to the medial face of the olecranon, behind the ulnar groove of the distal humerus. For this reason, aspiration is best done from the lateral side.

### STEP 1

Wear protective gloves at all times during this procedure and use sterile technique. This is important in aspirating an olecranon bursa because secondary infection may develop.

### STEP 2

Prep the skin with a bactericidal solution.

### STEP 3

Use a 27-gauge needle to infiltrate the skin over the lateral aspect of the bursa with 1 mL of 1% lidocaine.

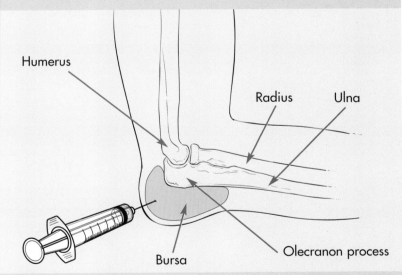

**Figure 1**
Location for needle insertion.

### STEP 4

Through the skin wheal, insert the 18-gauge needle attached to the 10-mL syringe into the enlarged bursa (**Figure 1**). Aspirate the contents until the bursa is flat. If there is any concern about infection, send the fluid for culture and sensitivity and do not inject the corticosteroid preparation into the cavity.

### STEP 5

If infection does not seem probable, a corticosteroid injection may be helpful. Remove the aspirating syringe and attach a 1-mL syringe containing 1 mL of a 40 mg/mL corticosteroid preparation. Inject this into the bursal cavity.

### STEP 6

Dress the puncture wound with a sterile adhesive bandage.

### STEP 7

Lightly wrap the elbow with an elastic dressing.

## ADVERSE OUTCOMES

Secondary infection is possible, though not likely if sterile technique is used. Recurrence of the bursal effusion is frequent but can be minimized by a compressive dressing and having the patient avoid direct trauma to the elbow (eg, resting the elbow on tabletops).

## AFTERCARE/PATIENT INSTRUCTIONS

Advise the patient to limit elbow motion for 1 or 2 days after the aspiration. If the patient has a recurrent bursitis, use a posterior plaster splint to limit elbow motion for 1 to 2 weeks after the aspiration.

# RUPTURE OF THE DISTAL BICEPS TENDON

## ICD-9 Code

**841.9**
Sprains and strains of elbow and forearm, unspecified site

## DEFINITION

Rupture of the distal biceps brachii tendon is uncommon, accounting for less than 5% of biceps tendon ruptures. However, in contrast to tears of the proximal biceps tendon, complete tears of the distal biceps tendon cause significantly greater weakness. If the lesion is not recognized and repaired in a timely fashion, strength of elbow flexion and forearm supination is decreased by 30% to 50%. Most often, ruptures occur in men older than 40 years of age who have preexisting degenerative changes in the biceps tendon.

These ruptures typically are located at the insertion of the biceps tendon into the radius (radial tuberosity). The rupture may be incomplete or complete. With complete ruptures, the biceps aponeurosis may remain intact initially.

## CLINICAL SYMPTOMS

Patients often report a history of sudden, sharp pain in the anterior elbow that followed an excessive extension force on the flexed elbow. The pain typically is severe for a few hours (acute inflammatory response), and then is followed by a chronic, dull ache in the anterior elbow region that is made worse by lifting activities.

## TESTS

### PHYSICAL EXAMINATION

Examination reveals tenderness and a defect in the antecubital fossa due to the absence of the usually prominent biceps tendon. Early on, ecchymosis will be present in the antecubital fossa and proximal forearm. With flexion of the elbow against resistance, the muscle belly retracts proximally (**Figure 1**).

If the rupture is incomplete, the defect will not be apparent, but the patient will exhibit pain and weakness on flexion of the elbow against resistance. If the rupture is complete but the bicipital aponeurosis is intact, the defect is not as obvious; however, comparison with the opposite side helps to confirm the diagnosis.

### DIAGNOSTIC TESTS

AP and lateral radiographs of the elbow usually are normal but may reveal an avulsion fracture of the bicipital tuberosity. MRI can be helpful in inconclusive cases.

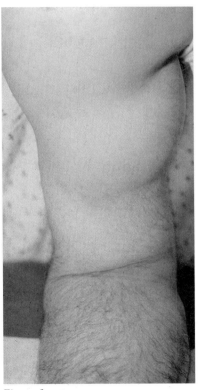

**Figure 1**
Clinical appearance of distal biceps tendon rupture.

Reprinted with permission from Ramsey ML: Distal biceps tendon injuries: diagnosis and management. J Am Acad Ortho Surg 1999;7:199-207.

## DIFFERENTIAL DIAGNOSIS

Bicipital tendinosis (tendon degenerative changes without rupture)

Cubital bursitis (enlargement of the bursa between the biceps tendon and radial tuberosity, may occur primarily or secondary to other conditions)

Entrapment of the lateral antebrachial cutaneous nerve (pain and dysesthesia lateral aspect proximal forearm)

## ADVERSE OUTCOMES OF THE DISEASE

Loss of elbow flexor strength is significant, particularly with the forearm in supination. Loss of forearm supination power (eg, turning a screwdriver) also occurs. With time, the muscle retracts and becomes fibrotic. In this situation, operative repair either is not possible or the results compromised with less return of muscle strength.

## TREATMENT

Most patients with complete ruptures do better with operative repair of the tendon. Partial ruptures can be managed nonoperatively with activity modification and intermittent splinting, but if this treatment fails, operative repair is indicated. Nonoperative management is used with older patients who are sedentary and do not require normal elbow flexor strength and endurance.

## ADVERSE OUTCOMES OF TREATMENT

Full return of muscle strength may not occur. Injury to the radial nerve is possible.

## REFERRAL DECISIONS/RED FLAGS

Due to the adverse and progressive effect on muscle strength, patients with rupture of the distal tendon of the biceps should be evaluated for possible operative repair.

# ULNAR NERVE COMPRESSION

## ICD-9 Code
354.2
Compression of the ulnar nerve

## SYNONYMS
Cubital tunnel syndrome
Tardy ulnar palsy
Ulnar nerve neuritis

## DEFINITION

Compression of the ulnar nerve at the elbow is second only to carpal tunnel syndrome as a source of nerve entrapment in the upper extremity. The nerve can be compressed at a number of sites from 10 cm proximal to the elbow to 5 cm below the joint. The most common sites are where the ulnar nerve passes in the groove on the posterior aspect of the medial epicondyle, in the so-called "cubital tunnel," and where it passes between the humeral and ulnar heads of the flexor carpi ulnaris muscle.

Ulnar nerve compression can develop acutely after a direct blow. Chronic symptoms occur in individuals who put prolonged pressure on the nerve by continuously leaning on the elbow or who keep the nerve on stretch by holding the elbows flexed for long periods during work or recreation (Figure 1). Ulnar nerve compression also can occur after trauma that results in osteophytes or scar tissue that encroach upon the nerve. Cubitus valgus (a carrying angle of more than 10°) places the nerve on stretch and over time also may cause ulnar neuritis. Instability of the ulnar nerve with repetitive subluxation or dislocation of the ulnar nerve on elbow flexion also can cause ulnar palsy.

## CLINICAL SYMPTOMS

Symptoms vary depending on the duration and severity of the nerve compression. Early symptoms include aching pain at the medial aspect of the elbow and numbness and tingling in the ring and little fingers. The paresthesias occasionally radiate proximally into the shoulder and neck. Weakness of the intrinsic muscles is a late finding and can interfere with activities of daily living, such as opening jars or turning a key in a door. Visible muscle wasting implies ulnar nerve compression of several months' to years' duration.

## TESTS

### PHYSICAL EXAMINATION

Inspect the elbow for deformity and measure the carrying angle. The nerve should be palpated for any mass lesions or localized tenderness. Lightly tapping on the nerve can cause pain and paresthesias over the ulnar border of the hand and the ring and little fingers (Tinel test).

Place your index finger over the ulnar groove as the elbow is flexed and extended to determine if the nerve slips out of the groove. The elbow flexion

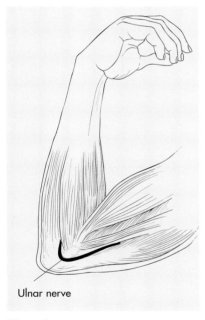

**Figure 1**
Ulnar nerve compressed during elbow flexion.

*Adapted with permission from Mackinnon SE, Dellon AL: Surgery of the Peripheral Nerve. New York, NY, Thieme Medical Publishers, 1988.*

Ulnar nerve

test is a provocative maneuver. The patient should flex the elbow as much as possible and then report any tingling or numbness in the hand as soon as it is felt (elbow flexion test). Record how quickly symptoms appear; when the symptoms do not develop within 60 seconds, the test is considered negative.

Assess sensation and muscle function of the ulnar nerve. Vibration and light touch perception are the first to be affected, and the little finger and the ulnar half of the ring finger are most likely to be involved. Two-point discrimination is affected when nerve compression has progressed to axonal degeneration.

Weakness is assessed by testing abduction and adduction of the little and index fingers, the ability to cross the index and middle fingers, and thumb-to-index pinch. With ulnar nerve entrapment and adductor muscle weakness, the interphalangeal joint of the thumb will flex (Froment sign) with thumb-to-index pinch. The ulnarly innervated extrinsic muscles are less commonly involved. Wasting of the intrinsic muscles is a late finding and produces a hollowed-out appearance between the metacarpals on the dorsal aspect of the hand.

## Diagnostic tests

Nerve conduction velocity studies provide an objective measurement of nerve compression. A reduction in velocity of 30% or more suggests significant compression of the ulnar nerve. Plain radiographs of the elbow are indicated when previous elbow trauma has occurred.

## Differential diagnosis

Carpal tunnel syndrome (numbness in thumb, index, and middle fingers; thenar muscle wasting)

Herniated cervical disk (rarely involves the C8 and T1 nerve roots)

Medial epicondylitis (tenderness over the medial epicondyle; no distal weakness, paresthesias, or numbness)

Thoracic outlet syndrome (normal nerve conduction velocity studies at the elbow; rarely, wasting in the hand)

Ulnar nerve entrapment at the wrist (strong wrist flexors and ulnar deviators, sensation intact over the dorsomedial hand and the dorsum of the little and ring fingers)

## Adverse outcomes of the disease

Loss of grip and pinch strength and loss of sensation in the ring and little fingers can be progressive and permanent in long-standing cases. Pain and tenderness at the elbow also can persist.

## Treatment

Modifying activities in the workplace to limit elbow flexion and direct pressure on the ulnar nerve is the most important step in treatment. At night, an elbow splint that keeps the elbow from flexing to a right angle can be worn. (A towel wrapped around the elbow is sufficient if a commercial splint is not available.) A sports elbow protector can be used at work to keep from bumping the elbow. NSAIDs can be of benefit for an acute, severe episode. Corticosteroid injections are not recommended.

Surgical decompression and transposition of the ulnar nerve should be considered for patients with bothersome symptoms or mild weakness that persists despite 3 to 4 months of nonoperative management or for patients with significant or progressive weakness.

## ADVERSE OUTCOMES OF TREATMENT

Care should be taken that any splint applied does not have straps across the medial elbow because this could increase nerve compression. NSAIDs can cause gastric, renal, or hepatic complications. Symptoms are not always improved after surgery.

## REFERRAL DECISIONS/RED FLAGS

Significant or progressive weakness or atrophy of the intrinsic muscles, or increasing numbness despite nonoperative treatment, indicates the need for further evaluation.

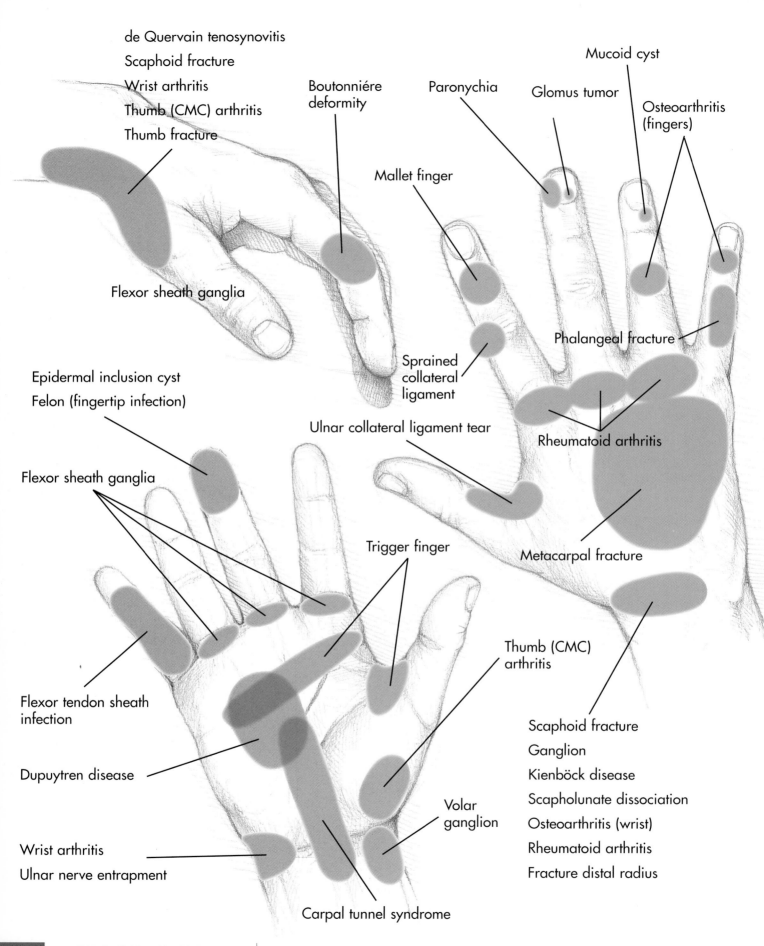

de Quervain tenosynovitis
Scaphoid fracture
Wrist arthritis
Thumb (CMC) arthritis
Thumb fracture

Boutonniére deformity

Paronychia

Mucoid cyst

Glomus tumor

Osteoarthritis (fingers)

Mallet finger

Flexor sheath ganglia

Phalangeal fracture

Sprained collateral ligament

Epidermal inclusion cyst
Felon (fingertip infection)

Ulnar collateral ligament tear

Rheumatoid arthritis

Flexor sheath ganglia

Trigger finger

Metacarpal fracture

Flexor tendon sheath infection

Thumb (CMC) arthritis

Dupuytren disease

Scaphoid fracture
Ganglion
Kienböck disease
Scapholunate dissociation
Osteoarthritis (wrist)
Rheumatoid arthritis
Fracture distal radius

Volar ganglion

Wrist arthritis
Ulnar nerve entrapment

Carpal tunnel syndrome

# HAND AND WRIST

**Section Editor**
Thomas R. Johnson, MD
Orthopedic Surgeons, PSC
St. Vincent Hospital and Health Center
Billings, Montana

William H. Anderson, Jr, MD
Department of Rehabilitation Medicine
St. Vincent Hospital and Health Center
Billings, Montana

W. Lea Gorsuch, MD
Great Falls Orthopaedic Associates
Great Falls, Michigan

Merlin L. Hamer, MD
LaJolla, California

Charles D. Jennings, MD
Great Falls Orthopaedic Associates
Great Falls, Michigan

Bert Jones, MD
Flathead Valley Orthopedics
Kalispell, Montana

James F. Schwarten, MD
Orthopaedic Surgeons, PSC
Yellowstone Medical Center
Billings, Montana

# HAND AND WRIST—AN OVERVIEW

Patients with chronic hand and wrist problems typically will have one (or more) of the following seven complaints: 1) pain, 2) instability, 3) stiffness, 4) swelling, 5) weakness, 6) numbness, or 7) a mass. Carpal tunnel syndrome, trigger finger, ganglia, carpometacarpal (CMC) arthritis of the thumb, and radiocarpal arthritis constitute more than 90% of the chronic problems in the hand and wrist.

Obtaining a complete history, including the patient's age, exact location of the pain, and whether the problem is acute or chronic, accompanied by a thorough physical examination, should result in making a correct diagnosis in more than 90% of patients. Because all of the structures in the hand and wrist are no more distant than 1.5 cm from the skin, palpation for swelling and tenderness is relatively easy (**Figure 1**). Diagnostic testing should be limited to plain radiographs in most patients.

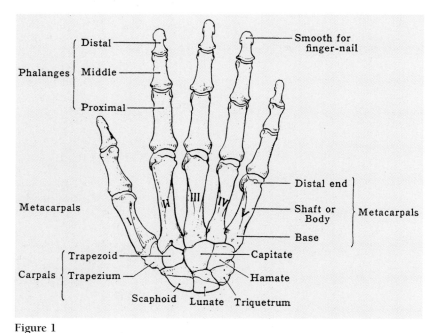

**Figure 1**
Bones of the hand: palmar view.

*Adapted with permission from Anderson JE: Grant's Atlas of Anatomy, ed 8. Baltimore, MD, Williams & Wilkins, 1983.*

## LOCATION OF PAIN

Localizing the patient's pain to one of the following four areas: radial; ulnar; volar; and dorsal; considerably reduces the list of possible diagnoses (**Figure 2**).

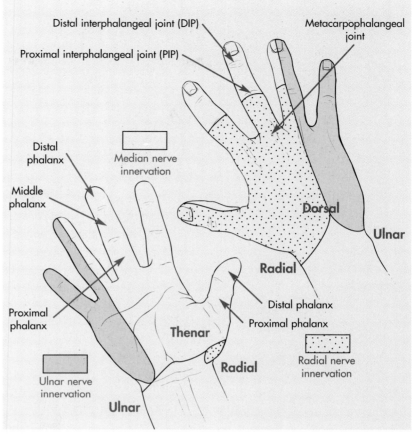

**Figure 2**
Regions of and sensory distribution in the hand.

## RADIAL PAIN

Wrist pain in patients younger than 30 years most commonly results from trauma. Posttraumatic tenderness and pain over the radial aspect of the wrist suggest a possible fracture of the scaphoid, which is the most commonly missed fracture in the wrist and hand. In the absence of trauma, pain associated with tenderness over the radial styloid is most likely de Quervain (wrist) tenosynovitis. Pain that occurs without numbness in patients older than 40 years is likely caused by posttraumatic arthritis or osteoarthritis. Pain at the base of the thumb in women in this age group is likely to be CMC arthritis.

## DORSAL PAIN

Pain in this region associated with a well-defined mass over the dorsoradial aspect of the wrist typically is a ganglion. Pain and loss of motion in the wrist in young adults is commonly Kienböck disease (osteonecrosis of the lunate). Plain radiographs easily confirm the diagnosis in the later stages of Kienböck disease.

## ULNAR PAIN

Pain in this region after trauma can be caused by a tear of the triangular fibro-cartilage complex, which is located distal to the ulnar styloid. Swelling and tenderness over the dorsoulnar or volar aspects of the wrist are likely caused by a tendinitis of the ulnar wrist extensor or flexor tendons.

## VOLAR PAIN

Carpal tunnel syndrome is by far the most common cause of volar wrist pain. Other causes include a volar ganglion, which should be easily palpable on the volar radial aspect of the wrist. Swelling over the volar region suggests inflammation of the finger flexor tendons. Patients with radiocarpal arthritis might have pain over both the dorsal and volar aspects of the wrist. Volar wrist pain also can be caused by arthritis between the pisiform and the triquetrum bones.

# INSTABILITY

Diagnosis of wrist instability is often quite complex, requiring considerable experience in interpreting radiographs, localizing signs and symptoms, and performing the physical examination. Typical symptoms are sensations of slipping, snapping, or clunking with certain wrist motions after an injury. The unstable structure might be a joint (following a tear of the supporting and stabilizing ligaments that hold together the carpal bones) or a subluxating tendon (following a tear of the restraining ligaments that guide the tendon). Plain posteroanterior radiographs of the wrist might show separation between the scaphoid and the lunate (Terry-Thomas sign), indicating a tear of the ligaments binding the scaphoid and the lunate (scapholunate dissociation).

# STIFFNESS

Morning stiffness is a common complaint with arthritis or tenosynovitis and also may be associated with carpal tunnel syndrome or trigger finger. Patients with trigger finger often have pain, as well, and localize the problem to the proximal interphalangeal (PIP) joint when it locks or "jumps" as the finger is flexed. In fact, the source of the problem is in the palm, where the thickened flexor tendon hangs up under the proximal tendon pulley at the distal palmar crease. Tenderness just distal to this crease confirms the diagnosis of trigger finger.

# SWELLING

Swelling in the joints of the hand and wrist is caused by synovitis, which can be secondary to infection or a systemic disease such as rheumatoid arthritis or gout. A history of penetrating trauma will help distinguish infection from systemic disease. Plain radiographs are useful in diagnosing osteoarthritis and rheumatoid arthritis. Swelling around the tendons can occur in association with rheumatoid arthritis and/or overuse syndromes such as de Quervain tenosynovitis. Pain and swelling around the wrist flexor or extensor tendons suggest calcific tendinitis; plain radiographs may show a calcific deposit in close proximity to the involved tendon.

## WEAKNESS

Weakness in the hand can be secondary to pain, as with CMC or radiocarpal arthritis. Weakness without pain suggests possible peripheral nerve entrapment. Ulnar nerve entrapment at the elbow will result in decreased grip and pinch strength in addition to loss of sensation in the little and ring fingers. A positive Finkelstein test and wasting of the intrinsic muscles is easily seen on physical examination in advanced cases.

## NUMBNESS

Figure 2 also shows the typical sensory distribution of the median, ulnar, and radial nerves; however, variability from this pattern can occur. Loss of sensation in some or all of the fingers should be considered indicative of carpal tunnel syndrome until proven otherwise. With carpal tunnel syndrome, the numbness characteristically occurs in the thumb, the index and long fingers, and the radial half of the ring finger; some patients report that the entire hand is numb.

Loss of sensation in the little and ring fingers usually is caused by entrapment of the ulnar nerve at the elbow (also possibly at the wrist, but this is rare). Patients with thoracic outlet syndrome often report symptoms at the ulnar side of the hand and forearm, but this condition is much less common than ulnar nerve entrapment at the elbow. Both the Tinel sign and elbow flexion tests will be negative with thoracic outlet syndrome.

Neck pain associated with loss of sensation in the thumb and index finger suggests a C6 radiculopathy, for which the Phalen test will be negative.

## MASSES

The most common mass in the hand and wrist is a ganglion cyst; these cysts most often occur in four locations: the dorsoradial and volar radial aspects of the wrist; the proximal finger flexor crease; and the distal interphalangeal joint. Multilobulated masses along the sides of the finger are most likely giant cell tumors. Nontender nodules in the palm and cords that cross both the metacarpophalangeal and PIP joints are consistent with Dupuytren disease. A hard mass at the dorsal base of the index metacarpal is a carpal boss—a bony mass consisting of spurs from the second and third metacarpals, the trapezoid, and the capitate.

# PHYSICAL EXAMINATION HAND AND WRIST

## Inspection/Palpation

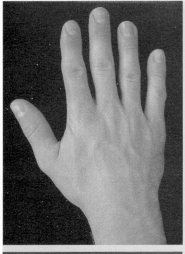

### Dorsum

Observe the alignment of the fingers. Inspect the nails for pitting and other evidence of systemic disorders. Look for swelling and synovitis of the finger and wrist joints. Note any osteophytes or bony prominences associated with degenerative arthritis. Atrophy between the metacarpals is caused by weakness of the intrinsic muscles.

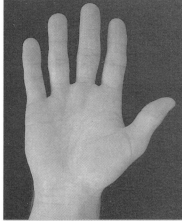

### Palm

Look for atrophy of the thenar muscles (median nerve innervated) and hypothenar muscles (ulnar nerve innervated). Note any thickening of the palmar fascia associated with Dupuytren contracture. Pain elicited by pressure over the thumb metacarpophalangeal (MP) joint suggests arthritis or instability of this joint.

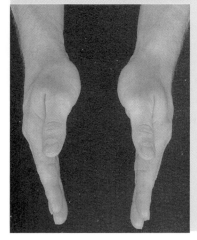

### Side view

Position the patient's hands with the palms facing each other to best visualize atrophy of the thenar muscles. Swelling in the joints of the thumb also is prominent in this position.

# Range of Motion

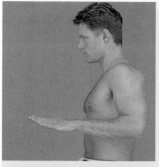

### Wrist flexion/extension: Zero Starting Position

Place the patient's forearm in the Zero Starting Position with forearm in pronation and the carpus aligned with the plane of the forearm. Place the goniometer on the dorsum of the wrist or on the radial side of the forearm to measure flexion and extension. Aligning the goniometer on the ulnar side may falsely elevate the measurement because of the mobility of the fifth metacarpal. Wrist motion occurs at the radiocarpal and midcarpal joints. Normal wrist flexion is 75° to 80°, and normal extension is 55° to 65°.

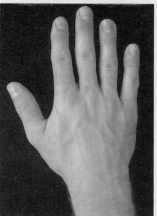

### Wrist radial/ulnar deviation

Place the patient's forearm in the Zero Starting Position with forearm in pronation and the carpus aligned with the plane of the forearm to measure radial and ulnar deviation. Align the goniometer with the third metacarpal and the axis of the forearm. In radial and ulnar deviation, the carpal rows rotate as linked segments. The buttress of the radial styloid limits radial deviation so that its arc of motion is significantly less. Normal radial deviation is 20° to 25°, and ulnar deviation is 35° to 40°.

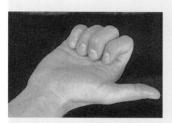

### Finger flexion/extension

Finger joint motion occurs primarily in the flexion-extension plane, with flexion accounting for most finger joint motion. From a functional perspective, finger flexion is a composite movement of motion of the MP, proximal interphalangeal (PIP), and distal interphalangeal (DIP) joints. Gender does not affect finger flexion in young adults; however, osteoarthritis often affects the DIP and PIP joints in older women; therefore, older men often demonstrate a greater range of finger joint motion. To evaluate whether flexion is impaired, measure the distance from the fingertip to the distal palmar crease. In young and middle-aged adults, the fingertip should touch the distal palmar crease. Flexion and extension also can be measured individually at the MP, PIP, and DIP joints. The wrist should be in neutral when measuring finger flexion. If the wrist is flexed, the extensor digitorum longus will be effectively tethered, thereby limiting finger flexion.

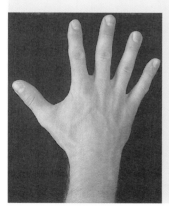

### Finger abduction/adduction

Abduction and adduction occur in the plane of the palm, primarily at the MP joints and centered on the long finger. Abduction is movement of the fingers away from the middle finger, while adduction is movement of the other fingers toward the long finger.

# Range of Motion

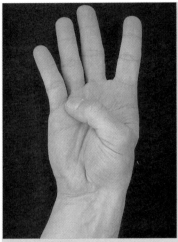

### Thumb opposition

Thumb motions are complex and reflect the overall importance of the thumb to the function of the hand. The principal thumb motions are abduction, adduction, opposition, flexion, and extension. Opposition is a composite motion created by movement at the carpometacarpal (CMC), MP, and IP joints and is valued as 50% to 60% of thumb function.

Measure opposition by asking the patient to touch the tip of the thumb to the base of the little finger. The amount of impairment can be assessed by measuring the distance from the tip of the thumb to the base of the little finger.

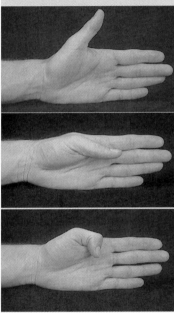

### Thumb flexion/extension

All thumb joints move in the plane of flexion-extension, but this movement is difficult to quantify at the CMC joint. Flexion at the thumb MP joint is typically 50° to 60°, but normal measurements also can be significantly less. Flexion at the IP joint ranges from 55° to 75° and depends on age and gender. Extension usually is not observed at the MP joint and is only 5° to 10° at the IP joint.

Measure thumb motion with the wrist in a neutral position. If the wrist is flexed, the extensor pollicis longus will be tethered, thereby limiting flexion at the MP and IP joints.

# Muscle Testing

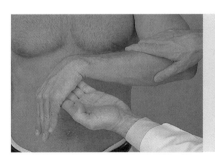

### Wrist flexion

To test the strength of the wrist flexors, the most powerful of which is the flexor carpi ulnaris, resist the patient's attempt to flex the wrist with the elbow fixed at 90°and the fingers extended (eliminates action of finger flexors). Weakness will be evident with fracture of the medial humeral condyle, tendinitis of the medial elbow, or lesions involving the median or ulnar nerve.

# Muscle Testing

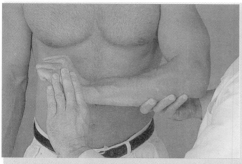

## Wrist extension

To test the strength of the wrist extensors, the most powerful of which are the extensor carpi ulnaris and extensor carpi radialis brevis, resist the patient's attempt to extend the wrist (eliminates action of finger extensors). Weakness will be evident with rupture of the extensor origin, fracture of the lateral humeral condyle, epicondylitis, or lesions involving the radial nerve or C6-C7 nerve roots.

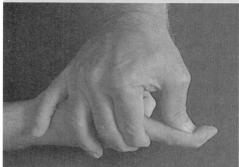

## Flexor digitorum profundus

Hold the PIP joint in extension and ask the patient to bend the finger. Inability to flex the DIP joint indicates an injury to the profundus tendon or injury to the median nerve or its anterior interosseous branch (innervates flexor digitorum profundus to index and often long finger), or to the ulnar nerve (innervates ring and little finger DIP joint).

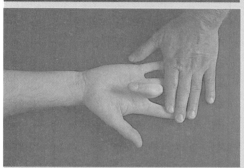

## Flexor digitorum sublimis

Hold all the fingers in full extension except for the finger being tested. Ask the patient to bend the fingers. The flexor digitorum profundus cannot independently flex the fingers when it is kept tethered by the other fingers being kept in extension. However, the flexor digitorum sublimis of each finger can work independently. A normal response is flexion at the PIP joint (figure). Inability to flex this finger indicates an injury to the sublimis tendon to that finger or injury to the median nerve.

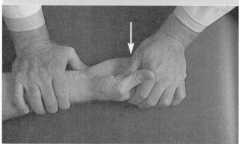

## Opponens strength

With the patient's hand palm up on the examining surface, ask the patient to abduct the thumb (place it straight up) and resist your attempt to push it down onto the table (abduction and extension). Weakness indicates damage to the motor branch of the median nerve, most commonly related to carpal tunnel syndrome.

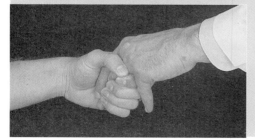

## Grip strength

A decrease in total grip strength reflects weakness of the finger flexors and/or intrinsic muscles of the hand.

# Sensory Testing

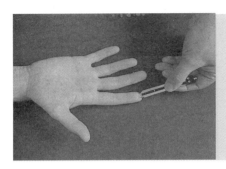

## Median, ulnar, and radial nerves

Assess median nerve sensation at the tip of the thumb, ulnar nerve at the tip of the little finger, and radial nerve at the dorsum of the thumb metacarpal. Check light touch and, for a more complete evaluation, assess two-point discrimination. Ask the patient to close both eyes as you lightly touch both points of an electrocardiogram caliper to the fingertip. Determine whether the patient is able to distinguish the two points 5-mm apart as separate points or a single point. Inability to discriminate the two points indicates diminished sensation.

# Special Tests

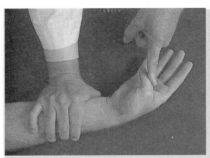

## Finkelstein test–de Quervain tenosynovitis

Flex and ulnarly deviate the wrist, then push the thumb into flexion. Pain at the dorsoradial aspect of the wrist indicates tenosynovitis of the first dorsal compartment (abductor pollicis longus and extensor brevis) tendons.

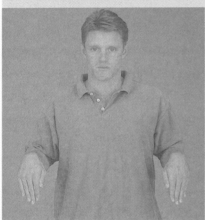

## Phalen test–Carpal tunnel syndrome

Ask the patient to hold both elbows with the forearms extending up perpendicular to the ground. Then have the patient let both wrists drop into flexion by gravity alone. Patients who experience numbness or tingling in the distribution of the median nerve within 60 seconds have a positive result.

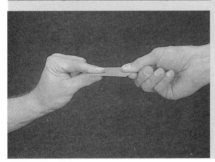

## Froment sign

Ask the patient to pinch a piece of paper between the thumb and index finger tip. If the adductor pollicis muscle is weak (ulnar nerve paralysis), the thumb IP joint will flex. Compare function with that of the opposite, normal thumb.

# Special Tests

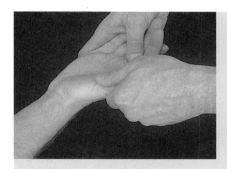

### Watson stress test—CMC arthritis

With the patient's palm up and the back of the hand resting on the table, and with the thumb in palmar abduction, push the thumb down toward the table with the MP and IP joints extended.

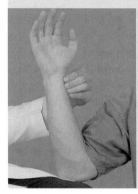

### Allen test—Arterial circulation to the hand

Ask the patient to open and close the hand three times, making a tight fist to exsanguinate the hand. Then compress the radial and ulnar arteries at the wrist with the fingers clenched. Release the ulnar artery while keeping the radial artery compressed. If the fingers and palm fill with blood (typically within 5 seconds), the ulnar artery is patent. Repeat these steps keeping the ulnar artery compressed but releasing the radial artery. Note the time for refilling of the hand. Commonly, one artery is dominant in supplying circulation to the hand.

# ANIMAL BITES

## ICD-9 Codes

882.0
    Open wound of hand, except
    fingers, without mention of
    complications
883.0
    Open wound of finger(s) without
    mention of complication
E906.0
    Dog bite
E906.3
    Cat bite

## DEFINITION

As many as 3 million people in the United States sustain animal bites each year. Animal bites most commonly occur on the fingers in the dominant hand of children. Dog bites account for up to 90% of animal bites; cat bites are second most common, constituting 5% of animal bites.

The risk of infection from a dog bite is 5% to 10%; the risk of infection from a cat bite is much higher (30% to 50%) because a cat's sharp teeth create deeper puncture wounds. The causative organism varies. *Pasteurella multocida* is a bacterium commonly associated with dog and cat bite wounds. Other bacteria isolated in dog bite wounds include α-hemolytic streptococci and *Staphylococcus aureus,* and anaerobic organisms such as *Bacteroides* and *Fusobacterium.*

Because rabies is a possibility as a result of the bite, it is important to be familiar with the status of rabies in your area. In the United States, more than 90% of rabies comes from wild animals, especially bats, skunks, raccoons, and foxes. However, outside the United States, the dog is the most common source of rabies. Approximately 50% of rabies cases reported to the Centers for Disease Control and Prevention in 1985 were from dog bites that occurred in foreign countries.

## CLINICAL SYMPTOMS

Pain, swelling, and redness around the puncture wound suggest an infection secondary to the bite. Loss of sensation and motion distal to the bite may indicate that a nerve or tendon is severed. Determine whether the bite was provoked by a sudden movement toward the animal. An animal that initiates an unprovoked attack is more likely to be rabid. The animal should be found, if possible, and observed for 10 days to determine whether it does or does not become ill.

## TESTS

### PHYSICAL EXAMINATION

Examination may reveal an irregular, jagged wound with devitalized tissue at the margins and swelling and redness around the wound. The depth of the wound and the time at which the patient was bitten should be determined. Purulent drainage may be present if the wound is more than 10 to 12 hours old. Sensation and tendon function should be tested in the affected hand or finger. Inspect the forearm for the presence of red streaks caused by lymphangitis. The inner aspect of the elbow and the axilla should be palpated for the presence of enlarged lymph nodes. Ensure that the patient's temperature is checked to rule out a fever.

## DIAGNOSTIC TESTS

AP and lateral radiographs of the affected part are necessary to rule out a fracture or presence of a foreign body. These views also may reveal gas in the soft tissues. Routine laboratory studies are not needed for wounds seen shortly after injury. However, if an infection is suspected, a swab of the wound should be sent for a Gram stain and aerobic and anaerobic cultures.

## DIFFERENTIAL DIAGNOSIS

Foreign body with secondary infection

## ADVERSE OUTCOMES OF THE DISEASE

Any of the following conditions could develop as a result of an untreated animal bite: sepsis in the joint, deep space infection, septic tenosynovitis, osteomyelitis, and/or rabies. Patients also may lose sensation and motion, and possibly their fingers, following an animal bite. Lymphedema with hand and finger stiffness is also possible.

## TREATMENT

Debridement, wound irrigation with 500 to 1,000 mL of saline solution, and outpatient antibiotics are appropriate for superficial wounds that do not have a nerve, tendon, or bony injury. Use of an anesthetic block will facilitate debridement of bite wounds on the finger. When the bite wound is on the back of the hand, 3 to 10 mL of local anesthetic should be infiltrated around the wound. Oral amoxicillin-clavulanate, 500 mg twice a day for 5 days, is a standard antibiotic regimen.

Primary suturing of animal bite wounds is controversial and hazardous. On occasion, some dog bite wounds might be sutured primarily as long as all necrotic tissue is debrided and the closure is loose over a Penrose drain. Because of a higher rate of infection associated with cat bites, these wounds should never be sutured primarily. In general, it is safest to leave animal bites open.

When there are signs of infection, closure should be delayed or the wound allowed to close by secondary intention. Intravenous antibiotics are indicated in this situation. Empiric therapy can be started with IV ampicillin-sulbactam, 1.5 to 3.0 g every 6 hours pending culture results and sensitivities. Tetracycline can be used in patients with a penicillin allergy. The patient can be switched to oral antibiotics in 24 to 48 hours if the wound is healing satisfactorily. Tetanus prophylaxis should be given, as outlined in Table 1.

When the animal is believed to be rabid, contact local or state public health officials regarding the need for rabies prophylaxis.

SECTION 4 | HAND AND WRIST

## Table 1
### Guide to Tetanus Prophylaxis in Wound Management

| History of tetanus toxoid (doses) | Clean, minor wound | | Contaminated wound | |
|---|---|---|---|---|
| | Td | TIG | Td | TIG |
| Unknown | Yes | No | Yes | Yes* |
| Fewer than 3 doses | Yes | No | Yes | Yes* |
| 3 or more | Yes, if more than 10 years since last dose | No | Yes, if more than 5 years since last dose | No |

Td = combined tetanus and diphtheria toxoid adsorbed (dose = 0.5 mL IM). TIG = tetanus immune globulin (dose = 250 IU IM).

* Td and TIG should be administered at different sites.

*Adapted with permission from the Centers for Disease Control and Prevention.*

## ADVERSE OUTCOMES OF TREATMENT

Infection secondary to primary wound closure can occur. Patients also can have allergic reactions to antibiotics.

## REFERRAL DECISIONS/RED FLAGS

Any patient with an animal bite that involves the tendon, nerve, joint capsule, or an underlying fracture requires further evaluation.

# Arthritis of the Hand

## Synonyms

Osteoarthritis

Rheumatoid arthritis

Degenerative joint disease

## Definition

Osteoarthritis and secondary degenerative joint disease are the most common causes of arthritis of the hand and wrist. These conditions are characterized by progressive loss of articular cartilage, possible reactive bony changes at the joint margins, and subchondral cyst formation. The etiology of primary osteoarthritis is unknown. Secondary osteoarthritis develops in joints affected by trauma, mechanical problems, or preexisting lesions.

Rheumatoid arthritis is a systemic condition that affects synovial tissue (**Figure 1**). All deformities, joint destruction, and pathologic anatomy that occur in patients with rheumatoid arthritis are a result of synovial hypertrophy and inflammation. The boggy synovium stretches the joint capsule and ligaments, causing deformity and joint instability. The articular cartilage also can be destroyed. Rheumatoid synovitis may surround and invade the flexor and extensor tendons, disrupting their motion and function.

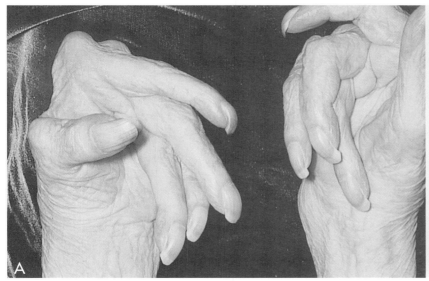
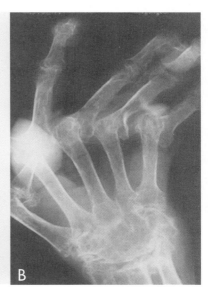

**Figure 1**
Advanced rheumatoid arthritis. A, Clinical appearance B, Radiographic appearance.

## CLINICAL SYMPTOMS

In osteoarthritis, the distal interphalangeal (DIP) and proximal interphalangeal (PIP) joints are most often involved. Patients report stiffness and loss of motion in the fingers. The wrist and metacarpophalangeal (MP) joints are most often involved in rheumatoid arthritis. Extensor or flexor tenosynovitis also is common. Patients with rheumatoid arthritis have increased pain in the morning and after extended activities.

## TESTS

### PHYSICAL EXAMINATION

Patients with rheumatoid arthritis involving the hands have fusiform swelling of multiple joints, with some joints swollen more than others. A boggy mass over the dorsum of the hand and crepitus with movement is quite common. Flexor tenosynovitis with crepitus at the wrist or in the fingers also is characteristic. Ulnar drift of the fingers may exist at the level of the MP joint. Other findings include contractures of the fingers at the PIP joints (boutonnière deformity) or hyperextension at the PIP joints with flexion at the DIP joints (swan-neck deformity).

Patients with osteoarthritis of the hand have bony nodules at the DIP joint (Heberden nodes). These nodules may be painful at first, but the pain usually resolves. Nodules also may occur at the PIP joints (Bouchard nodes). Involvement of the MP joints is much less common with osteoarthritis and, at this location, is often the result of previous trauma.

### DIAGNOSTIC TESTS

Posteroanterior (PA), oblique, and split finger lateral views are necessary. When a single digit is involved, isolated PA and true lateral views of the digit also are appropriate. Blood studies should be ordered for patients who have the characteristic changes of inflammatory arthritis but for whom the diagnosis has not been established.

## DIFFERENTIAL DIAGNOSIS

Pyogenic arthritis (may resemble the swollen joints of rheumatoid arthritis)

## ADVERSE OUTCOMES OF THE DISEASE

Rheumatoid arthritis can be slowly progressive, resulting in the typical rheumatoid hand deformity. Progressive osteoarthritis can cause joint destruction, particularly at the DIP, PIP, and wrist joints. Surgery for pain relief or stabilization may be necessary.

## TREATMENT

Rheumatoid arthritis has no cure. NSAIDs and other anti-inflammatory medications should be optimized. Cortisone injections can be extremely helpful for a severely inflamed joint or tendon sheath (see MP or PIP Joint Injection, p 216). Splinting for ulnar drift can slow a deformity but not prevent it from occurring.

Treatment of osteoarthritis typically includes NSAIDs and, occasionally, temporary splinting of an involved joint for pain relief.

## ADVERSE OUTCOMES OF TREATMENT

NSAIDs can cause gastric, hepatic, and renal complications. Other anti-inflammatory medications may adversely affect the immune system. Cortisone injections should be used very judiciously because tendon rupture, particularly of the extensor tendons, can occur. Infection also is a risk but largely can be avoided by careful use of sterile technique.

## REFERRAL DECISIONS/RED FLAGS

When a cortisone injection for extensor tenosynovitis is not effective, surgery to excise the inflamed synovium can prevent rupture of the tendon. Patients who cannot extend their fingers, especially the little finger, ring finger, or the thumb, could have ruptured the extensor tendon, and further evaluation is needed immediately.

Patients with rheumatoid arthritis who report increasing deformity and increasing pain in the hand may need reconstructive surgery.

Further evaluation also is needed for patients with osteoarthritis whose pain is no longer controlled with splinting and NSAIDs and who show radiographic evidence of joint destruction.

# PROCEDURE

# MP OR PIP JOINT INJECTION

## MATERIALS

Sterile gloves

Bactericidal skin preparation solution

Two 3-mL syringes with a 25-gauge needle

0.5 mL of a 1% local anesthetic solution without epinephrine

1 mL of a 40 mg/mL cortico-steroid preparation

Adhesive dressing

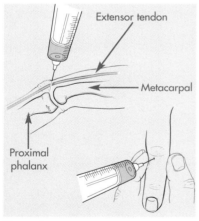

Extensor tendon

Metacarpal

Proximal phalanx

**Figure 1**
Location for needle insertion.

Injections are performed on the extensor aspect of either the metacar-pophalangeal (MP) or proximal interphalangeal (PIP) joint.

The entry site for the MP joint is the small sulcus just below the prominent metacarpal head that is most obvious with the finger flexed 20°. Identify this sulcus while moving the joint through a small amount of flexion and extension.

Identify the PIP joint in the same manner, although be aware that the dorsal rim of the middle phalanx often is more easily palpated with this joint in extension.

### STEP 1

Wear protective gloves at all times during this procedure and use sterile technique.

### STEP 2

Cleanse the skin with a bactericidal skin preparation solution.

### STEP 3

Insert the 25-gauge needle at the joint level on the dorsolateral side of the joint (**Figure 1**). Inject 0.5 mL of a 1% local anesthetic preparation into the joint, change syringes, and then with the new syringe inject 0.5 to 1.0 mL of 40 mg/mL corticosteroid preparation. Slight pressure against the syringe plunger should make the joint bulge slightly on either side.

### STEP 4

Dress the puncture wound with a sterile adhesive bandage.

## ADVERSE OUTCOMES

Although rare, infection is possible. Subcutaneous fat atrophy may occur if the corticosteroid preparation is injected external to the joint. This may produce a depressed area of thin, tender, and unsightly skin.

## AFTERCARE/PATIENT INSTRUCTIONS

The joint might be sore for 24 to 48 hours after injection. Instruct the patient to return to your office if undue swelling, pain, or redness occurs.

# ARTHRITIS OF THE THUMB CARPOMETACARPAL JOINT

## ICD-9 Codes

714.0
 Rheumatoid arthritis
715.14
 Osteoarthritis, primary, localized to the hand
715.24
 Osteoarthritis, secondary, localized to the hand
715.94
 Osteoarthritis, unspecified, localized to the hand
716.44
 Traumatic arthropathy of the hand
716.94
 Arthropathy, unspecified, hand

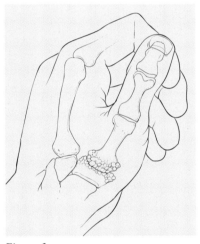

**Figure 1**
CMC arthritis of the thumb.

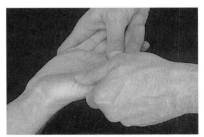

**Figure 2**
Watson stress test for CMC arthritis of the thumb.

## SYNONYMS

Carpometacarpal degenerative arthritis
Degenerative arthritis of the basal joint

## DEFINITION

Idiopathic degenerative arthritis of the thumb carpometacarpal (CMC) joint most commonly occurs in women between the ages of 40 and 70 years (**Figure 1**). In men, however, this condition usually results from previous trauma, either fracture-dislocation or dislocation. The idiopathic variety is thought to be caused by anatomic factors (joint configuration and ligamentous laxity) that predispose the joint to instability, shear forces, and subsequent degenerative change.

## CLINICAL SYMPTOMS

The most common symptom is pain at the base of the thumb that occurs with grip and pinch activities. The pain may radiate proximally into the wrist and forearm. Decreased pinch strength is a common complaint. Patients also may note instability, "catching," or "clicking" with certain movements. Late manifestations include stiffness of the CMC joint in adduction with secondary metacarpophalangeal (MP) hyperextension.

 Carpal tunnel syndrome may coexist with or mimic the symptoms of CMC arthritis.

## TESTS

### PHYSICAL EXAMINATION

The hallmark of this condition is tenderness over the palmar and radial aspects of the joint in the region of the base of the thumb. Manipulation of the CMC joint with simultaneous longitudinal loading (compression) causes pain and often some crepitation or instability. The Watson stress test readily reproduces the pain of CMC arthritis (**Figure 2**). With the palm facing up and the back of the hand resting on the table, the thumb is pushed down toward the table with the MP joint extended.

### DIAGNOSTIC TESTS

Posteroanterior and lateral radiographs of the thumb show joint space narrowing, subchondral sclerosis, and varying degrees of subluxation or dislocation at the CMC joint (**Figure 3**).

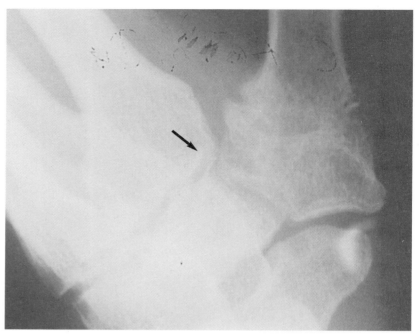

**Figure 3**
Radiographic appearance of CMC arthritis of the thumb.

## DIFFERENTIAL DIAGNOSIS

Arthritis of the wrist (evident on radiographs)

Carpal tunnel syndrome (positive Phalen test, decreased sensation in median nerve distribution)

de Quervain tenosynovitis (positive Finkelstein test)

Flexor carpi radialis tendinitis (pain with resisted wrist flexion, swelling over flexor carpi radialis tendon)

Fracture of the scaphoid (tenderness over the anatomic snuffbox)

Volar radial ganglion (palpable mass over the palmar surface of the wrist)

## ADVERSE OUTCOMES OF THE DISEASE

Chronic pain, loss of pinch and grip strength, and adduction contracture of the thumb (thumb held against the index finger) are all possible.

## TREATMENT

Initial treatment should consist of placing the thumb in a thumb spica splint for 3 weeks, with NSAIDs for pain relief. If symptoms recur, intermittent splinting that immobilizes the entire thumb should be continued. If splinting fails, a corticosteroid preparation should be injected into the joint (see Thumb Arthritis Injection, pp 220-221). Although injections do not alter the natural history of the disease, many patients report pain relief that lasts a few months with each injection. At least three injections can be given.

## ADVERSE OUTCOMES OF TREATMENT

NSAIDs can cause gastric, renal, or hepatic complications. Infection can develop after corticosteroid injection. Rapid progression of arthritis is possible as a result of multiple corticosteroid injections.

## REFERRAL DECISIONS/RED FLAGS

Failure of nonoperative treatment indicates the need for further evaluation.

# PROCEDURE
## THUMB (CARPOMETACARPAL) ARTHRITIS INJECTION

### MATERIALS

Sterile gloves

Bactericidal skin preparation solution

Two 3-mL syringes with a 25-gauge, ¾″ needle

0.5 mL of 40 mg/mL cortico-steroid preparation

2 mL of a 1% local anesthetic without epinephrine

Adhesive bandage

### STEP 1

Wear protective gloves at all times during this procedure and use sterile technique.

### STEP 2

Before putting on the gloves, mark the level of the carpometacarpal (CMC) joint on the dorsum of the hand with your thumbnail by gently indenting the skin at the interval between the base of the thumb metacarpal and the trapezium.

### STEP 3

Cleanse the skin over the CMC joint at the marked site with a bactericidal skin preparation solution.

### STEP 4

Insert the 25-gauge needle, attached to the syringe with the anesthetic solution, at the mark on the back of the CMC joint. Inject 0.5 mL of the 1% anesthetic subcutaneously.

### STEP 5

Next, pull on the end of the thumb to open the joint space. Advance the needle into the joint and inject 0.5 to 1 mL of the anesthetic solution (**Figure 1**). If resistance is encountered, redirect the needle and reinsert. After the anesthetic solution is injected, leave the needle in place and change syringes.

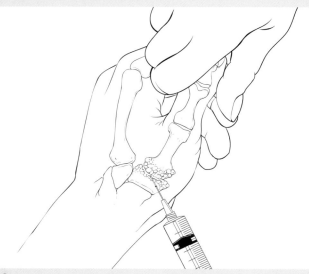

**Figure 2**
Injecting CMC joint of the thumb.

## STEP 6

Inject 0.5 mL of 40 mg/mL corticosteroid preparation through the same needle tract. The injection of fluid should meet little resistance if the needle is in the CMC joint.

## STEP 7

Dress the puncture wound with a sterile adhesive bandage.

## ADVERSE OUTCOMES

Depigmentation and fat atrophy at the site of injection, injury to sensory branches of the radial nerve, and joint space infection are possible.

## AFTERCARE/PATIENT INSTRUCTIONS

Advise the patient that 33% of patients may experience a "flare," manifested by increased joint pain, for 1 to 2 days. NSAIDs or an analgesic may be given to alleviate this pain. Also, ice can be helpful during the first 24 hours to decrease the pain. Also, the patient can wear a thumb spica splint for 2 or 3 days after the injection. The patient should experience relief within 5 to 7 days after the injection.

# ARTHRITIS OF THE WRIST

## ICD-9 Codes
712.23
   Pseudogout of the wrist
714.0
   Rheumatoid arthritis
715.13
   Osteoarthritis of the wrist, primary
715.23
   Osteoarthritis of the wrist, secondary
715.93
   Osteoarthritis of the wrist, unspecified
716.13
   Traumatic arthropathy of the wrist

## SYNONYM
Synovitis

## DEFINITION
Arthritis in the wrist is most commonly secondary to previous trauma, particularly fractures of the distal radius, or rheumatoid arthritis. Pseudogout also may cause arthritis of the wrist. Primary osteoarthritis and other arthritic conditions rarely affect the wrist.

## CLINICAL SYMPTOMS
Patients with rheumatoid arthritis typically report generalized swelling, tenderness, and limited motion. Hand function is often impaired by the synovitis and resultant instability of the carpal bones. The result is radial deviation of the wrist, ulnar deviation of the fingers, inefficient wrist and finger tendon function, decreased grip strength, and pain with daily activities.

Degenerative arthritis of the wrist is associated with swelling, pain, and limited motion of the wrist, but involvement of other joints is less common.

## TESTS

### PHYSICAL EXAMINATION
Examination reveals swelling, increased warmth, and limited motion. In patients with rheumatoid arthritis, involvement of the MP joints and deformity at the wrist and fingers also are common. The ulna appears prominent in these patients.

In posttraumatic degenerative arthritis, the finger joints usually appear normal.

### DIAGNOSTIC TESTS
Posteroanterior and lateral radiographs are helpful in distinguishing the various types of arthritis. Generalized thinning of bone structure (osteopenia) with erosions in the area of the joint surface is characteristic of rheumatoid arthritis. Subchondral sclerosis, joint space narrowing, spur formation, and, in some cases, erosion characterize primary or secondary osteoarthritis (Figure 1). Early calcification can indicate pseudogout, which can be confirmed by the presence of crystals in synovial fluid aspirate.

Laboratory studies, including erythrocyte sedimentation rate and tests for rheumatoid factor, antinuclear antibodies, and uric acid, may help confirm the diagnosis.

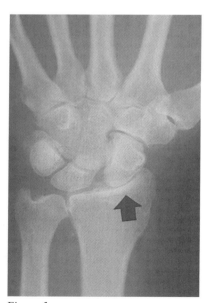

**Figure 1**
Radiograph showing osteoarthritis of the wrist (arrow).

## DIFFERENTIAL DIAGNOSIS

Septic arthritis of the wrist (acute onset, severe pain and restriction of wrist motion, systemic signs of infection)

Tenosynovitis (normal radiographs, swelling over the involved tendon)

## ADVERSE OUTCOMES OF THE DISEASE

Pain, loss of motion and/or strength, and impaired function in the fingers are possible.

## TREATMENT

Medical management depends on the etiology. Temporary immobilization in a splint can help relieve pain and swelling. In the absence of infection, injection of a corticosteroid may provide temporary pain relief (see Wrist Aspiration/Injection, p 224). Operative management usually is necessary when hand function decreases, when the joint becomes unstable, or when nonoperative treatment fails to relieve pain.

## ADVERSE OUTCOMES OF TREATMENT

Loss of motion and persistent pain can develop. NSAIDs can cause gastric, renal, or hepatic complications.

## REFERRAL DECISIONS/RED FLAGS

Patients with a possible wrist infection require immediate evaluation. Those with radiographic evidence of advanced disease and those who do not respond to splinting and NSAIDs also are candidates for further evaluation.

# PROCEDURE

# WRIST ASPIRATION/INJECTION

## MATERIALS

Sterile gloves

Bactericidal skin preparation solution

3-mL syringe with a 25-gauge needle

3-mL syringe with an 18-gauge needle

1-mL syringe

0.5 to 1 mL of 1% local anesthetic without epinephrine

0.5 to 1 mL of 40 mg/mL corticosteroid preparation (optional)

### STEP 1

Wear protective gloves at all times during this procedure and use sterile technique.

### STEP 2

Cleanse the area with a bactericidal skin preparation solution.

### STEP 3

Palpate the distal edge of the radius between the extensor carpi radialis brevis and extensor digitorum communis tendons. The depression just distal to the distal edge of the radius indicates the radiocarpal joint.

### STEP 4

Inject 2% local anesthetic in the subcutaneous tissue and joint capsule with the 25-gauge needle and then remove the needle.

### STEP 5

Insert the 18-gauge needle into the same site to aspirate the joint fluid. The joint fluid should be submitted for crystal analysis, cell count, smear Gram stain, and culture.

### STEP 6

If infection is not apparent, change the syringe and inject 0.5 to 1 mL of 40 mg/mL corticosteroid preparation. The corticosteroid preparation may be mixed with an equal amount of 2% local anesthetic for pain relief.

### STEP 7

Dress the puncture wound with a sterile adhesive bandage.

## ADVERSE OUTCOMES

Infection is possible because corticosteroids can mask the usual signs of infection.

## AFTERCARE/PATIENT INSTRUCTIONS

Instruct the patient to watch for signs of infection, such as increasing pain, swelling, heat, or redness, and to call your office if any of these signs occur.

# BOUTONNIÈRE DEFORMITY

| ICD-9 Code |
|---|
| 736.21 |
| Boutonnière deformity |

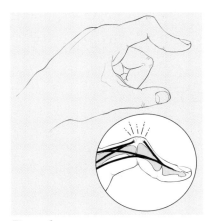

**Figure 1**
Boutonnière deformity.

*Adapted with permission from Steinberg GG, Akins CM, Baran DT: Ramamurti's Orthopaedics in Primary Care, ed 2. Philadelphia, PA, Williams & Wilkins, 1992, p 112.*

## SYNONYMS

Central slip extensor tendon injury
Jammed finger

## DEFINITION

Boutonnière deformity is caused by a rupture of the central portion of the extensor tendon at its insertion into the middle phalanx (**Figure 1**). The proximal interphalangeal (PIP) joint flexes from the unopposed pull of the flexor tendon. The head of the proximal phalanx "button holes" between the lateral bands of the extensor tendon mechanism. As a result, the lateral bands are displaced below the axis of rotation of the PIP joint, causing it to further flex. The lateral bands are displaced dorsal to the axis of the distal interphalangeal (DIP) joint, causing it to extend or hyperextend.

## CLINICAL SYMPTOMS

Patients typically report a history of trauma. The finger is held partially flexed at the PIP joint and extended or hyperextended at the DIP joint. With a recent injury, the PIP joint is painful and tender. Boutonnière deformity may not be apparent initially but can develop over 7 to 21 days as the intact lateral bands of the extensor tendon slip inferiorly.

## TESTS

### PHYSICAL EXAMINATION

Ask the patient to extend the injured finger and observe the position of the PIP and DIP joints. The PIP joint will be flexed more than 30° and the DIP joint will be extended or hyperextended. To demonstrate less severe or fixed deformities, hold the metacarpophalangeal and wrist joints in flexion and ask the patient to extend the PIP joint. Patients who lack 15° to 20° of extension at the PIP joint probably have a rupture of the central slip of the extensor tendon.

### DIAGNOSTIC TESTS

AP and lateral radiographs will rule out a fracture or a pseudo-boutonnière deformity (**Figure 2**).

## DIFFERENTIAL DIAGNOSIS

Fracture around the PIP joint (radiographs required to confirm)

Pseudo-boutonnière deformity (PIP joint is fixed in flexion and radiographs show calcification at the lateral aspect of the PIP joint) (see Figure 2)

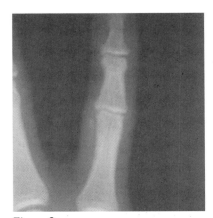

**Figure 2**
Pseudo-boutonnière deformity with lateral calcification.

Sprain of the PIP joint (may be difficult to differentiate on initial examination)

## ADVERSE OUTCOMES OF THE DISEASE

Flexion contracture of the PIP joint and extension contracture of the DIP joint are both possible.

## TREATMENT

The PIP joint should be splinted in extension for 6 weeks in a young patient and for 3 weeks in an elderly patient. The DIP joint is left free. Active and passive motion should be initiated at the DIP joint.

If the injury is more than 1 or 2 weeks old at presentation, it may not be possible to achieve full extension at the first visit. Use of a dynamic extension splint until full extension is achieved is required, followed by a static splinting program (**Figure 3**).

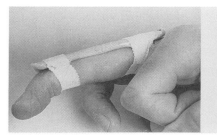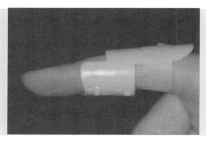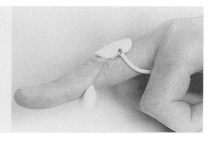

**Figure 3**
Static extension splint for the PIP joint (left), a commercial static splint (center) and a dynamic extension splint for the PIP joint (right).

*Reproduced with permission from Culver JE: Office management of athletic injuries of the hand and wrist, in Barr JS (ed): Instructional Course Lectures XXXVIII. Park Ridge, IL, American Academy of Orthopaedic Surgeons, 1989, pp 473–482.*

## ADVERSE OUTCOMES OF TREATMENT

Failure to achieve full extension, residual deformity, or both are possible.

## REFERRAL DECISIONS/RED FLAGS

Failure to achieve full extension, residual deformity, or both are indications for further evaluation.

# CARPAL TUNNEL SYNDROME

ICD-9 Code

354.0
Carpal tunnel syndrome

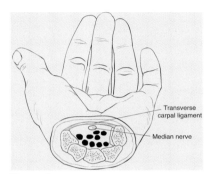

**Figure 1**
Cross-section of the carpal tunnel.

*Adapted with permission from Szabo RM, Steinberg DR: Nerve entrapment syndromes in the wrist. J Am Acad Orthop Surg 1994;2:116.*

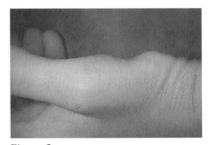

**Figure 2**
Thenar atrophy.

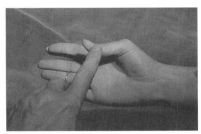

**Figure 3**
Testing for strength of opposition.

## SYNONYMS

Median nerve entrapment at the wrist

Median nerve compression

## DEFINITION

Carpal tunnel syndrome (entrapment of the median nerve at the wrist) is the most common compression neuropathy in the upper extremity. It most commonly affects middle-aged or pregnant women.

Any condition that reduces the size or space of the carpal tunnel can cause compression of the median nerve, resulting in paresthesias, pain, and sometimes paralysis (**Figure 1**). Common precipitating conditions include tenosynovitis of the adjacent flexor tendons (repetitive overuse trauma or rheumatoid arthritis), tumors, and medical conditions such as pregnancy or thyroid dysfunction that increase edema, or associated neuritis from diabetes.

## CLINICAL SYMPTOMS

Patients typically report a vague aching that radiates into the thenar area. Aching also may be perceived in the proximal forearm, and occasionally the pain can extend to the shoulder. The pain is typically accompanied by paresthesias and numbness in the median distribution (thumb and index, long, and radial half of ring fingers, or some combination thereof).

Patients report that they frequently drop objects, or that they cannot open jars or twist off lids. Pain or numbness sometimes is made worse by activities that require repetitive motion of the hand, repetitive activities, or stationary tasks done with the wrist held flexed or extended for long periods, such as when driving or reading. Patients often awaken at night with pain or numbness and typically report the need to rub or shake the hand to "get the circulation back." When the compression is severe and long-standing, persistent numbness and thenar atrophy can occur (**Figure 2**).

## TESTS

### PHYSICAL EXAMINATION

Inspect the hand for thenar atrophy. Check sensation of the median and ulnar nerves. Testing thumb opposition against resistance may reveal weakness of the thenar muscles (**Figure 3**).

The Phalen test is the most useful clinical test and is performed by placing the wrists in flexion. Aching and numbness in the distribution of the median nerve within 60 seconds (often within 15 seconds or less) is a positive test for carpal tunnel syndrome (**Figure 4**). Tapping over the median nerve at the wrist may produce tingling in some or all of the digits in the median nerve

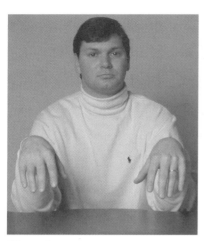

**Figure 4**
Phalen test.

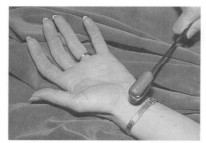

**Figure 5**
Median nerve percussion.

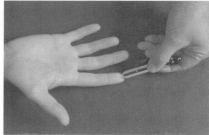

**Figure 6**
Testing for two-point discrimination.

distribution (Tinel sign) (**Figure 5**). Thumb pressure over the median nerve at the wrist for up to 30 seconds may elicit pain or paresthesias in the median distribution.

Patients with carpal tunnel syndrome may be unable to distinguish the two points of a caliper as separate points when they are closer than 5 mm together (**Figure 6**).

## DIAGNOSTIC TESTS

Radiographs of the wrist should be obtained if the patient has limited wrist motion. The most helpful objective diagnostic test is a median nerve conduction velocity study. These studies must be interpreted with caution, however. Some patients have no clinical signs or symptoms yet have abnormal nerve conduction velocity studies. Conversely, as many as 5% to 10% of patients with carpal tunnel syndrome have normal results.

## DIFFERENTIAL DIAGNOSIS

Arthritis of the carpometacarpal joint of the thumb (painful motion)

Cervical radiculopathy affecting C6 nerve (neck pain, numbness in the thumb and index fingers only)

Diabetes mellitus with neuropathy (history)

Flexor carpi radialis tenosynovitis (tenderness near the base of the thumb)

Hypothyroidism (abnormal results on thyroid function tests)

Median nerve compression at the elbow (tenderness at the proximal forearm)

Ulnar neuropathy (first dorsal interosseous weakness, numbness of the ring and little fingers)

Volar radial ganglion (mass near the base of the thumb above the wrist flexion crease)

Wrist arthritis (limited motion, evident on radiographs)

## ADVERSE OUTCOMES OF THE DISEASE

Permanent loss of sensation is possible, as are thenar atrophy and weakness of opposition.

## TREATMENT

For mild cases, splinting the wrist and a short-term course of NSAIDs or oral corticosteroids can be tried. The splint should be worn at night (at a minimum) and can be worn during the day if doing so does not interfere with the patient's work or daily activities. If these measures fail, consider injecting a corticosteroid into the carpal canal (see Carpal Tunnel Injection, pp 230-231). Injection has diagnostic as well as therapeutic benefits, but improvement may be only temporary. Care must be taken to avoid direct injection into the median nerve.

Work-related carpal tunnel syndrome may be improved with ergonomic modifications, such as using keyboard or forearm supports, adjusting the height of computer keyboards, and avoiding holding the wrist in a flexed position (as with dental hygienists). Patients with acute carpal tunnel syndrome may have wrist pain rather than the more typical signs of numbness and thenar weakness. These patients respond well to corticosteroid injection.

Carpal tunnel syndrome that occurs during pregnancy usually resolves when the pregnancy terminates; therefore, treatment should consist of splinting and other nonoperative measures, such as injection of corticosteroid.

Operative management is necessary for patients who have atrophy or weakness of the thenar muscles or decreased sensation, and for those who have intolerable symptoms despite a course of nonoperative treatment.

## ADVERSE OUTCOMES OF TREATMENT

NSAIDs can cause gastric, renal, or hepatic complications. Fluid retention, flushing of the skin, and shakiness can result from taking oral corticosteroids. Injecting corticosteroids is associated with the risk of an intraneural injection, which can have long-term adverse consequences. Prolonged nonoperative treatment can result in loss of sensation and thenar atrophy.

## REFERRAL DECISIONS/RED FLAGS

Failure of nonoperative treatment after 3 months warrants further evaluation. Persistent numbness, weakness, atrophy of the thenar muscles, or any combination of these are indications for further evaluation.

SECTION 4 | HAND AND WRIST

# PROCEDURE

## CARPAL TUNNEL INJECTION

### MATERIALS

Sterile gloves

Bactericidal skin preparation solution

Two 3-mL syringes with a 25-gauge, ¾" needle

2 to 5 mL of a 1% local anesthetic without epinephrine

1 mL of a 40 mg/mL corticosteroid preparation

Adhesive bandage

### STEP 1

Wear protective gloves at all times during this procedure and use sterile technique.

### STEP 2

Cleanse the volar aspect of the wrist with a bactericidal skin preparation solution.

### STEP 3

Insert the needle 1 cm proximal to the wrist flexion crease and 3 to 5 mm from the ulnar side of the palmaris longus. If the palmaris longus is absent, the direction of the needle may be aligned with the ring finger. Direct the needle toward the hand at an angle of 30° to 45° (**Figure 1**). Have the patient flex the fingers fully into the palm, then advance the needle approximately 1 to 1.5 cm until resistance is felt. If the patient reports paresthesias, redirect the needle.

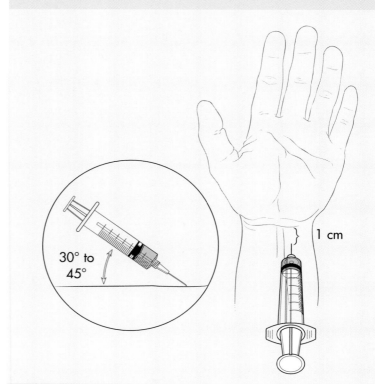

**Figure 1**
Location for needle insertion.

### STEP 4

Instruct the patient to slightly wiggle the tips of the ring and little fingers. If this causes slight movement of the tip of the needle, the needle is safely positioned.

### STEP 5

Ask the patient to extend the fingers as gentle pressure is applied to the syringe. The distal excursion of the flexor tendons of the ring and little fingers will carry the point of the needle into the carpal canal.

### STEP 6

If the patient reports any tingling, the needle has entered the nerve. If this occurs, do not continue with the injection. Otherwise, inject 1 to 2 mL of local anesthetic into the carpal canal. If resistance is encountered on attempting to inject the local anesthetic, the tip of the needle is embedded in the flexor tendons. Maintain some pressure on the syringe while slowly withdrawing the needle, until the anesthetic flows freely. Leave the needle in place and change syringes. Inject 1 mL of corticosteroid into the carpal canal, and then remove the needle.

### STEP 7

Dress the puncture wound with a sterile adhesive bandage.

## ADVERSE OUTCOMES

Infection or intraneural injection is possible.

## AFTERCARE/PATIENT INSTRUCTIONS

Advise the patient that occasional mild soreness may develop, that the hand and fingers may be numb for 1 to 2 hours following the injection, and that the injection could require 24 to 48 hours to take effect.

SECTION 4 | HAND AND WRIST

# DE QUERVAIN TENOSYNOVITIS

| ICD-9 Code |
|---|
| 727.04 de Quervain tenosynovitis |

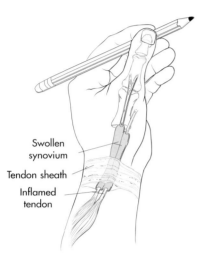

Swollen synovium

Tendon sheath

Inflamed tendon

**Figure 1**
de Quervain tenosynovitis of the first extensor compartment.

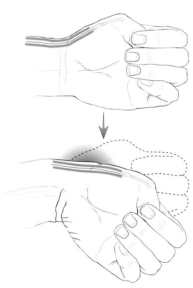

**Figure 2**
Finkelstein test.

*Adapted with permission from the American Society for Surgery of the Hand: Brochure: de Quervain's Stenosing Tenosynovitis. Englewood, CO, 1995.*

## SYNONYM
Stenosing tenosynovitis

## DEFINITION
de Quervain tenosynovitis is swelling or stenosis of the sheath that surrounds the abductor pollicis longus and extensor pollicis brevis tendons on the thumb side at the wrist (**Figure 1**). The inflammation thickens the tendon sheath (tenosynovium) and constricts the tendon as it glides in the sheath. This can cause pain, swelling, and a triggering phenomenon, with the tendon seeming to lock or stick as the patient moves the thumb. The disorder is more common in middle-aged women and is often precipitated by repetitive use of the thumb.

## CLINICAL SYMPTOMS
Patients report pain and swelling over the radial styloid that is aggravated by attempts to move the thumb or make a fist. They also may notice creaking as the tendon moves.

## TESTS
### PHYSICAL EXAMINATION
Examination reveals swelling and tenderness over the tendons in the region of the distal radius. Crepitus may be palpable as the patient flexes and extends the thumb. Full flexion of the thumb into the palm, followed by ulnar deviation of the wrist (Finkelstein test), will produce pain and is diagnostic for de Quervain tenosynovitis (**Figure 2**).

### DIAGNOSTIC TESTS
Even though this is largely a clinical diagnosis, posteroanterior and lateral radiographs of the wrist should be considered to rule out any bony abnormality, such as a deformed radial styloid process that might be a precipitating cause if there is a history of trauma. Calcification associated with tendinitis occasionally can be seen on radiographs.

## DIFFERENTIAL DIAGNOSIS
Carpometacarpal arthritis of the thumb (swelling over the joint, pain with joint compression)

Dorsal wrist ganglion (palpable mass)

Flexor carpi radialis tendinitis (pain and swelling over the tendon)

Fracture of the scaphoid (tenderness over the anatomic snuffbox)

Wrist arthritis (pain with movement, evident on radiographs)

## ADVERSE OUTCOMES OF THE DISEASE

Chronic pain, loss of strength, and loss of thumb motion can occur; tendon rupture is possible but is rare.

## TREATMENT

Initial treatment should consist of a thumb spica splint that immobilizes both the wrist and thumb. A 2-week course of NSAIDs also is helpful for pain relief. If immobilization fails, the tendon sheath should be injected with a corticosteroid preparation (see de Quervain Injection, p 234). The patient should have no more than three injections.

Operative treatment should be considered if corticosteroid injections are not successful.

## ADVERSE OUTCOMES OF TREATMENT

NSAIDs can cause gastric, renal, or hepatic complications. The patient can experience some discomfort from wearing the splint and will stop using it. Corticosteroids can sometimes cause subcutaneous atrophy and unslightly loss of pigmentation. Infection after corticosteroid injection also is a risk but largely can be avoided by careful use of sterile technique. Injury to the radial sensory nerve or incomplete release is possible with operative treatment.

## REFERRAL DECISIONS/RED FLAGS

Failure to respond to splinting and corticosteroid injections indicates the need for further evaluation.

# PROCEDURE

## DE QUERVAIN INJECTION

### MATERIALS

Sterile gloves

Bactericidal skin preparation solution

Two 3-mL syringes with a 27-gauge, $^7/_8$" needle

2 mL of 40 mg/mL corticosteroid preparation

2 mL of a 1% local anesthetic without epinephrine

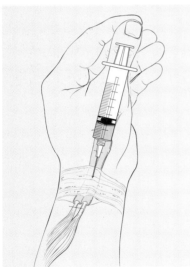

**Figure 1**
Location for needle insertion.

### STEP 1

Wear protective gloves at all times during this procedure and use sterile technique.

### STEP 2

Cleanse the skin with a bactericidal skin preparation solution.

### STEP 3

Insert the 27-gauge needle at a 45° angle to the skin in line with the two tendons (**Figure 1**). If the patient reports paresthesia into the thumb, the needle has pierced the sensory branch of the radial nerve. Move the needle 2 to 3 mm dorsal or volar.

### STEP 4

Create a skin wheal with 0.5 mL of 1% local anesthetic and advance the needle until it strikes one of the underlying tendons. Inject the remaining anesthetic while slowly withdrawing the needle, until the anesthetic flows freely. Leave the needle in place and change syringes.

### STEP 5

Ask the patient to move the thumb. Inject 2 mL of corticosteroid preparation into the tendon sheath. Palpation of the tendon sheath proximal to the point of injection should reveal swelling as the corticosteroid is injected.

### STEP 6

Dress the puncture wound with a sterile adhesive bandage.

### ADVERSE OUTCOMES

Subcutaneous fat atrophy can follow subcutaneous infiltration of the corticosteroid preparation, leading to a waxy appearing depression in the skin. In addition, although rare, infection is possible.

### AFTERCARE/PATIENT INSTRUCTIONS

Increased pain is not uncommon after the injection, especially in the first 24 to 48 hours. At least one third of patients will experience increased discomfort during this time.

# DUPUYTREN DISEASE

ICD-9 Code
728.6
    Dupuytren contracture

## SYNONYMS

Viking disease

Palmar fibromatosis

## DEFINITION

Dupuytren disease is a nodular thickening and contraction of the palmar fascia (**Figure 1**). The disease has a dominant genetic component, particularly involving people of northern European descent (ie, Viking disease). Dupuytren disease most commonly affects men older than age 50 years. Associated conditions include epilepsy, diabetes, pulmonary disease, alcoholism, and repetitive trauma (vibrational).

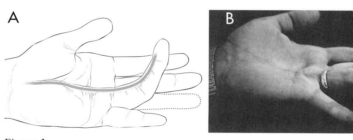

**Figure 1**

A, Dupuytren contracture of the ring finger. B, Clinical appearance of Dupuytren contracture.

*Adapted with permission from the American Society for Surgery of the Hand:* Brochure: Dupuytren's disease. *Englewood, CO, 1995.*

## CLINICAL SYMPTOMS

Patients initially notice one or more painless nodules near the distal palmar crease that are moderately sensitive to pressure. The nodule or nodules may gradually thicken and contract, causing the finger to flex at the metacarpophalangeal (MP) joint and, occasionally as the disease progresses, the proximal interphalangeal joint (PIP) joint. The ring finger is most commonly involved, followed by the small, long, thumb, and index fingers. Although extension is limited, finger flexion is usually normal. Invariably, the condition is painless in its later stages, but as the contractures increase, patients have trouble grasping objects, pulling on gloves, and putting the hand into a pocket. Sensation in the affected fingers usually is normal unless the patient has concomitant carpal tunnel syndrome.

## TESTS

### PHYSICAL EXAMINATION

Examination reveals a palmar skin nodule that in the early stages may resemble a callus. As the disease progresses, fascial bands (cords) extend distally and sometimes proximally to the nodule. These bands may cross the MP joint, which is most common, and the PIP joint, holding the finger in a contracted position. The bands are seldom tender unless the patient is in the early stages of the disease.

### DIAGNOSTIC TESTS

Diagnosis is made upon clinical examination. Radiographs are not needed.

## DIFFERENTIAL DIAGNOSIS

Flexion contracture secondary to joint or tendon injury (no cords or bands)

Locked trigger finger (no associated nodules)

## ADVERSE OUTCOMES OF THE DISEASE

Progressive flexion contracture of the fingers and limited function are possible.

## TREATMENT

Splinting or other nonoperative treatment is not curative, but night splints may slow the progression of the contractures. Surgery involves excising the thick soft-tissue bands and release of the joint contractures.

## ADVERSE OUTCOMES OF TREATMENT

Patients may experience nerve injury, skin slough, and recurrence of the disease postoperatively.

## REFERRAL DECISIONS/RED FLAGS

Patients with significant contractures (greater than 30°) of the MP joints who are troubled by their lack of extension are candidates for further evaluation. Likewise, patients with involvement of the PIP joint in association with Dupuytren disease require close follow-up.

# FINGERTIP INFECTIONS

## ICD-9 Codes
054.6
    Herpetic whitlow
681.01
    Felon
681.02
    Paronychia of finger

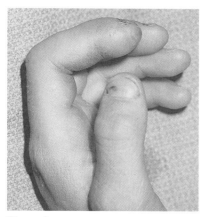

**Figure 1**
Felon.

*Reproduced with permission from Stern PJ: Selected acute infections, in Greene WB (ed): Instructional Course Lectures XXXIX. Park Ridge, IL, American Academy of Orthopaedic Surgeons, 1990, pp 539–546.*

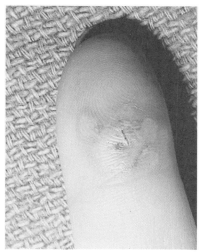

**Figure 2**
Herpetic whitlow.

*Reproduced with permission from Stern PJ: Selected acute infections, in Greene WB (ed): Instructional Course Lectures XXXIX. Park Ridge, IL, American Academy of Orthopaedic Surgeons, 1990, pp 539–546.*

## SYNONYMS

Felon

Paronychia

## DEFINITION

Infections of the fingertip typically occur in two locations: in the pulp or palmar tip of the finger (felon) and in the soft tissues directly surrounding the fingernail (paronychia). *Staphylococcus aureus* is the most common causative organism in both conditions.

Felons usually are caused by a puncture wound and most commonly occur in the thumb and index finger (**Figure 1**). A herpetic whitlow also causes swelling in the pulp of the finger (**Figure 2**). Differentiating a felon from herpetic whitlow is important, as incision and drainage of a felon usually is indicated, whereas incision of a whitlow is contraindicated and observation is sufficient. Health care workers who are frequently exposed to the herpes simplex virus from human saliva (ie, respiratory therapists, dental hygienists) are at increased risk for herpetic whitlow. Paronychia infections often occur after a manicure or the development of a nail deformity, such as a hangnail or an ingrown nail.

## CLINICAL SYMPTOMS

Felons are characterized by severe pain and swelling in the pad of the fingertip. With a felon, the entire pulp of the fingertip is swollen, tense, red, and very tender. Also, a puncture wound may be visible.

Paronychia infection is characterized by swelling of the tissues about the fingernail, usually along one side and about the base of the nail. Occasionally, the swelling can extend completely around the nail and is then referred to as a "run-around abscess." The pain associated with a paronychia is not as intense as that with a felon.

Swelling associated with a felon or paronychia should not extend proximal to the distal flexion crease. Any such extension suggests a deeper, more complex process, such as an infection in the flexor tendon sheath. Significantly increased pain with passive motion also may indicate flexor tendon sheath infection.

## TESTS

### PHYSICAL EXAMINATION

The fingertip should be examined for the location and extent of the swelling. The presence of small vesicles is a finding that suggests the diagnosis of herpetic whitlow.

## DIAGNOSTIC TESTS

Plain radiographs show soft-tissue swelling. Late in the course of infection, osteomyelitis of the distal phalanx may occur and is evident on radiographs as partial or complete resorption of the distal tuft of the phalanx. More aggressive surgical debridement is required in these cases.

## DIFFERENTIAL DIAGNOSIS

Chronic fungal infection (not responsive to antibiotics)

Epidermal inclusion cyst (dorsal swelling proximal to the nail, usually not very painful)

Herpetic felon (obvious vesicles)

Septic tenosynovitis (increased pain with active and passive motion of finger)

## ADVERSE OUTCOMES OF THE DISEASE

Untreated felons could lead to osteomyelitis of the distal phalanx. Nail deformities and progressive infection involving the distal joint and/or the flexor tendon sheath also may develop late in the course of these infections.

## TREATMENT

Most felons require surgical drainage under digital block anesthesia (see Digital Anesthetic Block [Hand], p 240) and tourniquet control. Either of two different incisions can be used: a central volar longitudinal incision or a dorsal midaxial or so-called "hockey stick" incision.

When a collection of pus can be seen under the skin on the pad side of the finger, use a central longitudinal incision, extending from the flexion crease to the fingertip (**Figure 3**). Culture the drainage for aerobic and anaerobic organisms. To allow drainage, keep the wound open, using a gauze packing strip, and remove it in 2 to 3 days. Allow the wound to close by secondary intention; never suture the wound.

When no collection of pus is readily visible under the skin, use a dorsal midaxial incision (**Figure 4**). For the thumb, make the incision on the radial (noncontact) side, and for the fingers, on the ulnar (noncontact) side. Extend the incision to the fingertip but do not wrap it around the tip. Make the incision down to the bone where the soft-tissue attachments to the bone can be separated by blunt dissection with a small hemostat. Use open packing gauze and then remove it in 2 to 3 days.

Treatment of an early-stage paronychia should be nonoperative. Application of warm, moist soaks for 10 minutes four times a day, combined with an oral antibiotic for 5 days, is usually adequate. Because *Staphylococcus aureus* is the most likely causative organism, an oral cephalosporin such as cephalexin, 250 mg four times a day, or dicloxacillin, 250 mg four times a day, is a good initial choice.

In later stages, when a purulent collection is noted at the nail bed margin or under the nail, drainage can be done by elevating the skin fold at the margin of the nail. More severe infections require partial or complete removal of

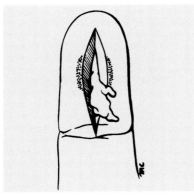

**Figure 3**
Central volar longitudinal incision of the pulp.

*Reproduced with permission from Stern PJ: Selected acute infections, in Greene WB (ed): Instructional Course Lectures XXXIX. Park Ridge, IL, American Academy of Orthopaedic Surgeons, 1990, pp 539–546.*

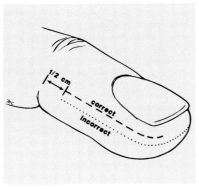

**Figure 4**
Dorsal midaxial "hockey stick" incision for drainage of a felon.

*Reproduced with permission from Stern PJ: Selected acute infections, in Greene WB (ed): Instructional Course Lectures XXXIX. Park Ridge, IL, American Academy of Orthopaedic Surgeons, 1990, pp 539–546.*

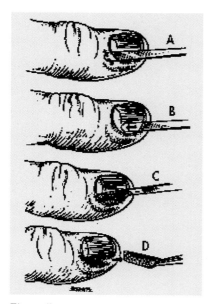

**Figure 5**
Portion of nail removed for paronychia.

*Reproduced with permission from American Society for Surgery of the Hand: Regional Review Course Manual. Rosemont, IL, American Society for Surgery of the Hand, 1998, pp 7/8–7/9.*

the nail (**Figure 5**). Under digital or metacarpal block anesthesia, the nail can be carefully elevated from the underlying sterile matrix using a hemostat or blunt metal probe. The nail can be completely removed by freeing the overlying cuticle, and the nail bed protected by a nonadherent gauze (Xeroform or Adaptic) carefully tucked underneath the cuticle and extending to the tip of the finger. The wound should be checked in 3 to 4 days, and the patient advised that the nail should grow out within several months.

## ADVERSE OUTCOMES OF TREATMENT

A painful scar may develop as a result of a misplaced incision, or a nail deformity can develop from injury to the germinal matrix. Inadequate drainage with persistent or recurrent infection may occur.

## REFERRAL DECISIONS/RED FLAGS

Persistent or progressive swelling or any evidence of an ascending infection, despite adequate antibiotic treatment and surgical decompression, is an indication for further evaluation.

SECTION 4 | HAND AND WRIST

# PROCEDURE

## DIGITAL ANESTHETIC BLOCK (HAND)

### MATERIALS

Sterile gloves

Bactericidal skin preparation solution

3-mL syringe with a 27-gauge needle

3 mL of 1% local anesthetic without epinephrine

Adhesive dressing

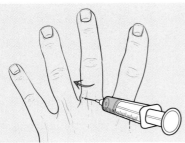

**Figure 1**
Location for needle insertion into the web space alongside the extensor tendon.

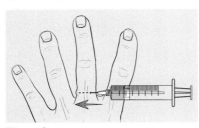

**Figure 2**
Location for needle insertion along the top of the extensor tendon.

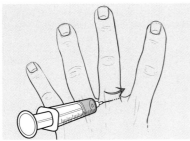

**Figure 3**
Location for needle insertion into the web space on the opposite side of the finger.

### STEP 1

Wear protective gloves at all times during this procedure and use sterile technique.

### STEP 2

Cleanse all surfaces of the base of the finger with a bactericidal skin preparation solution.

### STEP 3

Draw 3 mL of the local anesthetic into the syringe.

### STEP 4

Insert the 27-gauge needle into the web space alongside the extensor tendon (**Figure 1**). Advance the needle until it is almost at the volar skin and inject 1 mL of the local anesthetic.

### STEP 5

Withdraw the needle and insert it along the top of the extensor tendon (**Figure 2**). Inject 1 mL of the solution.

### STEP 6

Repeat the procedure in the web space on the opposite side of the finger (**Figure 3**).

### STEP 7

Dress the puncture wound with a sterile adhesive dressing.

### ADVERSE OUTCOMES

Although rare, infection is possible. Necrosis of a digit is possible if epinephrine is used in the anesthetic solution. Note that the agent should be injected on only three sides of the finger to avoid a circumferential nerve block that can cut off circulation to the finger from hydrostatic pressure.

### AFTERCARE/PATIENT INSTRUCTIONS

Advise the patient that local swelling at the site of the block should resolve in a few hours. Instruct the patient to call your office if the finger becomes dusky or completely white and to avoid touching hot surfaces or using sharp objects until all sensation has returned.

# FINGERTIP INJURIES/AMPUTATIONS

## ICD-9 Codes

883.0
Open wound of finger(s) without mention of complication
885.0
Traumatic amputation of thumb without mention of complication
886.0
Traumatic amputation of fingers without mention of complication
927.3
Crushing injury of finger(s)

## DEFINITION

Fingertip injuries and amputations are common. Some apparent amputations are actually crush injuries or lacerations. In addition to the soft tissue of the pulp, the distal phalanx and nail may be involved.

## CLINICAL SYMPTOMS

Patients report a history of a crush injury to the fingertip or a knife injury. The latter usually involves a finger in the nondominant hand.

## TESTS

### PHYSICAL EXAMINATION

The fingertip should be inspected carefully to determine the vascularity and sensation of the skin flaps and if bone is exposed. The orientation of the amputation also should be noted (**Figure 1**). The nail bed should be carefully examined for a painful subungual hematoma that should be drained and for lacerations of the nail bed that should be repaired. The vascularity of the tip, as well as the sensation, should be noted.

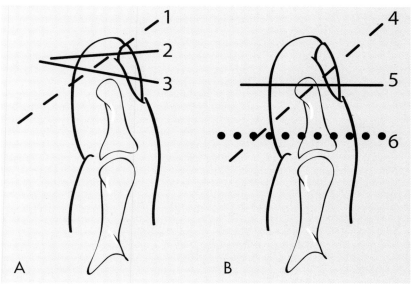

**Figure 1**
A, Levels of soft-tissue amputations that can be treated open and allowed to close by secondary intention. B, Levels of amputation that will require shortening of the bone.

### DIAGNOSTIC TESTS

If bone is exposed or if the finger is markedly swollen, AP and lateral radiographs of the finger should be obtained.

# Differential diagnosis

Amputation with injury to the nail matrix (evident on clinical examination)

Amputation with open fracture (evident on radiographs)

# Adverse outcomes of the disease

Painful amputation stump, dystrophic nail, loss of motion in the finger, and loss of grip and pinch strength are possible. Cold sensitivity/Raynaud phenomenon, a painful neuroma, or epidermal inclusion cyst also can develop. Complex regional pain syndrome also is possible.

# Treatment

The goals of treatment are to provide a tip with good soft-tissue coverage, adequate sensation, and to preserve as much length as is consistent with good function. Whether or not bone is exposed and the angle of the amputation relative to the long axis of the finger dictate the appropriate treatment options.

If no bone is exposed, the physician must decide if the skin can be closed without excess tension. If not, the wound should be allowed to close on its own. Initial treatment consists of thorough debridement and irrigation of the finger under a digital block and application of sterile dressings and a splint for comfort. The initial dressings should be changed after 24 to 72 hours. Wet to dry dressings using normal saline solution twice a day are then applied. The patient should be taught how to apply these dressings and the removable splint at home. The dressing changes are continued until the tip has healed. Finger range-of-motion exercises should begin after 48 hours. Once the wound has healed, tip desensitization techniques can be started. In most cases, allowing the wound to heal by secondary intention provides good function and acceptable cosmetic results while retaining maximum length of the finger.

If bone is exposed, a decision must be made whether to shorten the bone or to provide skin coverage by a reconstructive flap procedure. As a general guide, the exposed phalanx of any of the fingers can be shortened sufficiently to provide soft-tissue coverage without sacrificing function. Shortening the thumb is more controversial. Although retaining thumb length is desirable, maintaining length by covering exposed bone with an insensate flap or attenuated skin may compromise function of this important digit. Therefore, many thumb tip amputations with bone exposed can be treated by shortening the bone and closing the skin.

Associated nail bed injuries require special attention (see Nail Injuries, pp 273-275).

Treatment of amputation in children under age 6 years differs somewhat from the treatment in adults. After thorough debridement and defatting, the skin of a child's amputated fingertip can be sutured to the finger as a composite flap. Even if this tip does not survive (although many will), it serves as a biologic dressing until re-epithelialization of the tip occurs.

The tetanus immunization status of the patient must be checked and updated if necessary. If the wound is grossly contaminated and/or crushed, or if the patient has diabetes mellitus, prophylactic antibiotics are indicated for 5 days.

Replantation should be considered if thumb is amputated at or proximal to the interphalangeal (IP) joint, if a finger is amputated proximal to the middle of the middle phalanx, or when multiple fingers are amputated. A replantation center should be contacted for specific instructions. The amputated part is wrapped in a sterile gauze soaked in normal saline solution, placed in a plastic bag, and then the bag placed on ice.

Most patients, however, function quite well with single finger amputations. If cosmesis is a consideration, very life-like cosmetic finger prostheses are available.

## ADVERSE OUTCOMES OF TREATMENT

Necrosis of the fingertip and infection can develop. Cold sensitivity/Raynaud phenomenon, a painful neuroma, or epidermal inclusion cyst also can develop. Complex regional pain syndrome also is possible.

## REFERRAL DECISIONS/RED FLAGS

Patients with thumb amputations proximal to the IP joint and multiple finger amputations are suitable candidates for specialty evaluation. Patients with single finger amputations who desire replantation also should be referred to a replantation center.

# FLEXOR TENDON INJURIES

ICD-9 Codes

727.64
    Rupture of flexor tendons of hand
    and wrist, nontraumatic
842.1
    Tendon injuries of the wrist and
    hand, unspecified site

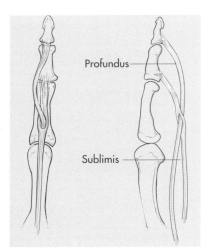

**Figure 1**
Extrinsic flexor tendons of the finger.

*Adapted with permission from Green DP (ed): Operative Hand Surgery, ed 2. New York, NY, Churchill Livingstone, 1988, p 1971.*

## SYNONYMS

Tendon laceration or rupture

Jersey finger

## DEFINITION

The flexor tendons of the hand are vulnerable to laceration or rupture. Complete lacerations of both the flexor digitorum sublimis (FDS) and flexor digitorum profundus (FDP) cause immediate loss of flexion at the proximal interphalangeal (PIP) and distal interphalangeal (DIP) joints. Incomplete or partial lacerations can be missed on initial examination, only to present several days later as a spontaneous rupture in the weakened tendon.

Ruptures of flexor tendons can be spontaneous, as in patients with rheumatoid arthritis, or traumatic. The latter type usually occurs during athletics (eg, football, wrestling, or rugby) when a player grabs another's jersey (thus the name jersey finger). When the fingers flex, the ring finger is most prominent and, therefore, the profundus tendon of the ring finger is most commonly ruptured during this activity.

## CLINICAL SYMPTOMS

Each finger is supplied with two flexor tendons: the FDP inserts into the distal phalanx and the FDS inserts into the middle phalanx (**Figure 1**). Therefore, if the FDP is cut but the FDS is intact, patients can flex the PIP and metacarpophalangeal (MP) joints, but not the DIP joint. If the FDS is cut but the FDP is intact, patients can flex the DIP, PIP, and MP joints (**Figure 2**). Because of

| Level of cut tendon | Tendon(s) cut | Loss of flexion joint(s) | Retained flexion joint(s) |
|---|---|---|---|
| (1) | FDP | DIP | MP & PIP |
| (2) | FDP & FDS | DIP & PIP | MP |
| (3) | FDS | NONE | MP, PIP, & DIP |

FDP = Flexor digitorum profundus tendon
PIP = Proximal interphalangeal joint
FDS = Flexor digitorum sublimis tendon
MP = Metacarpophalangeal joint
DIP = Distal interphalangeal joint

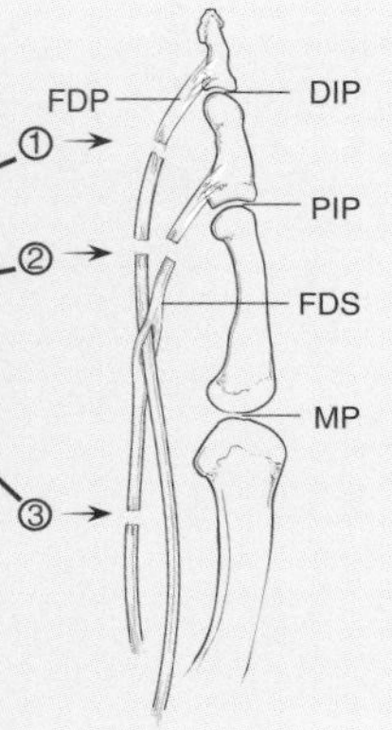

**Figure 2**
Effects of flexor tendon injuries on flexion of the finger joint.

*Adapted with permission from Green DP (ed): Operative Hand Surgery, ed 2. New York, NY, Churchill Livingstone, 1988, p 1971.*

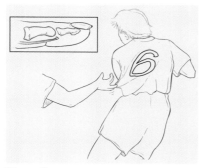

**Figure 3**
Mechanism of injury in rupture of the profundus tendon.

*Reproduced with permission from Carter PR: Common Hand Injuries and Infections: A Practical Approach to Early Treatment. Philadelphia, PA, WB Saunders, 1983.*

the close proximity of the digital nerves to the flexor tendons, open injuries to the flexor tendons are commonly associated with injuries to the digital nerves, as well. In this situation, patients will report numbness on one or both sides of the finger.

With traumatic rupture of the FDP, the ring finger becomes "caught" (**Figure 3**) and the profundus tendon is avulsed from its insertion, possibly accompanied by a bony fragment. This injury can be missed or diagnosed late because it is often considered to be a jammed finger. In patients with rheumatoid arthritis, ruptures usually are "silent," meaning that the patient notices that the finger will not bend but does not remember when the function was lost.

## TESTS

### PHYSICAL EXAMINATION

First, test for active flexion, then for strength of flexion. If the peritendinous structures are intact, the patient may retain flexion even in the presence of a complete laceration; however, flexion will be weak. Test flexion strength at both the DIP and PIP joints by asking the patient to flex the injured finger against your finger as you apply resistance.

Check flexion of the FDP by asking the patient to flex the fingertip at the DIP joint while the PIP joint is held in extension (**Figure 4**). To test the integrity of the FDS, hold the fingers straight, then have the patient flex each finger individually at the PIP joint (**Figure 5**). With a lacerated FDS but an intact FDP, PIP flexion will not occur when the other fingers are held extended. This is because the FDP tendons cannot function independently. This test is not reliable at the little finger because 20% to 30% of the population has a band connecting the ring and little fingers that prevents independent function of the sublimis to the little finger. In addition, in some patients, the FDP of the index finger can weakly flex the finger with the other fingers held extended.

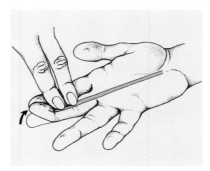

**Figure 4**
Test for function of the FDP.

*Reproduced with permission from American Society for Surgery of the Hand: The Hand: Examination and Diagnosis, ed 3. New York, NY, Churchill Livingstone, pp 18–19.*

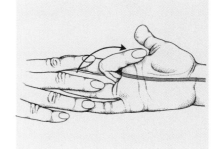

**Figure 5**
Test for function of the FDS.

*Reproduced with permission from American Society for Surgery of the Hand: The Hand: Examination and Diagnosis, ed 3. New York, NY, Churchill Livingstone, pp 18–19.*

Partial lacerations can pose a diagnostic challenge. Patients typically have full range of motion, but they have more pain with active flexion than would be expected. When the diagnosis is unclear, evaluation for possible surgical exploration should be considered.

Patients with a tendon rupture may have mild swelling over the flexion surface of the DIP joint and tenderness along the palmar surface of the finger. Test the strength of flexion at the DIP joint. When flexion is weak, rupture of the FDP must be considered a possibility. Patients with rheumatoid arthritis may not remember the point at which the tendon ruptured; they usually report only that the finger will not flex.

Sensation in the finger also should be evaluated because open tendon injuries are often accompanied by injuries to the nearby digital nerves. The vascular status of injured fingers should be checked and documented as well.

## DIAGNOSTIC TESTS

Posteroanterior and lateral radiographs of the involved finger may show a small avulsed fragment from the distal phalanx in an FDP rupture. These views also may identify a fracture.

## DIFFERENTIAL DIAGNOSIS

Anterior interosseous nerve paralysis (no laceration)

Partial tendon laceration (full flexion with pain and weakness)

Stenosing tenosynovitis with the finger locked in extension (no visible wound; tenderness over the proximal flexor pulley)

## ADVERSE OUTCOMES OF THE DISEASE

Loss of flexion and of grip and pinch strength in the involved and adjacent fingers is possible.

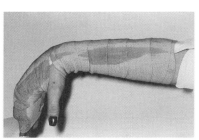

**Figure 6**
Splint for flexor tendon injury.

## TREATMENT

The principal goal of initial treatment is to correctly identify the condition and ensure that the patient is evaluated for surgical repair. Flexor tendon injuries ultimately require surgical repair. Initially, clean and repair superficial wounds and splint the hand in a position for flexor tendon injuries (**Figure 6**). Surgical exploration and repair should be done within a few days after injury.

## ADVERSE OUTCOMES OF TREATMENT

Postoperative infection or failure of the repair is possible.

## REFERRAL DECISIONS/RED FLAGS

Patients with any type of suspected flexor tendon injury (rupture or laceration) require further evaluation for surgical repair.

# FLEXOR TENDON SHEATH INFECTIONS

ICD-9 Code

727.89
Abscess of bursa or tendon

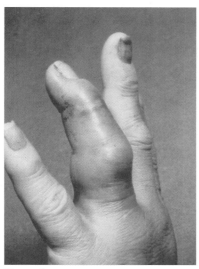

**Figure 1**
Septic tenosynovitis of the ring finger.

*Reproduced with permission from Stern PJ: Selected acute infections, in Greene WB (ed): Instructional Course Lectures XXXIX. Park Ridge, IL, American Academy of Orthopaedic Surgeons, 1990, pp 539–546.*

## SYNONYM
Septic tenosynovitis

## DEFINITION
The flexor tendons of the fingers and thumb are enclosed in a specialized tenosynovial sheath that extends from the distal palm to the distal joint (**Figure 1**). Infections within this space can develop from a puncture wound or can spread to the sheath from more superficial infection. These infections are, in essence, an abscess and are rapidly progressive, requiring prompt diagnosis and treatment.

## CLINICAL SYMPTOMS
Patients typically present with a history of a recent puncture wound to the flexor surface of the finger or thumb. Progressive swelling of the entire digit and significant pain develop 24 to 48 hours after injury.

## TESTS
### PHYSICAL EXAMINATION
Signs of a well-established septic flexor tenosynovitis include: 1) fusiform swelling of the finger; 2) significant tenderness along the course of the tendon sheath; 3) a marked increase in pain on passive extension; and 4) a flexed position of the finger at rest (**Figure 2**).

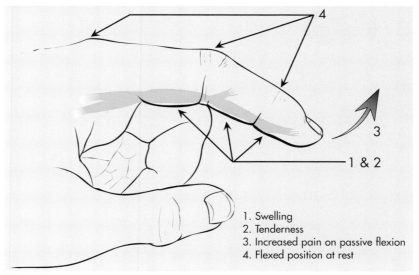

1. Swelling
2. Tenderness
3. Increased pain on passive flexion
4. Flexed position at rest

**Figure 2**
Signs of septic tenosynovitis.

*Adapted with permission from Carter PR: Common Hand Injuries and Infections: A Practical Approach to Early Treatment. Philadelphia, PA, WB Saunders, 1983, p 220.*

## DIAGNOSTIC TESTS

Plain radiographs may show soft-tissue swelling or, rarely, a foreign body or subcutaneous air.

## DIFFERENTIAL DIAGNOSIS

Aseptic flexor synovitis (swelling, tenderness, negative bacterial cultures)

Cellulitis (little or no pain with active motion of the finger)

## ADVERSE OUTCOMES OF THE DISEASE

These infections progress rapidly; therefore, complications such as skin loss or loss of the entire finger are possible. Other problems include significant stiffness from adhesions and ascending infection or involvement of the bone and joint.

## TREATMENT

If septic tenosynovitis is suspected but the swelling is not severe, parenteral antibiotics should be initiated and the patient reevaluated in 12 to 24 hours. Both *Staphylococcus* and *Streptococcus* should be covered. If the patient responds to parenteral antibiotics, these should be continued for 24 to 72 hours and then switched to oral antibiotics for an additional 7 to 14 days. If the patient has an established purulent flexor tenosynovitis or if the infection progresses or does not respond to antibiotic treatment, prompt referral for surgical drainage is indicated.

## ADVERSE OUTCOMES OF TREATMENT

Finger stiffness can persist, despite successful treatment of septic tenosynovitis.

## REFERRAL DECISIONS/RED FLAGS

Patients with well-established septic tenosynovitis and those who do not respond to antibiotic treatment require evaluation for possible surgery.

# FRACTURE OF THE DISTAL RADIUS

ICD-9 Codes
813.41
Colles fracture, Smith fracture
813.42
Other fractures of distal end of radius (alone)

## SYNONYMS

Colles fracture

Smith fracture

Barton fracture

Chauffeur's fracture

Die-punch fracture

## DEFINITION

Fractures involving the distal radius are the most frequently occurring fractures in adults (**Figure 1**). The most common type is the Colles fracture, in which the distal radius fracture fragment is tilted upward or dorsally. The articular surface of the radius may or may not be involved, and the ulnar styloid could be fractured. A Smith fracture is the opposite of a Colles fracture: the distal fragment is tilted downward or volarly. A Barton fracture is an intra-articular fracture associated with subluxation of the carpus, either dorsally or volarly, along with the displaced articular fragment of the radius. A chauffeur's fracture is an oblique fracture through the base of the radial styloid. A die-punch fracture is a depressed fracture of the articular surface opposite the lunate or scaphoid bone.

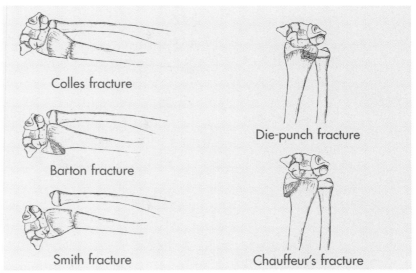

**Figure 1**
Types of fractures of the distal radius.

SECTION 4 | HAND AND WRIST

## CLINICAL SYMPTOMS

Patients have acute pain, tenderness, swelling, and deformity of the wrist, as well as a history of falling on the outstretched arm.

## TESTS

### PHYSICAL EXAMINATION

Look for swelling, deformity, and discoloration around the wrist and distal radius. Test for sensation in the hand over the median, radial, and ulnar nerve distribution. Also check the circulation to the fingertips. Examine the elbow for swelling and tenderness.

### DIAGNOSTIC TESTS

AP and lateral radiographs of the forearm, including the wrist, are necessary. Radiographs of the elbow should be obtained when elbow swelling and tenderness are present.

## DIFFERENTIAL DIAGNOSIS

Carpal fracture-dislocation (evident on radiographs)

Fracture of the scaphoid (tenderness over anatomic snuffbox, possibly evident on radiographs)

Tenosynovitis of the wrist (normal radiographs)

## ADVERSE OUTCOMES OF THE DISEASE

Malunion, loss of wrist motion, loss of finger motion, complex regional pain syndrome, decreased grip strength, posttraumatic arthritis, or (uncommonly) compartment syndrome can occur when a fracture of the distal radius is not treated.

## TREATMENT

The accuracy of reduction of distal radius fractures correlates with functional result. Anatomic reduction is the ideal, but less-than-perfect anatomic reduction sometimes can be accepted, depending on the comminution of the fracture and the patient's age and medical condition: older, less active persons are more tolerant of residual deformity than younger individuals.

Guidelines for acceptable alignment of distal radius fractures are as follows:

On the lateral view, no more than 5° of dorsal angulation is acceptable (**Figure 2**).

On the AP view, no less than 15° of radial inclination is acceptable.

Any overlap of the radial cortices should be reduced.

A step-off in the articular surface greater than 2 mm should be reduced.

AP and lateral radiographs of the fracture should be repeated each week for 2 weeks after the fracture because loss of alignment can occur.

For nondisplaced and minimally displaced, nonarticular fractures, a sugar tong splint should be applied for 2 to 3 weeks and a short-arm cast for an additional 2 to 3 weeks. (Two weeks in a sugar tong splint and 2 weeks in a

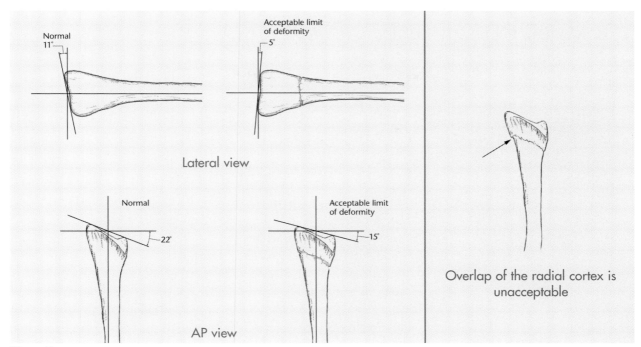

**Figure 2**
Guidelines for acceptable alignment of distal radius fractures.

short-arm cast are adequate for older, less active patients.) After the short-arm cast is removed, the patient should wear a removable splint for 3 weeks so that the splint can be removed for bathing and gentle exercise. The patient should be encouraged to move the shoulder of the injured arm through a full range of motion twice a day to prevent shoulder stiffness. Likewise, active and passive finger motion done in five sets four times a day should be encouraged.

Displaced fractures often are unstable and require additional internal and/or external fixation techniques.

## ADVERSE OUTCOMES OF TREATMENT

Recurrence of deformity, malunion, loss of wrist motion (flexion, extension, pronation, and supination), carpal tunnel syndrome, loss of finger motion, compartment syndrome, or paresthesias of the radial sensory nerve all can result following treatment.

## REFERRAL DECISIONS/RED FLAGS

Any displaced fracture that exceeds the parameters outlined above and any intra-articular fracture requires further evaluation. Patients with fractures that initially are nondisplaced but that show progressive collapse on radiographic follow-up require further evaluation.

# FRACTURE OF THE SCAPHOID

ICD-9 Code

814.01
Fracture of carpal bone, closed-
navicular (scaphoid) of wrist

## DEFINITION

The scaphoid spans the distal and proximal rows of the carpus and in that position is vulnerable to falls on the outstretched hand. The scaphoid is the most commonly fractured carpal bone. Young male adults are most commonly affected. These fractures are not common in children and older adults because the distal radius is the weak link in patients in these age groups. Of all scaphoid fractures, approximately 20% occur in the proximal pole, 60% in the middle or waist, and 20% in the distal pole.

In addition to their frequency, fractures of the scaphoid are important because their diagnosis is often delayed or missed. Patients may think they have a simple sprain and fail to seek medical attention. At the time of initial injury, routine radiographs may not demonstrate the fracture and, as a result, the fracture is inadequately immobilized.

Scaphoid fractures also have an increased incidence of nonunion and osteonecrosis. The blood supply to this bone is precarious because articular cartilage covers 80% of the scaphoid, and the major blood supply, which enters the bone in the distal third at the dorsal ridge, might be disrupted by the injury. Because of these anatomic features, displaced fractures of the scaphoid (more than 1 mm) have a nonunion rate of 55% to 90%. Fractures of the middle third are vulnerable to osteonecrosis, and fractures of the proximal third almost always result in osteonecrosis.

## CLINICAL SYMPTOMS

Pain and tenderness about the radial (thumb) side of the wrist are characteristic. Any type of wrist motion, such as gripping, is painful. Swelling about the back and radial side of the wrist is also common. If the patient reports a history of a high-energy injury, such as a car accident, ligamentous injuries and resultant carpal instability are possible in addition to the scaphoid fracture.

## TESTS

### PHYSICAL EXAMINATION

Palpation over the anatomic snuffbox reveals marked tenderness (Figure 1). The anatomic snuffbox area is defined by the abductor and long thumb extensor tendons just distal to the radial styloid. Likewise, pressure over the scaphoid tubercle on the underside of the wrist will produce pain with a scaphoid fracture. In addition, the patient may have decreased motion and grip strength. Assess function of the median, ulnar, and radial nerves, as well as circulatory status.

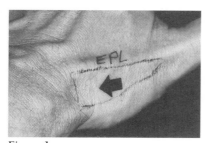

**Figure 1**
Anatomic snuffbox.

## DIAGNOSTIC TESTS

At the time of initial injury, scaphoid fractures may not be visible on posteroanterior (PA) and lateral radiographs of the wrist. Therefore, if these radiographs appear normal, obtain a PA view with the wrist in ulnar deviation and an oblique view to help visualize the fracture (**Figure 2**). If this series of initial radiographs is normal but the pain persists for 2 to 3 weeks, the PA and oblique views should be repeated. If the radiographs are still normal, a bone scan or MRI can be considered.

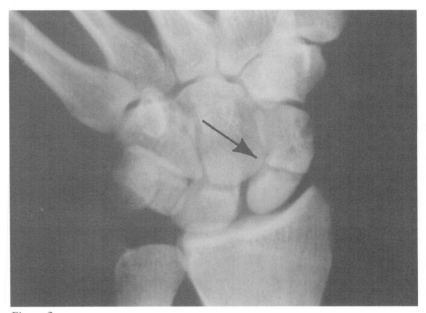

**Figure 2**
PA view of fracture (arrow) with the wrist in ulnar deviation.

## DIFFERENTIAL DIAGNOSIS

de Quervain tenosynovitis (positive Finkelstein test)

Fracture of the distal radius (evident on plain radiographs)

Scapholunate dissociation (increased gap between scaphoid and lunate [**Figure 3**])

Wrist arthritis (narrowing of joint space, evident on radiographs)

## ADVERSE OUTCOMES OF THE DISEASE

Nonunion, decreased grip strength and range of motion, and osteoarthritis of the radiocarpal joint are possible.

## TREATMENT

The treatment of acute nondisplaced fractures of the scaphoid is controversial because agreement is lacking on the optimum type of immobilization needed for these fractures. Conflicting data are reported regarding the optimum position of the wrist, whether the elbow should be immobilized, and whether the thumb should be included in the cast.

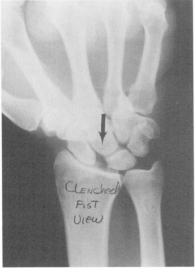

**Figure 3**
Scapholunate dissociation (arrow) with increased gap between the scaphoid and lunate.

Based on current data, immobilization for 6 weeks in a long-arm thumb spica cast with the wrist in a neutral position is recommended. If radiographs obtained after this time show that the fracture is healing, apply a short-arm thumb spica cast. However, if the fracture line appears to be getting wider, indicating absorption at the fracture site, or if the fracture shows any displacement, then further evaluation for possible surgery is indicated.

If the patient has pain over the region of the snuffbox but the initial radiographs are normal, place the hand and wrist in a thumb spica splint for 2 to 3 weeks, then repeat the radiographs. If the radiographs are still normal but tenderness over the scaphoid persists, order a bone scan or MRI. If the scan is positive, treat the hand as for an acute nondisplaced scaphoid fracture.

It may be difficult to determine on routine radiographs whether a scaphoid fracture has healed, and immobilization may be discontinued too soon. As a general rule, the closer the fracture line is to the proximal pole, the longer the time for healing. For fractures of the distal pole, the average time for healing is 6 to 8 weeks. Fractures of the middle third require 8 to 12 weeks to heal, and fractures of the proximal pole can take 12 to 24 weeks or longer. If plain radiographs do not clearly reveal that the fracture has healed, a tomogram can be ordered to better visualize the degree of healing.

## Adverse outcomes of treatment

Loss of motion from prolonged immobilization, and/or loss of grip strength can result.

## Referral decisions/Red flags

All patients with displaced fractures of the scaphoid need early further evaluation for possible operative treatment. Patients who show cystic absorption at the fracture site or displacement of the fracture after immobilization also need evaluation for surgical treatment. Patients with nondisplaced fractures that have not healed after 2 months of immobilization need further evaluation.

# Fracture of the Metacarpals and Phalanges

| ICD-9 Codes |
| --- |
| 815.00 |
|    Fracture of metacarpal bone(s), site |
|    unspecified, closed |
| 816.00 |
|    Fracture of one or more phalanges |
|    of hand, site unspecified, closed |

## Synonyms

Boxer's fracture

Fighter's fracture

## Definition

Metacarpal fractures are most common in adults (**Figure 1**). Fracture of the fifth metacarpal (boxer's fracture) is the most common fracture in the hand. A boxer's fracture is an injury of the distal metaphysis of the fifth metacarpal that results from a closed fist striking an object (**Figure 2**). In adult phalangeal fractures, the distal phalanx is the most commonly injured, followed by the proximal and the middle phalanges (**Figure 3**). Approximately 20% of these fractures are intra-articular.

Phalangeal fractures are more common in children. The most common fracture involves the physis of the little finger. Growth disturbances from physeal injuries of the phalanges are rare.

## Clinical symptoms

Patients typically have a history of trauma. Local tenderness, swelling, deformity, or decreased range of motion are common findings.

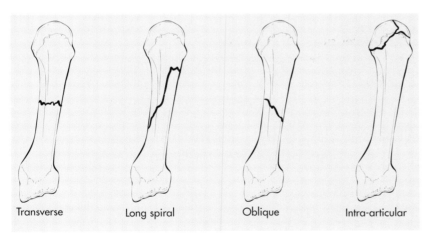

**Figure 1**
Types of metacarpal fractures.

*Adapted with permission from Dabezies EJ, Schutte JP: Fixation of metacarpal and phalangeal fractures with miniature plates and screws. J Hand Surg 1986;11A:283–288.*

Transverse    Long spiral    Oblique    Intra-articular

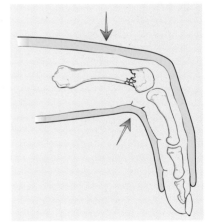

**Figure 2**
Fracture of the metacarpal neck (boxer's fracture).

*Adapted with permission from Green DP (ed): Operative Hand Surgery, ed 3. New York, NY, Churchill Livingstone, 1993.*

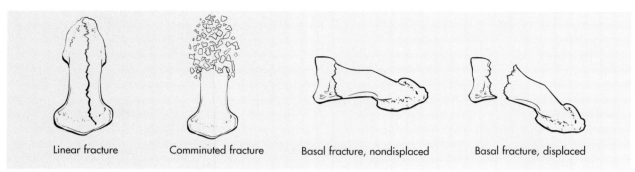

Linear fracture    Comminuted fracture    Basal fracture, nondisplaced    Basal fracture, displaced

**Figure 3**
Types of distal phalanx fractures.

*Adapted with permission from Rockwood CA, Green DP, Bucholz RW, et al (eds): Rockwood and Green's Fractures in Adults, ed 4. Philadelphia, PA, Lippincott-Raven, 1996, vol 2, pp 614, 627.*

## TESTS

### PHYSICAL EXAMINATION

Examination reveals swelling over the fracture site. The involved finger may appear shortened, or the knuckle may be depressed. The distal fragment may be rotated in relation to the proximal fragment. This is not easy to see with the fingers extended; however, when the patient makes a partial fist, the rotated fragments cause the involved finger to overlap onto its neighbor. Assess sensory function of the digital nerves.

### DIAGNOSTIC TESTS

Radiographs are always indicated for suspected fractures. For fractures of the phalanges, posteroanterior (PA) and true lateral views of the individual digits should be obtained. For metacarpal fractures, PA, lateral, and oblique views of the hand are indicated.

## DIFFERENTIAL DIAGNOSIS

Metacarpophalangeal (MP) and interphalangeal (IP) joint sprains (instability and joint tenderness)

MP and IP joint dislocations (evident on clinical examination)

## ADVERSE OUTCOMES OF THE DISEASE

Malunion, nonunion, and loss of finger motion are all possible.

## TREATMENT

### METACARPAL NECK FRACTURE

For a boxer's fracture, apply an ulnar gutter splint for 2 to 3 weeks in patients with 10° to 15° of angulation. With more than 15° of angulation but no extensor lag (the patient can fully extend the finger), use of an ulnar gutter cast or splint for 2 to 3 weeks also is appropriate. Advise the patient that although this fracture will not result in any functional deficit, there could be a loss of metacarpal prominence. If this is unsatisfactory to the patient, further evaluation is indicated.

With an extensor lag, or with more than 40° of angulation, referral for reduction is appropriate. Similar guidelines are appropriate for fractures of the metacarpal neck of the ring finger, although slightly less angulation is accepted because of prominence of the metacarpal head. The second and third metacarpals have less mobility and, therefore, less angulation is acceptable in these injuries. Use of a radial gutter splint is appropriate with less than 10° of angulation, but with greater angulation, functional loss could result and referral for reduction is appropriate.

## NONDISPLACED FRACTURES OF THE METACARPAL AND PHALANGEAL SHAFTS

Casting or splint immobilization for 3 weeks is indicated for phalangeal fractures and for 4 weeks for metacarpal fractures. When casting or splinting, always include the joint above and below the fracture and the adjacent digits. To avoid fixed contractures, the safe position of immobilization is with the MP joints held in approximately 70° of flexion and the proximal interphalangeal (PIP) and distal interphalangeal (DIP) joints held in extension. When loss of position is a possible problem, radiographs should be repeated 1 week after the injury.

Immobilization of phalangeal fractures for more than 3 to 4 weeks will result in stiffness. Do not wait for radiographic evidence of healing to begin exercises because full healing may not be apparent for 2 to 5 months. If the fracture seems clinically stable after cast removal, motion should be started.

## DISPLACED FRACTURES OF THE METACARPAL AND PHALANGEAL SHAFTS

Displaced transverse fractures of the metacarpals and phalanges tend to angulate (**Figure 4**). Spiral fractures tend to rotate, and oblique fractures tend to shorten. Patients with these types of fractures need further evaluation upon initial presentation.

SECTION 4 | HAND AND WRIST

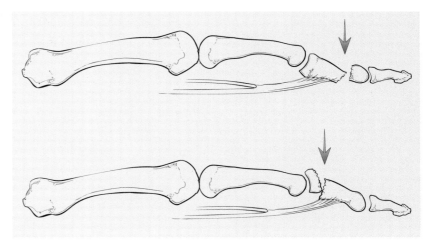

**Figure 4**
Phalangeal fractures angulate because of pull by the flexor tendons.

*Adapted with permission from Rockwood CA, Green DP, Bucholz RW, et al (eds): Rockwood and Green's Fractures in Adults, ed 4. Philadelphia, PA, Lippincott-Raven, 1996, vol 2, pp 614, 627.*

### INTRA-ARTICULAR FRACTURES

Splint nondisplaced intra-articular fractures with the MP joints in flexion and the PIP and DIP joints in extension. Repeat radiographs in 1 week to assess for continued articular congruity, then initiate active range of motion at 3 weeks. Displacement of intra-articular fractures greater than 1 mm is unacceptable because of loss of joint congruity; therefore, patients with displaced intra-articular fractures need further evaluation.

### ADVERSE OUTCOMES OF TREATMENT

Joint stiffness is the most common problem with hand fractures and is directly related to prolonged immobilization. Malunion caused by inadequate reduction also is possible.

### REFERRAL DECISIONS/RED FLAGS

Displaced fractures and intra-articular fractures usually require surgical pinning.

# FRACTURE OF THE BASE OF THE THUMB METACARPAL

| ICD-9 Code |
| --- |
| 816.00 |
| Fracture of one or more phalanges of hand, site unspecified, closed |

## SYNONYMS

Bennett fracture

Rolando fracture

## DEFINITION

A Bennett fracture is an oblique fracture of the base of the thumb metacarpal that enters the carpometacarpal (CMC) joint (**Figure 1**). This fracture has two pieces, one large, the other small. While the small volar fragment remains attached to the carpus, the major metacarpal fragment subluxates at the CMC joint (**Figure 2**).

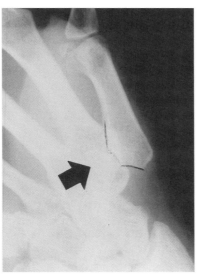

**Figure 1**
Radiograph showing Bennett fracture.

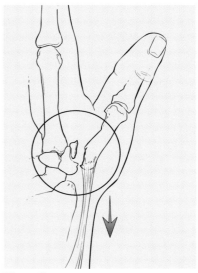

**Figure 2**
Fracture-subluxation of the base of the thumb metacarpal (Bennett fracture).

A Rolando fracture is less common than a Bennett fracture and is a Y-shaped intra-articular fracture at the base of the thumb metacarpal. A comminuted intra-articular fracture at the base of the thumb metacarpal also occurs.

## CLINICAL SYMPTOMS

Patients report pain and limited motion. Swelling and ecchymosis about the base of the thumb are common and are indicative of a metacarpal fracture or CMC dislocation.

## TESTS

### PHYSICAL EXAMINATION

Examination reveals that, when the tip of the thumb is held into the palm, the base of the thumb metacarpal is displaced radially and posteriorly. The patient cannot move the thumb without pain.

### DIAGNOSTIC TESTS

AP and lateral radiographs of the thumb will show these fractures.

## DIFFERENTIAL DIAGNOSIS

Arthritis of the CMC joint (narrow joint space evident on radiographs)

Dislocation of the CMC joint (evident on radiographs)

Fracture of the scaphoid (evident on radiographs)

Synovitis of the CMC joint (swollen joint, normal radiographs)

## ADVERSE OUTCOMES OF THE DISEASE

Posttraumatic arthritis of the CMC joint is possible, resulting in pain at the base of the thumb, along with loss of motion and pinch strength.

## TREATMENT

The goal of treatment is to restore the axial length of the thumb and to replace the metacarpal shaft fragment against the smaller volar lip fragment. Although anatomic reduction of the fracture is the goal, some offset can still produce a good functional outcome. A Bennett fracture almost always requires some form of surgical fixation to achieve stability in the joint.

Nondisplaced two-part fractures of the base of the thumb metacarpal can be treated in a thumb spica cast for 4 weeks.

## ADVERSE OUTCOMES OF TREATMENT

After surgery, pin tract irritation and infection can occur, as can tenderness around the surgical plates and screws. Displacement of the fracture (loss of position) and posttraumatic arthritis also are possible.

## REFERRAL DECISIONS/RED FLAGS

Patients with displaced fractures of the base of the thumb metacarpal need further evaluation.

# GANGLIA OF THE WRIST AND HAND

## ICD-9 Codes
727.41
    Ganglion of joint
727.42
    Ganglion of tendon sheath

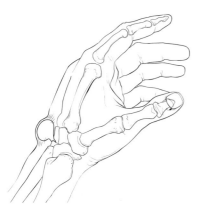

**Figure 1**
Clinical appearance of wrist ganglion.

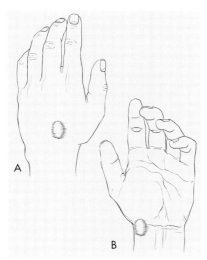

**Figure 2**
Clinical appearance of (A) dorsal and (B) volar wrist ganglia.

*Adapted with permission from the American Society for Surgery of the Hand: Brochure: Ganglion Cysts. Englewood, CO, 1995.*

## SYNONYMS

Synovial cyst

Mucous cyst

Volar retinacular ganglion

Flexor tendon sheath ganglion

## DEFINITION

A ganglion is a cystic structure that arises from the capsule of a joint or a tendon synovial sheath (**Figure 1**). The cyst contains a thick, clear, mucinous fluid identical in composition to joint fluid. Through degeneration or tearing of the joint capsule or tendon sheath, a connection to the joint or tendon sheath with a one-way valve is established. Thus, synovial fluid can enter the cyst but cannot flow freely back into the synovial cavity. Ganglia vary in size, and sometimes significant symptoms result from increased pressure on surrounding structures.

Ganglia are the most common soft-tissue tumors of the hand, generally affecting individuals between the ages of 15 and 40 years. These benign tumors typically develop and sometimes disappear spontaneously. Common locations include the dorsum of the wrist, the volar radial aspect of the wrist, and the base of the finger. The latter typically arises from the proximal annular ligament (A1 pulley) of the flexor tendon sheath. These also are known as volar retinacular ganglia.

Mucous cysts are a type of ganglion that develops from an arthritic distal interphalangeal (DIP) joint, most commonly in women between the ages of 40 and 70 years.

## CLINICAL SYMPTOMS

### WRIST

Patients typically have an unsightly lump, which may or may not be painful (**Figure 2**). The pain is described as aching and is aggravated by activities that require frequent movement of the wrist. Ganglia in the wrist often vary in size with an increase in size associated with times of increased activity. A history of variation in size is a key factor to distinguish a ganglion from other soft-tissue tumors.

Occasionally, a ganglion will occur in areas of the wrist that cause compression of the median or ulnar nerve. In this situation, sensory symptoms in the fingers and/or weakness of the intrinsic muscle develop.

### HAND AND FINGER

Patients with flexor tendon sheath cysts report tenderness when grasping and a bump at the base of the finger at the level of the proximal flexion crease

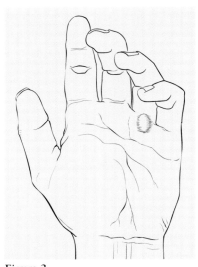

**Figure 3**
Flexor sheath ganglion.

*Adapted with permission from the American Society for Surgery of the Hand: Brochure: Ganglion Cysts. Englewood, CO, 1995.*

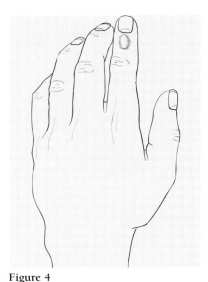

**Figure 4.**
Mucous cyst.

*Adapted with permission from the American Society for Surgery of the Hand: Brochure: Ganglion Cysts. Englewood, CO, 1995.*

(**Figure 3**). A tender mass in this area almost always is a flexor tendon sheath ganglion.

Patients with mucous cysts report swelling on the dorsum of the finger distal to the DIP joint (**Figure 4**). They also may report a cycle of the cyst breaking open, draining a clear, jelly-like fluid, and healing. Treatment often is sought when the cyst becomes painful, ulcerated, or infected, or is cosmetically displeasing. Patients also may have striations or furrowing of the fingernail because of pressure of the cyst on the nail matrix.

## TESTS

### PHYSICAL EXAMINATION—WRIST

A dorsal ganglion is typically a smooth, round or multilobulated structure on the dorsoradial aspect of the wrist that becomes more prominent with flexion. It usually is positioned directly over the scapholunate joint but can occur more distally even though its stalk usually emanates from the scapholunate joint.

A volar radial ganglion usually is a less well-defined mass situated between the flexor carpi radialis tendon and the radial styloid. It may extend underneath the radial artery and, in some cases, may adhere to the radial artery. On palpation, the ganglion may appear to pulsate and can be confused with an aneurysm. Symptoms also become more pronounced with extreme flexion or extension.

Ganglia usually are mildly tender with pressure. A prominent ganglion often will transilluminate when a penlight is placed at its side. Solid tumors will not transilluminate.

If a definite mass is not visible, the possibility of an occult ganglion should be considered. Swelling is more subtle with an occult ganglion. Palpation must be more thorough and careful in order to identify a small tender mass that is different from what is felt on the opposite wrist.

## PHYSICAL EXAMINATION—HAND AND FINGER

A volar retinacular ganglion of the flexor tendon sheath is characterized by a small, firm, tender mass at the base of the finger in the area of the metacarpophalangeal flexion crease, most often at the middle or ring fingers (see Figure 3). These ganglia are sometimes difficult to detect because of their small size; in fact, they may simply feel like a small seed; however, they are quite tender. These ganglia rarely affect motion and do not move with excursion of the tendon.

Mucous cysts are usually lying to one side of the extensor tendon (see Figure 4). Initial clinical findings include a mass or a blister. Arthritic nodules are associated with this joint.

## DIAGNOSTIC TESTS

Posteroanterior (PA), lateral, and oblique radiographs of the hand or PA and lateral radiographs of the wrist or the involved finger should be obtained to rule out bony pathology. In most cases, ganglia are not associated with radiographic changes. With a mucous cyst, degenerative changes and a small bony spur usually are seen rising from the dorsum of the distal phalanx at the DIP joint.

## DIFFERENTIAL DIAGNOSIS

### WRIST

Arthritis (evident on radiographs)

Bone tumor (evident on radiographs)

Intraosseous ganglion (evident on radiographs)

Kienböck disease (collapse of the lunate)

Soft-tissue tumor, benign or malignant (solid mass on palpation, rare)

### HAND AND FINGER

Dupuytren disease (presence of cords or bands)

Giant cell tumors (different locations, but usually about the phalanges)

Lipoma (larger in size, often in the palm)

## ADVERSE OUTCOMES OF THE DISEASE

### WRIST

Patients can experience a decrease in grip strength and painful wrist motion; they also may complain about the unsightly bump. On rare occasions, ganglia will cause significant compression on the median nerve.

### HAND AND FINGER

Patients often have pain in the hand and finger and an obvious deformity at the fingernail. Infection also can occur in association with a mucous cyst.

## TREATMENT

### WRIST

If the wrist ganglion is typical in presentation and physical findings, reassurance usually is adequate. When the patient has acute, severe symptoms, immobilizing the wrist will relieve symptoms and may cause the ganglion to decrease in size. However, immobilization is rarely a permanent solution. Occasionally, aspiration of a dorsal wrist ganglion will lead to resolution (see Ganglion Aspiration, p 265). Due to the proximity of the radial artery, volar wrist ganglia are rarely aspirated.

When the patient has significant symptoms or is seriously bothered by the appearance of the wrist ganglion, then surgical excision is indicated.

### HAND AND FINGER

Treatment of a ganglion of the tendon sheath consists of needle rupture followed by massage to disperse the contents of the cyst, or injection with 1% or 2% local anesthetic until the cyst pops. Exercise caution when performing a needle rupture because of the proximity of the neurovascular bundle. Operative management is occasionally required for painful flexor sheath ganglia.

Aspiration and/or rupture of a mucous cyst is not recommended because of the danger of introducing an infection into the DIP joint.

## ADVERSE OUTCOMES OF TREATMENT

### WRIST

Recurrence of wrist ganglia occurs in 5% to 10% of patients after surgical excision, and in up to 90% after needle aspiration. Injury to the radial artery can occur as a result of aspiration of a volar wrist ganglion.

### HAND AND FINGER

Recurrence of hand and finger ganglia also is quite common. Skin loss is possible, as is injury to the digital nerve.

## REFERRAL DECISION/RED FLAGS

### WRIST

Any mass with atypical findings should be evaluated with additional diagnostic tests or excisional biopsy. Recurrence after aspiration also is an indication for further evaluation.

### HAND AND FINGER

Persistence of a painful or bothersome cyst after one or two attempts at needle rupture or aspiration indicates that surgical excision should be considered. Increased erythema and pain in a mucous cyst suggests infection that may require operative treatment.

# PROCEDURE

## GANGLION ASPIRATION

### MATERIALS

Sterile gloves

Bactericidal skin preparation solution

3-mL syringe with a 27-gauge, ¾" needle

18-gauge needle

3 mL of a 1% local anesthetic without epinephrine

Elastic bandage

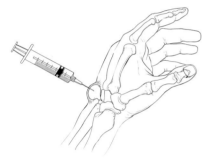

**Figure 1**
Location for needle insertion.

### STEP 1

Wear protective gloves at all times during this procedure and use sterile technique.

### STEP 2

Cleanse the area with a bactericidal skin preparation solution.

### STEP 3

Use a syringe with a 27-gauge needle to infiltrate 1% local anesthetic into the area immediately proximal to and surrounding the ganglion. Remove the 27-gauge needle and change to the 18-gauge needle.

### STEP 4

Penetrate the ganglion with the 18-gauge needle and attempt to withdraw as much fluid as possible (**Figure 1**). Injecting corticosteroid has not been shown to influence the recurrence rate and is not recommended.

### STEP 5

Apply a sterile dressing.

### ADVERSE OUTCOMES

Infection and recurrence of the ganglion are possible. Injury to the radial artery also can occur following attempts to aspirate volar wrist ganglia.

### AFTERCARE/PATIENT INSTRUCTIONS

Instruct the patient to wear the elastic bandage for 1 week, removing it only for bathing.

# HUMAN BITES

## ICD-9 Codes

882.0
  Open wound of hand except finger(s) alone, without mention of complication
883.0
  Open wound of fingers without mention of complication

## SYNONYMS
Clenched fist injury
Fight bite

## DEFINITION
Human bite wounds to the hand occur either directly from a bite (usually to the fingers) or indirectly when the hand strikes a tooth (clenched fist injury) (**Figure 1**). Few infections of the hand can progress more quickly or result in more significant complications. Early recognition and appropriate treatment are crucial, but because the laceration often is small and perhaps due to circumstances of the injury, these patients often do not seek medical attention until a serious infection has already developed (**Figure 2**).

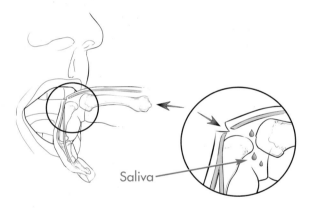

**Figure 1**
Mechanism of tendon laceration in human bite.

*Adapted with permission from Carter PR: Common Hand Injuries and Infections: A Practical Approach to Early Treatment. Philadelphia, PA, WB Saunders, 1983.*

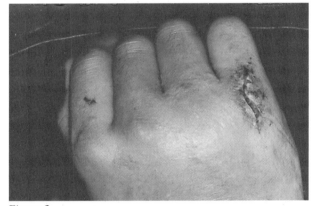

**Figure 2**
Possible tooth injury.

Human bite wounds contain greater concentrations of bacteria than animal bite wounds, especially anaerobic species. *Eikenella* species are associated with human bite wounds, but the most common organisms causing these infections are α-hemolytic streptococci and *Staphylococcus aureus*.

## CLINICAL SYMPTOMS
The history of the injury and a laceration is diagnostic but may be difficult to elicit from an embarrassed patient who has been in a fight. Warmth, swelling, pain, and a purulent discharge are often present. Examination may reveal evidence of damage to underlying structures, including lack of extension or flexion due to tendon damage (**Figure 3**) or a loss of sensation over the tip of the finger due to nerve injury.

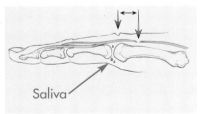

**Figure 3**
The tendon injury, cut in flexion, retracts as the joint extends.

*Adapted with permission from Carter PR: Common Hand Injuries and Infections: A Practical Approach to Early Treatment. Philadelphia, PA, WB Saunders, 1983.*

# TESTS

## PHYSICAL EXAMINATION

Measure and record the location of the laceration. A small laceration over the ring or little finger is a sign of a possible clenched fist injury. Beware of a tooth wound proximal to the metacarpophalangeal (MP) joint when the finger is extended but lies over the knuckle in a clenched fist. Document the location and severity of the swelling, erythema, and any purulent discharge. When the injury is on the dorsum of the hand, significant swelling may occur quickly (eg, when the injury is only 2 to 3 hours old). Assess function of the flexor and extensor tendons and sensory nerves distal to the laceration. Examine the forearm for signs of ascending infection (eg, lymphangitic streaks, enlarged epitrochlear nodes).

## DIAGNOSTIC TESTS

Posteroanterior, lateral, and oblique radiographs of the hand should be obtained to rule out an underlying fracture or presence of a foreign body. Aerobic and anaerobic cultures should be obtained when any drainage is present. A white blood cell count can serve as a baseline for following the clinical course, but this test may be within normal limits in the early phases after injury.

# DIFFERENTIAL DIAGNOSIS

Laceration from a sharp object (accurate history)

Septic joint caused by a retained foreign body (possibly evident on radiographs)

# ADVERSE OUTCOMES OF THE DISEASE

Tendon rupture and/or laceration can occur as a result of the bite. An abscess involving the deep palmar space, osteomyelitis, joint sepsis, joint stiffness, and possibly septic tenosynovitis can develop with delay in treatment.

# TREATMENT

Bite wounds can be treated on an outpatient basis if the joint has not been penetrated, if there has been no tendon or bony injury, and when medical treatment is sought within 8 hours of the injury.

Anesthetize the wound with a 1% plain lidocaine, carefully examine and debride the skin edges and any underlying necrotic tissue. The extensor mechanism over the MP joints should be examined with the finger flexed to assess for damage to the tendons or penetration of the underlying joint. Irrigate the wound with 1,000 mL of saline solution and apply saline-soaked gauze or a nonadherent dressing. Human bites should never be closed primarily.

Immobilize the hand in a bulky dressing that incorporates a dorsal plaster splint that holds the hand in a safe position (ie, with the MP joint at 60° to 90° of flexion and the interphalangeal joints in a resting, extended position).

## Table 1
### Guide to Tetanus Prophylaxis in Wound Management

| History of tetanus toxoid (doses) | Clean, minor wound | | Contaminated wound | |
|---|---|---|---|---|
| | Td | TIG | Td | TIG |
| Unknown | Yes | No | Yes | Yes* |
| Fewer than 3 doses | Yes | No | Yes | Yes* |
| 3 or more | Yes, if more than 10 years since last dose | No | Yes, if more than 5 years since last dose | No |

Td = combined tetanus and diphtheria toxoid adsorbed (dose = 0.5 mL IM). TIG = tetanus immune globulin (dose = 250 IU IM).

* Td and TIG should be administered at different sites.

*Adapted with permission from the Centers for Disease Control and Prevention.*

Appropriate tetanus prophylaxis should be given as outlined in Table 1, followed by antibiotics. Penicillin and a first-generation cephalosporin provide adequate coverage in most instances. Tetracycline can be used for patients who are allergic to penicillin.

Advise the patient to return within 24 hours for a recheck to confirm that infection has not developed. After the first 24 hours, daily whirlpool treatment or twice-daily dressing changes can be started. The wound should be allowed to close by secondary intention.

## ADVERSE OUTCOMES OF TREATMENT

Inadequate evaluation or treatment can lead to significant complications. Infection may develop with primary wound closure. Patients can experience sensitivity to antibiotics.

## REFERRAL DECISIONS/RED FLAGS

Wounds that involve the joint, tendon, nerve, or bone require further evaluation. A bite wound that becomes infected despite treatment with antibiotics also needs further evaluation.

# KIENBÖCK DISEASE

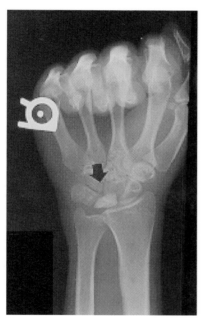

**Figure 1**
Radiograph showing Kienböck disease (arrow).

## SYNONYMS

Wrist sprain
Osteonecrosis of the carpal lunate

## DEFINITION

Kienböck disease is osteonecrosis of the carpal lunate that most commonly affects men between the ages of 20 and 40 years (**Figure 1**). Patients may have a history of trauma, but the cause of the disrupted blood supply is frequently difficult to establish. With progression of the disease, the lunate collapses and fragments ultimately lead to end-stage arthritis of the wrist.

## CLINICAL SYMPTOMS

Pain, stiffness, and diffuse swelling over the dorsal aspect of the wrist are common. Patients often report weakness or inability to grasp heavy objects.

## TESTS

### PHYSICAL EXAMINATION

Examination typically reveals tenderness, directly over the lunate bone (mid-dorsal wrist area, just distal to the radius). Grip strength usually is decreased. With progression of the disease, dorsal swelling and limited wrist motion is common.

### DIAGNOSTIC TESTS

Posteroanterior and lateral radiographs of the wrist are indicated. Failure to obtain radiographs is the most common reason for delay in diagnosis. In the early phase of Kienböck disease, radiographs show increased density or whiteness of the lunate bone compared with the surrounding carpal bones. In later stages, the dead bone will fragment and collapse, resulting in generalized degenerative arthritis of the wrist (**Figure 2**).

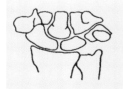
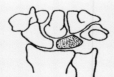
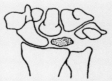
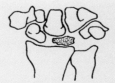
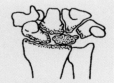

| Stage 1: No visible change in the lunate | Stage 2: Sclerosis of the lunate | Stage 3A: Sclerosis and fragmentation of the lunate | Stage 3B: Stage 3A with proximal migration of the capitate or fixed rotation of the scaphoid) | Stage 4: Stage 3A or 3B combined with degenerative changes at adjacent joints |

**Figure 2**
Lichtman's classification of Kienböck disease.

*Reproduced with permission from American Society for Surgery of the Hand: Hand Surgery Update. Rosemont, IL, American Academy of Orthopaedic Surgeons, 1994, p 86.*

# DIFFERENTIAL DIAGNOSIS

Fracture of the distal radius (evident on radiographs)

Fracture of the scaphoid (evident on radiographs)

Ganglion (discrete mass, normal radiographs)

Scapholunate dissociation (increased distance between the scaphoid and lunate on radiographs)

Tenosynovitis of the extensor tendon (diffuse swelling over extensor tendon extending onto the hand)

Wrist arthritis (narrowing of joint space but contour of lunate normal)

# ADVERSE OUTCOMES OF THE DISEASE

Untreated Kienböck disease almost always results in progressive arthritis.

# TREATMENT

When radiographs are normal, splint the wrist in a neutral position for 3 weeks. NSAIDs may make the patient more comfortable. If the pain persists after 3 weeks, further evaluation is indicated.

# ADVERSE OUTCOMES OF TREATMENT

Loss of motion, chronic pain, and decreased grip strength are possible.

# REFERRAL DECISIONS/RED FLAGS

Patients whose plain radiographs show any abnormality of the lunate need further evaluation. Persistent dorsal wrist pain, despite 3 weeks of immobilization, also is an indication for further evaluation.

# MALLET FINGER

ICD-9 Code
736.1
    Mallet finger

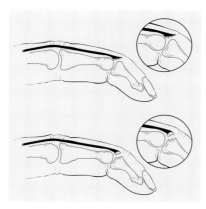

**Figure 1**
Mallet finger caused by rupture of the extensor tendon at its insertion (top); mallet finger caused by avulsion of a piece of distal phalanx (bottom).

*Adapted with permission from Rockwood CA, Green DP, Bucholz RW, et al (eds): Rockwood and Green's Fractures in Adults, ed 4. Philadelphia, PA, Lippincott-Raven, 1996, vol 2, p 617.*

## SYNONYMS

Baseball finger

Extensor tendon injury

## DEFINITION

A mallet finger deformity is caused by rupture or avulsion of the insertion of the extensor tendon at the base of the distal phalanx. Sometimes, instead of the tendon tearing, the injury avulses a fragment of the distal phalanx at the tendinous attachment (**Figure 1**). Laceration is a third mechanism of injury.

## CLINICAL SYMPTOMS

Patients report pain and an inability to straighten the fingertip.

## TESTS

### PHYSICAL EXAMINATION

Examination reveals that the distal interphalangeal (DIP) joint is in flexion and that the patient is unable to extend the joint. The dorsal area of the DIP joint initially is tender and slightly swollen, but about 2 weeks after the injury occurs, the fingertip usually is not painful.

## DIAGNOSTIC TESTS

AP and lateral radiographs may reveal a small bony avulsion from the dorsal side of the distal phalanx. With large dorsal avulsion fragments, the distal phalanx may subluxate in a volar direction from the unopposed pull of the flexor tendon.

## DIFFERENTIAL DIAGNOSIS

Fracture-dislocation of the DIP joint (evident on radiographs)

Fracture of the distal phalanx (evident on radiographs)

## ADVERSE OUTCOME OF THE DISEASE

Permanent flexion of the DIP joint is possible.

## TREATMENT

Continuous splinting of the DIP joint in extension is critical to restoring full function of the extensor tendon. The splint can be applied on either the volar or dorsal surface of the finger (**Figure 2**). With acute injuries, the splint should be worn for 6 weeks. If the injury is more than 3 months old, a splint should be worn for at least 8 weeks.

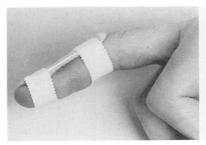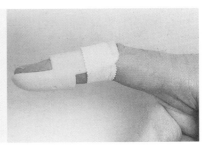

**Figure 2**
Types of splints used in treatment of mallet finger: dorsal aluminum (left), commercial splint (right).

*Reproduced with permission from Culver JE: Office management of athletic injuries of the hand and wrist, in Barr JS (ed): Instructional Course Lectures XXXVIII. Park Ridge, IL, American Academy of Orthopaedic Surgeons, 1989, pp 473-482.*

Advise patients to maintain the DIP joint in extension when the splint is removed for cleaning. If the fingertip droops at any time after the splint is applied, the healing process is disrupted and the period of splinting must be extended. Four or five days after the splint is applied, check the dorsal skin for maceration or pressure spots. If the joint does not come into full extension by the second visit, the patient should be evaluated for possible surgical pinning.

Weekly follow-up visits are helpful to monitor progress and usually lead to a better outcome than if the splint is applied and the patient is seen 6 to 8 weeks later. At the end of the splinting period, if there is no extensor lag evident, guarded active flexion is started with splinting continued at night for 2 to 4 weeks.

Certain occupations (eg, cooking, dishwashing, typing) make splint wear difficult, and patients doing these tasks repeatedly should be evaluated for possible surgical pinning.

## ADVERSE OUTCOME OF TREATMENT
Persistent deformity associated with flexion of the fingertip is possible, despite treatment.

## REFERRAL DECISIONS/RED FLAGS
Patients with volar subluxation of the distal phalanx and/or an avulsed bony fragment that involves more than one third of the joint surface need further evaluation.

# NAIL INJURIES

ICD-9 Code

883.0
　　Open wound of fingers without
　　mention of complication

## SYNONYMS

Subungual hematoma

Smashed finger

## DEFINITION

Many injuries to the fingertip are crushing in nature, resulting in various degrees of injury to the fingernail, nail bed, and distal phalanx (**Figure 1**). The types of nail bed injuries include simple lacerations, stellate lacerations, severe crush injuries, and avulsions. Approximately 50% will be associated with fractures of the distal phalanx.

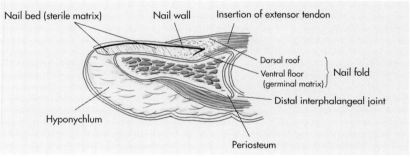

**Figure 1**
Anatomy of nail bed: Sagittal view.

## CLINICAL SYMPTOMS

Patients usually have pain and obvious injury to the fingertip.

## TESTS

### PHYSICAL EXAMINATION

Determine the extent of the injury, noting any subungual hematoma and its extent, avulsion or laceration of the nail, and whether an associated fracture of the distal phalanx is displaced or nondisplaced. When the fingernail is avulsed, note the extent of injury to the nail bed (both germinal and sterile matrices). Examine an avulsed fingernail for attached remnants of the nail bed. An avulsion of the fingernail in a child or infant may be associated with a physeal injury.

### DIAGNOSTIC TESTS

Posterolateral and lateral radiographs of the finger are necessary when a fracture of the distal phalanx is suspected.

## DIFFERENTIAL DIAGNOSIS

Mallet finger (unable to extend fully the distal interphalangeal joint)

## ADVERSE OUTCOMES OF THE DISEASE

If the patient has sustained damage to the nail bed, particularly the germinal matrix, a permanent nail deformity may result. This is often cosmetic but could be painful.

## TREATMENT

### SUBUNGUAL HEMATOMAS

Painful subungual hematomas can be treated with decompression. After scrubbing the finger, create a hole in the fingernail over the hematoma, using battery-operated microcautery, if available, or a heated paper clip or 18-gauge needle. The hole must be large enough to allow continued drainage.

### NAIL BED LACERATIONS

For lacerations of the nail bed with injury to the nail plate, the nail plate should be removed and the nail bed repaired. This should be done with adequate anesthesia (see Digital Anesthetic Block [Hand], p 240), with sterile preparation of the finger and the use of a finger tourniquet. Elevate all or part of the nail plate using a small scissors. The entire nail can be removed or just enough to allow visualization of the laceration and suture placement. Irrigate the wound, remove the hematoma, and meticulously suture the nail bed using 6-0 or 7-0 absorbable gut suture. After repair, if the nail plate is available, place it under the nail fold. Suture the nail to the fingertip with 5-0 nylon suture to keep it in place. If the nail is not available, place nonadherent gauze cut to conform to the nail bed underneath the fold. This gauze can be left in place because it will grow out with the new nail. An associated minimally displaced or nondisplaced fracture usually will be stabilized with the repair.

### NAIL AVULSIONS

The proximal portion of the nail bed (germinal matrix) may be avulsed and lying on top of the nail fold (**Figure 2**). This must be replaced underneath the nail fold and sutured in place. The sutures should be placed through the proximal fold to pull the nail bed into the fold. If the nail avulsion is associated with a fracture, the distal phalanx may need to be stabilized. Any nail bed tissue adherent to the fingernail should be gently removed with a scalpel and sewn in place in the nail bed defect using small absorbable suture. A large fragment of nail or the whole nail itself, when it has a large amount of nail bed still attached to it, should not have the tissue removed; rather, sew the entire fragment anatomically in place. Any injuries to the nail fold should be repaired with 5-0 nylon or monofilament suture.

### WOUND CARE

The finger should be dressed with antibacterial ointment, nonadherent gauze, sterile gauze, and an outer wrap. The finger should be splinted for protection.

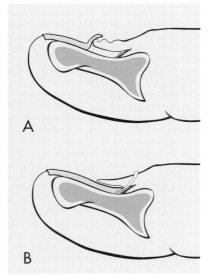

**Figure 2**
Detachment of the proximal portion of the nail bed (germinal matrix) (A) and replacement of the germinal matrix into the nail fold (B).

## ADVERSE OUTCOMES OF TREATMENT

Abnormal growth and subsequent deformity of the nail can occur.

## REFERRAL DECISIONS/RED FLAGS

Nail bed injuries with complex lacerations or loss of tissue or injury to the germinal matrix may require more involved operative treatment. Associated open fractures of the distal phalanx require further evaluation.

# PROCEDURE

## FISHHOOK REMOVAL

### MATERIALS

Sterile gloves

Bactericidal skin preparation solution

24" length of #0 or #1 nylon or silk suture

3-mL syringe with a 27-gauge needle

3 mL of a 1% local anesthetic without epinephrine

Wire cutter

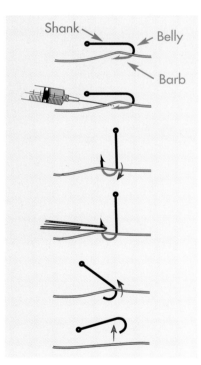

**Figure 1**
Technique 1 for removing a fishhook.

*Adapted with permission from Quadrant HealthCom, Barnett RC: Removal of fish hooks. Hosp Med 1980;16:56–57. Copyright © 1980 by Quadrant HealthCom, Inc.*

The presence of a barb in the fishhook makes retrograde extraction of the hook difficult. Most fishhook injuries involve the skin and subcutaneous tissues only. Although many techniques of fishhook removal have been described, only two will be discussed here (**Figures 1 and 2**). Remember to wear protective gloves at all times during this procedure and use sterile technique.

### FIRST TECHNIQUE

#### STEP 1

Cleanse the skin with a bactericidal skin preparation solution.

#### STEP 2

Use a 27-gauge needle to infiltrate the skin with 2 to 3 mL of 1% local anesthetic.

#### STEP 3

Grasp the exposed end of the hook (shank) with the thumb and index finger and rotate the hook to force the barb out through the skin.

#### STEP 4

Cut the barbed end of the hook with a wire cutter. Remove the rest of the hook retrograde. It will back out easily once the barb is gone.

### SECOND TECHNIQUE

#### STEP 1

Cleanse the skin with a bactericidal skin preparation solution.

#### STEP 2

Inject 2 to 3 mL of 1% local anesthetic about the hook.

#### STEP 3

Loop a size #0 or #1 nylon or silk suture around the belly of the hook at the point where it penetrates the skin.

#### STEP 4

Grasp the shank of the hook with your left thumb and long finger and press against the skin. At the same time, press gently downward on the belly of the hook with the left index finger to disengage the barb from the surrounding tissues.

### STEP 5

With your right hand, grasp the suture 10" to 12" from the hook and pull sharply to remove the hook. The hook often disengages with considerable velocity, so care must be taken that bystanders are not impaled by the flying fishhook.

### STEP 6

Dress the wound with a sterile adhesive bandage.

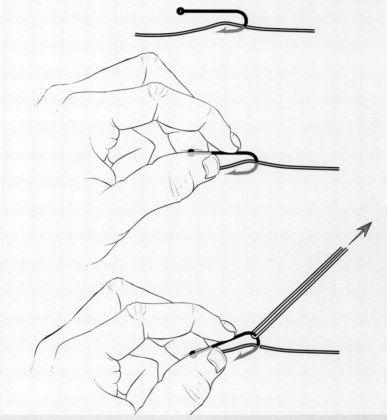

**Figure 2**
Technique 2 for removing a fishhook.

*Adapted with permission from Quadrant HealthCom, Barnett RC: Removal of fish hooks. Hosp Med 1980;16:56–57. Copyright © 1980 by Quadrant HealthCom, Inc.*

## ADVERSE OUTCOMES

Use of the first technique may inflict further soft-tissue damage by pushing the barb through the skin. Breakage of the hook or infection is possible.

## AFTERCARE/PATIENT INSTRUCTIONS

Check whether the patient has current tetanus prophylaxis. Advise the patient to keep the wound clean until it is healed, usually in 3 to 4 days. Instruct the patient to return to your office if redness, fever, or proximal swelling occur.

# Sprains and Dislocations of the Hand

ICD-9 Codes

834.00
Dislocation of finger or thumb, closed, unspecified site
842.10
Sprains and strains of hand, unspecified site

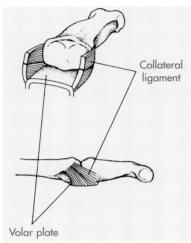

**Figure 1**
Collateral ligaments and volar plates of the PIP joint.

*Reproduced with permission from American Society for Surgery of the Hand: The Hand: Examination and Diagnosis, ed 3. New York, NY, Churchill Livingstone, p 54.*

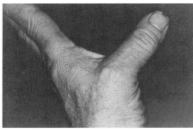

**Figure 2**
Clinical appearance of ulnar collateral ligament tear.

## Synonyms

Sprain

Jammed finger

Gamekeeper's thumb

Skier's thumb

## Definition

Sprains of the hand are common injuries characterized by a partial or complete tear of the collateral ligament and/or volar capsular ligament (eg, volar plate of either the metacarpophalangeal [MP], proximal interphalangeal [PIP], or distal interphalangeal [DIP] joint) (**Figure 1**). Most sprains of the hand are relatively straightforward injuries that can be managed nonoperatively. The exception is rupture of the ulnar collateral ligament of the thumb MP joint.

The ulnar collateral ligament of the thumb MP joint is an important stabilizer of the thumb. When this ligament is torn, the thumb deviates outward when the thumb and index finger pinch (**Figure 2**). The eponym gamekeeper's thumb originates from the chronic injury previously observed in English gamekeepers as a result of their method of killing rabbits. Today, a frequent cause of this injury is forced abduction of the thumb against a ski pole (skier's thumb); however, the injury also occurs with other ball-playing sports or with a fall.

Most dislocations in the hand are hyperextension injuries that result from a complete tear of the volar capsule that usually results in dorsal displacement of the distal element. Dislocation is most common at the PIP joint. Dorsal dislocations of the MP joint are either simple or complex. The latter is associated with interposition of the volar plate between the metacarpal head and the proximal phalanx (**Figure 3**). MP dislocations are more frequent in the thumb, and complex dislocations may require open reduction.

## Clinical symptoms

Patients almost always report a history of trauma and acute onset of pain. With a gamekeeper's thumb, pain and swelling is localized to the inside (ulnar aspect) of the thumb MP joint. With a dislocation, patients describe a deformity that developed immediately after the injury. The patient or a well-meaning friend may have reduced or attempted to reduce a dislocation before the patient seeks medical attention.

## Tests

### Physical examination

If the joint is swollen but not grossly deformed, palpate both sides of the joint for tenderness over the collateral ligaments (**Figure 4**). Radiographs should be

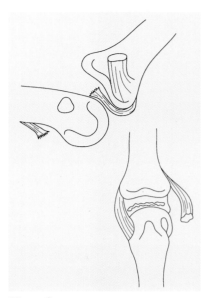

**Figure 3**
Interposition of the volar plate between metacarpal and proximal phalanx.

*Reproduced with permission from American Society for Surgery of the Hand: Hand Surgery Update. Rosemont, IL, American Academy of Orthopaedic Surgeons, 1994, p 22.*

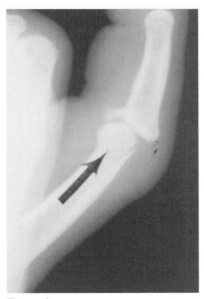

**Figure 6**
Fracture-dislocation of the PIP joint.

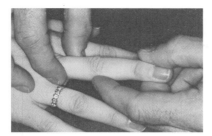

**Figure 4**
Palpation of the collateral ligaments.

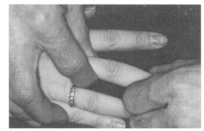

**Figure 5**
Applying medial and lateral stresses to the PIP joint.

obtained to rule out fractures, particularly nondisplaced fractures, which should not be stressed on examination. If there is no fracture, then joint stability should be tested by applying medial and lateral stresses to the joint (**Figure 5**). If the finger angulates under stress, it indicates a complete tear of the collateral ligament; if the patient has pain but no instability, assume there has been a sprain.

Dislocations usually are obvious on inspection. Complex dislocations of the MP joint are less apparent than simple dislocations. The latter have marked hyperextension of the proximal phalanx, but with complex dislocations, the MP joint is slightly hyperextended and the IP joints are slightly flexed.

## DIAGNOSTIC TESTS

AP and lateral radiographs are necessary to rule out a fracture or a fracture-dislocation (**Figure 6**).

## DIFFERENTIAL DIAGNOSIS

Extensor tendon rupture (boutonnière deformity, inability to extend the PIP joint)

Fracture (evident on radiographs)

## ADVERSE OUTCOMES OF THE DISEASE

Limited motion, stiffness, chronic pain, and swelling may persist. Chronic hyperextension of the PIP joint or flexion contracture can occur.

## TREATMENT

Most sprains of the collateral ligaments can be treated with splinting. The exception is an unstable, complete rupture of the ulnar collateral ligament of the thumb MP joint. These injuries may require surgical stabilization because interposition of the adductor pollicis tendon prevents adequate healing of the avulsed ligament. Buddy taping to an adjacent finger is effective treatment for collateral ligament injuries in the finger joints (**Figure 7**). Complete rupture of the volar plate can be treated by splinting the joint in 20° to 30° of flexion for 2 to 3 weeks or using buddy taping and early motion. Incomplete tears of the ulnar collateral ligament of the thumb MP joint can be treated in a thumb spica cast with the thumb slightly flexed for 4 weeks.

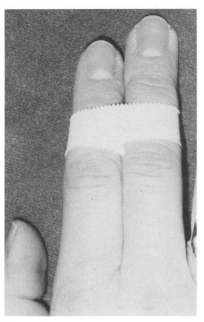

**Figure 7**
Buddy taping.

Closed reduction of a PIP or DIP joint dislocation should be done under a digital block anesthetic (see Digital Anesthetic Block [Hand]). To reduce the dislocation, grasp the distal portion of the finger and apply longitudinal traction while stabilizing the finger or hand proximal to the dislocation. Apply gentle pressure over the dorsum of the deformity to guide the reduction. After reduction, move the finger through a range of motion and then assess collateral ligament stability. If the joint seems stable, the finger can be buddy taped. If the joint has full range of motion after the reduction but tends to dislocate during the last 20° of extension, apply a dorsal extension block splint to allow healing of the volar plate (**Figure 8**). This type of splint blocks the last 20° to 30° of extension. Use the splint for 2 to 3 weeks, then buddy tape the finger to an adjacent finger for an additional 3 weeks.

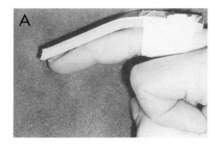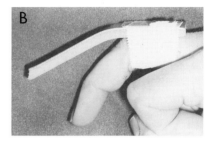

**Figure 8**
A, Dorsal extension block splint for PIP dislocations. B, Splint allows flexion but prevents excessive motion of the volar plate.

MP joint dislocations may be reduced with digital or regional nerve blocks. The latter may be more effective with complex MP dislocations. If the dislocation cannot be reduced with adequate anesthesia, soft tissue could be interposed, and open reduction may be necessary (**Figure 9**).

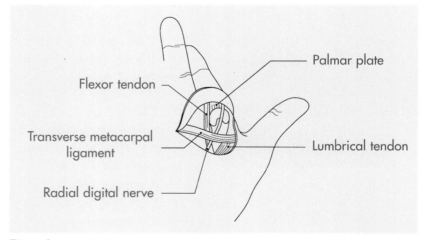

**Figure 9**
Entrapment of the metacarpal head between the lumbrical and extrinsic flexor tendon.

*Reproduced with permission from American Society for Surgery of the Hand: Hand Surgery Update. Rosemont, IL, American Academy of Orthopaedic Surgeons, 1994, p 22.*

DIP dislocations are typically dorsal or dorsolateral. With open injuries, suspect an associated tear of the extensor tendon. After adequate digital block anesthesia, apply longitudinal traction to reduce the dislocation. Open dislocations need appropriate debridement and irrigation but tend to be stable after reduction. Next, apply a dorsal aluminum splint over the middle and distal phalanges for 1 to 2 weeks. If the fingertip droops after the reduction and the patient cannot actively extend the distal phalanx, treat the injury as a mallet finger.

## Adverse outcomes of treatment

Instability, joint stiffness, persistent hyperextension deformity, and/or residual flexion deformity can develop. Arthritis also may develop with an inadequate reduction.

## Referral decisions/Red flags

Patients with an unstable thumb MP ulnar collateral ligament sprain need further evaluation for surgical stabilization. Patients whose dislocations cannot be reduced easily with digital anesthesia are candidates for open reduction. In addition, patients with fracture-dislocations and open dislocations need further evaluation. Open dislocations are best treated operatively to achieve adequate debridement and repair.

# TRIGGER FINGER

SECTION 4 | HAND AND WRIST

ICD-9 Code
727.03
    Trigger finger

## SYNONYMS
Locked finger
Stenosing tenosynovitis of the flexor tendons

## DEFINITION
The flexor tendons of the fingers glide back and forth under four annular and three cruciform pulleys that keep the tendons from bowstringing. The first annular pulley may become thickened and stenotic from chronic inflammation and irritation. As a result, motion of the tendon is limited and the finger may snap or lock during flexion of the finger or thumb (**Figure 1**). The long and ring fingers are most commonly affected, but any digit may be involved.

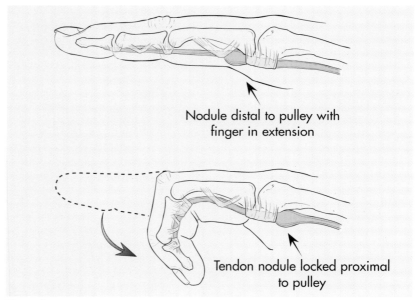

Nodule distal to pulley with finger in extension

Tendon nodule locked proximal to pulley

**Figure 1**
Nodule or thickening in flexor tendon, which strikes the proximal pulley, making finger extension difficult.

Trigger finger may be idiopathic or associated with rheumatoid arthritis or diabetes. The idiopathic type is more often observed in middle-aged women. A higher prevalence of trigger finger is observed in patients with carpal tunnel syndrome and de Quervain stenosing tenosynovitis.

## CLINICAL SYMPTOMS
Patients typically report pain and catching when they flex the finger and may describe the finger as going "out of joint." They may awaken with the finger locked in the palm, although the finger gradually unlocks during the day. The

proximal interphalangeal (PIP) joint may be identified as the source of the pain, but the stenosis is at the level of the metacarpophalangeal (MP) joint. Some patients have a painful nodule in the distal palm, usually at the level of the distal flexion crease, with no history of triggering. Other patients' only symptoms are swelling and/or stiffness in the fingers, particularly in the morning. Patients with rheumatoid arthritis or diabetes mellitus can have several fingers involved.

## TESTS

### PHYSICAL EXAMINATION

Examination reveals tenderness in the palm at the level of the distal palmar crease, usually overlying the MP joint. A nodule also may be palpable at this site. The nodule moves, and the finger may lock when the patient flexes and extends the affected finger. This maneuver is almost always painful for the patient. Full flexion of the finger may not be possible.

### DIAGNOSTIC TESTS

This is a clinical diagnosis; radiographs are not needed.

## DIFFERENTIAL DIAGNOSIS

Anomalous muscle belly in the palm (swelling more proximal in the palm)

Diabetes mellitus (single and multiple trigger fingers)

Dupuytren disease (palpable cord)

Ganglion of the tendon sheath (tendon mass at the base of the finger that does not move with flexion)

Rheumatoid arthritis (multiple joint involvement)

## ADVERSE OUTCOMES OF THE DISEASE

Flexion contracture of the PIP joint may develop, as could stiffness in extension.

## TREATMENT

Initial treatment can involve a short course of NSAIDs or injection of corticosteroid into the tendon sheath (see Trigger Finger Injection pp 285-286). If symptoms persist, a second injection in 3 to 4 weeks is indicated. However, because patients with rheumatoid disease are already at increased risk for tendon rupture, only one injection is indicated for these patients before surgical release should be considered. If two injections fail to resolve the trigger finger, surgical release should be considered.

## ADVERSE OUTCOMES OF TREATMENT

NSAIDs can cause gastric, renal, or hepatic complications. Repeated corticosteroid injections could lead to rupture of the flexor tendon and also can injure the digital sensory nerve. Infection also is a risk. In patients with diabetes, steroid injections can increase blood glucose levels.

## Referral decisions/Red flags

Failure of nonoperative treatment, development of contractures in the PIP joint, and/or a locked finger (in flexion or extension) indicate the need for further evaluation. Patients with rheumatoid arthritis whose problem does not resolve after a single injection also need additional evaluation. Patients with type 1 diabetes mellitus who do not tolerate steroid injection require specialty evaluation.

# PROCEDURE

## TRIGGER FINGER INJECTION

### MATERIALS

Sterile gloves

Bactericidal skin preparation solution

2 to 3 mL of a 1% local anesthetic without epinephrine

Two 3-mL syringes with a 25-gauge needle

1 mL of a 40 mg/mL corticosteroid preparation

Adhesive dressing

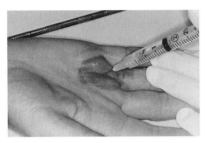

**Figure 1**
Location for needle insertion.

The flexor tendons pass beneath a pulley situated just distal to the distal palmar crease. Palpating this area as the patient flexes and extends the finger reveals a click or snapping sensation as the enlarged tendon passes beneath the pulley.

### MATERIALS

#### STEP 1

Wear protective gloves at all times during this procedure and use sterile technique.

#### STEP 2

Cleanse the palm with a bactericidal skin preparation solution.

#### STEP 3

Identify the lump on the tendon and infiltrate the skin at the distal palmar crease, which directly overlies the tendon, and inject the anesthetic at that level.

#### STEP 4

Inject 0.5 mL of a 1% anesthetic solution into the subcutaneous tissue (**Figure 1**), then advance the needle into the tendon sheath and inject the rest of the anesthetic (**Figure 2**). Continue to insert the needle as the patient moves the affected finger through a small arc of flexion and extension. When the needle touches the moving tendon, the patient will experience a scratchy sensation. If the needle moves, it has penetrated the tendon and should be partially withdrawn until the scratchy sensation occurs. At this point, the needle tip is inside the tendon sheath but external to the tendon.

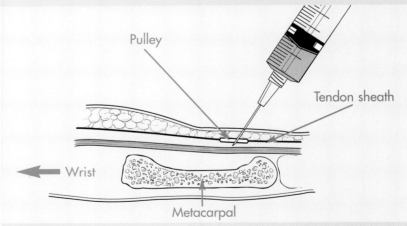

**Figure 2**
Insert the needle through the pulley.

SECTION 4 | HAND AND WRIST

## STEP 5

Leave the needle in place, change syringes, and then inject the corticosteroid preparation.

## STEP 6

Dress the puncture wound with a sterile adhesive bandage.

## ADVERSE OUTCOMES

Injection of corticosteroid into the subcutaneous tissues may lead to local fat atrophy and a tender, unsightly depression beneath the skin.

## AFTERCARE/PATIENT INSTRUCTIONS

Advise the patient of possible significant discomfort for 1 to 2 days following any injection of a corticosteroid. Also, the finger may be numb for 1 to 2 hours until the local anesthetic wears off. Instruct the patient to return to your office if swelling, redness, or inordinate pain occurs. The patient should be able to use the finger in a normal fashion after the injection.

# TUMORS OF THE HAND AND WRIST

ICD-9 Codes
195.4
    Malignant neoplasm, upper limb
213.5
    Benign neoplasms of short bones of
    upper limb
229.8
    Benign neoplasms of other and
    unspecified sites

## DEFINITION

Most tumors in the hand and wrist are benign, with primary malignant tumors and skeletal metastases accounting for less than 1% of these neoplasms. Ganglia, followed by giant cell tumors and epidermal inclusion cysts, are the most common benign soft-tissue tumors. Enchondromas are the most common benign neoplasm of the bones of the hand, accounting for 90%. Squamous cell carcinomas are the most common malignant neoplasm of the hand, and chondrosarcomas are the most common primary malignant bone tumor in the hand. Malignant melanomas are frequently seen in the upper extremity because of the exposure of the arm to sun.

## CLINICAL SYMPTOMS

Many tumors of the hand are painless. The exception is a glomus tumor, which characteristically is extremely painful and sensitive to cold. Enchondromas present with pain after a patient sustains a pathologic fracture through the weakened bone. Lipomas can cause pain and numbness in the fingers if the lesion is compressing an adjacent nerve. Masses located near joints can cause loss of motion.

## TESTS

### PHYSICAL EXAMINATION

Note the position, size, and characteristics of the mass. These factors help to narrow the diagnostic possibilities.

A ganglion cyst is characterized as a mass located over the dorsal or volar radial aspect of the wrist, the flexion crease of the finger at the level of the web space, or over the top of the distal interphalangeal (DIP) joint of the finger.

Epidermal inclusion cysts typically occur around the end of the finger (thumb and long) or at the end of an amputation stump. Pressing a small flashlight against an inclusion cyst will not transilluminate the mass, but this same maneuver will transilluminate a ganglion cyst.

A giant cell tumor is characterized by a multinodular, firm, nontender mass located around an interphalangeal (IP) joint, usually of the thumb or the index or long finger.

A blue or red area visible under the fingernail could be a glomus tumor, subungual hematoma, or foreign body. However, subungual discoloration in the absence of trauma should raise a suspicion of melanoma. Likewise, a mole (nevus) that changes shape or color can indicate a malignant melanoma.

Lipomas typically are superficial, soft, reasonably well defined, and nontender on palpation. A frequent location in the hand is the thenar eminence.

When lipomas are located on the palmar surface of the wrist, compression of the median or ulnar nerve may occur.

Recurrent paronychia infections and chronic nail deformities can be caused by underlying squamous cell carcinoma. A diagnosis of Kaposi sarcoma should be suspected in a patient with AIDS who develops skin nodules or red-brown plaques.

A symptomatic enchondroma is characterized by tenderness and swelling over the involved phalanx (usually the proximal). A pathologic fracture may be present.

A carpal boss is a dorsal prominence at the base of the third metacarpal or second metacarpal. These dorsal osteophytes may be confused with a neoplasm. A ganglion is sometimes associated with a carpal boss.

## DIAGNOSTIC TESTS

Posteroanterior (PA) and lateral radiographs of the involved finger or PA, lateral, and oblique views of the hand should be obtained.

## DIFFERENTIAL DIAGNOSIS

See Table 1 and Figure 1 for a complete listing.

## Table 1
### Common Benign Tumors of the Hand and Wrist

| Type of tumor* | Common location(s) | Patient age and gender | Signs and symptoms | Radiographic findings |
|---|---|---|---|---|
| Ganglion cyst (See Ganglia of the Wrist and Hand) | | | | |
| Epidermal inclusion cyst | Fingertip or anywhere from penetrating injury | Teens to middle age; more common in men | Painless, slow growing; does not transilluminate | Round soft-tissue mass, also in distal phalanx |
| Giant cell tumor of tendon sheath | Digits on palmar surface | > 30 years; ratio of men to women 2:3 | Slowly enlarging painless mass | 20% show cortical erosion |
| Glomus tumor | 50% occur under fingernail | 30-50 years; ratio of women to men 2:1 | Triad of symptoms: marked pain, cold intolerance, very tender, blue discoloration of nail | Some show erosion on lateral view |
| Lipoma | Thenar area in palm and first web space | 30-60 years; slight predominance in women | Painless, slow growing; might cause nerve entrapment | No bony involvement, soft-tissue mass |
| Enchondroma | In proximal phalanges or metacarpals | 10-60 years; affects men and women equally | Might become painful after trauma because of fracture | Radiolucent expansive lesion, cortex thin, fracture and areas of calcification possibly visible |

* See Figure 1.

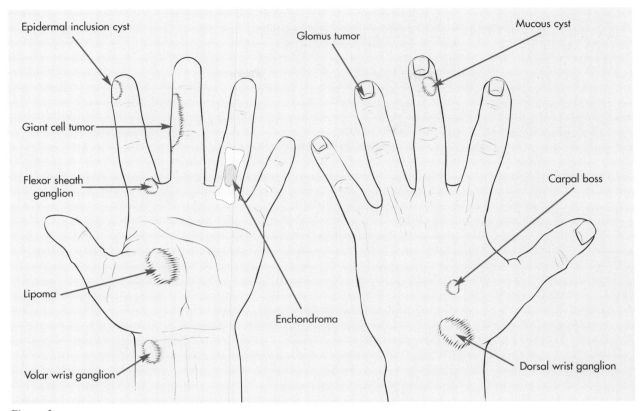

**Figure 1**
Typical locations and types of benign hand tumors.

## ADVERSE OUTCOMES OF THE DISEASE

Ganglia can result in limited joint motion. Nail changes, skin atrophy, and infection can develop as a result of a mucoid cyst. Drainage is a problem associated with epidermal mucoid cysts. Patients with giant cell tumors can have limited tendon function because of peritendinous adhesions. Nerve compression can develop as a result of lipoma. With an enchondroma, fracture can occur. Squamous cell carcinomas and malignant melanoma can metastasize and result in death.

## TREATMENT

Treatment is based on the diagnosis. Surgical excision and histologic examination are required for most expanding or symptomatic masses.

## ADVERSE OUTCOMES OF TREATMENT

Ganglia can recur at the same site in 5% to 10% of patients. The recurrence rate of giant cell tumors is relatively high after surgical excision. Joint stiffness can develop after treatment of pathologic fractures caused by enchondromas.

## REFERRAL DECISIONS/RED FLAGS

Patients with a painful or expanding mass, one that interferes with function, or one believed to be malignant need further evaluation.

# ULNAR NERVE ENTRAPMENT AT THE WRIST

| ICD-9 Code |
|---|
| 354.2 |
| Lesion of ulnar nerve |

## SYNONYM

Ulnar tunnel syndrome

## DEFINITION

Entrapment of the ulnar nerve at the wrist usually is caused by a space-occupying lesion such as a lipoma, ganglion, ulnar artery aneurysm, or muscle anomaly (**Figure 1**). Repetitive trauma, such as operating a jackhammer or using the base of the hand as a hammer, also may cause ulnar neuropathy at the wrist. Ulnar nerve entrapment at the wrist is less common than ulnar nerve entrapment at the elbow.

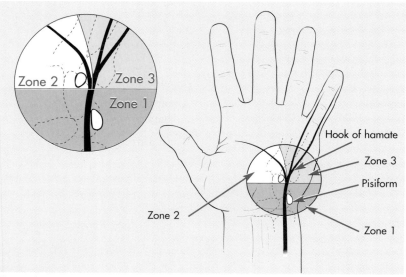

**Figure 1**
Distal ulnar tunnel showing the three zones of entrapment. Lesions in zone 1 cause both motor and sensory symptoms; lesions in zone 2 cause motor deficits; and lesions in zone 3 create sensory deficits.

## CLINICAL SYMPTOMS

Patients may or may not have pain, but they often report weakness and numbness.

## TESTS

### PHYSICAL EXAMINATION

Inspect the hypothenar eminence for atrophy. Assess sensory and motor function of the ulnar nerve In some patients, only the motor branch of the ulnar nerve may be affected, sparing the sensory branches; however, with sensory involvement, tapping over the ulnar nerve in the hypothenar region will pro-

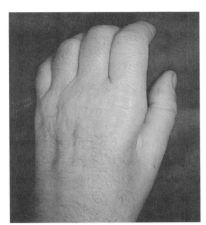

**Figure 2**
Intrinsic muscle wasting.

duce tingling in the ring and little fingers (Tinel sign). Sensation over the dorsal and ulnar aspects of the hand is normal. When the ulnar nerve is involved at the elbow, almost all patients will have both sensory and motor involvement, with numbness over the dorsal and ulnar sides of the hand. Motor weakness is detected by atrophy of the hypothenar and intrinsic muscles or weakness of the intrinsic muscles (finger spreaders) (**Figure 2**).

### DIAGNOSTIC TESTS

Results of nerve conduction velocity studies may be abnormal and may differentiate ulnar entrapment at the wrist from the more common entrapment at the elbow.

## DIFFERENTIAL DIAGNOSIS

Carpal tunnel syndrome (usually involves the thumb and index, long and ring fingers)

Cervical (C7-C8) radiculopathy (more proximal muscle involvement, numbness on the dorsum of the hand)

Peripheral neuropathy (from diabetes, alcoholism, or hypothyroidism; more generalized numbness)

Thoracic outlet syndrome (symptoms more diffuse)

Ulnar artery thrombosis in the hand (positive Allen test, firm cord on the ulnar side of the hand)

Ulnar neuropathy at the elbow (sensory changes on the dorsum of the hand)

Wrist arthritis (pain, limited motion, evident on radiographs)

## ADVERSE OUTCOMES OF THE DISEASE

Loss of intrinsic muscle function causes decreased grip strength and pinch. Sensory loss, when present, involves the ring and little fingers. In advanced disease, clawing of the ring and little fingers can develop.

## TREATMENT

Because the usual cause of ulnar entrapment at the wrist is extrinsic compression (because of a lipoma, ganglion, or tumor, for example), treatment is usually operative. When the obvious cause is external pressure, such as resting the hypothenar area on a keyboard or desk, then use of padding or a change in position could help.

## ADVERSE OUTCOMES OF TREATMENT

Postoperative infection, persistent symptoms, or both are possible.

## REFERRAL DECISIONS/RED FLAGS

Patients with ulnar weakness and neuropathy need further evaluation.

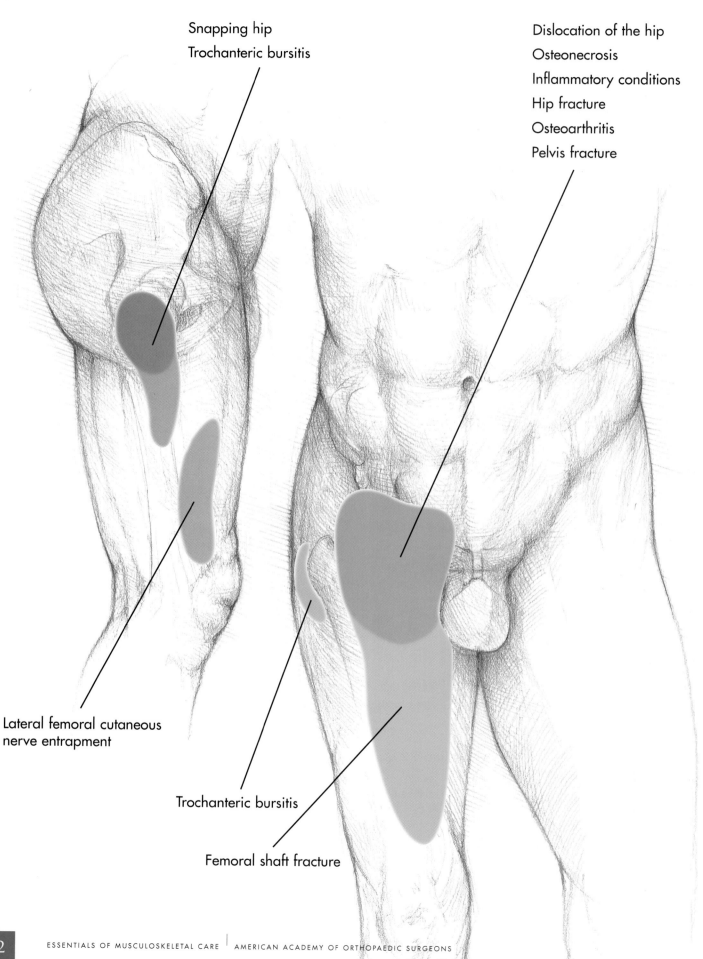

Snapping hip
Trochanteric bursitis

Dislocation of the hip
Osteonecrosis
Inflammatory conditions
Hip fracture
Osteoarthritis
Pelvis fracture

Lateral femoral cutaneous
nerve entrapment

Trochanteric bursitis

Femoral shaft fracture

# HIP AND THIGH

**Section Editor**
Jay R. Lieberman, MD
Associate Professor
Department of Orthopaedic Surgery
UCLA Medical Center
Los Angeles, California

Daniel J. Berry, MD
Associate Professor of Orthopedics
Mayo Medical School
Consultant in Orthopedic Surgery, Mayo Clinic
Department of Orthopedic Surgery
Mayo Foundation
Rochester, Minnesota

Kevin L. Garvin, MD, FACS
Professor and Chairman
Department of Orthopaedic Surgery and Rehabilitation
University of Nebraska Medical Center
Omaha, Nebraska

# HIP AND THIGH—AN OVERVIEW

When evaluating patients with hip or proximal thigh pain, you generally can assume that the pain comes from one of five likely sources: 1) the hip joint, 2) the soft tissues around the hip and pelvis, 3) the pelvic bones, 4) the sacroiliac joint, or 5) referred pain from the lumbar spine. Diagnosing pathology involving the hip joint and pelvis is often possible with a careful history and physical examination. In some cases, plain radiographs, a bone scan, or even MRI will be required.

The hip joint is just one part of the pelvic girdle. The pelvic girdle comprises three different bones (the ilium, pubic ramus, and sacrum) and two different joints (the hip joint and the sacroiliac joint). The hip joint refers specifically to the ball-and-socket joint that consists of the femoral head articulating with the acetabulum (**Figure 1**).

Radiographic examination of the hip should include an AP radiograph of the pelvis and either a frog-lateral view of the pelvis or an AP and lateral radiograph of the involved hip. All radiographs should be carefully evaluated for changes in bony architecture, including nondisplaced fractures as well as lytic and blastic lesions. The joint spaces (hip and sacroiliac) should be carefully assessed for narrowing.

## TYPE OF PAIN

Specific problems with the hip joint include osteoarthritis, osteonecrosis, inflammatory conditions, and fractures and dislocations. Other problems with the hip joint include developmental dysplasia, infection, and rheumatoid arthritis. Patients with these conditions usually report pain in the groin or anterior aspect of the proximal thigh. The hip joint is mobile; therefore, pathology affecting this joint also manifests as pain with ambulation, weight bearing, or limited motion.

The sacroiliac joint is practically immovable. Therefore, conditions such as seronegative arthritides or traumatic arthritis that involve the sacroiliac joint cause buttock and posterior thigh pain but are less likely to restrict function or motion.

Problems involving the bony pelvis include insufficiency fractures associated with osteoporosis, avulsion fractures from attached tendons, and primary or metastatic tumors. Problems involving both the hip joint and bony pelvis often manifest as pain in the groin, buttock, or lateral thigh.

Conditions that affect the soft tissues around the hip, such as trochanteric bursitis, lateral femoral cutaneous nerve impingement, and snapping hip syndrome, typically cause pain on the lateral or anterolateral aspect of the proximal thigh. Patients with an injury of the adductor muscles will note pain in

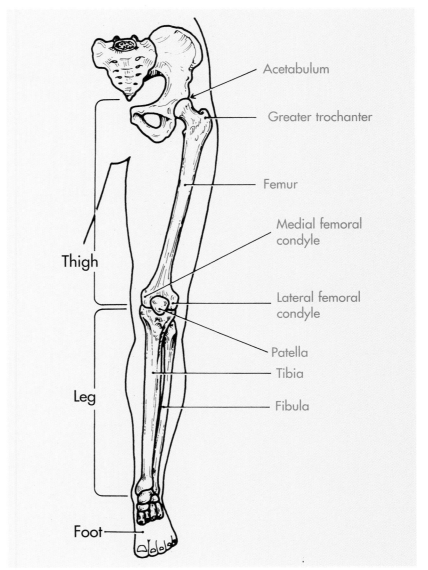

Acetabulum

Greater trochanter

Femur

Medial femoral condyle

Thigh

Lateral femoral condyle

Patella

Tibia

Leg

Fibula

Foot

**Figure 1**
Bones of the hip and leg.

the groin; hamstring injuries are associated with pain in the buttock or posterior aspect of the thigh.

Pathology in the lumbar spine can present as referred pain to the buttock and posterior thigh or even the lower leg. Patients with disk herniation, facet joint arthritis, and spinal stenosis may have pain limited to the buttock. However, these patients usually do not have anterior thigh pain, significant discomfort with either internal or external rotation of the hip, or limited range of motion of the hip joint.

# Gait

A brief examination of the patient's gait can be very helpful in making a diagnosis. Ask the patient to walk up and down the hall several times at a brisk pace. An abductor or gluteus medius lurch is manifested by a lateral shift of the body to the weight-bearing side with ambulation. This type of gait often occurs in patients who have intra-articular hip pathology (osteoarthritis, inflammatory arthritis, or osteonecrosis of the hip). Pain associated with a limp suggests pathology around the pelvis or hip and requires further investigation.

# PHYSICAL EXAMINATION
# HIP AND THIGH

## Inspection/Palpation

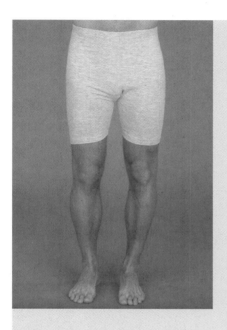

### Anterior view

With the patient standing, look for atrophy of the anterior thigh musculature and note the overall alignment of the hip, knee, and ankle.

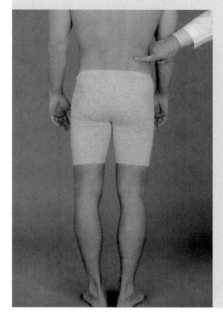

### Posterior view

With the patient standing, look for atrophy of the buttock and posterior
thigh musculature. Palpate the iliac crests (shown on figure), the posterior
iliac spine (deep to dimples of Venus), and the greater trochanter. Note
any pelvic obliquity (one iliac crest lower than the opposite side). Limb-
length discrepancy will cause an apparent pelvic obliquity that can be corrected by placing blocks under the shorter limb. Fixed pelvic obliquity
from a spinal deformity cannot be corrected by this maneuver. A
Trendelenburg test can be conducted at this time.

# Inspection/Palpation

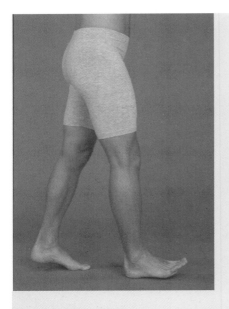

### Gait

Note how the patient walks across the room. Hip deformities often cause a limp that can range in severity from barely detectable to marked sway of the trunk and slowing of gait. If the problem is primarily arthritis without significant deformity, the patient will shorten the stance phase on the affected side. If the problem is primarily abductor muscle dysfunction, the patient will compensate by a marked Trendelenburg lurch.

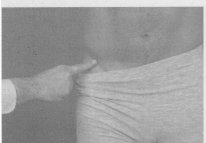

### Anterior view, supine

With the patient supine, palpate to identify any masses, abnormal adenopathy, or tenderness in the region of the anterior superior iliac spine (ASIS) (shown in figure) or greater trochanter. Patients with avulsion of the sartorius or rectus femoris will report tenderness at or directly inferior to the ASIS. Patients with meralgia paresthetica (entrapment of the lateral femoral cutaneous nerve) will report tenderness immediately medial to the ASIS and hypoesthesia over the distal lateral thigh.

Patients who report a popping sensation most likely have a thickened iliotibial band snapping over the greater trochanter that occurs as the hip moves into flexion and internal rotation. Ask the patient to recreate the snapping and palpate the iliotibial band as it snaps over the greater trochanter.

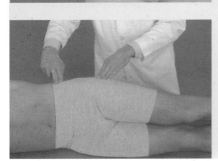

### Lateral view, side-lying

Place the patient in a side-lying position on the unaffected side to facilitate the examination. Structures in the region of the greater trochanter may be palpated in the supine position, but examination of this area is easier with the patient lying on the unaffected side. Tenderness directly over the trochanter reproduces pain with greater trochanteric bursitis. Tenderness at the proximal tip of the trochanter may indicate gluteus medius tendinitis. Tenderness at the posterior margin of the trochanter may indicate external rotator tendinitis.

# Range of Motion

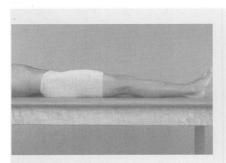

### Flexion: Zero Starting Position

Place the patient supine on a firm, flat surface with the opposite hip held in enough flexion to flatten the lumbar spine. Flattening the lumbar spine prevents excessive lordosis that can camouflage a hip flexion contracture.

Avoid positioning the opposite hip in excessive flexion, as this will rock the pelvis into abnormal posterior inclination, thereby creating a false-positive hip flexion contracture. Instead, flex the opposite hip to a position where the lumbar spine just starts to flatten or, more precisely, to a position where the inclination of the pelvis is similar to a normal standing posture (ie, the anterior superior iliac spine is inferior to the posterior iliac spine by only 2° to 3°).

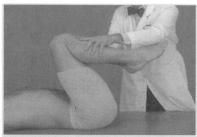

# Range of Motion

### Maximum flexion

Maximum flexion is the point at which the pelvis begins to rotate. Normal hip flexion in adults is 110° to 130°.

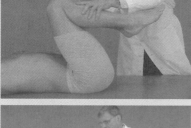

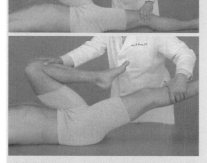

### Hip flexion contracture—Thomas test

With the opposite hip flexed as described in the Zero Starting Position, move the affected hip into flexion and then allow the hip to extend until the pelvis starts to rock. The patient in the top figure has no hip flexion contracture, whereas the patient shown in the bottom figure has a hip flexion contracture of 30°.

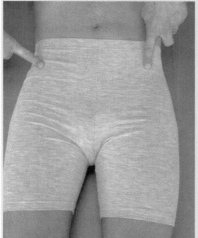

### Abduction and adduction: Zero Starting Position

The Zero Starting Position is with the pelvis level (ie, the limbs are at 90° angles to a transverse line across the anterior superior iliac spines).

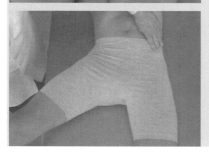

### Abduction

Measure abduction in degrees from the Zero Starting Position. Maximum abduction is reached when the pelvis begins to tilt, a movement that you can detect by keeping your hand on the patient's opposite ASIS when moving the leg. Normal hip abduction in adults is 35° to 50°.

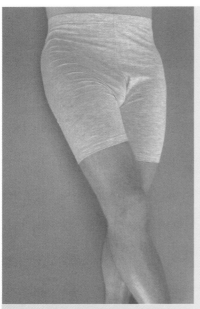

### Adduction

Elevate the opposite extremity to allow adduction. Maximum adduction is reached when the pelvis starts to rotate. If elevating the opposite extremity is impractical, measure adduction by moving the extremity over the top of the opposite limb. Normal hip adduction in adults is 25° to 35°.

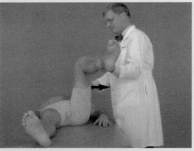

### Internal-external rotation in flexion

For adults, it is more practical to measure rotation with the hips in flexion. However, this approach should not be used in children or when it is necessary to assess femoral torsion or to obtain a more precise measurement of hip rotation in a "walking" position.

Flex the hip and knee to 90°, with the thigh held perpendicular to the transverse line across the anterior superior iliac spines. Measure internal rotation by rotating the tibia away from the midline of the trunk, thus producing inward rotation of the hip (top). Measure external rotation by rotating the tibia toward the midline of the trunk, thus producing external rotation at the hip (bottom). (See Intoeing/Outtoeing, pp 666-669.)

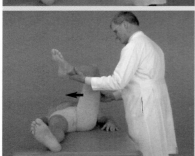

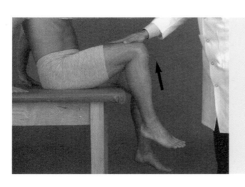

### Hip flexors

With the patient seated, ask him or her to flex the hip and then resist the effort to classify the grade of muscle strength.

# Muscle Testing

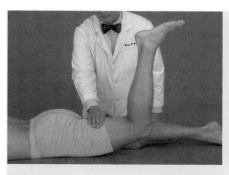

### Hip extensors

With the patient prone, place the knee in approximately 90° of flexion and ask the patient to extend the hip as you resist the effort with your hand by pushing against the thigh.

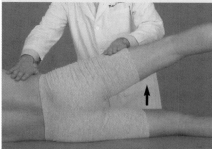

### Hip abductors

With the patient lying on the unaffected side, ask him or her to abduct the hip as you resist the effort. Note that hip abductor strength also can be assessed by the Trendelenburg test.

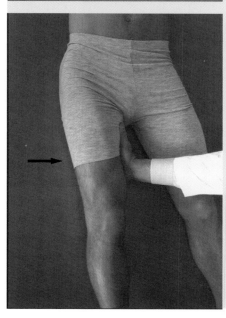

### Hip adductors

With the patient supine, place your hand on the medial thigh and ask the patient to adduct the hip as you resist the effort.

# Special Tests

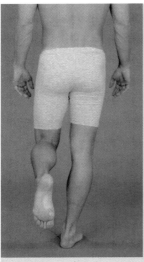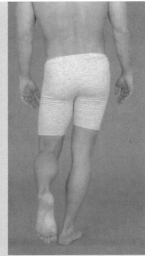

### Trendelenburg test

Ask the patient to stand on one leg. With normal hip abductor strength, the pelvis will stay level (left). If hip abductor strength is inadequate on the stance limb side, the pelvis will drop with the iliac crest becoming lower on the opposite side (positive Trendelenburg test) (right).

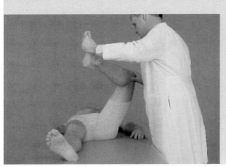

### FABER test

The FABER (flexion-abduction-external rotation) maneuver, sometimes called the figure-of-4 test, is a stress maneuver to detect hip and sacroiliac pathology. With the patient supine, place the affected hip in flexion, abduction, and external rotation (as shown in figure) and then press the hip back into extension by placing the foot on the opposite tibia. If the maneuver is painful, then the hip or sacroiliac region may be affected. Increased pain with this test also may be a nonorganic finding.

# DISLOCATION OF THE HIP

ICD-9 Codes
835.01
    Posterior dislocation
835.02
    Anterior dislocation

## DEFINITION

Dislocation of the hip occurs when the femoral head is displaced from the acetabulum. Because of its strong capsule and deep acetabulum, the hip is rarely dislocated in adults. The causative injury usually is high-energy trauma, such as a motor vehicle accident or fall from a considerable height. Posterior dislocations (femoral head posterior to the acetabulum) are more common, accounting for more than 90% of these injuries.

## CLINICAL SYMPTOMS

Patients have severe pain, are unable to move the lower extremity, and may experience numbness throughout the lower limb. Patients often have multiple injuries and may be unconscious from associated head trauma.

## TESTS

### PHYSICAL EXAMINATION

With a posterior dislocation, the affected limb is short and the hip is fixed in a position of flexion, adduction, and internal rotation (**Figure 1**). Assess the status of distal pulses and function of the femoral, posterior tibial, and peroneal nerves. Sciatic nerve injuries are common (8% to 20% incidence). Of note, neurologic dysfunction may be isolated to the peroneal or posterior tibial component of the sciatic nerve.

With anterior dislocations, the hip assumes a position of mild flexion, abduction, and external rotation. Femoral nerve palsy may be present, but nerve injuries are less frequent with anterior dislocations.

Abrasions or swelling around the knee may indicate significant knee ligament injury because most hip dislocations typically occur from a direct blow to the flexed hip and knee. An associated ipsilateral fracture of the femur or acetabulum will alter the typical findings in hip dislocations.

### DIAGNOSTIC TESTS

An AP radiograph of the pelvis, and AP and lateral views of the femur to include the knee, should be obtained. On the AP radiograph, the femoral heads and joint spaces should appear symmetric in size. With a posterior hip dislocation, the affected femoral head appears smaller than the contralateral femoral head (**Figure 2**). With an anterior hip dislocation, the femoral head appears larger than the femoral head on the opposite, normal hip. Look for fractures of the acetabulum or femoral head. If these fragments are entrapped within the joint, the joint space may be widened.

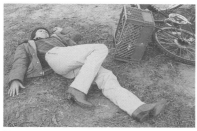

**Figure 1**
The clinical appearance of a posterior dislocation of the right hip.

*Reproduced with permission from Heckman JD (ed): Emergency Care and Transportation of the Sick and Injured, ed 4. Park Ridge, IL, American Academy of Orthopaedic Surgeons, 1987, p 208.*

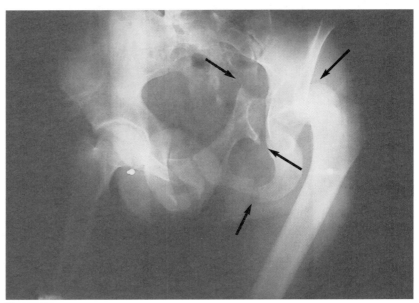

**Figure 2**
Posterior dislocation of the left hip (arrow, top right) with associated fractures of the acetabulum and the pubic rami.

*Reproduced with permission from Kasser JR (ed): Orthopaedic Knowledge Update 5. Rosemont, IL, American Academy of Orthopaedic Surgeons, 1996, pp 365–378.*

## DIFFERENTIAL DIAGNOSIS

Central fracture-dislocation of the hip (pain in the groin and/or buttock)

Fracture of the hip or shaft of the femur (pain in the groin, buttock, and thigh)

Fracture of the posterior acetabular rim (pain in the groin and/or buttock)

## ADVERSE OUTCOMES OF THE DISEASE

Osteonecrosis of the femoral head occurs in approximately 10% of patients because the dislocation tears the hip capsule and disrupts the blood supply to the femoral head. Delay in reduction increases the risk of osteonecrosis. The osteonecrosis may not be apparent for as long as 2 or 3 years after the injury; therefore, these patients need ongoing evaluation. Posttraumatic arthritis, chondrolysis (dissolution of articular cartilage), limp, sciatic or femoral nerve injury, and chronic pain also can occur.

## TREATMENT

A hip dislocation is an emergency. A reduction should be performed as soon as possible to decrease the risk of osteonecrosis. The reduction should be performed in an atraumatic fashion to avoid damage to the articular cartilage or fracture of the femoral head or acetabulum. Associated fractures of the femoral head or intra-articular loose bodies should be ruled out before the reduction is performed. Repeat radiographs and postreduction CT are necessary to identify unrecognized intra-articular bony fragments and to confirm reduction. In addition, nerve and vascular function should be evaluated both before and after reduction. The postreduction treatment of an uncomplicated dislocated hip is early crutch-assisted ambulation with weight bearing as tolerated until the patient is free of pain, usually 2 to 4 weeks after the injury. Patients should then begin hip abduction and extension exercises and use a walking aid in the hand opposite the involved hip until they can walk without a limp.

## ADVERSE OUTCOMES OF TREATMENT

Redislocation, osteonecrosis, posttraumatic arthritis, and a missed loose body or fracture are all possible.

## REFERRAL DECISIONS/RED FLAGS

All traumatic dislocations of the hip are serious injuries requiring immediate attention.

# FRACTURES OF THE FEMORAL SHAFT

ICD-9 Code
821.01
    Fracture of the femoral shaft, closed

## DEFINITION

The shaft or diaphysis of the femur is defined as that portion between the regions of the proximal subtrochanteric region and the distal supracondylar area of the knee. In most adults, fractures of the femoral shaft are caused by high-energy trauma such as a motor vehicle accident. As such, this injury is severe and is associated with potentially life-threatening pulmonary and vascular complications. Pathologic fractures of the femoral shaft are less common, occur in bone weakened by osteopenia or tumors, result from low-energy injuries such as a simple fall, and have a much lower incidence of vascular and pulmonary complications.

## CLINICAL SYMPTOMS

Severe pain in the thigh and inability to move the leg are striking. Patients who have sustained the injury as a result of high-energy trauma are likely to have multisystem injuries and may not be alert or even responsive to questioning. In these patients, conducting a thorough, sequential examination from the head to the toes according to the ATLS protocol for life-threatening injuries is essential.

## TESTS

### PHYSICAL EXAMINATION

Inspect for deformity, swelling, and open injuries. Palpate for areas of tenderness along the thigh and adjacent joints. Evaluate vascular status of the limb distal to the fracture. Assess function of the femoral, peroneal, and posterior tibial nerves. In the presence of deformity and vascular compromise, simple manual longitudinal traction should be applied to determine whether the deformity is the cause of the ischemia.

### DIAGNOSTIC TESTS

Fracture is confirmed by AP and lateral radiographs of the femur (**Figure** 1). High-energy trauma can disrupt adjacent joints, and radiographs of the hip, knee, and pelvis must be obtained (**Figure** 2). When vascular compromise is identified, arterial studies are required.

## DIFFERENTIAL DIAGNOSIS

Fractures of other adjacent areas (evident on radiographs)

Malignant or metastatic lesion of the femur (pain in the thigh with activity or at rest, evident on radiographs)

Osteomyelitis with bone destruction (pain in the thigh, evident on radiographs)

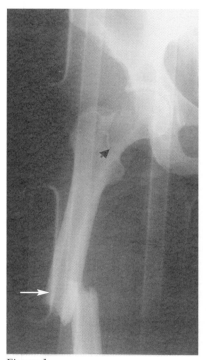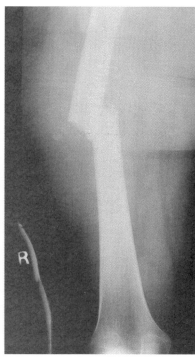

**Figure 1**
Femoral shaft fracture (arrow, left; and right) with ipsilateral femoral neck fracture (solid arrowhead, left).

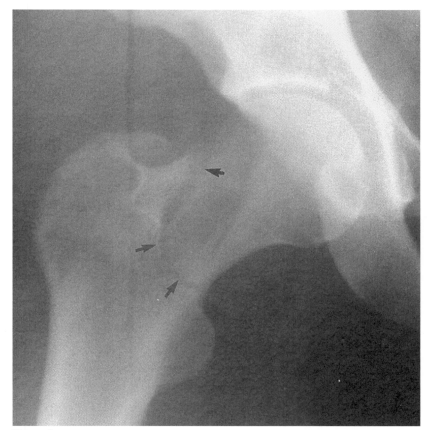

**Figure 2**
An ipsilateral femoral neck shaft fracture caused by high-energy trauma.

Soft-tissue injury without fracture (pain, swelling, ecchymosis of the thigh, pain with knee motion)

Stress fractures of the femur (pain in the thigh that increases with weight bearing, may be evident on plain radiographs, but MRI may be needed to confirm the diagnosis)

## ADVERSE OUTCOMES OF THE DISEASE

The most significant adverse outcomes are those associated with violent trauma or long-bone fractures, such as fat embolism, adult respiratory distress syndrome, and multisystem organ failure. Acute arterial injury also is life threatening and requires immediate recognition and treatment. Complications of open fractures, such as infection, can result in sepsis and therefore emphasize the need for appropriate emergent wound care.

## TREATMENT

Immediate splinting and traction should be applied for comfort, with the understanding that operative treatment of almost all fractures is indicated to lessen the risk of pulmonary and other systemic complications. Open fractures require operative treatment as soon as the patient is medically stabilized.

## ADVERSE OUTCOME OF TREATMENT

Nonunion, malunion, infection, venous thrombosis, fat embolism syndrome, and adult respiratory distress syndrome are potential problems even with expeditious treatment.

## REFERRAL DECISIONS/RED FLAGS

All femoral long bone fractures require further evaluation.

# FRACTURE OF THE PELVIS

## DEFINITION

Pelvic fractures include fractures of the pelvic ring and acetabulum. These injuries range in severity from stable, low-energy fractures that heal readily and allow early, assisted ambulation to severe, life-threatening, unstable fractures associated with massive blood loss and hemodynamic instability. Stable pelvic ring fractures are generally those that involve only one side of the ring. For example, a unilateral fracture of the superior and inferior pubic ramus is a stable injury. Unstable pelvic ring fractures disrupt the ring at two sites. For example, a fracture of a superior and inferior pubic ramus combined with a fracture of the sacrum or ilium is considered an unstable pelvic fracture. Another unstable pattern is disruption of the symphysis pubis combined with a fracture of the sacrum or disruption of one or both sacroiliac ligaments (**Figure 1**).

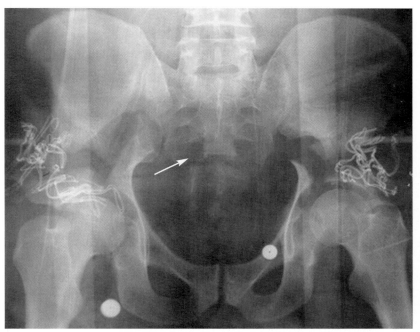

**Figure 1**
Radiograph showing bilateral open acetabular fractures and a transverse sacral fracture.

*Reproduced with permission from Routt MLC Jr: Fixation of pelvic ring disruptions, in Levine AM (ed): Orthopaedic Knowledge Update: Trauma. Rosemont, IL, American Academy of Orthopaedic Surgeons, 1996, pp 241-248.*

## CLINICAL SYMPTOMS

Patients have pain in the region of the pelvis, groin, ilium, or buttock. Patients with high-energy injuries can present in shock and often have associated musculoskeletal or multisystem injuries.

# Tests

## Physical examination

Inspect for swelling and ecchymosis. Palpation and gentle compression of the pelvis often will localize the area of injury. Evaluate the patient's hemodynamic status and the neurovascular status of the lower extremities, including the status of the femoral, peroneal, and posterior tibial nerves. Unstable fractures are associated with genitourinary injuries and injuries of the perineum and rectum. The possibility of these injuries should be considered.

## Diagnostic tests

An AP radiograph of the pelvis identifies most fractures. Special views, CT, and/or MRI may be needed to define the extent of injury or identify an occult fracture.

# Differential diagnosis

Hip arthritis (pain in the groin or buttock, limited hip motion, evident on radiographs)

Hip fracture (pain in the groin or buttock, shortened and externally rotated leg)

Hip strain (pain in the groin or buttock)

Tumors involving the bony pelvis or sacrum (pain in the low back, groin, rectum, and/or buttock, evident on radiographs)

# Adverse outcomes of the disease

For high-energy injuries and open pelvic fractures, death can occur from shock, associated injuries, or multisystem failure. Associated genitourinary injuries and neurovascular injuries can cause adverse outcomes. Malunion of the pelvis can lead to deformity of the pelvis and/or limb-length discrepancy. Nonunion of pelvic fractures is uncommon. Acetabular fractures are intra-articular injuries that can lead to arthritis and long-term pain. For several months after the fracture, patients are at increased risk for venous thromboembolic disease.

# Treatment

Treatment of pelvic fractures is determined by the degree of pelvic instability and the presence of associated injuries. Pelvic fractures associated with minor injuries, such as falls in the elderly patient, are common and typically have a stable pattern. Treatment consists of analgesics, gait training for protected weight bearing with a walker, and protection against complications related to immobility, such as venous thromboembolism and skin breakdown. Most patients require protected weight bearing for about 6 weeks until the pain has subsided and the fractures demonstrate early healing.

Pelvic fractures sustained in high-energy injuries often are life threatening. Initial treatment focuses on hemodynamic resuscitation. Definitive treatment of unstable pelvic and acetabular fractures usually requires operative intervention.

## ADVERSE OUTCOMES OF TREATMENT

Degenerative arthritis of the sacroiliac or hip joint, heterotopic ossification, malunion, nonunion, or neurovascular injury can occur.

## REFERRAL DECISIONS/RED FLAGS

High-energy displaced pelvic fractures and open pelvic fractures are best managed in association with a trauma team because there can be life-threatening injuries. Fractures involving the acetabulum or sacroiliac joint require evaluation for possible reduction and fixation. Fractures that fail to heal and pain that persists for more than 12 weeks after injury require further evaluation.

# FRACTURE OF THE PROXIMAL FEMUR

## ICD-9 Codes

820.00
  Femoral neck (transcervical) fracture
820.21
  Intertrochanteric femur fracture

## DEFINITION

Hip fractures are a common problem in elderly individuals with osteoporosis. These fractures generally involve either the femoral neck, which is susceptible to a twisting injury, or the intertrochanteric region, which is susceptible to a fall on the greater trochanter. Both types occur with approximately the same frequency and affect the same patient population.

Age is the most important risk factor for a hip fracture. The frequency of hip fractures generally doubles with each decade beyond age 50 years. White women are two to three times more likely to be affected than black or Hispanic women. Other risk factors include sedentary lifestyle, smoking, alcoholism, use of psychotropic medication, dementia, and living in an urban area.

Decreased proprioceptive function and loss of protective responses increase the likelihood that elderly patients will fall, and when they fall, the lateral thigh and hip region often will strike the ground first. Dizziness, stroke, syncope, peripheral neuropathies, and medications are other factors that can compromise balance and predispose elderly patients to hip fractures.

## CLINICAL SYMPTOMS

Most patients report a fall followed by the inability to walk. A few can walk with assistance (crutches, cane, or walker) but have groin or buttock pain on weight bearing that seems to get worse as they walk. Occasionally, patients report pain referred to the knee. Elderly patients with hip pain after a fall should be treated as if they have a hip fracture until proven otherwise.

## TESTS

### PHYSICAL EXAMINATION

Patients with a displaced femoral neck or intertrochanteric fracture lie with the limb externally rotated, abducted, and shortened. Patients with stress fractures or nondisplaced fractures of the femoral neck may have no obvious deformity. Attempts to log roll the limb (as a rolling pin) are painful.

### DIAGNOSTIC TESTS

AP pelvis and cross table lateral radiographs of the involved hip usually reveal most hip fractures (**Figure 1**). MRI is useful to visualize acute occult hip fractures in patients with a typical history and examination but negative radiographs (**Figure 2**).

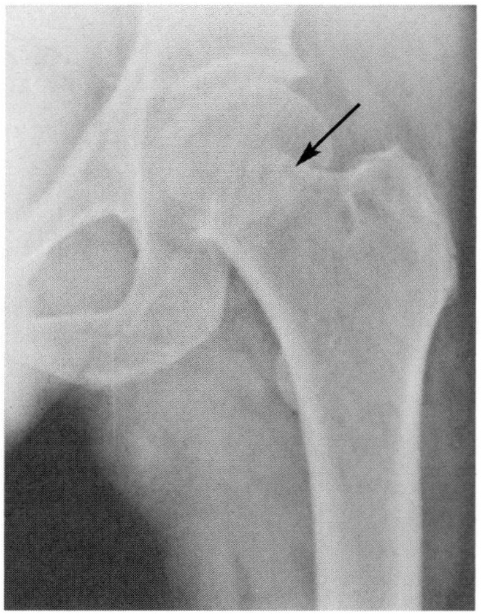

## DIFFERENTIAL DIAGNOSIS

Pathologic fracture (underlying or associated tumor, benign or malignant)

Pelvic fracture (normal hip-joint motion, pain on external rotation)

**Figure 1**
An impacted fracture of the femoral neck.

*Reproduced with permission from Callaghan JJ, Dennis DA, Paprosky WG, Rosenberg AG (eds): Orthopaedic Knowledge Update: Hip and Knee Reconstruction. Rosemont, IL, American Academy of Orthopaedic Surgeons, 1995, pp 97–108.*

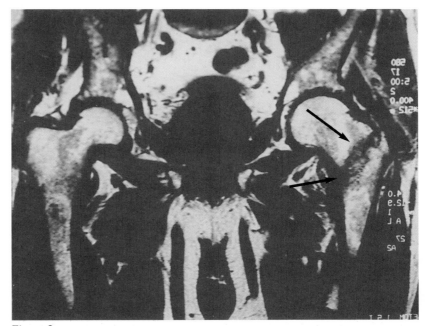

**Figure 2**
MRI scan of hips demonstrating increased signal (arrows) along intertrochanteric line (left hip) consistent with a fracture.

*Reproduced with permission from Callaghan JJ, Dennis DA, Paprosky WG, Rosenberg AG (eds): Orthopaedic Knowledge Update: Hip and Knee Reconstruction. Rosemont, IL, American Academy of Orthopaedic Surgeons, 1995, pp 97–108.*

## ADVERSE OUTCOMES OF THE DISEASE

Thrombophlebitis, limp, inability to walk, pneumonia, painful nonunion of the fracture, osteonecrosis of the femoral head, decubitus ulcer, and even death are possible.

## TREATMENT

Treatment is determined primarily by location (femoral neck versus intertrochanteric), degree of displacement, and the age of the patient. Operative management is required for most patients. In the older population, nondisplaced or minimally displaced fractures of the femoral neck usually are stabilized with internal fixation devices, whereas displaced fractures are treated by replacement arthroplasty. Intertrochanteric hip fractures are generally fixed using a compression screw and side plate.

A small number of patients are best managed nonoperatively. For example, patients with end-stage Alzheimer's disease who were not walking before injury and who have minimal pain are at increased risk for anesthesia and postoperative complications. These patients do better with nonoperative management that includes analgesics and mobilization as quickly as possible into an upright sitting position to decrease the risk of pulmonary problems associated with prolonged bed rest.

The timing of the surgery depends on the fracture type and the health of the patient. Patients with multiple medical conditions require a thorough preoperative medical evaluation, but complications associated with bed rest are decreased if the fracture can be stabilized within the first 24 to 48 hours after injury. Femoral neck fractures in young and middle-aged adults occur with high-energy trauma and have a high rate of osteonecrosis that can be lessened by emergency surgery.

## ADVERSE OUTCOMES OF TREATMENT

Osteonecrosis of the femoral head, malunion, and failure of fixation of the surgical device (especially in patients with severe osteoporosis) are possible. Other complications include thrombophlebitis, infection, and decubitus ulcer; death is also a possibility.

## REFERRAL DECISIONS/RED FLAGS

A femoral neck fracture in a patient younger than age 60 years constitutes a surgical emergency. Because all nondisplaced hip fractures have the potential to displace, they require surgical evaluation. Hip fractures in alert, ambulatory patients are best treated surgically when a patient's medical condition allows.

# INFLAMMATORY ARTHRITIS

## ICD-9 Codes
710.05
    Systemic lupus erythematosus
714.05
    Rheumatoid arthritis
720.05
    Ankylosing spondylitis

## SYNONYM
Synovitis of the hip

## DEFINITION
Most inflammatory conditions that involve the hip are local manifestations of systemic disorders; however, these conditions may first present with symptoms referable to the hip. Although any of the inflammatory arthritides listed in the differential diagnosis may involve the hip, the prevalence of hip involvement is highest in rheumatoid arthritis and ankylosing spondylitis. End-stage arthritis of the hip also is commonly observed in patients with systemic lupus erythematosus, but this is usually secondary to osteonecrosis.

With few exceptions, the pathophysiology of inflammatory arthropathies results from an immunologic host response to antigenic challenge. The exact cause of many inflammatory conditions remains unclear, but epidemiologic and genetic evidence supports a genetic component to many inflammatory arthritides.

## CLINICAL SYMPTOMS
Inflammatory arthritis of the hip is characterized by a dull, aching pain in the groin, lateral thigh, or buttocks region. The pain is often episodic, with patients experiencing morning stiffness, improvement with moderate activity, and increased pain and stiffness following more vigorous activity.

## TESTS

### PHYSICAL EXAMINATION
Antalgic gait (short stance phase on the affected side) or a limp is common. Hip motion is variably restricted. Loss of internal rotation typically is the most sensitive finding in adults with hip joint disease (see Physical Examination–Hip and Thigh). Synovial inflammation can be detected by placing the patient in a prone position with the knee flexed and applying gentle rotation (as moving a rolling pin) to the extremity, moving only the hip.

### DIAGNOSTIC TESTS
AP pelvis and groin lateral or frog-lateral radiographs obtained in the early stages of inflammatory conditions may show osteopenia and/or a joint effusion in the affected hip. In later stages of inflammatory conditions, symmetric joint space loss and periarticular bone erosions are typical (**Figure 1**).

For a patient with acute synovitis, laboratory studies should include complete blood count, acute phase reactants (erythrocyte sedimentation rate or C-reactive protein), rheumatoid factor, and antinuclear antibody test. When an effusion is present, aspiration performed with radiographic assistance can be

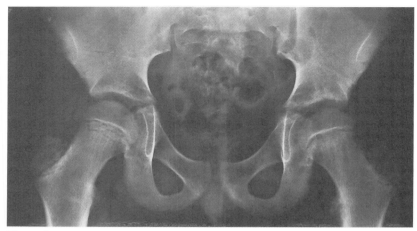

**Figure 1**
AP radiograph of the pelvis (note symmetric joint space commonly seen in rheumatoid arthritis of the hip joint and reduced density of the femoral head on the right side of the radiograph).

*Reproduced with permission from Orthopaedic In-Training Examination 1996. Rosemont, IL, American Academy of Orthopaedic Surgeons, 1996.*

considered. The aspirate should be sent for culture, cell count with differential analysis, and inspection for crystalline deposits.

## DIFFERENTIAL DIAGNOSIS

Ankylosing spondylitis (stiffness of the spine and hips, low back pain, evident on radiographs)

Calcium pyrophosphate deposition disease (uncommon in the hip)

Gout (rare in hip, previous diagnosis of gout most probable, pain in groin or buttock)

Hemophilic arthropathy (previous diagnosis of hemophilia, pain with motion, evident on radiographs)

Infection (acute onset, pain in the groin, fever, marked restriction of motion)

Inflammatory bowel disease (previous diagnosis of bowel disease most probable, groin and buttock discomfort)

Osteoarthritis of the hip (pain in the groin or buttock, limited range of motion)

Osteonecrosis (dull ache in groin or buttock, evident on radiographs and/or MRI)

Reiter syndrome (arthritis, conjunctivitis, pain in the hip, urethritis)

Rheumatoid arthritis (pain in the groin or buttock, decreased range of motion, evident on radiographs)

Stress fracture (pain in the groin or buttock with activity, evident on MRI)

Systemic lupus erythematosus (pain in the groin or buttock, limited range of motion)

Trochanteric bursitis (pain in the lateral aspect of the thigh)

## ADVERSE OUTCOMES OF THE DISEASE

Adverse outcomes include a limp, severe generalized disability and immobility when the disease is systemic, and complete destruction of the joint.

## TREATMENT

Treatment depends on the individual diagnosis. Infection in the hip joint mandates immediate operative drainage. For noninfectious inflammatory arthritis, first-line agents and second-line medications may be useful. A physical therapy program emphasizing range of motion and judicious strengthening exercises may be helpful. Most patients with hip pain and a limp benefit by use of a cane in the hand opposite the symptomatic hip. Bilateral pain may require the use of a walker or bilateral crutches. In addition, these patients often have multiple joint involvement and difficulty doing routine activities. Devices such as a long shoehorn (facilitates putting on shoes) may facilitate daily activities.

Synovectomy may be effective if erosion of cartilage has not occurred; however, the indications for this procedure in hip disease remain controversial. Total hip arthroplasty remains a highly successful method of relieving pain and restoring function in patients with advanced disease.

## ADVERSE OUTCOMES OF TREATMENT

NSAIDs can cause gastric, renal, or hepatic complications. Osteonecrosis of the femoral head and worsening of osteoporosis may develop after treatment with oral corticosteroids. Thrombophlebitis, postoperative infection, and loosening of prosthetic implants may occur after total joint arthroplasty.

## REFERRAL DECISIONS/RED FLAGS

Septic arthritis requires emergent consideration of operative drainage. For noninfectious arthritis, development of severe pain, pain at rest, night pain, severe limp, or osteonecrosis indicates the need for further evaluation.

# LATERAL FEMORAL CUTANEOUS NERVE SYNDROME

| ICD-9 Code |
| --- |
| 355.1 |
| Meralgia paresthetica |

## SYNONYM

Meralgia paresthetica

## DEFINITION

Compression or entrapment of the lateral femoral cutaneous nerve is characterized by pain, burning (dysesthesia), or hypoesthesia over the lateral thigh. Motor nerve dysfunction does not occur because the lateral femoral cutaneous nerve is a sensory nerve. The nerve is most susceptible to compression as it exits the pelvis just medial to the anterosuperior iliac spine. This syndrome can be caused by a number of factors, including obesity, compression from tight clothing or straps around the waist (eg, tool belt, backpack), scar tissue from previous operations, significant trauma (especially involving hip extension), or mild repetitive trauma over the course of the nerve. Pathologic intrapelvic or abdominal processes (cecal tumors) can cause compression in this syndrome, but this is rare.

## CLINICAL SYMPTOMS

Symptoms associated with this condition include pain and dysesthesia in the anterolateral or lateral thigh that sometimes extends to the lateral knee. Uncommonly, patients may report aching in the groin area and, if the condition is acute, pain radiating to the sacroiliac joint area. Joggers describe the pain as an "electric jab" each time the affected hip extends, usually after running a short distance.

## TESTS

### PHYSICAL EXAMINATION

Hypoesthesia or dysesthesia in the distribution of the lateral femoral cutaneous nerve is typical, with the most reproducible spot of hypoesthesia above and lateral to the knee (**Figure 1**). Burning is most consistent in this area. Pressure over the nerve as it exits the pelvis just medial to or directly over the anterosuperior iliac spine can produce tenderness or reproduce paresthesias along the distribution of the nerve. Muscle weakness and reflex changes are absent. Abdominal and pelvic examinations are needed to exclude intra-abdominal problems.

### DIAGNOSTIC TESTS

An AP pelvis radiograph will rule out any abnormality, and AP and lateral radiographs of the hip may be appropriate when the patient has restricted internal rotation of the hip and groin pain. CT or MRI is appropriate to investigate a suspected intrapelvic mass.

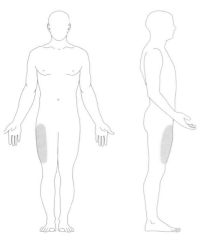

**Figure 1**
Hypoesthesia or dysesthesia associated with lateral femoral cutaneous nerve entrapment.

## DIFFERENTIAL DIAGNOSIS

Diabetes mellitus or other causes of peripheral neuropathy (numbness in the feet)

Hip arthritis (limited internal rotation, a limp)

Intra-abdominal tumor (pelvic or abdominal mass, hematochezia, weight loss)

Lumbar disk herniation (L1-4 motor and sensory changes, positive prone rectus femoris stretch test)

Trochanteric bursitis (tenderness over trochanter, stiffness when rising)

## ADVERSE OUTCOMES OF THE DISEASE

Pain and dysesthesia will continue if the patient is not treated.

## TREATMENT

Numbness is often well tolerated, but burning dysesthesia can become intolerable. Removing the source of compression, such as a tight waistband or mild repetitive trauma to the nerve, can relieve the symptoms of burning. In obese patients, significant weight loss often relieves symptoms. Infiltration of the area around the nerve as it exits the pelvis near the anterosuperior iliac spine with a corticosteroid preparation may reduce symptoms. Operative release of the nerve is most commonly needed in patients with persistent burning dysesthesia.

## ADVERSE OUTCOMES OF TREATMENT

In some instances, symptoms persist despite treatment.

## REFERRAL DECISIONS/RED FLAGS

A suspected pelvic or abdominal mass signals the need for immediate further evaluation. The presence of intolerable symptoms that have failed to respond to nonoperative treatment also indicates the need for further evaluation.

# OSTEOARTHRITIS OF THE HIP

## ICD-9 Codes

**715.15**
Primary (idiopathic) osteoarthritis of the hip

**715.25**
Secondary osteoarthritis of the hip (eg, Legg-Calvé-Perthes disease)

**716.15**
Traumatic arthritis of the hip

## SYNONYMS

Degenerative arthritis of the hip
Osteoarthrosis of the hip

## DEFINITION

Osteoarthritis of the hip is characterized by loss of articular cartilage of the hip joint. The osteoarthrosis may be primary (idiopathic) or secondary to hip diseases during childhood, trauma, osteonecrosis, previous joint infection, or other conditions.

## CLINICAL SYMPTOMS

The classic presentation is a gradual onset of anterior thigh or groin pain. Some patients have pain in the buttock or the lateral aspect of the thigh. The pain may be referred to the distal thigh (knee) and may be perceived only in the knee. Initially, pain occurs only with activity, but gradually the frequency and intensity of the pain increases to the point that even rest does not relieve the pain. Pain that wakes a patient from sleep (night pain) is associated with severe arthritis. As osteoarthritis progresses, patients have limited motion and a limp. Occasionally, patients will have a severe limp and stiffness but little pain.

A careful history is necessary to determine whether the patient had hip problems as an infant or toddler (developmental dysplasia of the hip), as a child (Legg-Calvé-Perthes disease), or as an adolescent (slipped capital femoral epiphysis). Patients with osteoarthritis of the hip can have other coexisting conditions, as listed in the differential diagnosis.

## TESTS

### PHYSICAL EXAMINATION

The earliest sign of osteoarthritis of the hip is loss of internal rotation. Gradually, as the arthritis worsens, patients will lose flexion and extension. Flexion contractures make gait more awkward because the patient must sway the back to get the hip straight. In addition, an antalgic gait (short stance on the painful leg) and an abductor lurch (swaying the trunk far over the affected hip) develop as the body tries to compensate for the pain and secondary weakness in the hip abductor muscles.

### DIAGNOSTIC TESTS

AP and lateral radiographs of the hip are indicated for patients with pain and limited internal rotation of the hip. The classic radiographic features of osteoarthritis of the hips are joint space narrowing, osteophytes, cyst formation, and subchondral sclerosis (**Figure 1**).

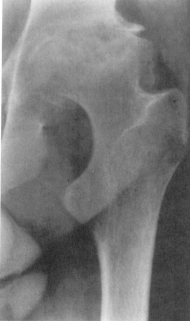

**Figure 1**
Radiograph of left hip with severe joint space narrowing, osteophytes, and cyst formation.

*Reproduced with permission from Callaghan JJ, Dennis DA, Paprosky WG, et al (eds): Orthopaedic Knowledge Update: Hip and Knee Reconstruction. Rosemont, IL, American Academy of Orthopaedic Surgeons, 1995, pp 79–86.*

# DIFFERENTIAL DIAGNOSIS

Degenerative lumbar disk disease (normal hip motion)

Femoral cutaneous nerve entrapment (sensory changes, burning, normal motion)

Herniated lumbar disk (diminished knee reflex, sensory changes)

Inflammatory arthritis of the hip (rheumatoid arthritis, systemic lupus erythematosus, ankylosing spondylitis)

Osteonecrosis of the femoral head (evident on radiographs)

Trochanteric bursitis (local tenderness, normal motion)

Tumor of the pelvis or spine (back pain, night pain, normal motion)

## ADVERSE OUTCOMES OF THE DISEASE

Osteoarthritis of the hip is a progressive condition that has no cure. The usual clinical course is deteriorating gait, increasing pain and stiffness, and, eventually, pain at rest and at night.

## TREATMENT

Treatment depends on the stage of the disease and the age of the patient. Initial treatment includes acetaminophen or NSAIDs and physical therapy to improve strength and range of motion. As the disease progresses, patients will benefit from use of a cane held in the hand opposite the affected hip.

Patients between the ages of 20 and 50 years who have hip pain often will have hip dysplasia, residual effects of developmental hip dysplasia, Legg-Calvé-Perthes disease, or slipped capital femoral epiphysis. These patients may benefit from an early realignment osteotomy, which can alter the progression of the disease or fusion of the hip.

When pain persists in older patients, a total hip replacement arthroplasty is indicated.

## ADVERSE OUTCOMES OF TREATMENT

NSAIDs can cause gastric, renal, or hepatic problems. Postoperative thrombophlebitis, infection, and failure of the prosthetic components are complications associated with total hip arthroplasty. Younger patients may require multiple revisions during their lifetimes. Osteoarthritis at the spine or knee joint may develop over time after hip fusion. Patients with osteotomies can have persistent hip pain and a limp.

## REFERRAL DECISIONS/RED FLAGS

Younger patients require further evaluation because an osteotomy could slow progression of the disease. All patients with hip pain at rest require further evaluation.

# OSTEONECROSIS OF THE HIP

## Outline 1
### Risk Factors for Osteonecrosis

Alcohol

Caisson disease

Chronic pancreatitis

Corticosteroid use

Crohn disease

Gaucher disease

Myeloproliferative disorders

Radiation treatment

Rheumatoid arthritis

Trauma

Sickle cell disease

Systemic lupus erythematosus

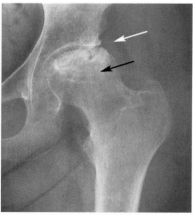

**Figure 1**
Sclerosis (black arrow) and collapse of the femoral head (white arrow).

*Reproduced with permission from Cabanela ME: Hip arthroplasty in osteonecrosis of the femoral head, in Jones JP, Urbaniak M (eds): Osteonecrosis. Rosemont, IL, American Academy of Orthopaedic Surgeons, 1997, pp 385-390.*

## SYNONYMS

Avascular necrosis of the hip

Aseptic necrosis of the hip

## DEFINITION

Osteonecrosis of the hip results from the death of varying amounts of bone in the femoral head. The causative event may be traumatic disruption of the vascular supply to the femoral head or deficient circulation from other causes, (eg, microvascular thrombosis in patients with sickle cell anemia). Initially, only the osteocytes and other cells are affected, but with time the bone structure fragments and collapses. As a result, the articular surface is disrupted and progressive arthritis develops.

Osteonecrosis affects 10,000 to 20,000 new patients per year in the United States, occurs with greater frequency in the third through fifth decades, and often is bilateral. Risk factors include trauma (hip dislocation or femoral neck fracture), history of corticosteroid use, alcohol abuse, sickle cell disease, rheumatoid arthritis, and systemic lupus erythematosus. A list of common clinical entities associated with osteonecrosis appears in Outline 1. Of note, the association with corticosteroids generally is associated with the amount and duration of medication; however, osteonecrosis can develop after only one or two doses of intravenous corticosteroids.

## CLINICAL SYMPTOMS

Patients usually report an indolent onset of a dull ache or a throbbing pain in the groin, lateral hip, or buttock. However, the pain can begin suddenly with collapse of the necrotic femoral head. Thus, the patient's complete history must be obtained. Some patients have a tendency to minimize their use of alcohol.

## TESTS

### PHYSICAL EXAMINATION

Patients report pain with internal and external rotation and usually have diminished internal rotation, flexion, and abduction of the joint. They often have an antalgic gait (short stance phase). The degree of symptoms largely depends on the degree of arthritis (how much and which part of the articular surface is disrupted).

### DIAGNOSTIC TESTS

AP pelvis and frog-lateral radiographs of the pelvis should be obtained first. One of the earliest signs of osteonecrosis is sclerosis of the femoral head (**Figure 1**). However, in the early stage of the disease, radiographs may appear normal (symptoms in this situation are most likely associated with subtle collapse of the subchondral bone and subsequent shift or wrinkle of the articular surface). MRI of the pelvis to examine both femoral heads is indicated when the patient has risk factors for osteonecrosis but no changes in the femoral head, when only sclerotic changes are seen in the femoral head on plain radiographs, or when osteonecrosis of the opposite hip is suspected. A single band-like area of low intensity on the T1-weighted image or double-line signs on the T2-weighted image confirm the diagnosis (**Figure 2**). When the radiographs demonstrate evidence of significant collapse of the femoral head or degenerative arthritis of the hip joint, MRI is not necessary.

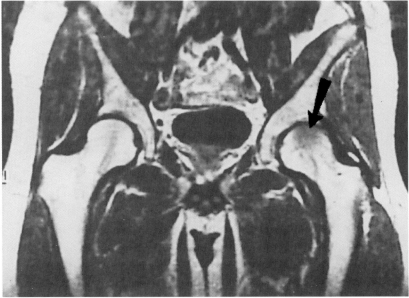

**Figure 2**
MRI scan of hips consistent with osteonecrosis of the left hip (arrow). This AP view reveals significant involvement of the weight-bearing surface. The opposite hip is normal.

*Reproduced with permission from Poss R (ed): Orthopaedic Knowledge Update 3. Park Ridge, IL, American Academy of Orthopaedic Surgeons, 1990, p 540.*

## DIFFERENTIAL DIAGNOSIS

Fracture of the femoral neck (evident on radiographs, MRI)

Lumbar disk disease (back pain, reflex changes, radiation below knee)

Muscle strain or groin pull (normal radiographs, intermittent limp)

Osteoarthritis of the hip (no risk factors, absence of sclerosis within the femoral heads on radiographs)

Septic arthritis of the hip (fever, constitutional symptoms)

Transient osteoporosis of the hip (disabling pain without previous trauma, osteopenia, in women in third trimester of pregnancy or middle-aged men)

## Adverse outcomes of the disease

Pain, limp, collapse of the femoral head, secondary osteoarthritis, and disability can occur.

## Treatment

The prognosis depends on the extent of the osteonecrosis and its location (degree of involvement of weight-bearing surface). Protective weight bearing should be considered only as a temporary treatment until a more definitive work-up and treatment plan can be established. The appropriate reconstructive procedure for a hip that has not collapsed is controversial. Once collapse occurs, a hip arthroplasty is the procedure of choice for relieving pain and restoring function. The timing of this procedure depends on the patient's age, diagnosis, and symptoms.

## Adverse outcomes of treatment

Reconstructive procedures may not prevent collapse of the femoral head and may actually accelerate collapse of the femoral head. Fracture of the proximal femur can follow any procedure that invades the femoral cortex. Postoperative infection and/or thrombophlebitis also can develop.

## Referral decisions/Red flags

Suspicion or confirmation of osteonecrosis indicates the need for immediate further evaluation. A patient with one of the risk factors and hip pain requires evaluation of the hip.

# SNAPPING HIP

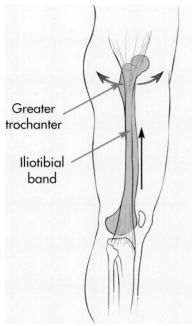

**Figure 1**
Iliotibial band slips anteriorly and posteriorly over the prominent greater trochanter.

Greater
trochanter

Iliotibial
band

## DEFINITION

Snapping hip is characterized by a snapping or popping sensation that occurs as tendons around the hip move over bony prominences. The most common site is the iliotibial band snapping over the greater trochanter. Snapping also can occur when the iliopsoas tendon slides over the pectineal eminence of the pelvis or from intra-articular tears of the acetabular labrum (fibrocartilage rim at the periphery of the acetabulum).

## CLINICAL SYMPTOMS

Iliotibial band subluxation usually occurs with walking or rotation of the hip. Patients will point to the trochanteric area (**Figure 1**). Some patients notice the snapping when they lie with the affected side up and rotate the leg. If a trochanteric bursitis subsequently develops, patients will report increased pain when first rising in the morning, pain at night, and difficulty lying on the affected side.

Snapping caused by subluxation of the iliopsoas tendon usually is felt in the groin as the hip extends from a flexed position, as when rising from a chair. Many patients feel the snapping but have no disability. In a few patients, the snapping is either annoying or painful.

Snapping from intra-articular causes is more disabling and more likely to cause patients to grab for support.

## TESTS

### PHYSICAL EXAMINATION

Iliotibial band subluxation can be recreated by having the patient stand and then rotate the hip while holding it in an adducted position. A snap can be palpated as the iliotibial band slides over the greater trochanter. Snapping of the iliopsoas tendon may be palpated as the hip extends from a flexed position and the tendon moves over the pectineal eminence of the pelvis. Restricted internal rotation of the involved hip, a limp, or shortening of the limb suggests problems within the hip joint.

### DIAGNOSTIC TESTS

AP pelvis and lateral hip radiographs can exclude bony pathology or intra-articular hip disease. Radiographs typically are normal for patients with a snapping hip. A CT arthrogram may be necessary to rule out intra-articular loose bodies. An MRI with gadolinium may be necessary to rule out a labral tear.

## DIFFERENTIAL DIAGNOSIS

Osteoarthritis of the hip (limited internal rotation)

Osteochondral loose body (a fragment of bone and cartilage within the joint, pain with hip motion)

Osteonecrosis of the femoral head (compromised blood supply of the femoral head, groin pain)

Tear of the acetabular labrum (pain or instability with hip motion)

## ADVERSE OUTCOMES OF THE DISEASE

Pain and annoyance are the two most common complaints.

## TREATMENT

Snapping hip is often painless, and once the diagnosis is made with certainty, patients often require only an explanation of the source of the symptoms for reassurance. Patients who are significantly bothered by the symptoms should be advised to avoid provocative maneuvers and activities so that the symptoms can subside. Physical therapy consisting of stretching exercises (ie, iliotibial band, hip abductors, hip adductors, and hip flexors) and a short course of NSAIDs may reduce the discomfort associated with tendon snapping and secondary bursitis. Corticosteroid injection into the greater trochanteric bursa (for snapping iliotibial band) or into the psoas sheath (for snapping iliopsoas tendon) can reduce pain.

Surgery is reserved for the uncommon disabling cases that fail to resolve with nonoperative management.

## ADVERSE OUTCOMES OF TREATMENT

NSAIDs can cause gastric, renal, or hepatic complications. Postoperative infection or persistent pain also is possible.

## REFERRAL DECISIONS/RED FLAGS

Unclear diagnosis, intra-articular pathology, and/or failure of nonoperative measures indicate the need for further evaluation.

# STRAINS OF THE HIP

ICD-9 Code

843.9
    Strains and sprains of hip and
    thigh, unspecified site

## DEFINITION

Hip strain is a general term applied to injured muscle-tendon units around the hip. Vigorous muscular contraction while the muscle is on stretch frequently causes the injury. For example, forceful hip flexion can strain the iliopsoas muscle, as when a soccer player forcibly flexes the hip to kick a ball and the leg is blocked or forcefully extended by an opponent. Overuse injuries are a second cause of hip strains. Several muscles, including the abdominals, hip flexors (iliopsoas, sartorius, or rectus femoris), and adductors, should be considered when a patient has pain around the hip after an acute or overuse injury (**Figures 1 and 2**).

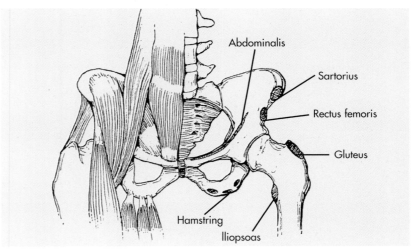

**Figure 1**
Anterior view of pelvis: muscle origins and insertions.

*Reproduced with permission from Delee JC, Drez D Jr (eds): Orthopaedic Sports Medicine: Principles and Practice. vol 2, Philadelphia, PA, WB Saunders, 1994, pp 1063–1085.*

## CLINICAL SYMPTOMS

The most common presenting symptom is pain over the injured muscle that is exacerbated when that area continues to be used during strenuous activities.

## TESTS

### PHYSICAL EXAMINATION

The deep location of the hip muscles compromises the examination, and precise localization of the injured muscle is not always possible. Strain of the hip adductors is identified by tenderness in the groin and increased pain with passive abduction. Injury to the abdominal muscles is increased when the patient

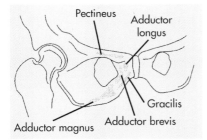

**Figure 2**
Anterior view of pelvis: adductor muscle insertions.

does a sit-up. When a hip flexor is injured, the pain is worse with flexion of the hip against resistance. Strain of the rectus femoris is delineated by increased pain when putting the rectus femoris on stretch (see Physical Examination–Knee and Lower Leg). Injury to the iliopsoas typically causes pain in the deep groin or inner thigh, while pain from a proximal sartorius strain is more superficial and lateral.

## DIAGNOSTIC TESTS

AP radiographs of the pelvis and a frog-lateral view of the involved hip can rule out a fracture or bony lesion. A bone scan or MRI can contribute useful information to help the physician arrive at the correct diagnosis, but these studies are rarely necessary except in the elite athlete (**Figure 3**).

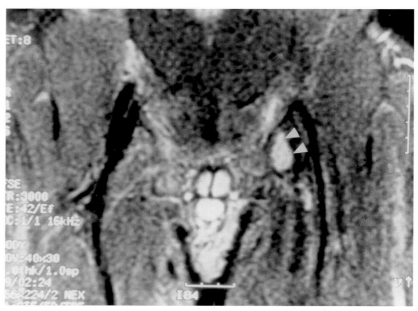

**Figure 3**
AP pelvic MRI of a 21-year-old man with a several-month history of groin pain and difficulty running. He was diagnosed with an adductor muscle tear (arrowheads).

## DIFFERENTIAL DIAGNOSIS

Hip avulsion fractures (may be seen with strains of the sartorius, eg, avulsion fracture of the anterior superior iliac spine; rectus femoris, eg, avulsion fracture of the anterior inferior iliac spine)

Osteonecrosis of the hip (chronic dull ache in groin, inner thigh, or buttock; evident on radiographs, MRI)

Pelvic or proximal femoral tumors (pain at rest or at night, increased pain with weight bearing)

## ADVERSE OUTCOME OF THE DISEASE

Chronic injury can be debilitating and threaten athletic performance. If pain persists, the patient's gait can be altered, resulting in secondary injuries.

# TREATMENT

Rehabilitation enhances full recovery and should be initiated after confirmation of the injury. For most patients, modification of activities, followed by a home exercise program, is sufficient. Elite athletes usually are treated with a more aggressive and costly regimen (**Table 1**). Rehabilitation can be divided into five phases that generally are completed within approximately 6 weeks. Phase I includes rest, ice, compression, and protected weight bearing with the use of crutches (48 to 72 hours). Phase II includes active and passive range-of-motion exercises, accompanied by heat or ultrasound (72 hours up to 1 week). The final three phases include different isometric exercises and sport-specific training. The purpose of the final phases is to increase strength and flexibility and focus on returning the patient to the preinjury level of activity. If pain is exacerbated during the rehabilitation process, the patient should return to the phase of treatment before symptoms recurred.

## Table 1
### Rehabilitation Guidelines for Muscle Injuries in Elite Athletes

|  | Goals | Treatment | Time frame |
|---|---|---|---|
| Phase I | Reduce pain, inflammation, and bleeding | Rest, ice, and compression; crutches if needed | 48 to 72 hours |
| Phase II | Regain range of motion | Passive range of motion, heat, ultrasound, electrical muscle stimulation | 72 hours to week 1 |
| Phase III | Increase strength, flexibility, and endurance | Isometrics, well-leg cycling | Weeks 1 to 3 |
| Phase IV | Increase strength and coordination | Isotonic and isokinetic exercises | Weeks 3 to 4 |
| Phase V | Return to competition | Sport-specific training | Weeks 4 to 6 |

*Reproduced with permission from Delee JC, Drez D Jr (eds): Orthopaedic Sports Medicine: Principles and Practice. vol 2, Philadelphia, PA, WB Saunders, 1994, pp 1063–1085.*

## ADVERSE OUTCOMES OF TREATMENT

Recalcitrant pain can indicate a more serious injury or tendinous disruption that requires further evaluation. Recurrent injuries also are possible and more likely to occur in competitive or weekend athletes who fail to maintain flexibility of the affected muscle.

## REFERRAL DECISION/RED FLAGS

Patients who do not respond to treatment require further evaluation to ensure that a more serious injury has not occurred and that a malignancy or osteonecrosis of the hip is not mimicking symptoms of hip strain.

# STRAINS OF THE THIGH

| ICD-9 Code |
| --- |
| 843.9 |
| Sprains and strains of hip and thigh, unspecified site |

## DEFINITION

Injury to the thigh muscles can be temporarily painful and devastating to the avid elite or weekend athlete. The posterior thigh muscles (hamstring muscles) are injured more often than the anterior thigh muscles (quadriceps). Most hamstring strains occur when one of these muscles (biceps femoris, semimembranosus, or semitendinosus) is put on stretch during an active contraction. The strain or tear usually occurs at the musculotendinous junction. The quadriceps may sustain a similar injury; however, the quadriceps is more often injured by a direct blow.

## CLINICAL SYMPTOMS

A patient with a hamstring strain typically reports a sudden onset of posterior or thigh pain that occurred while running, water skiing, or some other rapid movement. A "pop" may have been perceived at the onset of pain. Quadriceps contusions are associated with a direct blow during contact sports.

## TESTS

### PHYSICAL EXAMINATION

Physical examination reveals local tenderness at the site of the injured muscle. With time, the inflammation spreads and the tenderness can become less localized. Muscle injury and associated hemorrhage may be evident by ecchymosis located in the posterior thigh. The hamstrings span two joints, originating above the hip on the ischial tuberosity and inserting below the knee on the tibia and fibula. Therefore, placing the hamstring on stretch to confirm the diagnosis requires flexion of the hip followed by extension of the knee. Three components of the quadriceps muscle (vastus medialis, vastus intermedius, and vastus lateralis) only span one joint. Therefore, pain associated with strain or contusion of this part of the quadriceps muscle is exacerbated by flexion of the knee and is not related to the position of the hip. However, the rectus femoris component of the quadriceps muscle spans the hip and knee. To put this muscle on stretch, perform the prone rectus femoris test (see Physical Examination–Knee and Lower Leg) by flexing the knee with the hip in extension.

### DIAGNOSTIC TESTS

Radiographs or other specialized imaging studies typically are not needed in patients with a typical history and examination. Suspicion of a fracture or bony avulsion injury can be confirmed by plain radiographs. MRI can confirm the thigh strain but is rarely indicated because a history and physical examination can adequately provide a correct diagnosis (**Figure 1**).

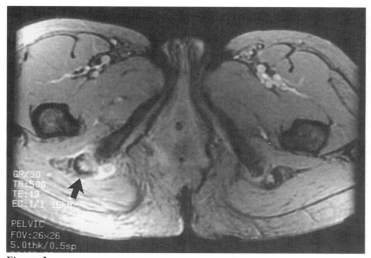 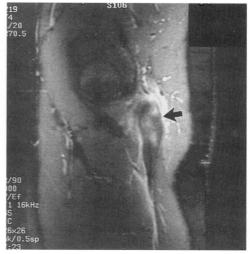

**Figure 1**
Axial MRI of a 39-year-old woman who sustained an acute injury (arrow) to the hamstring while water skiing (left), and sagittal MRI of the injury (arrow) (right).

## DIFFERENTIAL DIAGNOSIS

Adductor injuries (pain in the groin and inner thigh, ecchymosis, occasional sharp, stabbing pain)

Iliopsoas strains (pain in the groin with hip flexion)

Muscle strain of other pelvic/hip muscles (pain with ambulation)

Pelvic avulsion fractures (pain and ecchymosis over the anterosuperior iliac spine, evident on radiographs)

Proximal femoral tumor (pain in the groin or thigh at rest or at night, pain with weight bearing, evident on radiographs)

## ADVERSE OUTCOMES OF THE DISEASE

Chronic hamstring injuries are debilitating and can be career ending for an elite athlete. Contusion (hemorrhage) in the quadriceps muscle may progress to myositis ossificans with a resulting restriction of knee flexion and a possible diagnostic dilemma (the clinical appearance may simulate malignant tumor).

## TREATMENT

Initial treatment includes prevention of further swelling and hemorrhage by having the patient rest and elevate the limb while applying ice and compressive wraps as needed. As time passes, the patient should begin a program of rehabilitation with stretching and strengthening of the injured muscle. The degree of rehabilitation necessary depends on the patient's general activity level and the severity of the injury. Most patients can be treated with a home exercise program. Elite athletes usually are treated with a more aggressive and costly regimen. The long-term results are generally similar. If myositis ossificans develops in the quadriceps muscle, the rehabilitation process is typically longer. However, operative excision of the ossific mass is rarely needed.

**Protocol for Treatment of Hamstring Injuries in Elite Athletes**

Phase I (Days 1 to 5)
Rest, ice, compression, elevation (RICE)

Phase II (Weeks 2 and 3)
Ice
Stretching exercises
NSAIDs
Electrical stimulation
Isometric exercises
Isotonic exercises*
Conditioning exercises

Phase III (Weeks 4 through 6)
Ice
Stretching exercises
NSAIDs
Electrical stimulation*
Isotonic exercises
Isokinetic exercises*†
Conditioning exercises

Phase IV (Weeks 7 and 8)
Ice
Stretching exercises
Isokinetic exercises†
Running
Sport-specific training

Phase V
Return to sports

*Optional
†Concentric high speeds at first, proceeding to eccentric slow speeds.
*Reproduced with permission from Delee JC, Drez D Jr (eds): Orthopaedic Sports Medicine: Principles and Practice. vol 2, Philadelphia, PA, WB Saunders, 1994, pp 1063–1085.*

## Adverse outcome of treatment

NSAIDs can cause gastric, renal, or hepatic complications. Failure to rehabilitate the injury adequately can result in chronic problems.

## Referral decisions/Red flags

Patients who fail to respond to appropriate rehabilitation require further evaluation.

# Transient Osteoporosis of the Hip

ICD-9 Code

733.09
Osteoporosis not elsewhere classified or drug-induced

## Synonym

Bone marrow edema syndrome

## Definition

Transient osteoporosis of the hip is an uncommon idiopathic condition characterized by spontaneous onset of hip pain associated with radiographic osteoporosis of the femoral head and neck. The condition is most frequent in middle-aged men and in women during the third trimester of pregnancy. Resolution is spontaneous, usually within 6 to 12 months.

## Clinical symptoms

Patients typically have spontaneous onset of hip area pain in the anterior thigh (groin), lateral hip, or buttock. Pain is usually worse with weight bearing and less prominent at rest. Symptoms typically worsen for the first several months, then gradually abate.

## Tests

### Physical examination

Patients usually have an antalgic gait and pain at the limits of hip motion.

### Diagnostic tests

Plain radiographs of the hip typically demonstrate diffuse osteoporosis of the femoral head and neck. However, in the early phase of the disease, osteoporosis may not be evident. MRI is helpful to rule out other diagnoses and help confirm the diagnosis of transient osteoporosis. The typical MRI findings are of bone marrow edema of the femoral neck with a diffusely decreased signal on T1-weighted images and a diffusely increased signal on T2-weighted images. The signal change usually extends into the intertrochanteric region.

## Differential diagnosis

Infections involving the proximal femur or hip joint (pain, constitutional symptoms)

Osteonecrosis of the femoral head (pain in the groin or buttock, sclerosis on radiographs)

Pigmented villonodular synovitis of the hip (pain in the groin or buttock, evident on MRI and biopsy)

Stress fracture of the femoral neck (pain in the groin or buttock, evident on radiograph or MRI)

Tumors involving the proximal femur (pain in the groin, buttock, or thigh, evident on radiograph or MRI)

Section 5 | Hip and Thigh

## ADVERSE OUTCOMES OF THE DISEASE

Fracture of the femoral neck can occur during the time the bone is weakened by osteoporosis. Pregnant women with the disease appear to be at higher risk for femoral neck fracture.

## TREATMENT

The disease is a self-limited process that typically resolves spontaneously within 6 to 12 months after onset of symptoms. After other diseases have been excluded and a firm diagnosis is established (usually plain radiographs and MRI are sufficient), the treatment is supportive. Patients are provided with mild analgesics and placed on crutches to limit weight bearing until symptoms resolve and radiographs demonstrate reconstitution of normal bone density.

## REFERRAL DECISIONS/RED FLAGS

The diagnosis may be difficult to make with certainty. Women in the third trimester of pregnancy are at risk for the disease. Decisions regarding imaging studies and choice of analgesics should be made in consultation with the patient's obstetrician. Pregnant women with the disease appear to be at greater risk for femoral neck fracture.

# TROCHANTERIC BURSITIS

### ICD-9 Code
726.5
Enthesopathy of hip region

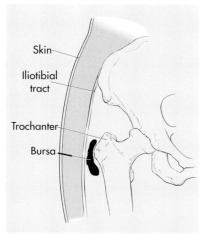

**Figure 1**
Relationship of trochanteric bursa between the iliotibial band and the greater trochanter.

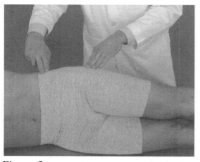

**Figure 2**
Palpate the greater trochanter with the patient in the lateral decubitus position.

## SYNONYM
Greater trochanteric bursitis

## DEFINITION
Inflammation and hypertrophy of the greater trochanteric bursa may develop without apparent cause or in association with lumbar spine disease, intra-articular hip pathology, significant limb-length inequalities, inflammatory arthritis, or previous surgery around the hip (particularly when internal fixation devices are placed in or near the greater trochanter) (**Figure 1**).

## CLINICAL SYMPTOMS
Patients usually have pain and tenderness over the greater trochanter. The pain may radiate distally to the knee or ankle (but not onto the foot) or proximally into the buttock. The pain is worse when first rising from a seated or recumbent position, feels somewhat better after a few steps, and recurs after walking for half an hour or more. Patients report night pain and are unable to lie on the affected side. Inflammation (tendinitis) of the gluteal tendons can cause a similar pain pattern.

## TESTS
### PHYSICAL EXAMINATION
Point tenderness over the lateral greater trochanter is the essential finding (**Figure 2**). Tenderness above the trochanter suggests tendinitis of the gluteus medius tendon. Patients report increased discomfort with adduction of the hip or adduction combined with internal rotation.

### DIAGNOSTIC TESTS
AP pelvis and lateral hip radiographs are necessary to rule out bony abnormalities and intra-articular hip pathology. Occasionally, rounded or irregular calcific deposits may be seen above the trochanter at the attachment of the gluteus medius. Bone scans and MRI rarely are needed to make the diagnosis but occasionally may be helpful to rule out uncommon conditions such as occult fractures, tumors, or osteonecrosis of the femoral head.

## DIFFERENTIAL DIAGNOSIS

Metastatic tumor (evident on radiographs, weight loss, constitutional symptoms)

Osteoarthritis of the hip (painful internal rotation, evident on radiographs)

Sciatica (pain posteriorly, pain radiating to the foot, motor and sensory changes, reflex changes)

Septic arthritis of the hip (fever, severe pain with motion)

Snapping hip (obvious snap of the iliotibial band)

Trochanteric fracture (evident on radiographs, persistent limp when walking, positive Trendelenburg sign)

## ADVERSE OUTCOMES OF THE DISEASE

Chronic pain, a limp, and/or complaints of sleep disturbance are possible.

## TREATMENT

NSAIDs, activity modifications, and short-term use of a cane are sufficient for most patients. Injection of a local anesthetic and corticosteroid preparation into the greater trochanteric bursa (see Trochanteric Bursitis Injection) can be helpful in relieving symptoms. Occasionally, repeat injections are required for symptomatic relief. Surgery is indicated only rarely for intransigent cases.

## ADVERSE OUTCOMES OF TREATMENT

NSAIDs can cause gastric, renal, or hepatic complications. In some patients, pain may persist. Although rare, infection from the injection can develop. Infection largely can be avoided by the careful use of sterile technique.

## REFERRAL DECISIONS/RED FLAGS

Failure of treatment, diagnostic uncertainty, and/or suspected fracture are indications for further evaluation.

# PROCEDURE

## TROCHANTERIC BURSITIS INJECTION

### MATERIALS

Sterile gloves

Bactericidal skin preparation solution

10-mL syringe

20-gauge or 22-gauge, 1½" needle (use a spinal needle in larger patients)

3 to 5 mL of 1% lidocaine

40 to 80 mg of a corticosteroid preparation

Adhesive dressing

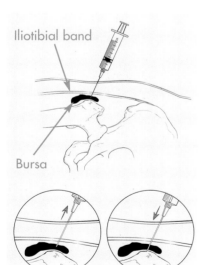

**Figure 1**
Location for needle insertion.

*Adapted with permission of the Mayo Foundation, Rochester, MN.*

**STEP 1**

Wear protective gloves at all times during the procedure and use sterile technique.

**STEP 2**

Ask the patient to lie in the lateral decubitus position with the affected hip turned upward. Place a pillow between the patient's knees to relax the iliotibial band and reduce the pressure required to inject the solution.

**STEP 3**

Cleanse the skin with a bactericidal skin preparation.

**STEP 4**

Draw lidocaine into a 10-mL syringe.

**STEP 5**

Draw the chosen dose of corticosteroid preparation into the same syringe and mix the two solutions.

**STEP 6**

Palpate the greater trochanter and identify the point of maximum tenderness.

**STEP 7**

Insert the needle until it contacts bone, then withdraw it 1 or 2 mm so that the tip is in the bursa and not in the bone (**Figure 1**). Usually, a 1½" needle is sufficient, but for larger patients a spinal needle might be needed to reach the trochanteric bursa. Do not withdraw the needle too far or it will be outside the trochanteric bursa.

**STEP 8**

Aspirate to ensure that the needle is not in an intravascular position, then inject the corticosteroid preparation/local anesthetic mixture in 1- to 2-mL aliquots.

**STEP 9**

Partially withdraw the needle, then reinsert it and inject another aliquot. Continue this to infiltrate the entire bursa, an area of several square centimeters around the point of maximum tenderness.

**STEP 10**

Withdraw the needle completely and apply gentle pressure over the injection site.

SECTION 5   HIP AND THIGH

## STEP 11

Dress the puncture wound with a sterile adhesive bandage.

## ADVERSE OUTCOMES

Although rare, infection or allergic reactions to the local anesthetic or corticosteroid preparation are possible. Always query the patient about medication allergies before the procedure. In some patients with diabetes, poor control of blood glucose levels may occur, but this is usually temporary. A minority of patients requires more than one injection to achieve lasting pain relief; however, repeated injections with corticosteroids should be avoided.

## AFTERCARE/PATIENT INSTRUCTIONS

Advise the patient that as the local anesthetic wears off, pain often persists or becomes worse for a few days until the corticosteroid takes effect. Instruct the patient to attempt weight bearing as tolerated and to contact you if symptoms recur or if redness, fever, immobilizing pain, or any other evidence of a local problem related to the injection occurs.

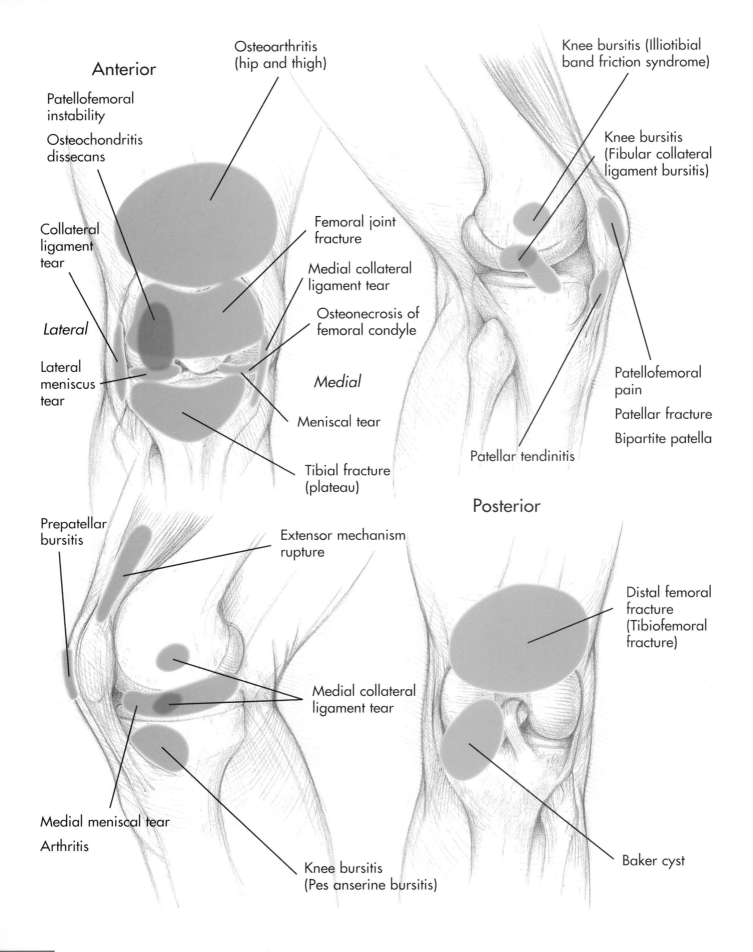

Anterior

Patellofemoral instability

Osteochondritis dissecans

Osteoarthritis (hip and thigh)

Collateral ligament tear

*Lateral*

Lateral meniscus tear

Femoral joint fracture

Medial collateral ligament tear

Osteonecrosis of femoral condyle

*Medial*

Meniscal tear

Tibial fracture (plateau)

Knee bursitis (Illiotibial band friction syndrome)

Knee bursitis (Fibular collateral ligament bursitis)

Patellofemoral pain

Patellar fracture

Bipartite patella

Patellar tendinitis

Prepatellar bursitis

Extensor mechanism rupture

Medial collateral ligament tear

Medial meniscal tear

Arthritis

Knee bursitis (Pes anserine bursitis)

Posterior

Distal femoral fracture (Tibiofemoral fracture)

Baker cyst

# KNEE
# AND LOWER LEG

## Section Editor
Kenneth E. DeHaven, MD
Professor, Associate Chair for Clinical Affairs
Director of Athletic Medicine
Department of Orthopaedics
University of Rochester School of Medicine
and Dentistry
Rochester, New York

Kevin P. Black, MD
Associate Professor and Vice Chairman
Department of Orthopaedics and Rehabilitation
Penn State University College of Medicine
Hershey, Pennsylvania

Robert D. Bronstein, MD
Associate Professor
Department of Orthopaedics
University of Rochester School of Medicine and
Dentistry
Rochester, New York

Andrew J. Cosgarea, MD
Associate Professor
Department of Orthopaedic Surgery
Johns Hopkins University
Baltimore, Maryland

Michael D. Maloney, MD
Assistant Professor
Department of Orthopaedics
University of Rochester School of Medicine and
Dentistry
Rochester, New York

Wayne Joseph Sebastianelli, MD
Associate Professor
Department of Orthopaedics and Rehabilitation
Director of Athletic Medicine
Penn State University College of Medicine
Hershey, Pennsylvania

# KNEE AND LOWER LEG—AN OVERVIEW

Most knee problems can be diagnosed by obtaining an appropriate medical history, performing a thorough examination of the knee, and taking appropriate radiographs. Patients with knee problems often report pain, instability, stiffness, swelling, locking, or weakness. These findings can occur in or around any aspect of the knee. Careful localization of the pain and tenderness will significantly limit the different diagnostic possibilities. Examination of patients with knee problems also includes a screening evaluation of hip joint rotation because patients with intrinsic hip problems might present with distal thigh pain and other symptoms that mimic knee disorders.

Radiographic examination of the knee should include AP and lateral radiographs. When the patient is able to stand, obtain weight-bearing AP radiographs of both knees so that the injured knee can be compared with the opposite, uninjured knee. When symptoms are localized to the patellofemoral joint, a patellofemoral view is helpful. All radiographs should be evaluated for changes in bony architecture, including lytic and blastic lesions.

AP radiographs are best used to evaluate medial and lateral compartment arthritis, fractures of the distal femur and proximal tibia, and alignment of the femur to the tibia. A lateral radiograph is helpful in assessing the patella for fractures and malposition and in analyzing the bony architecture of the distal femur and proximal tibia. Axial patellofemoral views are best used to assess subluxation of the patella and arthritis of the patellofemoral joint.

MRI rarely is needed in the initial diagnostic work-up but might play an important role in surgical planning.

## ACUTE PAIN

Possible diagnoses fall into six basic categories, any of which can be painful: 1) fractures, 2) meniscal injuries, 3) ligamentous injuries, 4) musculotendinous strains, 5) extensor mechanism injuries, and 6) contusions.

Fractures can involve the distal femur, patella, proximal tibia, and fibula. Inspect for swelling and deformity, palpate for tenderness in the bone itself, and obtain appropriate radiographs. Patellar fractures can result from indirect forces, such as falls, but fractures of the tibia and femur at the knee usually result from major trauma. Patellar dislocations are often reduced at the scene when a helper extends the knee for transportation.

Obtaining a history of the mechanism of injury is key in diagnosing meniscal tears. A history of a twisting injury sustained with the foot planted on the ground and locking (inability to extend the knee completely) with localized pain and tenderness along the joint line are indicative of meniscal pathology. Some patients report that manipulating or pushing on the knee enabled them to "unlock it."

Patients with ligamentous injuries have acute pain, swelling, and instability. Strains of various musculotendinous structures around the knee also cause acute pain and swelling, but most do not result in instability. Patients with injuries to the extensor mechanism report a fall with sudden weakness or collapse. Contusions are from direct blows and cause localized pain and tenderness.

## CHRONIC PAIN

Conditions that cause chronic knee pain include arthritis, tumors, sepsis, and overuse syndromes (including bursitis/tendinitis and anterior knee pain). Arthritis is relatively easy to diagnose because symptoms localize to the joint line and are associated with loss of motion and radiographic changes.

Tumors are characterized by night pain (relentless pain in which the patient is unable to sleep) and often can be palpated or identified on radiographs. The most common malignant tumors are osteosarcoma (in adolescents) and chondrosarcoma (in adults). The most common benign tumor is giant cell tumor, which typically occurs in adults aged 20 to 30 years. Metastatic disease to the knee region is uncommon.

Sepsis in the knee joint is rare in adults; it is more commonly located in the prepatellar bursa. Inspection and palpation of the involved area easily determine the location of the infection. Although swelling, erythema, and loss of knee motion are characteristic of either condition, infection in the prepatellar bursa causes swelling over the patella. With sepsis in the knee joint, swelling occurs around (medial, lateral, and suprapatellar regions) but not over the patella.

Bursitis/tendinitis and anterior knee pain have similar characteristics: both usually are chronic, often secondary to overuse, and often bilateral. The pain typically is worse with rising or walking after sitting, at night, and with prolonged exercise or use.

## LOCATION OF PAIN

### ANTERIOR KNEE PAIN
Tenderness at the upper pole of the patella indicates a tendinitis or partial tear of the quadriceps insertion on the patella. Pain localized to the superior lateral portion of the patella suggests a bipartite patella. Tendinitis or overuse injury of the patellar tendon (also called the patellar ligament) produces pain at the inferior pole of the patella or at the tibial tubercle.

### MEDIAL KNEE PAIN
Pain at the medial joint line, midway between the front and back of the knee, is common with a torn meniscus, especially with degenerative tears that occur

as the result of minor trauma such as twisting or rising from a squat. When the meniscal tear is sufficiently large or loose, patients also might report catching or locking. Tenderness in this area also is common with arthritis that affects the medial compartment of the knee. Pain proximal to and/or at the medial joint line, with localized swelling and a history of recent injury, usually indicates a sprain or tear of the medial collateral ligament either at its origin from the medial femoral epicondyle or in the midsubstance of the ligament.

Distal to the medial joint line lies the insertion of the pes anserinus tendons (composed of the sartorius, gracillus, and semitendinosus tendons, and so named because they resemble the foot of a goose) and the superficial portion of the medial collateral ligament. Pain in this area, in the absence of trauma, suggests a bursitis under the pes anserine tendons. This condition often is associated with osteoarthritis of the medial knee joint.

## LATERAL KNEE PAIN

Pain over the lateral femoral condyle suggests an iliotibial band friction syndrome, usually associated with overuse or erratic exercise habits. Pain over the lateral joint line usually indicates a disorder of the lateral meniscus or osteoarthritis of the lateral joint (more common in women or obese patients).

## POSTERIOR KNEE PAIN

Pain at the posteromedial corner of the knee can indicate a tear of the medial meniscus (at the joint line), a Baker (popliteal) cyst, or both. Popliteal aneurysms also can be painful in the popliteal area. Patients with knee effusions may perceive popliteal pain from the distention of the joint capsule.

# INSTABILITY

The knee joint is actually two joints: one between the tibia and the femur (tibiofemoral joint) and one between the patella and the femur (patellofemoral joint). True instability means one bony component moves on another in an abnormal fashion, such as the patella sliding laterally on the femur in recurrent subluxation of the patella, or the tibia moving anteriorly on the femur in the anterior cruciate–deficient knee. Patients typically use the terms "giving way," "slippage," or "buckling," which can refer to true instability or to collapse of the knee (often secondary to pain or muscle weakness in the axis of the quadriceps mechanism).

## TIBIOFEMORAL INSTABILITY

Differentiating instability caused by specific ligament injury can be difficult in a painful, traumatized knee because of muscle guarding. During examination, four ligament complexes should be gently assessed with the patient as relaxed as possible: 1) anterior cruciate ligament, 2) posterior cruciate ligament, 3) medial collateral ligament, and 4) lateral collateral ligament. Although several different tests can evaluate specific ligament integrity, the following are the most specific and reliable:

- Lachman test for the anterior cruciate ligament;

- Posterior drawer test and thumb sign for the posterior cruciate ligament;

- Varus and valgus stress testing for the medial and lateral collateral ligaments.

Complete descriptions and illustrations of these tests are included in the Physical Examination portion of this section. Varus and valgus stress testing should be performed in full extension to assess the cruciate ligaments (which support the collateral ligaments in full extension) and the more posterior structures and in slight flexion (25°) to specifically evaluate the medial and lateral collateral ligaments. Any increased recurvatum (back knee) compared with the opposite knee suggests injury to the posterior structures, as well.

Chronic instability of the knee also occurs with severe arthritis because, with the loss of articular cartilage and bone height from the arthritis (relative laxity), the ligaments are not at full tension.

### PATELLOFEMORAL INSTABILITY

Instability in the extensor mechanism is usually caused by a lateral dislocation or subluxation of the patella. The diagnosis is made by palpation. When the patella remains dislocated, the patient's knee often will be locked in approximately 45° of flexion with an obvious deformity present. Following an acute subluxation or dislocation that has spontaneously reduced, the patient usually exhibits dramatic apprehension when an attempt is made to displace the patella laterally.

## STIFFNESS

Stiffness of the knee is the most common complaint that accompanies an effusion. The distention of the knee cavity prevents full flexion, and the patient feels that the knee is "stiff" but might not notice that it is also swollen.

Arthritis is the other common cause of stiffness. Patients with arthritis often report that the knee sticks or locks momentarily as they walk. This occurs because the articular surfaces are rough and incongruous and act like two pieces of sandpaper rubbing together.

Stiffness also can result from any inflammatory condition at the knee, including arthritis, overuse syndromes, and traumatic effusion.

## SWELLING

When patients report swelling, they are most often talking about soft-tissue puffiness in the infrapatellar bursa. This bursa is located behind and to either side of the patellar tendon (infrapatellar tendon). Think of this structure as the knee's thermometer: it swells with a variety of knee disorders and is obvious to patients because it feels tense when they kneel, is prominent when they rub their knees, and is obvious when they look at their knees in the mirror.

With an intra-articular effusion, distention occurs around and above the patella in the knee cavity. Patients often notice this as stiffness; they cannot fully flex the knee because the knee cavity is filled with synovial fluid or blood and therefore cannot be compressed.

## LOCKING

True locking occurs when a torn meniscus prevents the knee from extending fully. The knee can flex from the stuck position (although the range of flexion also is typically limited). Patients also note that the knee is stiff after prolonged sitting, with the stiffness gradually loosening when they start moving. Often patients are able to "unlock" their knee by forcefully flexing or extending or by some other maneuver they have learned works for them.

Pseudolocking occurs with arthritis, when the adjacent rough surfaces stick momentarily as they glide onto one another. It also can occur with minor knee conditions such as a medial synovial plica, when the synovial tissue becomes momentarily stuck under the patella as the knee extends.

## WEAKNESS

Weakness of the muscles around the knee can occur acutely or gradually. Acute catastrophic weakness usually occurs as a result of disruption of the extensor mechanism in one of three locations: 1) a tear of the patellar tendon below the patella, 2) a tear of the quadriceps tendon above the patella, or 3) a fracture through the patella. With partial ruptures, the extensor mechanism might continue to function, but without proper protection, the tear could become complete.

# PHYSICAL EXAMINATION
# KNEE AND LOWER LEG

## Inspection/Palpation

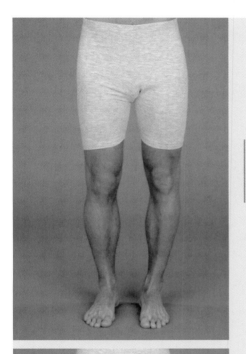

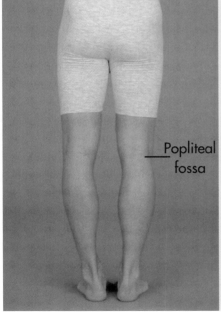

Popliteal fossa

### Anterior view

With the patient standing, look for valgus (knock-knee) or varus (bowleg) deformities, asymmetry of alignment, and thigh atrophy. Internal femoral torsion will rotate the knees so that the patellae point inward when the feet are straight ahead.

### Posterior view

With the patient standing, look for atrophy of the thigh and calf muscles. Swelling in the popliteal fossa suggests a Baker cyst that will be better delineated by palpation with the patient supine and the muscles relaxed.

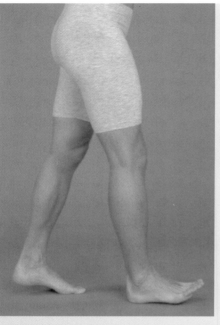

### Gait

Watch the patient walk. With arthritic knee conditions, the patient will limit motion and shorten the duration of the stance phase on the affected side.

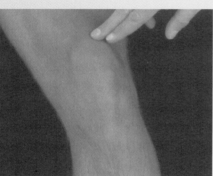

### Patellar tracking

Palpate the patella as the patient flexes and extends the knee. Crepitus is noted with patellofemoral arthritis; however, the degree of crepitus does not correlate with the severity of the arthritis.

Watch movement of the patella while the patient flexes and extends the knee. As the knee moves from extension to flexion, the patella normally moves in a gentle arc from a relatively lateral position when the knee is extended, to a more medial position during early flexion, and then back to a relatively lateral position as flexion continues. With patellar instability, this arc of movement is increased and may make an inverted "J- shaped" motion as the patella moves proximally.

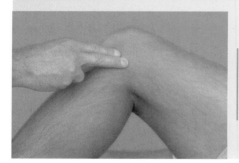

### Joint line tenderness

Flex the patient's knee and identify the joint line (soft spot between the femur and tibia). Tenderness is associated with a torn meniscus. Feel along the joint margin on both the medial and lateral sides of the knee. (Only lateral is shown here.) An area of increased tenderness supports the diagnosis of a torn meniscus.

# Inspection/Palpation

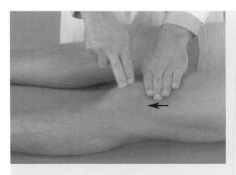

## Knee effusion

Inspect the suprapatellar region. A large knee effusion will be readily visible in this region. Subtle knee effusions can be demonstrated by "milking down" joint fluid from the suprapatellar pouch. Hold the fluid wave in place with one hand and ballott the patella. Excessive fluid will create a spongy feeling as the patella is pushed down.

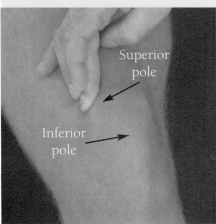

Superior pole

Inferior pole

## Patella

Palpate the superior and inferior poles of the patella. Quadriceps tendinitis or rupture causes tenderness at the superior pole, while patellar tendinitis (jumper's knee) or rupture creates tenderness at the inferior pole. Displace the patella laterally to palpate the lateral facet on the undersurface of the patella. Reverse the displacement to assess the medial facet.

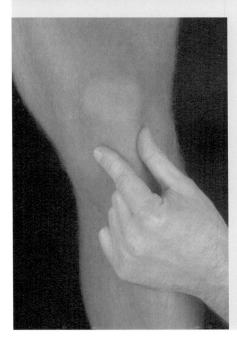

## Infrapatellar bursa

Palpate below the patella, on either side of the patellar tendon, for swelling. Often this condition is visible with a dumbbell-like swelling on either side of the tendon. The asymmetry is easily seen with the patient seated or standing.

# Range of Motion

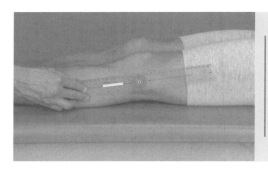

### Flexion–extension: Zero Starting Position

Knee motion is primarily flexion and extension. Knee extension (sometimes called hyperextension) is more often seen in young children. It is normal for adults to have a slight 5° flexion contracture. In adults, knee flexion normally ranges from 135° to 145°.

Measure flexion using the Zero Starting Position, with the knee straight. Extension or hyperextension is motion opposite to flexion at the Zero Starting Position.

# Muscle Testing

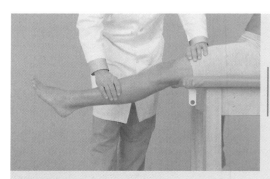

### Quadriceps

With the patient seated, ask him or her to extend the knee as you resist the effort by pushing against the tibia after the knee is in full extension.

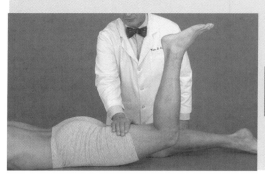

### Hamstrings

With the patient prone, place the knee in approximately 90° of flexion and ask the patient to extend the hip as you resist the effort with your opposite hand by pushing against the thigh.

# Special Tests

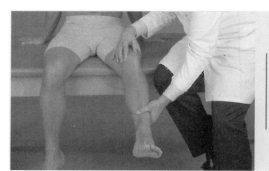

### Patellar instability—Apprehension sign

With the patient seated and the quadriceps relaxed, place the knee in extension. Displace the patella laterally and then flex the knee to 30°. With instability, this maneuver displaces the patella to an abnormal position on the lateral femoral condyle. The patient often perceives pain and becomes apprehensive.

# Special Tests

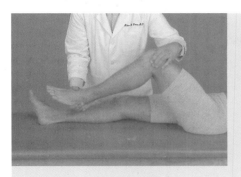

### Meniscal tear—McMurray circumduction test

Flex the knee to the maximum pain-free position. Hold that position while externally rotating the foot, and then gradually extend the knee while maintaining the tibia in external rotation. This maneuver stresses the medial meniscus and often elicits a localized medial compartment click and/or pain in patients with a posterior horn tear. The same maneuver performed while rotating the foot internally will stress the lateral mensicus. Pain-free flexion beyond 90° is necessary for this test to be useful.

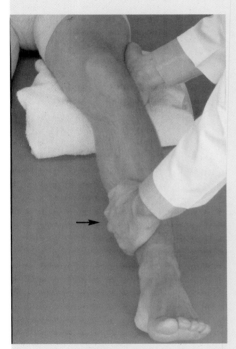

### Medial collateral ligament—Valgus stress test

Assess medial collateral ligament (MCL) stability with the thigh supported to relax the quadriceps muscle. Apply stress initially with the knee extended and then flexed to 25°. With the thigh supported and the knee extended, place one hand on the lateral side of the knee, grasp the medial distal tibia with the other hand, and abduct the knee. If the knee opens up in a valgus direction more than the opposite knee, the patient has either a complete or partial tear of the MCL. If the knee opens up in full extension, the patient has a severe injury involving more than the MCL.

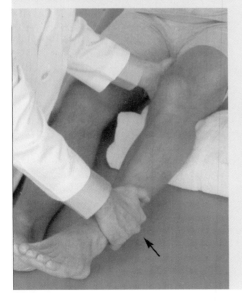

### Lateral collateral ligament—Varus stress test

Assess lateral collateral ligament (LCL) stability with the knee in extension and 25° of flexion by reversing the stress pattern used for the MCL. If the knee opens up more than the opposite knee in a varus direction, the patient has either a complete or partial tear of the LCL. If the knee opens up in full extension, the patient has a severe injury involving more than the LCL.

### Anterior cruciate ligament—Lachman test

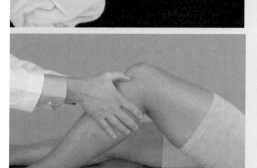

With the thigh supported and the thigh muscles relaxed, flex the knee to 25° and grasp the distal femur from the lateral side with one hand and the proximal tibia from the medial side with the other hand. Maintain the knee in neutral rotation, then initiate a "shucking" motion by pulling anteriorly on the tibia while pushing posteriorly on the femur, focusing on the amount of bony translation of the tibia relative to the femur. Increased anterior translation indicates a partial or complete tear of the anterior cruciate ligament. (*Note: To allow effective photography, the examiner's hands are placed on the medial aspect of the femur. See diagram on p 361 for correct position of the hands while performing the Lachman test.*)

### Posterior cruciate ligament—Thumb sign

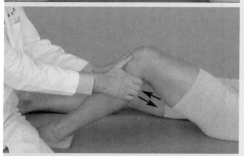

With the patient supine, flex the knee to 90° with the foot supported on the table. Normally, the anterior tibial plateaus sit 1 cm anterior to the femoral condyles, and you may place your thumbs on top on the medial and lateral tibial plateaus. If the posterior cruciate ligament (PCL) is injured, the proximal tibia falls back and the area available to place your thumbs decreases. When the tibial plateaus are flush with the femoral condyles, there is 10 mm or more of posterior laxity, consistent with a complete tear of the PCL.

### Anterior and posterior drawer test

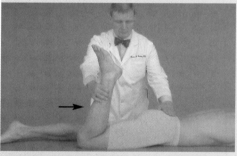

The drawer test of anterior and posterior cruciate ligament instability is easier to perform but is not as sensitive as the Lachman test or thumb sign. With the knee flexed to 90°, stabilize the leg by sitting on the patient's foot. Grasp the proximal tibia with both hands. Palpate the hamstring tendons to ensure that they are relaxed. Slide the tibia anteriorly for an anterior drawer test and posteriorly for a posterior drawer test. Compare the results with the uninjured knee, which should always be examined first.

### Prone rectus femoris test

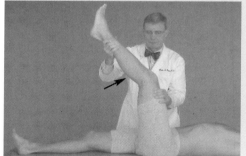

Assess tightness or contracture of the rectus femoris by placing the rectus femoris on stretch. With the patient prone, flex the knee. Limited knee flexion in this position, compared with supine flexion, indicates tightness of the rectus femoris portion of the quadriceps muscle. With severe tightness, the pelvis will elevate as the hip moves into flexion.

### Hamstring tightness—Popliteal angle

The hamstrings require special positioning to assess tightness because they also cross two joints (originate on the pelvis and insert on the tibia). To place the hamstrings on stretch, flex the hips to 90° and then extend the knee. The degree of knee flexion contracture in this position, referred to as the popliteal angle, is a measurement of hamstring tightness. The popliteal angle in children is normally 10° to 30° but is often more in adults.

# Leg Pain: Acute

## Definition

Acute leg pain usually occurs secondary to an injury. With the exception of a compartment syndrome, the different causes of acute leg pain are painful temporarily but resolve without sequelae.

### Compartment syndrome

The muscles of the leg are divided by fibrous septae into four compartments: anterior, lateral, posterior, and deep posterior (**Figure 1**). Compartment syndrome of the leg may affect one or more of the four compartments. The anterior compartment is the most frequently involved.

Compartment syndromes are characterized by an elevation of intracompartmental pressure to a degree that compromises blood flow to the involved muscles and nerves. Although acute compartment syndromes most often develop after fractures of the tibia, any condition that has the potential to cause significant swelling, such as contusions, muscle strains, or crush injuries, also can result in this limb-threatening condition.

The hallmark symptom of an acute compartment syndrome is severe leg pain that is out of proportion to what would otherwise be expected. As the condition progresses, patients also may experience paresthesias or numbness on the dorsum of the foot (with anterior or lateral compartment involvement) or on the plantar aspect (with involvement of the deep posterior compartment).

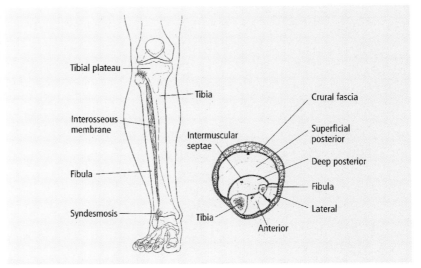

**Figure 1**
Cross-sectional view of leg showing compartmental anatomy.

*Reproduced with permission from Sullivan JA, Anderson SJ (eds): Care of the Young Athlete. Rosemont, IL, American Academy of Orthopaedic Surgeons, 1999, p 406.*

Acute compartment syndromes cause marked swelling, tenseness, and tenderness of the involved compartment. Increased pain with passive stretching of the muscles of the involved compartment is characteristic. For example, with an anterior compartment syndrome, passive stretch of the extensor hallucis longus (eg, flexing the great toe) causes marked pain. With involvement of the lateral compartment, inversion of the foot will passively stretch the peroneus longus and brevis. With a deep posterior compartment syndrome, extension of the great toe will place the flexor hallucis longus on stretch. Superficial compartment muscles are put on stretch by dorsiflexing the ankle. Decreased sensation of the involved nerves is often present at onset of the syndrome, but paralysis and loss of dorsalis pedis and posterior tibial pulses are late findings.

A clinically significant compartment syndrome is present when the diastolic pressure minus the compartment pressure is less than 30 mm Hg.

*Acute compartment syndromes are surgical emergencies.* Failure to diagnose and immediately treat a compartment syndrome can result in tissue necrosis and permanent muscle contracture, pain, weakness, and neurologic injury. Do not be misled by the presence of intact pulses or intact sensation.

## CONTUSIONS

Contusions are injuries to the leg sustained from a direct blow. Although the resulting disability usually is minor, contusions can be quite painful, with significant swelling and tenderness. Excessive swelling can result in a compartment syndrome, which therefore should be considered in the clinical evaluation.

Contusions cause swelling, tenderness, and ecchymosis of the involved muscle. Active muscle contraction and passive stretch will be painful.

Contusions are treated with minor analgesics, rest, ice, elevation, and range-of-motion, calf stretching, and strengthening exercises (bilateral heel raises, heel raises with weights, single-leg heel raises).

## MEDIAL GASTROCNEMIUS TEARS

Acute strains or ruptures of the medial head of the gastrocnemius muscle usually occur at the muscle-tendon junction. The patient typically feels a pulling or tearing sensation in the calf. Most of the pain is located proximally and medially.

This injury can result in diffuse calf pain, swelling, and tenderness. The pain is located primarily over the medial aspect of the proximal calf. The patient holds the ankle in plantar flexion to avoid placing tension on the injured muscle and typically ambulates with the ankle in a plantar flexed position. The patient is unable to perform a single-leg toe raise. Ecchymosis can develop in the calf over 24 hours.

Medial gastrocnemius strains are treated with minor analgesics, rest, ice, elevation and range-of-motion, calf stretching, and strengthening exercises.

## RUPTURE OF POPLITEAL CYST

Ruptures of popliteal cysts usually occur in older patients with degenerative arthritis or rheumatoid arthritis. Fluid from the cyst can extravasate down the leg and over 24 hours cause diffuse calf pain and swelling. The condition can closely mimic a deep vein thrombosis.

The patient will have no history of trauma. Usually, patients have been diagnosed as having a popliteal cyst in the past, or they have noticed an uncomfortable fullness in the popliteal fossa.

Although usually not necessary, MRI can help confirm the presence of a ruptured popliteal cyst by showing both the cyst and fluid extravasation.

Ruptured popliteal cysts are treated symptomatically with minor analgesics, rest, and elevation. Long-term treatment is directed at the etiology of the popliteal cyst. Detailed information on popliteal cysts is provided on pp 397-398.

# Leg Pain: Chronic

## Definition

Chronic leg pain is defined as pain that has been present for more than 2 or 3 weeks. The etiology includes a spectrum of disorders. In addition to the unique conditions discussed in this chapter, chronic pain in the calf region also may be secondary to infection (osteomyelitis or pyomyositis), tumors (soft-tissue or bone), and other general disorders.

### Stress fracture

Stress fractures of the tibia and fibula typically follow a relatively rapid increase in exercise intensity. The pain initially occurs only in association with exercise, but with continued activity, the pain also is noted with normal walking or even at rest. Tenderness is localized to the affected area of bone, typically 4 to 6 cm in length. Six or more weeks after the onset of symptoms, swelling secondary to the bony callus may be palpable.

AP and lateral radiographs of the tibia should be obtained; however, stress fractures may not be visible on plain radiographs for 3 weeks or longer after injury. When the pain is not severe and when the patient is not involved in an occupation or athletic activity that puts him or her at risk for further injury, then radiographs can be repeated 3 to 4 weeks after initial examination. However, when immediate confirmation of the suspected diagnosis is necessary, a bone scan will show increased uptake at the location of the stress fracture (**Figure 1**). Correlating these findings with the area of pain and tenderness is important because bone scans of athletes placing repetitive stresses on their legs often show areas of increased uptake in asymptomatic locations.

In most situations, the pain of a stress fracture limits participation in competitive or recreational activities and thus prevents further injury, although a stress fracture in a patient who continues activity can become a displaced fracture. Prolonged healing time is a more likely outcome of delaying diagnosis of a painful stress fracture.

When diagnosed early, most patients with stress fractures of the tibia and fibula respond well to a period of rest. Mild pain can be treated with activity modifications. Long leg pneumatic splints or other removable fracture braces may be useful for moderate pain in the early healing process. When significant pain occurs with walking, initial treatment is cast immobilization and limited weight bearing. Low-impact exercise, such as bicycling and swimming, can be substituted to maintain cardiovascular conditioning. Return to activity depends on the severity and duration of symptoms before diagnosis, but averages about 2 months.

Patients whose symptoms do not significantly improve after 2 to 3 weeks of rest require further evaluation.

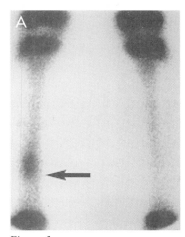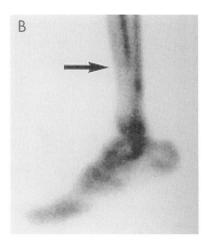

**Figure 1**
Bone scans. A, Stress fracture with focal uptake. B, Medial tibial stress syndrome with more diffuse uptake along the posteromedial shaft of the tibia.

*Reproduced with permission from Sullivan JA, Anderson SJ (eds): Care of the Young Athlete. Rosemont, IL, American Academy of Orthopaedic Surgeons, 1999, p 408.*

Menstrual cycle (frequency) and dietary habits (calcium intake) should be discussed with women.

An unusual and difficult stress injury to diagnose is a fatigue fracture of the anterior cortex of the midshaft of the tibia, referred to as the "dreaded black line." Treatment of this injury is controversial and ranges from cast immobilization with no weight bearing to intramedullary rod insertion.

## EXERTIONAL COMPARTMENT SYNDROME

Exertional compartment syndrome of the leg, sometimes called chronic compartment syndrome, is an exercise-induced pathologic increase in tissue pressure (typically greater than 40 mm Hg) in one or more of the four muscle compartments. The result is leg pain and occasionally paresthesias radiating into the foot. This syndrome is associated with prolonged walking or running activity. Symptoms gradually develop with exercise, but with cessation of the activity, the compartment tissue pressure returns to normal (less than 10 mm Hg), and symptoms gradually resolve within 30 minutes. Patients with an exertional compartment syndrome do not experience pain at rest.

The anterior compartment is most commonly involved, and patients may note weakness of the foot dorsiflexors and paresthesias in the dorsum of the first web space. Deep posterior compartment syndromes can result in paresthesias on the plantar aspect of the foot secondary to tibial nerve involvement.

Most patients have no abnormal physical findings when they are not exercising, although some will have defects of the anterior compartment fascia. In a patient who is examined during exercise, the involved compartment musculature can appear swollen and tense and may be tender to palpation.

The best way to confirm the diagnosis is to measure compartment pressures (anterior, lateral, superficial, and deep posterior) using an indwelling catheter. Patients with exertional compartment syndromes develop pressures that exceed 40 mm Hg with exercise and which remain elevated for a prolonged period after activity, taking 30 minutes or longer to return to normal.

In rare situations, a patient with a chronic exertional compartment syndrome will develop an acute compartment syndrome. Presumably, this occurs when the swelling and pressure increase to such an extent that they do not return to normal after cessation of exercise. This condition requires emergent treatment.

Nonoperative treatment of exertional compartment syndromes requires discontinuing an activity or decreasing its intensity to an asymptomatic level. Surgical treatment is fasciotomy of the involved compartment.

## SHIN-SPLINTS

Shin-splints are a poorly understood condition characterized by the gradual onset of posteromedial pain in the distal third of the leg. This condition commonly develops in response to exercise and probably represents inflammation of the periosteum secondary to repetitive muscle contraction. Examination shows tenderness along the posterior medial crest of the tibia in the middle or distal thirds of the leg. Conditions such as stress fractures and exertional compartment syndromes must be ruled out before a diagnosis of shin-splints is made.

No adverse outcomes of shin-splints are known.

## CLAUDICATION

Claudication is discomfort in the legs associated with activity that is secondary to a neurogenic or vascular etiology. Claudication can lead to paresthesias and dysesthesias. Neurogenic claudication is associated with spinal stenosis. Ischemia to the cauda equina is the underlying pathology, induced by postures that mechanically compress the nerve roots with resultant paresthesias and dysesthesias. Vascular claudication is secondary to peripheral vascular disease and compromised blood flow with walking activities. It can result in a similar type of leg pain.

Patients with neurogenic claudication experience vague pain that begins in the buttocks and spreads to the legs while walking. Walking down inclines significantly increases symptoms secondary to the associated increased lordotic posture. Symptoms typically resolve after sitting or lying down. In general, the pain of neurogenic claudication tends to progress from proximal to distal in the lower extremity, whereas the pain of vascular claudication tends to start distally and radiate proximally. Pain and paresthesias do not resolve immediately on cessation of walking in patients with neurogenic claudication. This differs from the pain associated with vascular claudication, which typically subsides when walking stops.

Patients with neurogenic claudication may have no abnormal physical findings at rest, but weakness and reflex changes can develop after activities that provoke leg pain. Patients with vascular claudication have diminished or absent pulses below the waist, along with redness and pallor changes with elevation.

AP and lateral radiographs of the spine in patients with neurogenic claudication show degenerative changes. MRI and CT can define the pathology, although neither imaging study is necessary as a primary screening tool.

Doppler studies and arteriography will demonstrate vascular disease in patients with vascular claudication.

Patients with either vascular or neurogenic claudication can experience significant compromise in quality of life because of their inability to walk. Patients with neurogenic claudication can be treated with over-the-counter analgesic medications, intermittent NSAIDs, epidural corticosteroid injections, flexion exercises for the lumbar spine, and surgical decompression. Patients with vascular claudication require evaluation by a vascular surgeon.

# ANTERIOR CRUCIATE LIGAMENT TEAR

## ICD-9 Codes
717.83
Chronic disruption of anterior cruciate ligament
844.2
Acute anterior cruciate ligament tear

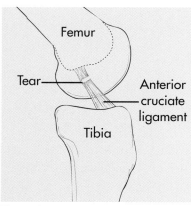

**Figure 1**
Complete ACL tear.

## SYNONYMS
Torn cruciate
Crucial ligament tear
ACL tear
Anterior cruciate insufficiency

## DEFINITION
The anterior cruciate ligament (ACL) is a primary stabilizer of the knee (**Figure 1**). A tear of the ACL results from a rotational (twisting) or hyperextension force applied to the knee joint that overcomes the strength of the ligament. Although partial tears can occur, injuries involving the ACL more often result in complete tears. About half the time, an ACL tear is accompanied by a significant meniscal tear. An ACL tear also can occur in association with a tear of the medial collateral ligament or, more rarely, with tears of the lateral ligaments or the posterior cruciate ligament. While uncommon, knee injuries that disrupt multiple ligaments also can injure the popliteal artery and result in a limb-threatening emergency.

## CLINICAL SYMPTOMS
Patients with ACL tears usually report sudden pain and giving way of the knee from a twisting or hyperextension-type injury. One third of patients report an audible pop as the ligament tears. A patient who sustains an ACL tear during athletic activity usually is unable to continue participating because of pain and/or instability. The pain increases because an effusion caused by bleeding into the joint (hemarthrosis) develops over the ensuing 24 hours.

As the swelling resolves, the patient temporarily may have no trouble moving the knee; however, if the tear is left untreated, recurrent instability develops, particularly with attempts to return to agility sports. Chronic knee instability from an untreated ACL tear can lead to further meniscal and articular cartilage damage, with resulting degenerative arthritis.

## TESTS
### PHYSICAL EXAMINATION
The most sensitive test for ACL insufficiency is the Lachman test, in which the knee is flexed to 25° and the tibia is gently pulled forward while the femur is stabilized (**Figure 2**). Because of the subcutaneous location of the medial tibia, it is easier to grasp the tibia on the medial side (right hand for right knee, left hand for left knee) while stabilizing the femur from the lateral side with the

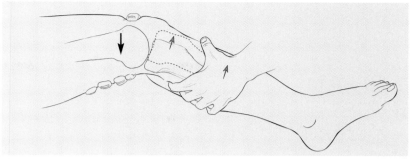

**Figure 2**
Correct position for the Lachman test. The knee is flexed approximately 25° while the examiner gently pulls the tibia forward with the medial hand while stabilizing the distal femur with the lateral hand. In a relaxed patient, increased anterior translation of the tibia with a soft end point constitutes a positive test.

opposite hand. Increased motion of the tibia with no solid end point indicates a tear of the ACL. The anterior drawer test, performed with the knee flexed 90°, is negative in 50% of acute ACL tears and so is less helpful.

## DIAGNOSTIC TESTS

Plain radiographs taken in the AP, lateral, and tunnel views are optimal for every patient with a suspected ACL tear. Usually these radiographs are positive only for an effusion and possibly an avulsion fracture of the lateral capsular margin of the tibia (lateral capsular sign or Segond fracture); however, radiographs are helpful in ruling out other pathology.

MRI, although quite sensitive at detecting ACL tears, is expensive and rarely necessary. Usually the diagnosis can reliably be made on physical examination by an experienced examiner.

## DIFFERENTIAL DIAGNOSIS

Fracture (tenderness over the bone, evident on radiographs)

Meniscal tear (continued tenderness along the joint line, pain or trapping with circumduction)

Patellar dislocation/subluxation (positive apprehension sign when displacing the patella laterally)

Patellar tendon or quadriceps rupture (inability to perform straight-leg raise)

Posterior cruciate ligament tear (posterior drawer test, abnormal thumb sign, firm end point on Lachman test)

## ADVERSE OUTCOMES OF THE DISEASE

Untreated, the recurring instability resulting from ACL instability can cause subsequent meniscal tears and degenerative disease. The instability also makes successful return to participation in agility sports unlikely.

## TREATMENT

Initial treatment of an acute ACL injury includes rest, ice, and use of crutches until the patient is able to ambulate without a limp. If the knee effusion (hemarthrosis) is tense, aspiration may be indicated to relieve symptoms (see Knee Joint Aspiration, pp 371-372). A knee immobilizer or range-of-motion brace may be used for comfort when necessary until acute pain subsides.

Early range-of-motion exercises are important. With the patient sitting, the injured knee should be actively extended and flexed as comfort allows. Exercises should be performed repeatedly for several minutes four or five times daily. Full extension and flexion should be regained as soon as pain and swelling permit.

Definitive treatment of an ACL injury depends on the patient's age, desired activity level, and any associated injuries. For young, active patients, ACL reconstruction offers the best chance for a successful return to agility sports. Older or less active individuals can be treated with physical therapy aimed at controlling the instability. ACL functional bracing, although controversial, also may be helpful with older or less active patients.

## ADVERSE OUTCOMES OF TREATMENT

Nonoperative treatment carries the risk of recurrent instability, meniscal tears, and degenerative joint disease. Scarring of the knee joint (arthrofibrosis) with loss of motion can occur after ACL injury or postoperatively after ACL reconstruction. Surgical reconstruction carries the usual risks of surgery, and the ACL can tear again. Fracture of the femur or patellar graft site also may occur after ACL reconstruction when a portion of the patellar tendon is used for the ACL graft.

## REFERRAL DECISIONS/RED FLAGS

Patients with suspected ACL tears and/or with posttraumatic knee effusions require further evaluation and treatment. Even patients who are not candidates for ACL reconstruction can benefit from regular monitoring of the ACL tear.

# ARTHRITIS OF THE KNEE

## ICD-9 Codes

274.0
  Gouty arthropathy
710.05
  Systemic lupus erythematosus
712.96
  Unspecified crystal arthropathy, lower leg
714.06
  Rheumatoid arthritis, lower leg
715.16
  Osteoarthrosis, localized, primary, lower leg
715.26
  Osteoarthrosis, localized, secondary, lower leg
716.16
  Traumatic arthropathy, lower leg

## SYNONYMS

Osteoarthritis
Degenerative joint disease
"Wear and tear" arthritis
Rheumatoid arthritis

## DEFINITION

Osteoarthritis (OA) is the most common form of knee arthritis and can involve each of the three compartments of the knee individually or in combination. The knee can be divided into the medial compartment, including the medial tibial plateau and the medial femoral condyle; the lateral compartment, including the lateral tibial plateau and lateral femoral condyle; and the patellofemoral joint, including the patella and the femoral trochlear groove. Statistically, the medial compartment of the knee is the area most frequently involved in OA, resulting in a bowleg or genu varum deformity. Knock-knees or genu valgum occurs when the lateral compartment is primarily involved with the destructive arthritic process. Isolated patellofemoral arthritis can exist; however, it is most frequently associated with concomitant tibial femoral arthritis.

Secondary knee arthropathy usually occurs in individuals with a strong history of trauma, including fractures, meniscal tears, and/or meniscectomy, or with chronic ligament insufficiencies, such as anterior cruciate ligament-deficient knees. Arthritis of the knee also may occur secondary to intra-articular fractures (posttraumatic) and inflammatory arthritides such as rheumatoid arthritis.

## CLINICAL SYMPTOMS

Statistically, OA affects patients older than age 55 years, particularly those who are obese and genetically predisposed. Insidious onset of pain is common.

As the arthritis progresses, the patient will have pain on weight bearing, regardless of the initial cause. Common complaints include buckling or giving way, which is caused by bony areas impinging upon each other. The patient will likely report a history of difficulty climbing and descending stairs. Stiffness and intermittent joint swelling can limit motion at the extremes of flexion and extension. Symptoms of locking or catching, often mimicking a meniscal tear, can result from the impingement or sticking of rough joint surfaces and reflexive dysfunction of the quadriceps muscle or the impingement of inflamed synovial tissue between the joint surfaces. With severe arthritis, pain can occur when the patient is resting or even sleeping.

## TESTS

### PHYSICAL EXAMINATION

Examination will commonly reveal an angular deformity through the knee, that is, a varus or valgus deformity, which can be confirmed by a weight-bearing examination. At times the opposite knee can be used for comparison; however, it is not uncommon for a patient to have windswept deformities (one knee valgus, one knee varus). The osteoarthritic knee often will have a mild effusion, with diffuse tenderness along the joint lines at times extending into the medial hamstring tendon insertion on the anteromedial tibia. Careful palpation may reveal thickening and osteophytes along the articular margin of the femur. Crepitus around the patellofemoral joint is often present. Loss of range of motion often parallels progression of the arthritis.

### DIAGNOSTIC TESTS

Weight-bearing AP radiographs with both knees in full extension will show narrowing of the joint space (**Figure 1**). Radiographic findings of degenerative arthritis include asymmetric joint narrowing, bone sclerosis, periarticular cysts, and osteophytes. Radiographic findings of inflammatory arthritis include symmetric joint narrowing, disuse osteopenia, and bony erosions at the articular margins. The overall condition of the patellofemoral and the tibial femoral joints can be further assessed with lateral and patellofemoral views. In addition, weight-bearing AP radiographs with the knee in approximately 40° of flexion also can help identify narrowing of the articular surface because they profile different weight-bearing areas of the tibia and femur. The intercondylar notch view or tunnel view often will reveal osteophytes, as well as demonstrate osteochondral loose bodies.

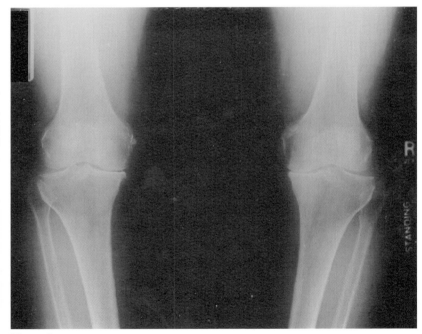

**Figure 1**
Weight-bearing AP radiograph of both knees showing substantial collapse of the medial joint space. Note the subchondral sclerosis.

## DIFFERENTIAL DIAGNOSIS

Herniated L3 or L4 disk with radiculopathy (diminished knee reflex, numbness)

Meniscal tear (history of trauma and/or locking and catching)

Osteonecrosis of the femur or tibia (over age 50, women more often than men; history of steroid use, blood dyscrasia)

Pigmented villonodular synovitis (unexplained recurring hemarthrosis)

Primary hip pathology (dermatomal referred pain to the knee, limited range of hip motion)

Septic arthritis (fever, malaise, abnormal joint fluid)

Tendinitis/bursitis (tenderness directly over a tendon or bursa)

## ADVERSE OUTCOMES OF THE DISEASE

Chronic pain may ensue, with substantial loss of knee function. Weight-bearing activity and walking can produce significant discomfort. The overall physical condition of the patient declines because a high level of activity cannot be maintained. Weight gain also often occurs.

## TREATMENT

Nonoperative management includes NSAIDs and perhaps the use of intra-articular injections (corticosteroids or viscosupplementation). Concomitant use of acetaminophen is often helpful. Modality treatments including ice, heat, and liniments also may temporarily relieve stiffness and aching. Mechanical aids such as neoprene sleeves and elastic bandages can help control swelling that occurs with activity. Maintenance of muscle tone can be assisted by the use of gravity-eliminating exercises such as water aerobics and recumbent cycles. Progressive resistive exercises (weight training) in pain-free arcs of motion can help diminish muscle atrophy and improve muscle endurance. Use of a cane or single crutch in the hand opposite the painful limb (so that the limb can be protected when it is in heel-strike phase) can help decrease pain while ambulating. A patient with poor balance or a history of falling should use an ambulatory assistive device, such as a walker. Severe functional limitations and pain at rest or at night indicate the failure of nonoperative management and the need for surgical treatment.

## ADVERSE OUTCOMES OF TREATMENT

Gastrointestinal or hepatic complications can result from chronic use of NSAIDs, as well as concomitant fluid retention and diminished renal function, which can lead to edema and hypertension. Repeated intra-articular injections of corticosteroids typically will provide only temporary relief and can result in iatrogenic sepsis and/or accelerated destruction of cartilage.

## REFERRAL DECISIONS/RED FLAGS

Any patient with pain at rest, decreased range of motion, or significant functional limitations requires further evaluation.

# BIPARTITE PATELLA

ICD-9 Codes

732.4
Juvenile osteochondrosis of lower extremity, excluding foot
755.64
Congenital deformity of knee joint
822.0
Fracture of patella

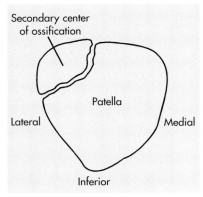

**Figure 1**
The most common location of bipartite patella.

## DEFINITION

A bipartite (or occasionally tripartite) patella results when one or more secondary centers of ossification of the patella fail to fuse (**Figure 1**). Most commonly the superolateral pole does not unite; sometimes the lateral and occasionally the inferior pole of the patella fails to unite. Thick fibrous tissue joins the unfused ossification center to the remainder of the patella. Although a bipartite patella usually is asymptomatic and an incidental radiographic finding, it can become symptomatic, causing anterior knee pain.

## CLINICAL SYMPTOMS

Symptoms can follow direct or indirect trauma to the knee or can develop in the absence of trauma as the gradual onset of anterior knee pain. Symptoms most often develop with some stretching or tearing of the fibrous union. Patients report increased discomfort with activities that increase stress or force of the quadriceps muscle on the patella (eg, using stairs, playing sports–especially those involving jumping) or when squatting or rising to a standing position.

## TESTS

### PHYSICAL EXAMINATION

Examination may reveal a prominence over the superolateral pole of the patella. When symptomatic, the area over the unfused fragment will be tender.

### DIAGNOSTIC TESTS

The unfused ossification center is best seen on AP and axial views. The fragments have rounded edges, and the orientation of the lucency dividing the fragments from the major patellar fragment is usually oblique.

## DIFFERENTIAL DIAGNOSIS

Asymptomatic bipartite patella (lack of tenderness over fragment)

Patellar fracture (sharp radiographic appearance of the fragment edges, knee effusion from bleeding into the joint)

Patellofemoral pain (lack of tenderness over the anterior surface of patella)

## ADVERSE OUTCOMES OF THE DISEASE

Continued pain and limited function are possible.

# TREATMENT

The goal of nonoperative treatment of a symptomatic bipartite patella is decreasing the stress across the fibrous union to allow renewed maturation and strength of this tissue. Most patients with a symptomatic bipartite patella will respond to a period of activity modifications. This may require a period of protected weight bearing with crutches and a knee immobilizer. The immobilizer is removed several times a day for range-of-motion exercises. With the patient sitting, the injured knee should be actively extended and flexed through the range of motion that comfort allows.

Surgery to excise the superolateral fragment is rarely necessary because most patients respond to nonoperative treatment.

## ADVERSE OUTCOMES OF TREATMENT

Persistent pain may occur with nonoperative treatment. Postoperative infection and continued pain can occur with surgical management.

## REFERRAL DECISIONS/RED FLAGS

Confirmation of diagnosis or the failure of nonoperative treatment are indications for further evaluation.

# BURSITIS OF THE KNEE

## ICD-9 Codes
726.60
    Enthesopathy of knee, unspecified
726.61
    Pes anserinus tendinitis or bursitis
726.65
    Prepatellar bursitis

## SYNONYMS
Prepatellar bursitis
Pes anserine bursitis
Iliotibial band syndrome

## DEFINITION
Bursae lie between the skin and bony prominences or between tendons, ligaments, and bone. They are lined by synovial tissue, which produces a small amount of fluid to decrease friction between adjacent structures. Chronic pressure or friction (overuse) causes thickening of this synovial lining and subsequent excessive fluid formation, thereby leading to localized swelling and pain.

The prepatellar bursa on the anterior aspect of the knee is superficial and lies between the skin and the bony patella. When this bursa becomes inflamed and filled with fluid, it forms a domed-shaped swelling over the anterior aspect of the knee. The condition often develops secondary to chronic kneeling (housemaid's knee). Persons who work at installing carpets or tile floors also are susceptible.

The pes anserinus bursa lies under the insertion site of the sartorius, gracilis, and semitendinosus muscles on the medial flare of the tibia just below the tibial plateau. The bursa may become inflamed with overuse, but more commonly, pes anserine bursitis occurs in patients with early osteoarthritis in the medial compartment of the knee. Pes anserine bursitis also can be confused with medial meniscal pathology because the bursitis pain is located along the anteromedial aspect of the proximal tibia (**Figure 1**).

The iliotibial band crosses the lateral aspect of the knee and may become irritated with repetitive movement over the lateral femoral condyle as the knee is flexed and extended (**Figure 2**). Long-distance runners are particularly susceptible.

## CLINICAL SYMPTOMS
At first, pain will be present only with activity or direct pressure. The pain often is more severe after the patient has been sedentary for some time, and patients will notice a limp when first arising from a chair. Patients also note localized swelling over the involved structure. This is most marked with prepatellar bursitis.

## TESTS
### PHYSICAL EXAMINATION
Inspect the knee for areas of swelling, and palpate structures for localized ten-

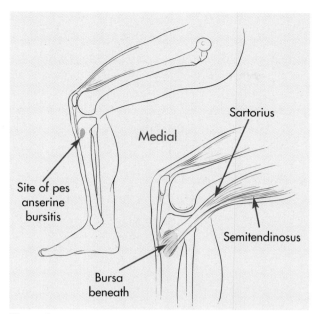

**Figure 1**
Region of pes anserine tenderness–medial view.

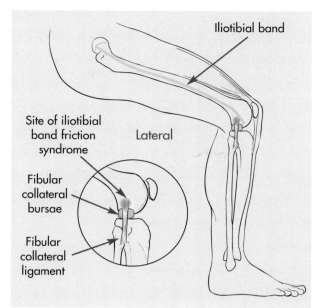

**Figure 2**
Region of iliotibial band bursitis–lateral view.

derness. Compression of the saphenous nerve and its infrapatellar branch by swelling of the pes anserinus bursa may cause numbness below the patella. Measure range of knee motion and then watch the patient walk. An antalgic gait suggests osteoarthritis of the knee. An abnormal thrust at the knee or ankle can cause irritation of the iliotibial band.

## DIAGNOSTIC TESTS

AP and lateral radiographs should be obtained in patients with chronic pain to rule out bony conditions.

## DIFFERENTIAL DIAGNOSIS

Inflammatory arthritis (polyarticular, abnormal laboratory studies)

Medial meniscal tear (catching, locking, and effusions)

Osteoarthritis of the knee (intra-articular effusion, osteophytes)

Patellar fracture (trauma, intra-articular hemarthrosis)

Patellar tendinitis (jumper's knee) (tenderness at the inferior pole of the patella)

Saphenous nerve entrapment (numbness over the medial shin, dysesthesia)

Septic knee (flexion contracture, pain with knee motion, intra-articular swelling)

Tumor (pain, mass)

## ADVERSE OUTCOMES OF THE DISEASE

Chronic bursitis leads to continued pain and antalgic gait. Pressure from continued swelling can cause weakening of overlying ligaments and/or tendons that can lead to partial tearing and spontaneous rupture.

## TREATMENT

Most patients respond to nonoperative treatment, including a short-term course of NSAIDs, ice, and activity modifications. Therapeutic modalities such as ultrasound and phonophoresis may help. Patients with identifiable tightness should perform quadriceps, hamstring, or iliotibial band stretching/flexibility exercises to assist recovery. Injection of a corticosteroid preparation is appropriate in recalcitrant cases. Surgical treatment for bursitis of the knee is the exception rather than the rule.

## ADVERSE OUTCOMES OF TREATMENT

NSAIDs can lead to concomitant gastric, renal, or hepatic complications. Infection from corticosteroid injection is possible. Tendon or ligament weakening as a result of corticosteroid injection theoretically could lead to spontaneous rupture.

## REFERRAL DECISIONS/RED FLAGS

Any patient who does not respond to nonoperative treatment or who has signs of ligament or tendon insufficiency requires further evaluation. The associated osteoarthritis in recurrent pes anserine bursitis requires evaluation.

# PROCEDURE

## KNEE JOINT ASPIRATION/INJECTION

### MATERIALS

Sterile gloves

Bactericidal skin preparation solution

25-gauge needle

30-mL or 60-mL syringe with an 18-gauge, 1½" needle

5 mL of a local anesthetic

Corticosteroid or viscosupplement preparation (optional)

Adhesive dressing

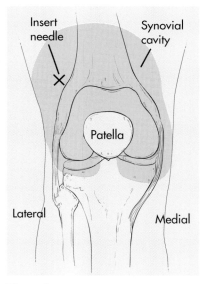

**Figure 1**
Location for needle insertion.

Aspiration of the knee joint can serve both diagnostic and therapeutic purposes. Traumatic injuries such as single- or multiple-ligament injuries, chondral or osteochondral injuries, or other fractures can produce large effusions around the knee. Pain can be relieved by draining a tense hemarthrosis. Aspiration also can help identify the etiology of an effusion. Gram stain, culture, and crystal analysis helps differentiate infectious from inflammatory processes. With an injury, place bloody aspirates in a small cup. Fat droplets from the bone marrow will accumulate on the surface if an intra-articular fracture (distal femur, patella, or tibial plateau) is present.

Injection into the knee joint is the method commonly used to administer corticosteroids or other medications to an inflamed joint. Patients with an arthritic condition of the knee can obtain improvement of symptoms for significant periods with the appropriate administration of a corticosteroid or viscosupplement preparation (hyaluronic acid).

### STEP 1

Wear protective gloves at all times during this procedure and use sterile technique.

### STEP 2

Have the patient lie supine on the examining table with the abdominal and lower extremity muscles as relaxed as possible.

### STEP 3

Mentally or with a marking pen, outline the landmarks for entry into the joint. Understand that the knee joint will extend almost one handwidth above the superior aspect of the patella, especially when a joint effusion is present. Typical entry will occur from the lateral aspect of the knee either at the level of the proximal third of the patella or just superior to the patella (**Figure 1**).

### STEP 4

Prepare the skin with a bactericidal solution.

### STEP 5

Use the 25-gauge needle to infiltrate the skin with 3 to 5 mL of local anesthetic at the point of entry.

# Knee Joint Aspiration/Injection (continued)

## Step 6

Using an 18-gauge, 1½" needle attached to a 30-mL or 60-mL syringe, enter the knee joint at the anesthetized site. Penetration of the joint capsule will be felt as a give or "pop." Withdraw the plunger of the syringe to aspirate the fluid; in a large effusion, the flow should be easy. If establishing flow is difficult, a slight change in the needle's path can be made; the needle might be within a fat pad or thick synovium. Manual pressure can be applied to the suprapatellar region to milk more fluid out of the knee. As fluid is withdrawn, the needle may become blocked with synovium; again, a slight change in direction, with the application of forward pressure to the plunger, will usually free the needle tip and allow flow to continue.

## Step 7

Once the aspiration is complete, inject medication or local anesthetic into the joint if indicated. The aspirating syringe can be removed from the needle while maintaining the needle within the knee, and a syringe with the solution to be injected can be attached.

## Step 8

When the aspiration and/or injection is complete, apply a sterile dressing.

## Adverse outcomes

As with any invasive procedure, extreme care should be taken to use sterile technique. Infection, although not common, can be introduced into the knee. Be sure that the needle's path to the knee joint does not pass through any area of the skin that appears to be compromised or potentially colonized.

## Aftercare/Patient instructions

When a large effusion is removed, apply a compressive wrap to minimize reaccumulation of fluid. In addition, rest and elevation of the lower extremity are recommended. Instruct the patient to notify you immediately at any sign of infection, rapid reaccumulation of fluid, or severe pain.

# COLLATERAL LIGAMENT TEAR

ICD-9 Codes
717.81
    Old disruption of lateral collateral ligament
717.82
    Old disruption of medial collateral ligament
844.0
    Acute lateral collateral ligament sprain
844.1
    Acute medial collateral ligament sprain

## DEFINITION

The shape of the knee provides limited inherent stability. Stability of the knee joint is largely dependent on its ligaments and periarticular muscles. Therefore, injuries to knee ligaments are common. Four ligaments provide primary stabilization of the knee. The medial and lateral collateral ligaments are outside the joint and stabilize the knee against valgus and varus stresses (Figure 1). The anterior and posterior cruciate ligaments are inside the joint and stabilize the knee against anterior and posterior stresses.

The mechanism of injury in a medial collateral ligament (MCL) tear (or sprain) is commonly a valgus (abduction) force without rotation, such as in a football clipping injury. The less common lateral collateral ligament (LCL) tear is the result of a pure varus (adduction) force to the knee. Variable external rotation stress frequently occurs with MCL sprains. Injuries to the collateral ligaments can occur alone or in association with a meniscal tear or an anterior or posterior cruciate ligament tear.

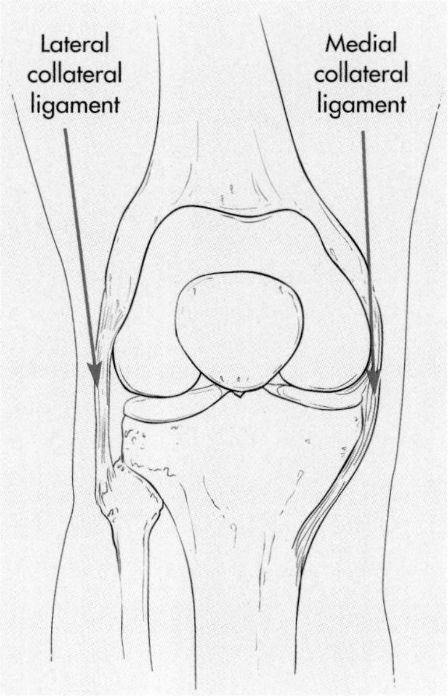

## CLINICAL SYMPTOMS

Most patients are able to ambulate after an acute injury and may be able to return to play for the remainder of the game. Patients report localized swelling or stiffness and medial or lateral pain and tenderness, but instability and mechanical symptoms, such as locking or popping, are infrequent after an isolated collateral ligament injury. Within 24 to 48 hours, localized ecchymosis and a small effusion develop.

## TESTS

### PHYSICAL EXAMINATION

The uninjured knee should be examined first to understand what is normal for the patient. This also reduces the patient's fears about examining the painful limb. Patients often have swelling in and around the injured ligament, but the presence of a significant knee effusion might indicate an associated intra-articular injury.

The MCL may be tender along its entire course, from the medial femoral condyle to its tibial insertion. Isolated tenderness at the most proximal or distal extent of the MCL can signify an avulsion-type injury. The LCL may be tender anywhere along its course, from the lateral femoral epicondyle to its insertion on the fibular head. The MCL is best palpated in slight flexion, but the LCL is best examined in the "figure 4" position.

Apply a varus and then a valgus stress with the knee first in full extension and then at 25° of flexion (to relax the cruciate ligaments and posterior capsule). (See Physical Examination—Knee and Lower Leg). Laxity in full exten-

**Figure 1**
Medial and lateral knee structures.

sion indicates a more extensive injury (to the anterior and posterior cruciate ligaments plus posterior capsule rather than to just the MCL or LCL). These injuries are knee dislocations with spontaneous reduction in which there may be a major neurovascular injury.

Increased joint space opening of less than 5 mm compared with the normal knee is considered a grade I (interstitial) tear, whereas increased opening of more than 10 mm is considered a grade III (complete) tear. A grade II (partial) tear falls between these extremes. The degree of instability may be masked in a patient with significant pain and involuntary muscle contraction. Be aware of the possibility of a false-negative examination for laxity because of muscle guarding.

### DIAGNOSTIC TESTS

AP and lateral radiographs, although usually negative, may reveal an avulsion from the femoral origin of the MCL or the fibular insertion of the LCL.

## DIFFERENTIAL DIAGNOSIS

Anterior cruciate ligament tear (moderate to marked knee effusion, positive Lachman test)

Epiphyseal fracture of the distal femur (tenderness at epiphyseal plate, evident on radiographs)

Meniscal tear (mild to moderate knee effusion, joint line tenderness)

Osteochondral fracture (radiographic evidence of loose osteochondral fragment)

Patellar subluxation or dislocation with spontaneous reduction (positive apprehension sign)

Posterior cruciate ligament tear (positive posterior drawer test or thumb sign)

Tibial plateau fracture (bony tenderness and radiographic evidence of fracture)

## ADVERSE OUTCOME OF THE DISEASE

Although instability of the knee is rare, it can occur in association with disruption of the anterior and/or posterior lateral ligament. Lateral instability can occur after isolated LCL tears in patients with varus alignment.

## TREATMENT

Treatment of isolated MCL tears, even when complete, usually is nonoperative. Grade I sprains with no effusion likely will resolve within a couple of weeks. Rest, ice, compression, and elevation (RICE), coupled with crutches and a short-term course of NSAIDs, usually are adequate. With grade II sprains, use of a hinged brace and weight bearing as tolerated are appropriate. For grade III injuries, use of a hinged brace with gradual return to full weight bearing over the course of 4 to 6 weeks is indicated. Rehabilitation includes early range-of-motion exercises (including bicycling) and quadriceps and hamstring progressive resistance exercises. Grade III injuries frequently require 3 to 4 months of protective bracing before the patient can return to unrestricted activity.

Although grade I and II LCL tears also should be treated nonoperatively, grade III LCL tears invariably involve a tear of the posterolateral capsular complex and are best treated surgically to avoid late instability, especially in varus knees.

## ADVERSE OUTCOMES OF TREATMENT

Frank instability is very uncommon after an isolated collateral ligament injury, but chronic pain and recurrence are possible. Patients are vulnerable to recurrence for 6 months; therefore, bracing for high-risk activities (contact sports) is recommended. Missed associated diagnoses, such as of meniscal and anterior cruciate ligament tears, can complicate the course of nonoperative treatment, and patients may ultimately require surgical intervention.

## REFERRAL DECISIONS/RED FLAGS

Patients with hemarthrosis, significant joint effusion, or instability need further evaluation. Failure to respond to nonoperative treatment could mean a missed diagnosis, such as an associated cruciate or posterior capsule rupture or meniscal tear.

# FRACTURES ABOUT THE KNEE

ICD-9 Codes

821.2
　Fracture of other and unspecified parts of femur, lower end, closed
823.0
　Fracture of tibia and fibula, upper end, closed

## DEFINITION

Distal femur fractures can be classified as supracondylar, condylar involving the medial or lateral femoral condyle, or combinations of these injuries (Figure 1). They account for 4% to 7% of all femur fractures. Fractures of the proximal tibial metaphysis are called tibial plateau fractures (Figure 2).

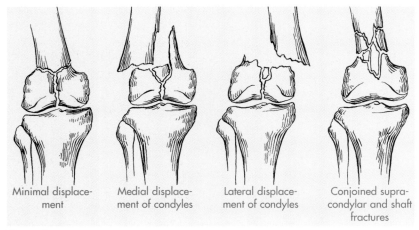

Minimal displacement　　Medial displacement of condyles　　Lateral displacement of condyles　　Conjoined supracondylar and shaft fractures

**Figure 1**
Supra- and intercondylar fracture patterns of the distal femur.

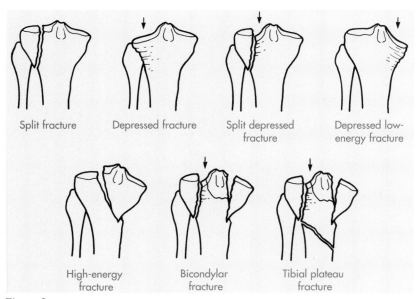

Split fracture　　Depressed fracture　　Split depressed fracture　　Depressed low-energy fracture

High-energy fracture　　Bicondylar fracture　　Tibial plateau fracture

**Figure 2**
Tibial plateau fracture patterns.

*Adapted with permission from Perry CR: Fractures of the tibial plateau, in Schafer M (ed): Instructional Course Lectures 43. Rosemont, IL, American Academy of Orthopaedic Surgeons, 1994, pp 119–126.*

In young patients, these fractures usually occur as a result of high-energy trauma and are often associated with other injuries. In elderly patients with osteoporosis, these fractures occur as a result of a low-energy force. Tibial plateau fractures often result from a valgus force (lateral plateau fracture) or varus force (medial plateau fracture).

Many of these fractures are intra-articular, ie the fracture extends into the joint.

## CLINICAL SYMPTOMS

Patients report an injury with immediate onset of pain and swelling.

## TESTS

### PHYSICAL EXAMINATION

Swelling of the knee is often marked because bleeding from intra-articular fractures extends into the joint. Inspect for skin integrity. Assess function of deep peroneal, superficial peroneal, and posterior tibial nerves, as well as distal pulses. Inspect for other injuries, particularly in the patient who has sustained high-energy trauma.

### DIAGNOSTIC TESTS

Initial radiographic examination should include AP and lateral views of the knee. Oblique radiographs and CT tomograms may be necessary for preoperative planning. When distal pulses are absent, Doppler examination also is useful.

## DIFFERENTIAL DIAGNOSIS

Cruciate ligament disruption (no fracture on radiographs)

Knee dislocation (evident on radiographs)

Quadriceps rupture (no fracture on radiographs, inability to extend the knee against gravity)

Thigh contusion and/or compartment syndrome (negative radiographs, compartment pressure measurements if in question)

## ADVERSE OUTCOMES OF THE DISEASE

Nonunion, or malunion of the fracture is possible, with resultant loss of function and the need for surgical salvage procedures. The instability of an unrecognized fracture also can cause neurovascular injury or skin breakdown. Uncorrected intra-articular step-off (articular surface displacement) can lead to arthritic changes.

## TREATMENT

For patients with tense, painful knee effusions, consider arthrocentesis for pain relief (see Knee Joint Aspiration pp 371-372). Nonoperative treatment is often indicated for nondisplaced or minimally displaced fractures. Displaced fractures usually require open reduction and internal fixation. With intra-articular fractures, the goal of surgical treatment is restoration of joint alignment and congruity. Emergent treatment is required for open fractures, vascular injuries requiring repair, and compartment syndrome.

## ADVERSE OUTCOMES OF TREATMENT

Complications of treatment include stiffness of the knee, nonunion, failure of fixation, malunion, infection, and injury to neurovascular structures.

## REFERRAL DECISIONS/RED FLAGS

These injuries typically require further evaluation. Even nondisplaced fractures in this region are at increased risk for displacement.

# MENISCAL TEAR

### ICD-9 Codes

**717.3**
Old tear of medial meniscus, unspecified

**717.40**
Old tear of lateral meniscus, unspecified

**717.9**
Unspecified internal derangement of knee

**836.0**
Acute tear of medial meniscus of knee

**836.1**
Acute tear of lateral meniscus of knee

## SYNONYMS

Torn cartilage

Locked knee

## DEFINITION

The medial and lateral menisci are fibrocartilaginous pads that function as shock absorbers between the femoral condyles and tibial plateaus. Meniscal tears can occur alone or in association with ligament injuries such as anterior cruciate ligament tears. Meniscal tears disrupt the mechanics of the knee, leading to varying degrees of symptoms, and predisposing the knee to degenerative arthritis.

## CLINICAL SYMPTOMS

Patients with traumatic tears typically report a significant twisting injury to the knee. Older patients with a degenerative tear may have a history of minimal or no trauma, such as simply rising from a squatting position. Patients usually can ambulate after an acute injury and frequently may be able to continue to participate in athletics.

Traumatic tears are typically followed by the insidious onset of knee swelling and stiffness over 2 to 3 days. Mechanical symptoms such as locking, catching, and popping can then develop. Patients usually experience pain on the medial or lateral side of the knee, particularly with twisting or squatting activities. In some cases, large unstable fragments of meniscal tissue can become incarcerated in the knee joint, leading to a "locked knee." More frequently, motion is limited by a feeling of tightness in the knee secondary to the effusion. The mechanical symptoms and degree of pain tend to wax and wane.

## TESTS

### PHYSICAL EXAMINATION

The most common finding on physical examination is tenderness over the medial or lateral joint line. Young patients who have traumatic tears that disrupt the peripheral blood supply typically present with a large effusion or hemarthrosis. In degenerative tears or tears that involve the avascular central body of the meniscus, effusions are typically small or absent. Knee motion may be limited secondary to pain or an effusion. During provocative testing, forced flexion and circumduction (internal and external rotation of the foot) frequently elicit pain on the side of the knee with the meniscal tear. The McMurray test is positive when the flexion-circumduction maneuver is associated with a painful click.

**SECTION 6 | KNEE AND LOWER LEG**

## Diagnostic tests

AP, lateral, tunnel, and axial views are indicated for patients with a history of trauma or an effusion. For patients with chronic conditions, the AP and lateral views should be weight bearing. A weight-bearing PA view with the knees flexed 45° is sensitive for early degenerative arthritis and is recommended in older patients. MRI is highly specific and sensitive for meniscal pathology. Knee aspiration is indicated when a diagnosis of infection or crystal arthropathy is considered.

## Differential diagnosis

Anterior cruciate ligament tear (hemarthrosis, positive Lachman test)

Crystal disease (aspiration)

Loose body (fragment evident on radiographs)

Medial collateral ligament tear (pain and instability with valgus stress)

Osteoarthritis (joint space narrowing on weight-bearing radiographs)

Osteochondritis dissecans (evident on radiographs, especially medial femoral condyle)

Osteonecrosis of the femoral condyle (patient age over 50 years, pain, evident on radiographs or MRI)

Patellar subluxation or dislocation (tender medial patella, apprehension sign)

Pes anserine bursitis (tender distal to medial joint line)

Saphenous neuritis (tender to palpation along the course of the saphenous nerve)

Tibial plateau fracture (bony tenderness, evident on radiographs)

## Adverse outcomes of the disease

Recurrent episodes of locking and damage to the adjacent articular cartilage with subsequent osteoarthritis are possible, particularly with a delay in definitive treatment. With the exception of the outer rim, the blood supply to the meniscus is poor. Although small peripheral tears can heal, most tears are more central and cannot heal. Patients with recurrent stiffness, locking, or pain have a mechanically significant tear, which suggests ongoing internal damage. Failure to recognize and treat a traumatic tear can lead to progressive damage and a lost opportunity for surgical repair.

## Treatment

In the absence of mechanical symptoms and particularly when a degenerative tear is present, initial treatment should consist of rest, ice, compression, and elevation (RICE). A short course of oral analgesics, such as acetaminophen or ibuprofen, can facilitate return to normal activity. Traumatic tears in younger patients should be evaluated and treated aggressively. Sports activity should be restricted until MRI evaluation is made or symptoms resolve. Surgical debridement or repair is indicated in younger patients with significant tears and in older patients who do not respond to nonoperative treatment.

## ADVERSE OUTCOMES OF TREATMENT

NSAIDs can cause gastric, renal, or hepatic complications. Meniscal repair has a 10% to 30% failure rate, sometimes necessitating subsequent re-repair or partial meniscectomy. Persistent pain after a partial meniscectomy can occur secondary to concomitant pathology, such as osteoarthritis or saphenous neuritis. Traumatic osteoarthritis may be a late complication in the involved compartment following partial meniscectomy. Postoperative infection is rare.

## REFERRAL DECISIONS/RED FLAGS

A patient with a traumatic effusion, mechanical symptoms, or ligamentous instability requires further evaluation. Patients who do not respond to nonoperative treatment and have persistent joint line tenderness or effusions also may require further evaluation.

SECTION 6 | KNEE AND LOWER LEG

# OSTEOCHONDRITIS DISSECANS

| ICD-9 Code | |
|---|---|
| 732.7 | Osteochondritis dissecans |

## DEFINITION

Osteochondritis dissecans (OCD) is osteonecrosis of subchondral bone. This disorder most commonly occurs in the knee but also may develop in other locations such as the talus and distal humerus. The most common location in the knee is the lateral side of the medial femoral condyle (**Figure 1**), but it also can be found in other areas of the distal femur and, uncommonly, in the patella.

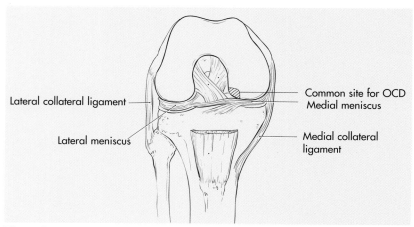

**Figure 1**
The most common location for osteochondritis dissecans of the knee.
*Adapted with permission from Mercler LR: Practical Orthopedics, ed 4. St. Louis, MO, Mosby Year Book, 1995, p 208.*

The lesion is thought to result from repetitive small stresses to the subchondral bone that disrupt the blood supply to an area of bone. The osteonecrotic bone becomes separated from surrounding viable bone by fibrous tissue. Over time, the resultant osteonecrosis weakens the involved area, and shear forces gradually fracture (dissect) the articular cartilage surface. Ultimately the osteonecrotic fragment can completely fragment and become loose bodies in the joint.

## CLINICAL SYMPTOMS

Patients usually report the gradual onset of knee pain. They also may report knee effusions and catching or locking symptoms, particularly when the overlying articular cartilage has been disrupted. Walking with the foot rotated outward may relieve the pain.

# TESTS

## PHYSICAL EXAMINATION

Examination will reveal tenderness with palpation of the involved area. The most common site on the medial femoral condyle is palpated with the knee flexed 90°. Pressure is directed over the medial femoral condyle, just medial to the inferior pole of the patella. The Wilson test may be positive and is performed with the patient supine, flexing the hip and knee 90° and internally rotating the tibia. The knee is then slowly extended. The Wilson test is positive when the patient reports pain as the knee reaches approximately 20° to 30° and when pain is relieved with external rotation of the tibia while maintaining the same flexion angle (as the tibial spine abuts and is rotated away from the OCD lesion on the medial femoral condyle).

## DIAGNOSTIC TESTS

The lesion is best seen on tunnel and lateral views, although it can also usually be seen on an AP view. MRI can help in visualizing the integrity of the overlying articular cartilage and in staging the lesion.

# DIFFERENTIAL DIAGNOSIS

Cruciate ligament injury (positive diagnostic tests, negative radiographs)

Meniscal tear (joint line tenderness, negative radiographs)

# ADVERSE OUTCOMES OF THE DISEASE

Untreated or unsuccessfully treated OCD lesions can fragment, forming loose bodies and leaving defects in the articular cartilage that can lead to degenerative joint disease.

# TREATMENT

The goal of treatment is to obtain healing of the lesion. If shear forces are minimized, new bone formation can replace the osteonecrotic bone. This process requires creeping substitution of new bone formation. Whether treated nonoperatively or by surgery, healing of OCD lesions takes 8 months or more.

Patients can be treated nonoperatively when the overlying articular cartilage is intact; however, nonoperative treatment is not likely to succeed after skeletal maturity. Nonoperative treatment includes activity modifications to the point that symptoms are relieved—specifically, avoiding running and jumping activities and possibly a period of crutch ambulation. Immobilization is reserved for refractory symptoms or noncompliant patients.

Surgical treatment is necessary after skeletal maturity and in children whose lesion has progressed to the stage that the articular cartilage has partially or totally separated. If the lesion is intact (still in place), drilling the lesion to promote vascular ingrowth and creeping substitution is performed. Unstable lesions require temporary internal fixation to promote healing. When the fragment is loose, treatment consists of removing the free fragment and debriding the articular surface defect.

## ADVERSE OUTCOMES OF TREATMENT

Unsuccessful treatment of OCD can lead to a defect in the joint surface, with progressive osteoarthritis. This may require a cartilage replacement procedure. Possible complications of surgical treatment are infection or further damage to the joint caused by the hardware or failure of the hardware.

## REFERRAL DECISIONS/RED FLAGS

Children with lesions < 1 cm in width usually do well with nonoperative treatment; however, those with lesions > 2 cm usually have progressive problems. Children with lesions between 1 and 2 cm should be treated based on symptoms and radiographic findings. After the physis has closed, the prognosis for healing is significantly less, and these patients require further evaluation.

# OSTEONECROSIS OF THE FEMORAL CONDYLE

## ICD-9 Code

733.43
   Aseptic necrosis of bone, medial
   femoral condyle

## SYNONYM

Avascular necrosis

## DEFINITION

Osteonecrosis literally means "bone death" and occurs in the femoral condyle when a segment of bone loses its blood supply. The etiology is unknown but may begin as a stress fracture and probably involves some combination of trauma and altered blood flow. A portion of the weight-bearing surface of the medial femoral condyle is most often involved. The typical patient is a woman (female-to-male ratio is 3:1) who is over 60 years of age.

Osteonecrosis of the femoral condyle may be idiopathic or may be associated with chronic steroid therapy, renal transplantation, systemic lupus erythematosus, sickle cell anemia, and Gaucher disease. Microfracture of the subchondral bone occurs along with segmental collapse. Ultimately, progression to osteoarthritis is likely.

## CLINICAL SYMPTOMS

Patients typically describe a sudden, sharp pain localized to the medial compartment. This pain probably develops when a shear force causes a subchondral fracture or disruption of the articular surface. An effusion may be present, and the patient may limit motion secondary to pain. Bilateral complaints occur in less than 20% of patients.

## TESTS

### PHYSICAL EXAMINATION

Physical examination will reveal an effusion, some loss of motion, and oftentimes a flexion contracture when the condition is unrecognized. Pain to palpation over the medial femoral condyle also is common.

### DIAGNOSTIC TESTS

Radiographically, osteonecrosis of the medial femoral condyle has been divided into stages to better define the extent of the pathology and outline appropriate care. These signs begin with flattening of the convexity of the condyle and progress through joint space narrowing, sclerosis, and osteophyte formation. The two determinants for accurate diagnosis are the area of the lesion and the percentage of involvement of the condyle. MRI or a bone scan can be helpful in making the diagnosis and determining the extent of involvement.

## DIFFERENTIAL DIAGNOSIS

Meniscal tears (evident on MRI)

Osteoarthritis (tricompartmental involvement)

Osteochondritis dissecans (location, gender and age predilection)

Pes anserine bursitis (location)

## ADVERSE OUTCOME OF THE DISEASE

Unrecognized or untreated symptomatic osteonecrosis will progress to osteoarthritis. Current treatment seeks to slow this progression.

## TREATMENT

Nonoperative management can include an unloading brace, NSAIDs, pain medication, and a conditioning program to restore quadriceps strength and endurance with modifications as necessary to avoid knee pain when exercising. Surgical intervention can include debridement and drilling, procedures to alter the weight-bearing axis and unload the medial compartment, and finally—for advanced cases—total knee replacement.

## ADVERSE OUTCOMES OF TREATMENT

Surgical complications can occur. The results of procedures that alter the weight-bearing axis are mixed: risk to neurovascular structures and overcorrection are the two main concerns. Total knee replacement provides excellent pain relief and improved function but carries the possible need for future revision.

## REFERRAL DECISIONS/RED FLAGS

Failure to improve with nonoperative treatment warrants consideration of surgical intervention. Disproportionate pain, which can indicate complex regional pain syndrome, also indicates the need for further evaluation.

# PATELLOFEMORAL INSTABILITY AND MALALIGNMENT

## ICD-9 Codes

718.36
Recurrent dislocation of joint, lower leg
836.3
Dislocation of patella, closed

## SYNONYMS

Patellar subluxation

Patellar dislocation

Miserable malalignment syndrome

## DEFINITION

Patellofemoral instability and malalignment encompass a spectrum of pathologic conditions that range from abnormal motion of the patella as it glides over the distal femur, to recurrent subluxation of the patella, and to recurrent dislocation of the patella. Patellofemoral instability usually occurs in a lateral direction (**Figure** 1). Medial patellar instability is quite rare. The term "patellofemoral malalignment" indicates that the patella is tilted laterally or predisposed to lateral subluxation, usually because of one or more anatomic factors.

Subluxation or dislocation can be caused by direct trauma or, more frequently, by an indirect mechanism of injury. A common history is that of a right-handed softball player who dislocates the right patella while swinging the baseball bat. When the right foot is planted firmly on the ground as the torso rotates to the left, the patella lags behind, resulting in a lateral dislocation.

## CLINICAL SYMPTOMS

Patients usually describe severe pain, sometimes report hearing a pop, and occasionally see a deformity of the knee. Patients frequently believe that the kneecap has dislocated medially because of the unusual prominence of the medial femoral condyle, which is no longer covered by the patella. The knee is usually maintained in a flexed position. The patella often reduces spontaneously, although sometimes a manual reduction is required.

Subluxation or dislocation of the patella causes tearing of the restraining medial retinacular tissue and the medial patellofemoral ligament, leading to pain, hemarthrosis, and loss of knee motion. Patients who have sustained one episode of instability are likely to sustain additional episodes, particularly when the medial soft tissues have healed in a "stretched out" position and when the patients have anatomic predisposing factors. Recurrent episodes of instability tend to be less traumatic than the initial episode, with patients experiencing milder symptoms.

In contrast to patients with patellar instability, the primary complaint of patients with symptomatic malalignment is retropatellar pain. This type of anterior knee pain usually is exacerbated by the use of stairs, especially

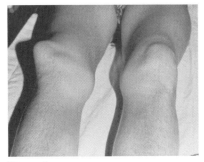

**Figure 1**
Acute lateral patellar dislocation.

*Reproduced with permission from Crosby LA, Lewallen DG (eds): Emergency Care and Transportation of the Sick and Injured, ed 6. Rosemont, IL, American Academy of Orthopaedic Surgeons, 1995, p 555.*

descending stairs. Patients also may describe pain with prolonged sitting (theater sign) or during squatting. With long-standing maltracking, progressive degenerative changes may occur, leading to patellofemoral arthrosis.

## TESTS

### PHYSICAL EXAMINATION

Patients with acute patellar instability show apprehension at attempts to manipulate the patella, demonstrating fear and anxiety (apprehension sign) when the patella is translated laterally. Range of motion may be limited in extension and flexion because of pain or fluid in the joint. If the retinaculum is torn, there will be tenderness along the medial edge of the patella, or just proximal to the medial femoral epicondyle when the medial patellofemoral ligament is torn at its origin. Patients with chronic instability exhibit the apprehension sign but may not have tenderness.

The physical examination of patients with malalignment is more subtle. The gait pattern may demonstrate a tendency for the patellae to point inward (femoral anteversion, tibial torsion) or knock-knee alignment (genu valgum). Genu valgum may be increased, and the distal portion of the vastus medialis may be dysplastic or atrophied. Increased patellar mobility also is common (lateral translation greater than one half the width of the patella), along with tightness of the lateral retinaculum (inability to elevate the lateral edge of the patella to a horizontal position). A high-riding patella (patella alta) and abnormal tracking (positive J sign) also may be observed.

### DIAGNOSTIC TESTS

AP, lateral, tunnel, and axial views are necessary. The axial or sunrise view shows the relationship of the patella to the femoral trochlea. Normally, the patella is centered in the trochlea. Patients with malalignment or previous episodes of instability may demonstrate lateral tilt or subluxation of the patella (**Figure 2**). In patients with excessive lateral pressure syndrome that has progressed to frank patellofemoral arthrosis, radiographs reveal joint space narrowing and other degenerative changes, especially in the lateral articulation. Axial CT can be useful in better delineating the exact nature of the patellar and trochlear relationship, particularly when surgical treatment is considered.

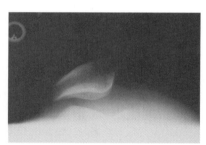

**Figure 2**
Axial view of the knee showing patellar tilt and subluxation.

## DIFFERENTIAL DIAGNOSIS

Anterior cruciate ligament tear (increased anterior laxity with Lachman test)

Medial collateral ligament tear (pain and laxity with valgus testing)

Medial meniscal tear (medial joint line tenderness)

Patellofemoral pain syndrome (pain without malalignment or instability)

## ADVERSE OUTCOMES OF THE DISEASE

Anterior knee pain secondary to patellar instability or maltracking can lead to secondary quadriceps weakness, further compromising stability and exacerbating the underlying problem. Recurrent episodes of patellar instability and prolonged maltracking can limit daily and sports activities and also lead to patellofemoral arthrosis.

## TREATMENT

The initial treatment of an acute patellar subluxation or dislocation includes application of a compressive dressing and protective splint with the knee in extension. These measures approximate the torn medial supporting structures. Aspiration of the knee should be considered in patients who have a significant effusion. Adjunctive measures include the use of oral analgesics, frequent application of ice in the first 24 to 48 hours and modified weight bearing. The patient is instructed in isometric exercises of the quadriceps that are done initially with the splint on. The patient is reevaluated every 2 weeks. When tenderness has resolved over the medial structures, range-of-motion and more vigorous strengthening exercises are started. The total duration of immobilization varies, depending on symptoms, but should not exceed 6 weeks. Loose bodies seen on radiographs after patellar reduction may need to be removed.

Initial treatment of patients with chronic recurrent maltracking or instability should include exercises emphasizing quadriceps strengthening and flexibility. An elastic brace with a lateral buttress can facilitate the return to occupational or recreational activities. Occasionally, physical therapy modalities such as electrical stimulation or taping can be useful.

When nonoperative measures fail, proximal or distal realignment of the extensor mechanism may be indicated.

## ADVERSE OUTCOMES OF TREATMENT

The most common adverse outcome after treatment is residual patellofemoral pain. Patellar instability can recur after lateral retinacular release or proximal realignment, but instability is unlikely after distal bony realignment. Even when successful stabilization of the patella is achieved, patellofemoral pain may persist, particularly with concomitant degenerative articular cartilage. Postoperative infection is rare.

## REFERRAL DECISIONS/RED FLAGS

Patients with a significant effusion after a traumatic knee injury require further evaluation, as do patients with an osteochondral fracture from an acute patellar dislocation. Patients with patellofemoral malalignment or pain that fails to respond to nonoperative measures also require further evaluation.

# PATELLOFEMORAL PAIN

## ICD-9 Codes
717.7
Chondromalacia of patella
719.46
Pain in joint, knee

## SYNONYMS
Patellofemoral pain syndrome
Anterior knee pain
Chondromalacia

## DEFINITION

Patellofemoral pain syndrome refers to a constellation of problems characterized by a diffuse, aching anterior knee pain that increases with activities that place additional loads across the patellofemoral joint, such as running, climbing up or down stairs, kneeling, and squatting. Forces on the articular surface of the patella in a typical 200-lb man can vary from 600 to 3,000 lb per square inch in activities ranging from walking to running. The etiology of this syndrome is multifactorial and in many situations related to overuse and overload of the patellofemoral joint. Although patellar malalignment can cause anterior knee pain, it is not a necessary component.

The term chondromalacia should not be used to describe this condition because chondromalacia indicates that pathologic changes are present in the articular surface of the patella, which may not necessarily be true. In addition, many patients who undergo arthroscopy have degenerative changes on the undersurface of the patella consistent with chondromalacia, yet they have no symptoms referable to the patellofemoral joint. For this reason, the terms patellofemoral pain syndrome or anterior knee pain are preferable.

## CLINICAL SYMPTOMS

Patients most commonly report a diffuse aching anterior knee pain that is worse after prolonged sitting (theater sign), climbing stairs, jumping, or squatting. Some patients report a sense of instability or a retropatellar catching sensation. Usually no history of swelling is reported. Often the pain develops after an increase in activity level or in weight training. In most instances, patients will report no preexisting trauma but on occasion there may be a history of a direct blow to the patella.

## TESTS

### PHYSICAL EXAMINATION

When the patellofemoral joint is thought to contribute to the patient's pain, it should be deferred until the end of the examination; otherwise, the patient likely will resist the entire examination.

The patient should first be examined in weight-bearing stance. Watch the patient walk to see whether the patellae point toward each other (a sign of increased femoral anteversion). Look for genu valgum (knock-knees) and for inadequate development of the vastus medialis obliquus muscle at the distal and medial thigh.

The Q angle, which is the angle constructed by a line drawn from the anterosuperior iliac spine to the center of the patella, and from there to the center of the tibial tubercle, should be measured next (**Figure 1**). In women, the Q angle should be less than 22° with the knee in extension and less than 9° with the knee in 90° of flexion. In men, the Q angle should be less than 18° with the knee in extension and less than 8° with the knee in 90° of flexion.

Excessive femoral anteversion in which internal rotation of the hip exceeds external rotation by more than 30° should be checked. Tracking of the patella as the knee moves through flexion and extension also should be observed. As the knee nears full extension, the patella may move laterally more than 1 cm or might even subluxate (a sign of instability). Soft-tissue restraints to medial and lateral patellar translation also should be evaluated. With the knee fully extended, the lateral patellar facet should be elevated to at least a neutral position. At 30° of flexion, the patella should be translated to at least one quadrant medially but not more than two quadrants laterally.

The patellar apprehension sign is a test performed to evaluate the possibility of patellar instability. With the knee extended, translate the patella laterally and then flex the knee to 30°. Marked discomfort or apprehension by the patient suggests instability. Palpate the patella as the patient places the knee through a range of motion to determine whether crepitus is present and, if so, at what position. Hamstring and quadriceps muscle tightness also should be evaluated.

## DIAGNOSTIC TESTS

AP, lateral, and bilateral axial views are necessary. The axial view helps to rule out malalignment and arthritis (**Figures 2, 3**).

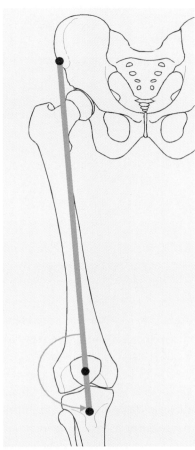

**Figure 1**
Diagram of the Q angle.

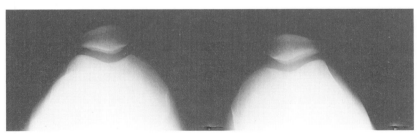

**Figure 2**
Axial view showing the patella aligned well in the femoral groove.

**Figure 3**
Axial view showing bilateral patellar subluxation.

SECTION 6 | KNEE AND LOWER LEG

## DIFFERENTIAL DIAGNOSIS

Meniscal tear (with or without locking, joint line tenderness)

Patellar malalignment (clinical and radiographic malalignment)

Patellar osteoarthritis (in older patients; effusion, crepitus, and evidence on axial radiograph)

Patellar tendinitis (jumper's knee) (inferior pole tenderness, local tenderness at patellar tendon)

Pathologic plica (medial parapatellar pain and tenderness, palpable cord in the medial parapatellar region)

Quadriceps tendinitis (local tenderness at insertion)

## ADVERSE OUTCOMES OF THE DISEASE

Pain and dysfunction are the principal problems.

## TREATMENT

Activity levels should be adjusted to a pain-free level. A program of quadriceps strengthening and quadriceps and hamstring flexibility should be initiated. Quadriceps exercises need to be individually modified as necessary to avoid causing knee pain (short-arc open or closed chain, or isometric). Use of a simple knee sleeve with a patellar cutout or strap may help. Some patients benefit from intermittent, short-term use of acetaminophen or NSAIDs. Weight loss is recommended when a patient is obese. Patients with persistent pain despite nonoperative treatment may be candidates for surgery.

## ADVERSE OUTCOMES OF TREATMENT

NSAIDs can cause gastric, renal, or hepatic complications. Aggressive full-arc quadriceps exercises typically aggravate the symptoms.

## REFERRAL DECISIONS/RED FLAGS

Persistent symptoms, including pain or recurrent effusions, or findings suggestive of patellar instability indicate the need for further evaluation.

# PATELLAR/QUADRICEPS TENDINITIS

ICD-9 Codes
726.60
    Enthesopathy of knee, unspecified
726.64
    Patellar tendinitis

## SYNONYMS

Extensor mechanism tendinitis
Jumper's knee

## DEFINITION

Extensor mechanism tendinitis is an overuse or overload syndrome involving either the quadriceps tendon at its insertion on the superior pole of the patella or the patellar tendon at the inferior pole of the patella or its insertion at the tibial tubercle. Younger adults (under age 40 years) with this condition often engage in jumping sports (jumper's knee) or have erratic exercise habits. Patellar or quadriceps tendinitis also can develop in older patients after a lifting strain or a significant change in exercise level. Weight gain is sometimes a factor.

## CLINICAL SYMPTOMS

Anterior knee pain is the hallmark. Patients often point to a tender spot where symptoms concentrate. The pain is often noted immediately at the end of exercise or following sitting that has been preceded by exercise. Pain also may be reported with prolonged sitting, squatting, or kneeling. Climbing or descending stairs, running, and, of course, jumping often increase the pain.

## TESTS

### PHYSICAL EXAMINATION

Palpate for tenderness at the bony attachment of the quadriceps tendon or the infrapatellar tendon. Increased heat, mild swelling, and soft-tissue crepitus also may be evident in the tender region. Examination in the area of the infrapatellar bursa (below the patella and behind the infrapatellar tendon) often reveals puffiness (**Figure 1**). Knee motion is normal but frequently is painful with resisted full extension. Pain is most exacerbated by hyperflexion of the knee, which increases the stresses on the extensor mechanism. When the condition is long-standing, 2 cm or more of quadriceps atrophy may be evident. Other general knee tests are negative in isolated cases.

### DIAGNOSTIC TESTS

AP and lateral radiographs of the knee typically are negative but may show small osteophytes or heterotopic ossification at the upper or lower pole of the patella (lateral views). MRI is reserved for recalcitrant cases for which surgical treatment is being considered or for cases in which partial rupture is possible (significant weakness in extension but no palpable defect).

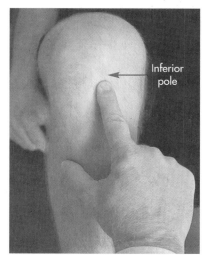

Inferior pole

**Figure 1**
Palpation of the inferior pole of the patella.

## Differential Diagnosis

Anterior or posterior cruciate ligament injury (positive Lachman or posterior drawer test)

Inflammatory conditions (systemic disorders)

Partial rupture of the extensor mechanism (weakness, palpable defect, difficulty with straight-leg raising test)

Patellofemoral pain syndrome (anterior knee pain, other abnormal patellofemoral signs but not superior or inferior pole tenderness)

Septic arthritis of the knee (fever, warmth, painful motion, elevated erythrocyte sedimentation rate)

## Adverse Outcomes of the Disease

Pain and rarely spontaneous rupture of the quadriceps or infrapatellar tendon can occur.

## Treatment

Treatment is primarily symptomatic but involves three critical aspects. First is a period of relative rest from aggravating activities. Depending on the severity of the condition, this period can vary from 3 to 5 days to as long as 3 weeks. In some instances, patients may need to use a knee immobilizer intermittently. NSAIDs can help control symptoms, but local injections of corticosteroids should be avoided because these injections significantly increase the risk of rupture of the extensor mechanism.

The second phase of treatment focuses on regaining a pain-free range of motion, flexibility of the quadriceps and hamstrings, and strength. Exercises focusing on pain-free quadriceps strengthening and flexibility should be initiated, often in conjunction with ultrasound and phonophoresis. Use of a knee sleeve with a patellar cutout or a compression strap at the level of the patellar tendon is sometimes helpful.

The third phase of treatment is gradual resumption of the activities that caused the symptoms while continuing the exercises that have restored strength and flexibility. Use of heat before activity and ice after also is often helpful.

## Adverse Outcomes of Treatment

NSAIDs can cause gastric, renal, or hepatic complications. Pain is possible, and occasionally spontaneous rupture of the tendon can occur. Persistent functional impairment is the most common disability.

## Referral Decisions/Red Flags

Patients with a possible rupture of the extensor mechanism need further evaluation as soon as possible. Cases recalcitrant to nonoperative management also require further evaluation.

# PLICA SYNDROME

ICD-9 Codes

717.9
Unspecified internal derangement of knee

727.00
Synovitis and tenosynovitis, unspecified

## DEFINITION

A plica is a normal fold in the synovium. The synovium of the knee joint has five basic plicae. Three of them (suprapatellar, medial, and infrapatellar) are considered distinct structures, and two are considered minor folds. The suprapatellar plica extends from the undersurface of the quadriceps tendon to the medial or lateral capsule of the knee. The medial plica extends from the medial joint capsule to the medial anterior fat pad. The infrapatellar plica (ligamentum mucosa) can cover the anterior cruciate ligament as it extends anterior to this structure.

A plica that becomes inflamed and thickened from trauma or overuse can interfere with normal joint motion as the pathologic structure "bowstrings" over the femoral condyle or other structures. Plica syndromes usually result from a combination of trauma and mechanical malalignment and can occur at any age. The medial plica most often becomes pathologic.

## CLINICAL SYMPTOMS

The onset of pain is often insidious but may be related to a fall or injury. Patients most often describe aching in the anterior or anteromedial aspect of the knee that is activity related. Some patients note a painful snapping or popping in the knee. Buckling or a sense of instability may occur, but true giving way, locking, or obvious effusion is uncommon.

## TESTS

### PHYSICAL EXAMINATION

Inspect the knee for tenderness. With a pathologic medial plica, tenderness is localized to the medial aspect of the patella. With the knee flexed, a pathologic plica may be palpated as a thickened band. Place the knee in 90° of flexion and then extend the knee. With a pathologic plica, a pop may occur at about 60° of flexion.

Other conditions such as patellofemoral disorders may present with similar symptoms and should be excluded.

### DIAGNOSTIC TESTS

AP, lateral, tunnel, and axial views are normal but should be obtained to rule out other conditions.

## DIFFERENTIAL DIAGNOSIS

Meniscal tear (giving way, joint line tenderness, pain with circumduction)

Osteochondritis dissecans (spontaneous onset, evident on radiographs)

Patellofemoral instability (positive apprehension sign)

SECTION 6 | KNEE AND LOWER LEG

Prepatellar bursitis (location)

Quadriceps or patellar tendinitis (tenderness at tendon insertion sites)

Septic arthritis (severe pain, febrile, effusion, diagnostic joint aspiration)

## ADVERSE OUTCOMES OF THE DISEASE

Continued discomfort and interference with running activities can occur, as can erosive changes in the femoral condyle cartilage as the thickened plica snaps over the condyle.

## TREATMENT

Initial management is aimed at decreasing inflammation and thickening of the plica. Activity modifications and NSAIDs should be considered. An injection of local anesthetic and corticosteroid preparation into the plica can be both diagnostic and therapeutic. Based on the physical examination, an appropriate flexibility and strengthening program should be initiated. With persistent symptoms, and no other evidence of other intra-articular disorders, arthroscopic resection of the plica should be considered.

## ADVERSE OUTCOMES OF TREATMENT

NSAIDs can cause gastric, renal, or hepatic complications. Repeated intra-articular injections of corticosteroid can lead to accelerated destruction of articular cartilage and/or iatrogenic sepsis. Surgical resection can be ineffective or complicated by infection and stiffness.

## REFERRAL DECISIONS/RED FLAGS

Continued discomfort and symptoms of instability indicate the need for further evaluation.

# POPLITEAL CYST

| ICD-9 Code |
|---|
| 727.51 |
| Popliteal cyst |

## SYNONYMS

Baker cyst
Synovial cyst

## DEFINITION

A popliteal cyst, commonly known as a Baker cyst, is the most common synovial cyst in the knee and develops in the popliteal bursa located at the posteromedial aspect of the knee joint. This normally thin bursa communicates with the knee joint and becomes more prominent (cystic) when synovitis or trauma creates excessive joint fluid that then tracks into the popliteal bursa.

Popliteal cysts are associated with degenerative meniscal tears and systemic inflammatory conditions such as rheumatoid arthritis. These cysts fluctuate in size and symptoms. When they rupture, these cysts can cause severe calf pain and swelling and can be mistaken for a deep venous thrombosis.

## CLINICAL SYMPTOMS

Patients present with swelling or fullness in the popliteal fossa with accompanying pain or tenderness. Mechanical complaints referable to the knee are common. Smaller cysts may be asymptomatic, but change in size is common. Larger cysts can dissect down the posterior calf and/or rupture, resulting in severe calf pain and decreased motion at the ankle.

## TESTS

### PHYSICAL EXAMINATION

Inspect the popliteal fossa and compare it with that of the opposite leg. Palpate the area to determine the size, consistency, and amount of tenderness. Cyst locations vary, but most commonly are found to course between the semimembranosus muscle and the medial head of the gastrocnemius muscle. Examine the knee for signs of meniscal or other pathology. Effusion and accompanying mechanical signs indicate an intra-articular irritant causing the generation of excessive joint fluid. Examine the leg to determine whether the cyst has extravasated, causing swelling and tenderness in the calf.

Popliteal cysts may be identified as an incidental finding on a symptomatic knee examination.

### DIAGNOSTIC TESTS

Radiographs of the knee are usually negative but may show the outline of the cyst or show calcification present in the cyst or within the knee. MRI usually

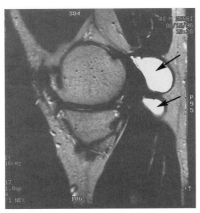

**Figure 1**
MRI showing the cystic nature of a popliteal cyst (arrows).

is not necessary but can demonstrate both the location and character of the cystic fluid, as well as determine the presence of intra-articular pathology (Figure 1).

Cyst aspiration should be approached with caution because of the close proximity of neurovascular structures in the popliteal fossa. Furthermore, the cyst fluid may be gelatinous and not easily retrievable with a standard-bore needle.

## DIFFERENTIAL DIAGNOSIS

Deep venous thrombosis (evident on ultrasound or venogram)

Exertional compartment syndrome (physical examination)

Inflammatory arthritis (serologic studies)

Medial gastrocnemius strain (physical examination)

Soft-tissue tumor (evident on MRI)

Superficial phlebitis (superficial tenderness, negative ultrasound or venogram)

## ADVERSE OUTCOMES OF THE DISEASE

A cyst rupture can cause severe pain in the posterior calf that, with the swelling, can mimic a deep venous thrombosis. Mass effect of a cyst can cause compression of surrounding neurovascular structures with sensory or motor changes or venous occlusion.

## TREATMENT

Aspiration has been suggested, but this provides only transient relief because the cyst lining remains intact and the fluid commonly reaccumulates. Treatment should be directed at the cause of increased synovial fluid. When intra-articular lesions resulting in increased production of synovial fluid can be successfully treated (usually by arthroscopic excision of a torn medial meniscus), the cyst usually resolves spontaneously and excision is unnecessary. Cysts associated with severe arthritis typically resolve after knee replacement. Cyst excision may be required in some patients.

## ADVERSE OUTCOMES OF TREATMENT

Open excision carries the risk of injury to neighboring nerves and blood vessels; dissection should be performed with caution. Recurrence rate, combined with resolution of any internal derangement, is low (around 5%).

## REFERRAL DECISIONS/RED FLAGS

Night pain, weight loss, fever and/or chills, or other constitutional symptoms indicate the possibility of a neoplastic process and therefore the need for further evaluation.

# POSTERIOR CRUCIATE LIGAMENT SPRAIN

ICD-9 Codes
717.84
    Old disruption of posterior cruciate
    ligament
844.2
    Acute posterior cruciate ligament
    tear

## SYNONYM
PCL tear

## DEFINITION
The posterior cruciate ligament (PCL) is considered the strongest ligament in the knee and serves as the primary restraint to posterior translation of the tibia relative to the femur. Anatomically, it originates on the medial intercondylar wall of the femur and inserts on the posterior aspect of the tibia, running in an oblique direction. Injury to the PCL can be either a stretch injury or a complete rupture, is less common than injuries to the anterior cruciate ligament (ACL), and is often overlooked. Isolated PCL injuries occur less frequently than combined ligament injuries (PCL with ACL and/or collateral ligament injury).

## CLINICAL SYMPTOMS
Four injury patterns suggest the possibility of a PCL injury:

- a dashboard injury—a posteriorly directed force to the anterior knee with the knee in flexion, as in a motor vehicle accident

- a fall onto a flexed knee with the foot in plantar flexion results in impact to the tibial tubercle; in comparison, the foot in dorsiflexion results in patellofemoral impact

- a pure hyperflexion injury to the knee

- a hyperextension injury to the knee–typically, the ACL ruptures first, then with sufficient force, injury to the PCL follows. This combination most commonly occurs in contact sports and a direct load on the anteromedial proximal tibia with the knee in extension. This mechanism of injury frequently results in a knee dislocation with or without spontaneous reduction.

An effusion commonly develops within the first 24 hours after injury, and range of motion usually is limited. Patients also may report pain and feelings of instability with weight bearing, especially with combined ligamentous injuries.

## TESTS

### PHYSICAL EXAMINATION
Examination typically reveals a significant effusion and decreased range of motion. Pain to palpation may not be exhibited. A thorough examination for knee stability is needed because PCL injuries are often a component of a com-

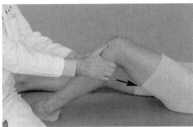

**Figure 1**
Posterior drawer test.

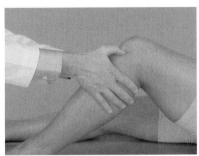

**Figure 2**
Thumb sign.

bined ligamentous injury. In the acute setting, the physical examination can be difficult because of loss of motion and muscle guarding, which can mask increases in translation. Therefore, reexamining the patient once swelling has decreased is often helpful.

The most sensitive test is the posterior drawer test performed with the patient supine and the knee in 90° of flexion (**Figure 1**). However, increased posterior translation of the tibia relative to the femur is easily misinterpreted as a positive anterior drawer sign as the tibia is pulled back to the anterior position. This misinterpretation is further complicated by the frequent co-existence of an ACL tear. The thumb sign will clarify the situation. With a PCL injury, the tibia is in a posterior position relative to the femur because of gravity, and there will be no place to sit your thumbs on the anterior tibial plateaus (**Figure 2**). The true neutral position of the tibia also can be best judged by the thumb sign. Pull the tibia forward enough to have the normal space to sit your thumbs. Anterior displacement beyond this position indicates abnormal anterior instability from an ACL tear.

Finally, in acute multiple ligament disruption, with or without spontaneous reduction, distal neurovascular status should be assessed because deficits can be seen.

### DIAGNOSTIC TESTS

AP and lateral radiographs of the knee obtained in the acute setting can identify bony pathology, aid in diagnosis, and alter surgical management. MRI can be useful in confirming PCL tears, as well as any concomitant injuries to ligaments, menisci, and articular cartilage.

### DIFFERENTIAL DIAGNOSIS

ACL tear (positive Lachman test, pivot shift)

Articular cartilage injury (pain on palpation, evident on radiographs or MRI)

Combined ligament injury (laxity in multiple directions, evident on MRI)

Medial or lateral collateral ligament tear (pain on palpation and varus/valgus laxity)

Meniscal tear (joint line tenderness)

Patellar or quadriceps tendon rupture (inability to achieve straight-leg raise)

Patellofemoral dislocation (apprehension with lateral patellar displacement)

Tibial plateau fracture (evident on radiographs)

### ADVERSE OUTCOMES OF THE DISEASE

Limb-threatening vascular injury may be present if a dislocated knee with spontaneous reduction has not been recognized and fully evaluated. Recurrent instability, subsequent meniscal tears, and osteoarthritis of the knee are all possible.

## TREATMENT

Isolated PCL injuries typically are treated with a structured program that initially concentrates on resolving swelling and restoring range of motion. Once these goals have been achieved, progression to strengthening exercises can be initiated, with an emphasis on the quadriceps (short-arc terminal extension exercises from 30° of flexion to 0°). Functional bracing can be helpful when the patient returns to contact sports.

Failure of nonoperative treatment typically manifests as recurrent instability and/or subsequent meniscal tears. These patients require PCL reconstruction to restore functional stability. After reconstructive procedures, instability is improved but translation usually remains increased relative to the normal side.

## ADVERSE OUTCOMES OF TREATMENT

Osteoarthritic changes involving the medial and patellofemoral compartments are a well-documented sequela to both nonoperative and surgically reconstructed knees. Surgical reconstruction may be complicated by infection, graft failure, and recurrent instability.

## REFERRAL DECISIONS/RED FLAGS

Neurovascular compromise or deficits indicate the possibility of a knee dislocation. Any patient with a PCL injury and the possibility of damage to other ligamentous structures requires specialty evaluation.

# PREPATELLAR BURSITIS

ICD-9 Codes
682.6
    Other cellulitis and abscess, leg,
    except foot
726.65
    Prepatellar bursitis

## DEFINITION

The prepatellar bursa is located between the skin and the patella. This bursa can become inflamed (bursitis) or infected (septic bursitis) as a result of trauma to the anterior knee, such as a direct blow, or from chronic irritation from activities that require extensive kneeling, such as wrestling or carpet installation. Bacterial infections typically result from direct penetration that may be an unrecognized event in patients who kneel extensively. *Staphylococcus aureus* and *Streptococcus* species are the most common infecting organisms.

## CLINICAL SYMPTOMS

Patients report pain and swelling at the front of the knee.

## TESTS

### PHYSICAL EXAMINATION

A patient with bursitis or septic bursitis will have swelling, increased warmth, and erythematous changes over the patella. These changes are more severe with septic bursitis, and in these patients, the swelling is such that the patella will not be palpable in its subcutaneous position (**Figure 1**). The knee is held straight or only slightly flexed. Flexion of the knee is painful because this motion puts stretch on the inflamed prepatellar bursa. Systemic signs usually are not as dramatic with an infected prepatellar bursa as they are with septic arthritis of the knee.

### DIAGNOSTIC TESTS

Radiographs will be normal with the exception of anterior soft-tissue swelling. Aspiration of prepatellar septic bursitis can obtain purulent or seropurlent material. This aspiration should be done in a manner that does not seed the knee joint.

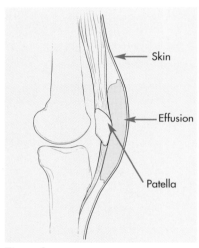

**Figure 1**
Involved region with septic prepatellar bursitis.

## DIFFERENTIAL DIAGNOSIS

Septic arthritis of the knee (effusion of the joint but the patella can be palpated in its subcutaneous position, knee held in more flexion)

## ADVERSE OUTCOMES OF THE DISEASE

Progression of a septic bursitis can result in chronic drainage or can spread to the knee joint.

## TREATMENT

A noninfected, inflamed bursa can be treated with activity modifications and temporary immobilization. Early-onset, mild septic bursitis can be treated with oral antibiotics. More severe infections require initial treatment with intravenous antibiotics. Repeat aspiration may help in decompressing the bursa. Surgical drainage may be necessary but is not often required.

## ADVERSE OUTCOMES OF TREATMENT

Chronic or recurrent infection, septic arthritis, or emergence of resistant organisms can occur.

## REFERRAL DECISIONS/RED FLAGS

Prepatellar bursa infections can require surgical treatment when they cannot be aspirated, do not respond to antibiotics, or become recurrent.

# QUADRICEPS AND PATELLA TENDON RUPTURES

## ICD-9 Codes

822.0
  Fracture of patella
844.8
  Sprains and strains of knee and
  leg, other specified sites
959.7
  Injury, other and unspecified, knee,
  leg, ankle, and foot

## DEFINITION

A rupture of the quadriceps or patella tendon, as well as a fracture, will disrupt the extensor mechanism of the knee. Quadriceps and patellar tendon disruptions typically occur with a fall on a knee that is partially flexed. When the quadriceps muscle forcibly contracts to break the impact of the fall, the quadriceps or patellar tendon may overwhelmed. Fractures of the patella more often result from a direct blow from a motor vehicle accident but also may occur by the indirect mechanism of a fall.

Most patients with ruptures of the quadriceps or patellar tendon are between 30 and 60 years old. A history of previous quadriceps or patellar tendinitis is surprisingly uncommon.

## CLINICAL SYMPTOMS

Patients report significant pain and swelling after an acute injury. Walking may be possible, but patients note a sense of instability with ambulation.

## TESTS

### PHYSICAL EXAMINATION

A large effusion is usually present. Palpate the knee for defects indicating the area of rupture (**Figure 1**). Fractures of the patella are usually obvious, but ruptures of the quadriceps or patellar tendon can be missed. The key to diagnosis is the patient's inability to extend the knee against gravity or perform a straight-leg raising test.

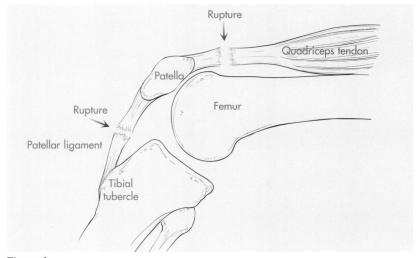

**Figure 1**
Common areas of rupture. These should be palpated during the physical examination.

## DIAGNOSTIC TESTS

Plain radiographs are appropriate to rule out a patellar fracture. The lateral view may show that, with rupture of the patellar tendon, the patella is in a higher than usual location or that, with rupture of the quadriceps tendon, the patella is in a slightly lower than usual location. MRI will confirm rupture of a tendon, but this is rarely necessary in the presence of the strong clinical findings.

## DIFFERENTIAL DIAGNOSIS

Collateral ligament tear (varus or valgus injury, medial or lateral tenderness and instability)

Cruciate ligament disruption (effusion may be similar, but the patient is able to extend the knee)

Meniscal tear (effusion relatively small, joint line tenderness, circumduction pain)

## ADVERSE OUTCOMES OF THE DISEASE

Unless the rupture is surgically repaired, marked disability will develop secondary to the deficient extensor mechanism. Delay in treatment significantly increases the difficulty of surgery and may compromise the outcome.

## TREATMENT

Surgical repair is the treatment of choice for a complete rupture of the quadriceps or patellar tendon and for a displaced fracture of the patella. The uncommon partial tears of the tendons and nondisplaced fractures can be treated by immobilization.

## ADVERSE OUTCOMES OF TREATMENT

Postoperative infection, pain, and weakness of the extensor mechanism are possible.

## REFERRAL DECISIONS/RED FLAGS

All patients with a history and physical examination that suggest extensor mechanism rupture require further evaluation for surgery.

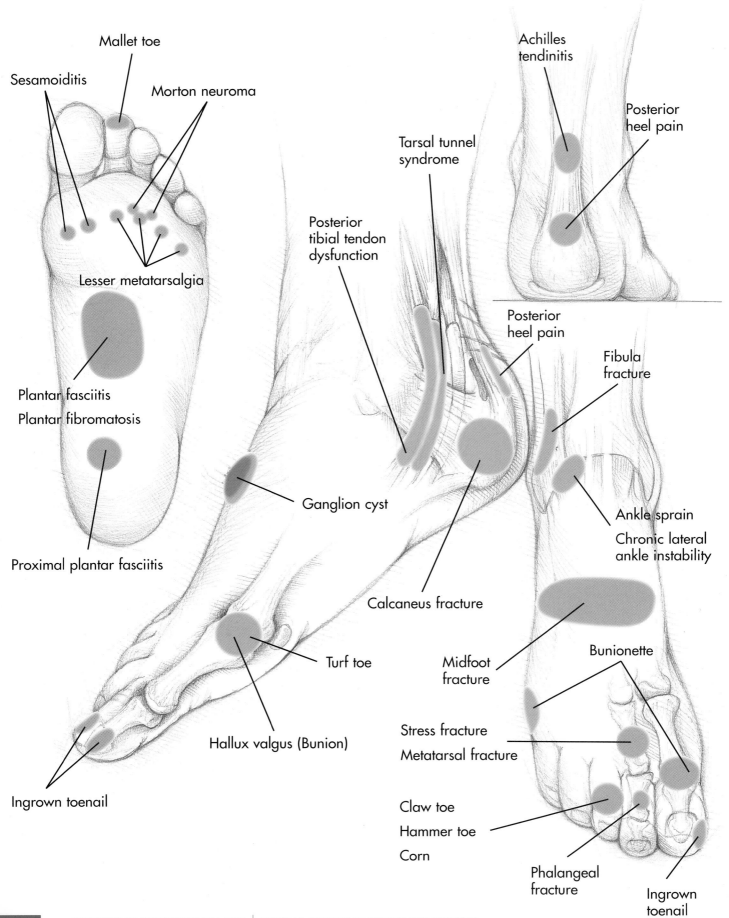

Mallet toe

Sesamoiditis

Morton neuroma

Achilles tendinitis

Posterior heel pain

Tarsal tunnel syndrome

Lesser metatarsalgia

Posterior tibial tendon dysfunction

Posterior heel pain

Fibula fracture

Plantar fasciitis

Plantar fibromatosis

Ganglion cyst

Proximal plantar fasciitis

Ankle sprain

Chronic lateral ankle instability

Calcaneus fracture

Midfoot fracture

Bunionette

Turf toe

Stress fracture

Metatarsal fracture

Hallux valgus (Bunion)

Claw toe

Hammer toe

Corn

Ingrown toenail

Phalangeal fracture

Ingrown toenail

ESSENTIALS OF MUSCULOSKELETAL CARE | AMERICAN ACADEMY OF ORTHOPAEDIC SURGEONS

# FOOT AND ANKLE

## Section Editor

Glenn B. Pfeffer, MD
California Pacific Medical Center
San Francisco, California
Assistant Clinical Professor
Department of Orthopaedics
University of California School of Medicine
San Francisco, California

Richard A. Balderston, MD
Philadelphia, Pennsylvania

Judith F. Baumhauer, MD
Associate Professor
Chief, Division of Foot and Ankle Surgery
Department of Orthopaedics
University of Rochester School of Medicine and Dentistry
Rochester, New York

Thomas H. Lee, MD
Clinical Assistant Professor
Director, Division of Foot and Ankle
Department of Orthopaedics
The Ohio State University Medical Center
Columbus, Ohio

Martin J. O'Malley, MD
Assistant Professor of Orthopaedic Surgery
Department of Surgery
Weill Medical College of Cornell University
Hospital for Special Surgery
New York, New York

# FOOT AND ANKLE– AN OVERVIEW

One mile of walking generates more than 60 tons of stress on each foot. Therefore, it is not surprising that more than 20% of musculoskeletal problems affect the foot and ankle. Most of these disorders can be treated in the office setting.

The key to the successful diagnosis of a foot problem is to determine the exact location and duration of symptoms. A pertinent medical history also should be obtained because various systemic illnesses increase the foot's susceptibility to injury. Diabetes, peripheral vascular disease, neuropathy, and inflammatory arthritis can affect the foot. A history of bilateral foot pain should prompt a search for a possible systemic or spinal etiology.

Most patients with foot problems report pain. Chronic pain is more common and is defined as more than 2 weeks' duration. Acute pain is an unusual presentation unless a fracture, sprain, or infection is present. Always consider a stress fracture when a patient reports recent onset of pain over the metatarsals, especially in the distal aspects of the second or third metatarsals.

When radiographs are necessary, obtain standing AP and lateral radiographs because standing views show the effect of weight bearing, a source of important information. An oblique view is obtained in a supine position.

## FOREFOOT PROBLEMS

Forefoot problems occur nine times more often in women than in men, an association that is directly attributable to wearing high-heeled, pointed-toe shoes. Shoe modification (lower heels, wider shoes) is always the first line of treatment. Bunions, hammer toes, claw toes, ingrown toenails, metatarsalgia, and interdigital neuromas account for most instances of forefoot pain, and these problems are detailed in subsequent chapters.

Other common problems in the forefoot are hallux rigidus (arthritis of the metatarsophalangeal joint of the great toe) and stress fractures. Limited extension (dorsiflexion) of the great toe is consistent with hallux rigidus. Pain and tenderness directly over the second or third metatarsals suggest a stress fracture.

## MIDFOOT PROBLEMS

Chronic dorsal pain at the midfoot most commonly occurs secondary to degenerative arthritis involving one or more of the midfoot joints. Patients are often able to pinpoint the exact location of the pain. A bony prominence, referred to as dorsal bossing, can be palpated and corresponds to the underlying arthritic joint. Pain on the plantar aspect of the midfoot is unusual and occurs with midfoot plantar fasciitis or plantar fibromas.

# HINDFOOT PROBLEMS

Plantar heel pain secondary to plantar fasciitis is the most common problem in the hindfoot. The pain associated with this condition is often severe with the first few steps out of bed; patients normally are pain-free during rest. Patients have focal tenderness directly over the plantar medial heel; often, on examination, considerable pressure must be applied in this area to duplicate the patient's symptoms.

Posterior heel pain usually is indirectly related to irritation from shoes and directly associated with a prominent superior process of the calcaneus (Haglund deformity) and/or dystrophic changes in the Achilles tendon at its insertion. Often an associated superficial bursitis of the posterior heel is present. When evaluating a patient with posterior heel pain, make sure that the problem is not more proximal within the Achilles tendon; otherwise, a partial or even complete rupture of the tendon could be missed.

A commonly overlooked problem in the hindfoot is posterior tibial dysfunction. This condition is characterized by pain and tenderness posterior and distal to the medial malleolus in the region of the posterior tibial tendon. Progressive dysfunction results in an acquired flatfoot that can give rise to additional pain on the lateral side of the ankle as the tip of the fibula abuts the collapsing foot.

# ANKLE PROBLEMS

More than 25,000 individuals sprain an ankle each day in the United States. Acute anterolateral ankle pain, swelling, and frequently ecchymosis are the hallmarks of this condition.

Chronic ankle pain commonly occurs at the anterolateral aspect of the ankle. A history of intermittent giving way suggests a diagnosis of ankle instability. Chronic low-grade pain and swelling are consistent with injury to the peroneal tendons or an occult fracture (osteochondral lesion) of the ankle joint. Subtalar synovitis or arthritis also can present in a similar fashion.

Arthritis of the ankle is most commonly secondary to previous trauma or rheumatoid arthritis. Tarsal tunnel syndrome can cause chronic medial ankle pain but almost always is associated with neurogenic symptoms that radiate into the plantar aspect of the foot.

# PHYSICAL EXAMINATION
# FOOT AND ANKLE

## Inspection/Palpation

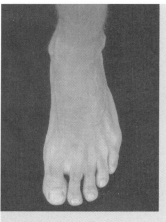

### Anterior view, standing

Inspect the foot and ankle from the front and look at alignment of the great and lesser toes, position of the foot in relation to the limb, and medial curvature of the forefoot (metatarsus adductus).

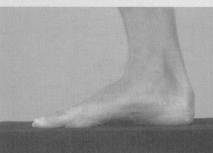

### Medial view

Inspect for a high arch (cavus foot) or flatfoot posture (pes planus), or undue prominence of the medial midfoot (accessory navicular). The arches of both feet should be symmetric.

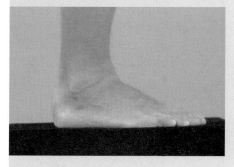

### Lateral view

Inspect for callosities, ankle swelling, or prominence of the posterior calcaneus.

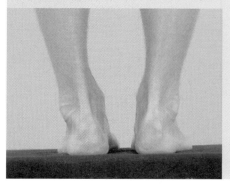

### Posterior view

Assess heel alignment from the back. Normal is neutral or slight valgus (turned-out heel), with no more than one or two lateral toes visible from behind. A patient with an acquired flatfoot from posterior tibial tendon dysfunction will have increased valgus of the calcaneus and more than two visible toes ("too many toes" sign). A varus calcaneus (turned-in heel) occurs with a cavus foot. An inflamed prominence of the posterior heel is called a "pump bump." Patient in figure has mild varus of the heel.

# Inspection/Palpation

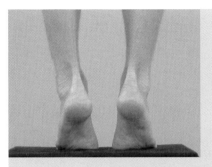

### Standing on toes

With the patient standing on the toes, look to see that the heels move into a normal varus position.

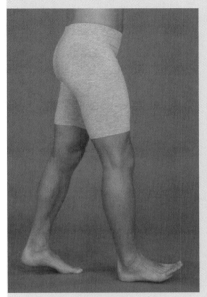

### Gait

Look for deviations from normal while the patient walks. Analyze alignment of the foot during the different phases of gait: heel strike, midstance, toe-off, swing phase. With a static or other upper motor neuron disorder, the plantar flexors may be overactive and cause the foot to drop during swing phase. Weakness or paralysis of the ankle dorsiflexors from peroneal nerve dysfunction causes similar abnormalities.

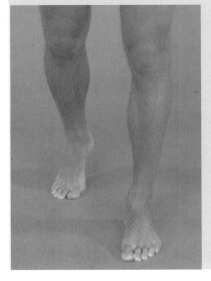

### Angle of gait

Assess the angle of gait, which is the angle of the foot in relation to the axis of the limb when a patient is walking, to identify problems of intoeing and outtoeing. When walking, the foot is normally positioned in 0° to 20° of external rotation. Because tibial torsion is typically asymmetric, one foot is normally positioned in more external rotation.

# Inspection/Palpation

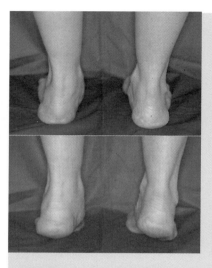

### "Too many toes" sign

View the feet of a patient with an acquired flatfoot from posterior tibial tendon dysfunction from behind. In the normal weight-bearing position, the patient will appear to have too many toes in the affected foot, as this patient does in the left foot (top). When the same patient attempts to rise on her toes, her left heel does not move into a normal varus position as her right heel does (bottom).

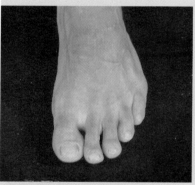

### Anterior view, supine

Inspect the top of the foot for a bunion and associated hallux valgus at the great toe metatarsophalangeal (MP) joint, or bunionette at the fifth MP joint. Inspect the lesser toes for abnormalities in alignment (eg, hammer toe, mallet toe, claw toe). Claw toe commonly occurs in patients with diabetes, rheumatoid arthritis, Charcot-Marie-Tooth disease, or cavus foot deformities. The MP joint is extended and the proximal interphalangeal (PIP) and distal interphalangeal (DIP) joints are flexed. Multiple toes tend to be involved and often a corn (hard callus) is apparent over the PIP joint. Inspect the nails for poor techniques in trimming and associated infection.

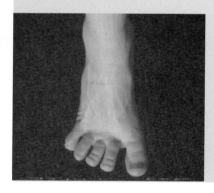

### Spread toes

Ask the patient to spread or fan the toes as widely as possible. Look for corns or ulcerations between the toes. Inability to actively spread the toes may indicate loss of intrinsic muscle function.

# Inspection/Palpation

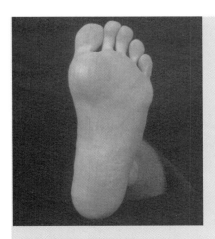

## Plantar surface

With the patient supine, inspect the bottom of the foot for plantar warts (which usually do not occur beneath the metatarsal head), a plantar callus (which occurs beneath the metatarsal head), prominence of the metatarsal heads, or ulceration (especially in diabetic feet).

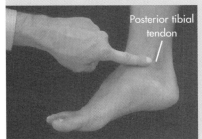

Posterior tibial tendon

## Medial malleolus

Palpate the area posterior and inferior to the medial malleolus in the region of the posterior tibial nerve. In patients with tarsal tunnel syndrome, percussion over the nerve should reproduce symptoms, often described as "shooting" pains (paresthesias) in the heel and plantar aspect of the foot. Patients with posterior tibial dysfunction will have swelling and tenderness along the course of the tendon.

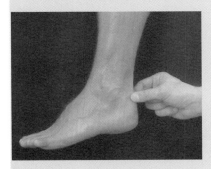

## Posterior heel

Palpate both sides of the Achilles tendon insertion to identify swelling or tenderness. Positive findings are signs of retrocalcaneal bursitis, a condition that is often associated with a prominence of the posterior superior calcaneus (pump bump or Haglund deformity). Swelling and tenderness of the Achilles tendon at its insertion is associated with tendinitis or calcific dystrophic tendinosis.

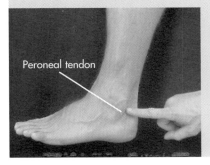

Peroneal tendon

## Peroneal tendons

Palpate behind and below the fibular malleolus for tenderness or swelling associated with peroneal tenosynovitis or for subluxation of the tendons during active dorsiflexion and plantar flexion of the ankle.

SECTION 7 | FOOT AND ANKLE

# Inspection/Palpation

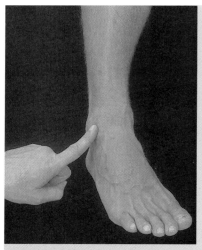

### Anterior ankle

Palpate over the anterior talofibular ligament and/or calcaneofibular ligament for tenderness associated with sprain, often the result of an acute inversion injury. In patients with chronic ankle pain, palpate at the anterolateral corner of the ankle joint (soft junction of the tibia, fibula, and talus) for synovitis.

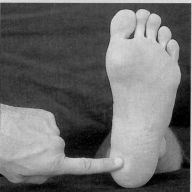

### Plantar fascia

Palpate the plantar fascia for tenderness or swelling. With plantar fasciitis, tenderness is noted with considerable pressure over the medial proximal aspect of the plantar fascia. Rupture of the plantar fascia is associated with tenderness and swelling in the middle third of the plantar fascia. Plantar fibromatosis causes swelling and thickening of the plantar fascia that typically begins in the middle portion.

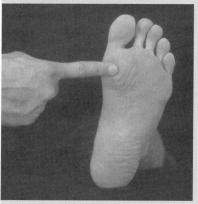

### Sesamoid

Palpate the area beneath the first metatarsal head for tenderness. If the sesamoids are involved, the tender spot will move as the toe is flexed and extended. The medial sesamoid is more commonly injured or inflamed.

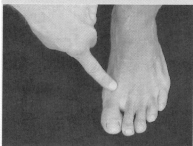

### MP joint

Palpate the top of the foot for tenderness and swelling of the MP joints that may be present with rheumatoid arthritis, idiopathic synovitis, Freiberg infraction, or metatarsalgia. Dorsal osteophytes are present at the great toe MP joint with hallux rigidus.

# Range of Motion

### Ankle motion: Zero Starting Position

Ankle motion is primarily extension (usually termed dorsiflexion) and flexion (usually termed plantar flexion). Dorsiflexion is movement of the foot toward the anterior surface of the tibia, and plantar flexion is movement of the foot in the opposite direction. Active ankle motion typically is greater than passive motion. Normal ankle dorsiflexion is 10° to 20°, and plantar flexion is 35° to 50°.

As the foot moves from dorsiflexion to plantar flexion, much of the motion occurs at the ankle joint, but other joints in the foot also contribute to this movement as well. Distinguishing the dorsiflexion/plantar flexion motion that occurs at the ankle joint from that at other joints is difficult and not critical. The total arc of motion is more important from a functional standpoint. Therefore, it is understood that clinical measurements of ankle motion also record motion of other joints of the foot.

The Zero Starting Position is with the foot perpendicular to the tibia. Align the goniometer with the axis of the leg and the lateral side of the plantar surface of the foot. To relax the gastrocnemius, measure ankle motion with the knee flexed. To assess heel cord tightness, measure ankle motion with the knee extended.

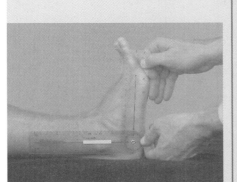

### Inversion and eversion

Inversion (turning the heel inward) and eversion (turning the heel outward) primarily reflect motion at the talocalcaneal (subtalar) joint. Precise measurements are difficult with standard techniques; therefore, in the clinical setting, these motions usually are estimated visually. The Zero Starting Position is with the ankle in slight dorsiflexion. This position limits lateral motion at the ankle joint and, therefore, provides better assessment of talocalcaneal mobility.

Restricted motion may be seen in patients with subtalar arthritis, end-stage posterior tibial tendon dysfunction, or tarsal coalition (bony connection between talus and calcaneus).

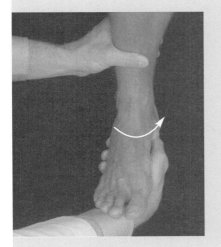

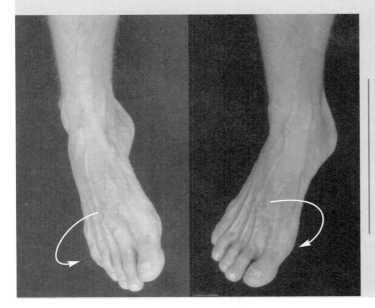

### Supination and pronation

Supination and pronation refer to rotation of the foot about an anterior/posterior axis. Supination includes inversion of the heel, as well as adduction and plantar flexion of the midfoot.

Pronation is the opposite motion and includes eversion of the heel and abduction and dorsiflexion of the midfoot.

Supination and pronation of the foot are difficult to quantify. Compare motion of the affected foot with that on the unaffected side for the most useful information.

# Range of Motion

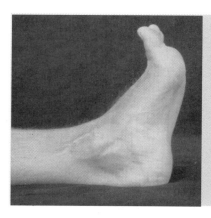

### Great toe: Zero Starting Position

Motion at the MP and interphalangeal (IP) joints occurs in the dorsiflexion/plantar flexion plane. Dorsiflexion (extension) is the primary motion of the MP joint, but this plane of motion is virtually nonexistent at the IP joint.

The Zero Starting Position for measuring motion at the MP joint is the functional neutral position. This position aligns the great toe with the plantar surface of the foot. This position, in contrast to the anatomic neutral position, is easier to measure and facilitates description of toe movement during walking. Reduced motion at the MP joint may indicate hallux rigidus.

# Muscle Testing

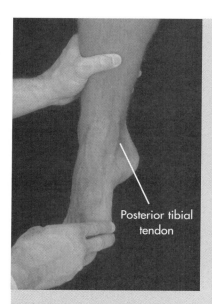

Posterior tibial tendon

### Posterior tibialis

To test the strength of the posterior tibialis muscle or integrity of the posterior tibial tendon, stabilize the tibia and with the foot in plantar flexion (to eliminate activity of the tibialis anterior) resist the patient's attempt to invert the foot. Weakness indicates injury or dysfunction of the posterior tibialis or a lesion involving the posterior tibial nerve or L5 nerve root.

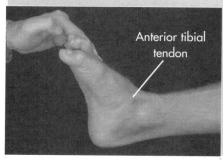

Anterior tibial tendon

### Anterior tibialis

To test the strength of the anterior tibialis muscle, ask the patient to flex the toes (to eliminate activity of the toe extensors) and then invert and dorsiflex the foot against resistance. Weakness indicates a lesion involving the L4 nerve root or deep peroneal nerve.

# Muscle Testing

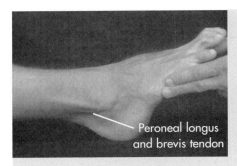

## Peroneus longus and brevis

To test the strength of the peroneus longus and brevis muscles, stabilize the tibia and position the foot in plantar flexion (to eliminate activity of the lateral toe extensors). Resist the patient's attempt to evert the foot. Weakness indicates injury or dysfunction of the peroneal tendons or a lesion involving the superficial peroneal nerve.

Peroneal longus and brevis tendon

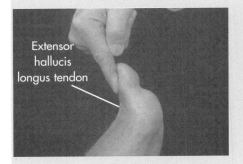

Extensor hallucis longus tendon

## Extensor hallucis longus

With the ankle in neutral, ask the patient to extend the great toe against resistance. Weakness indicates deep peroneal weakness. Note that the extensor hallucis muscle is the easiest and most specific muscle to assess for L5 nerve root dysfunction.

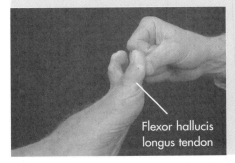

## Flexor hallucis longus

With the ankle in neutral, ask the patient to flex the great toe against resistance. Weakness indicates posterior tibialis weakness. The flexor hallucis muscle is the easiest and most specific muscle to assess for S1 nerve root dysfunction.

Flexor hallucis longus tendon

# Special Tests

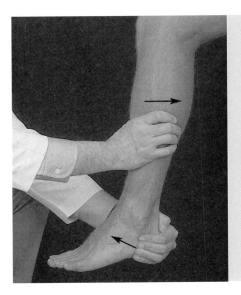

## Anterior drawer test

To test stability of the anterior talofibular ligament, place the ankle in approximately 20° of plantar flexion. Stabilize the tibia, grasp the hindfoot, and pull forward. Asymmetric or excessive motion will occur with chronic ankle laxity and severe acute ankle sprains.

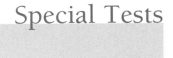

SECTION 7 | FOOT AND ANKLE

# Special Tests

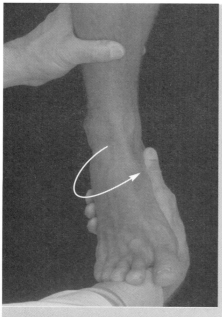

## Varus stress test

With the tibia stabilized and the ankle in neutral, grasp the calcaneus and invert the hindfoot. Excessive or asymmetric motion will occur with chronic laxity of the calcaneofibular ligament.

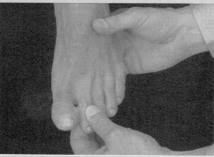

## MP instability

With the patient sitting, stabilize the foot, then grasp the proximal phalanx of each toe and move the joint in a dorsal (up) and plantar (down) direction. Instability is often present after chronic synovitis or a long-standing claw toe deformity. The second toe is most often affected.

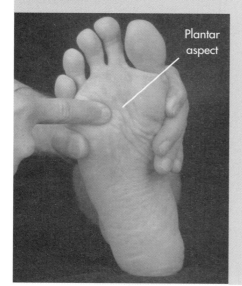

Plantar aspect

## Interdigital (Morton) neuroma test

Apply upward pressure between adjacent metatarsal heads, and then compress the metatarsals from side to side with the free hand. The upward pressure places the neuroma between the metatarsal heads, allowing it to be compressed during side-to-side compression. Interdigital neuromas are almost always located either between the second and third or between the third and fourth metatarsal heads.

# Sensory Testing

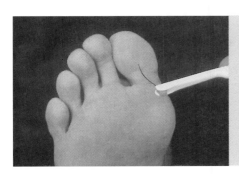

*Sensitivity test*
Use a 0.10-g, 5.07-diameter filament to identify protective sensation in a patient with diabetes.

# ACHILLES TENDON RUPTURE

**ICD-9 Code**

845.09
Sprains and strains of ankle and
foot; Achilles tendon

## SYNONYMS

Heel cord rupture

Tendoachilles rupture

## DEFINITION

Disruption of the Achilles tendon (heel cord) usually occurs 5 to 7 cm proximal to the insertion of tendon into the calcaneus. This condition commonly affects middle-aged men who play tennis, squash, basketball, or other quick, stop-and-go sports.

## CLINICAL SYMPTOMS

The sudden, severe calf pain typically is described as a "gunshot wound" or as a "direct hit from a racquet." The severe acute pain can resolve quickly and the injury can be misdiagnosed as an ankle sprain. When the rupture is missed, significant weakness that impairs ambulation will develop.

## TESTS

### PHYSICAL EXAMINATION

Swelling in the lower calf is common. The patient often has difficulty bearing weight and often has a palpable defect in the tendon. With the patient lying prone, the injured foot will rest 90° to the tibia, whereas a foot with an intact Achilles tendon will be in slight plantar flexion because of the resting tension in the tendon. Perform the Thompson test by placing the patient prone with the knee and ankle at 90°. The test also can be done with the patient kneeling on a chair. A squeeze of the calf normally results in passive plantar flexion of the ankle (**Figure 1**); a positive test is the absence of plantar flexion. The Thompson test is most reliable within 48 hours of the rupture.

### DIAGNOSTIC TESTS

None usually are needed.

## DIFFERENTIAL DIAGNOSIS

Achilles tendinitis (inflammation of the Achilles tendon without disruption)

Deep vein thrombosis (no history of injury, negative Thompson test)

Medial gastrocnemius tear (proximal partial tear of muscle and fascia of the medial head of the gastrocnemius-soleus complex)

Plantaris rupture (little evidence that this exists as an isolated entity)

Stress fracture of the tibia (constant pain over a localized area of the tibia)

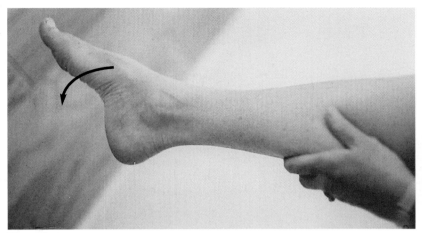

**Figure 1**
Squeezing the calf normally results in passive plantar flexion of the ankle.

*Reproduced with permission from Lutter LD: Hindfoot problems, in Heckman JD (ed): Instructional Course Lectures 42. Rosemont, IL, American Academy of Orthopaedic Surgeons, 1993, p 196.*

## ADVERSE OUTCOMES OF THE DISEASE

Weakness during the stance phase of gait and decreased athletic function are possible. Patients note that when they are walking, they feel as if they are on soft beach sand.

## TREATMENT

Nonoperative treatment consists of a graduated program of casting or bracing with the foot in plantar flexion. Surgical repair also requires cast immobilization. Choosing nonoperative or surgical treatment is based on the patient's level of activity, age, medical condition, and surgical risk. Delay in initiating either type of treatment complicates therapy because muscle contraction widens the gap at the tendon rupture. When either treatment is delayed beyond a few days, Achilles tendon rupture becomes more complicated to treat because retraction of the proximal muscle widens the gap. Whatever treatment modality is selected, stretching and strengthening exercises should be emphasized during the rehabilitation phase.

## ADVERSE OUTCOMES OF TREATMENT

Surgical risks include infection. A second rupture can occur with either type of treatment.

## REFERRAL DECISIONS/RED FLAGS

History of a sudden pop with pain and swelling in the calf indicates probable rupture of the Achilles tendon and the need for further evaluation within 24 hours.

# ANKLE SPRAIN

## ICD-9 Code
845.00
    Sprains and strains of the ankle
    and foot

## SYNONYMS
Inversion injury
Lateral collateral ligament tear

## DEFINITION
Approximately 25,000 people sprain an ankle every day. Ankle sprains are not always simple injuries. Residual symptoms occur in up to 40% of patients.

The lateral ligaments (anterior talofibular and calcaneofibular) are the only structures injured most of the time, but other ligament tears can occur with an inversion injury (**Figure 1**). Additional injury to the syndesmosis, the thick ligaments connecting the distal tibia and fibula, also may occur. This combined injury, referred to as a "high" ankle sprain, increases recovery time. Less common are associated injuries to the medial deltoid ligament.

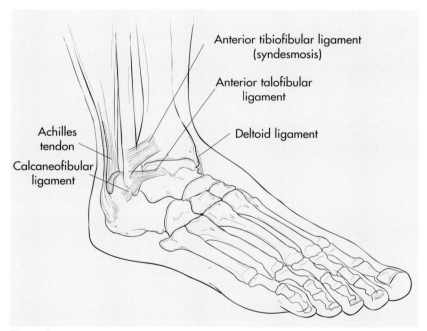

**Figure 1**
Ligaments of the ankle.
*Adapted with permission from The Physician and Sportsmedicine. McGraw Hill Companies, 1992.*

## CLINICAL SYMPTOMS
Pain over the injured ligaments, swelling, and loss of function are common. A severe sprain is more common in patients who report feeling a pop, followed

by immediate swelling and the inability to walk. Determine whether the patient has a history of ankle sprains and giving way; this history identifies an acute injury superimposed on chronic ankle instability.

## TESTS

### PHYSICAL EXAMINATION

Examination often reveals ecchymosis and swelling around the entire ankle joint, not just the lateral side. Tenderness on palpation over the anterior talofibular and calcaneofibular ligaments can help identify which ligaments are injured. Palpate the lateral and medial malleoli and the base of the fifth metatarsal for crepitation or tenderness caused by a fracture.

Injury to the syndesmosis is suggested by two tests: the squeeze test and the external rotation test. The squeeze test is performed by compressing the tibia and fibula at the midcalf. The external rotation test is performed by placing the ankle in dorsiflexion and then externally rotating the foot. A positive result is indicated by the presence of pain over the distal tibiofibular junction (syndesmosis).

### DIAGNOSTIC TESTS

When tenderness is present over the distal fibula, ankle joint, syndesmosis, or other bony structure, radiographs of the ankle and/or foot are needed to rule out a fracture. Radiographs also are indicated when the patient has marked swelling and cannot bear weight on the affected extremity.

## DIFFERENTIAL DIAGNOSIS

Fracture of the calcaneus, talus, lateral malleolus, or base of the fifth metatarsal (focal tenderness over the fractured anatomic structure, evident on radiographs)

Fracture of the lateral process of the talus (focal tenderness, swelling below the fibula)

Fracture of the proximal fibula (Maisonneuve fracture associated with tear of deltoid and disruption of syndesmotic ligament)

Osteochondral fracture of the talar dome (evident on ankle radiographs, bone scan, or by MRI)

Peroneal tendon tear or subluxation (retrofibular tenderness and swelling)

## ADVERSE OUTCOMES OF THE DISEASE

An untreated severe sprain can result in chronic pain, instability, and the possibility of ankle arthritis. Chronic instability may be secondary to incomplete rehabilitation.

## TREATMENT

The goal of treatment is to prevent chronic pain and instability. Phase 1 consists of NSAIDs, ice, compression, and elevation. The use of a brace or air stirrup is indicated for protection and to promote soft-tissue healing (**Figure 2**). Encourage weight bearing as tolerated, with the use of crutches as needed. Forty-eight hours after the injury, contrast baths can help decrease swelling

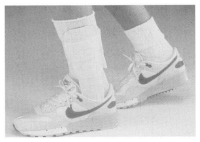

**Figure 2**
An air stirrup-type ankle brace.

(see Contrast Baths). For severe sprains, the use of a cast or cast boot for 3 weeks may facilitate walking and healing.

Phase 2 begins when the patient can bear weight without increased pain or swelling, usually 2 to 4 weeks after the injury. Continue use of the air stirrup or brace. Begin exercises to increase peroneal and dorsiflexor strength; stretching the Achilles tendon also should be done. Continue this phase until the patient has full range of motion and 80% of normal ankle strength. Plantar flexion exercises are not included in the exercise program because they place the ankle in a position of least stability.

Phase 3 usually begins 4 to 6 weeks after injury. This phase of functional conditioning includes proprioception, agility, and endurance training. Exercises that are helpful for proprioception include standing on the sprained ankle with the opposite foot elevated and the eyes closed. Running in progressively smaller figures-of-8 is excellent for agility and peroneal strength. During this time, the patient should be weaned from the air stirrup or ankle brace.

This three-phase treatment program can take only 2 weeks to complete for minor sprains or up to 6 to 8 weeks for severe injuries. For athletes with moderate to severe sprains who are returning to sports, the use of a functional brace or air stirrup, or taping on a long-term basis, will help prevent recurrent injury. The use of a brace is particularly indicated for athletes in sports associated with a high risk for ankle sprains, such as basketball, volleyball, and soccer. Exercises during this final phase should include peroneal strengthening in both dorsiflexion and plantar flexion, as well as continued Achilles tendon stretching.

## ADVERSE OUTCOMES OF TREATMENT

NSAIDs can cause gastric, renal, or hepatic complications. Most ankle sprains can be treated with functional immobilization, such as an air stirrup. Casting and ankle immobilization for more than 3 weeks may cause stiffness and a slower return to normal activity.

## REFERRAL DECISIONS/RED FLAGS

Fractures of the foot and ankle, tears or subluxation of the peroneal tendons, nerve injury, a history of repeated giving way (chronic instability), and failure to improve in 6 weeks with appropriate treatment all indicate serious injury and the need for further evaluation.

# PROCEDURE

## CONTRAST BATHS

*MATERIALS*

Two buckets

Ice

Warm water

*STEP 1*

To decrease inflammation in the foot, ankle, or hand, first soak the affected area in a cold-water bath. The water temperature should be as cold as can be tolerated; adding several small ice cubes is usually the best method of cooling the water. Soak for 30 seconds.

*STEP 2*

Immediately place the affected area into a second bucket filled with water that is as warm as tolerated, generally around 104°F (40°C). Soak for 30 seconds.

*STEP 3*

Place the affected area back into the cold water for 30 seconds. Continue to alternate between the cold and warm water for a total of 5 minutes. The first and last soaks should be in the cold water.

### AFTERCARE/PATIENT INSTRUCTIONS

Advise the patient that, ideally, the contrast baths should be repeated three times a day. If that is not possible, then once in the morning and once in the evening usually is sufficient. Patients with a peripheral neuropathy, decreased sensibility, or vascular insufficiency should be careful to avoid injury from water of extreme temperature.

SECTION 7 | FOOT AND ANKLE

# ARTHRITIS OF THE FOOT AND ANKLE

## ICD-9 Codes

714.0
　Rheumatoid arthritis
715.17
　Osteoarthritis, localized, primary, ankle and foot
715.27
　Osteoarthritis, localized, secondary, ankle and foot
716.17
　Traumatic arthritis

## SYNONYMS

Osteoarthritis

Posttraumatic arthritis

## DEFINITION

The most common types of arthritis of the foot and ankle are osteoarthritis (degenerative arthritis) and traumatic arthritis. Frequent locations of arthritis in the foot and ankle are the first metatarsophalangeal (MP) joint of the great toe, the midfoot (metatarsocunieform or Lisfranc joint), the talonavicular joint, the subtalar (talocalcaneal) joint, and the ankle joint (**Figure 1**).

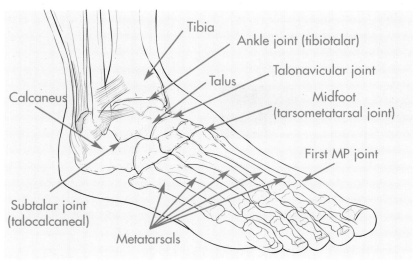

**Figure 1**
Common sites of foot and ankle arthritis.

## CLINICAL SYMPTOMS

Patients with arthritis of the first MP joint report pain, loss of dorsiflexion, and swelling of the great toe joint (see Hallux Rigidus, pp 463-465).

Midfoot osteoarthritis commonly occurs in older patients and also after a Lisfranc (tarsometatarsal) dislocation. The patient usually reports diffuse aching in the midfoot foot that worsens with prolonged walking or standing and difficulty pushing off with the foot.

Talonavicular arthritis causes focal pain over the joint (medial aspect of the hindfoot). This is a common site for arthritis in patients with rheumatoid arthritis.

Subtalar arthritis produces pain below the medial malleolus and distal fibula and frequently is a result of calcaneal fractures. Difficulty walking on uneven surfaces (such as sand or rocky terrain) results because this joint motion is primarily inversion and eversion of the foot.

Most patients with ankle arthritis have a history of trauma. Pain, swelling, and stiffness in the anterior ankle are the common complaints. Patients with ankle arthritis have difficulty moving the ankle up and down and tend to walk with the leg externally rotated.

## TESTS

### PHYSICAL EXAMINATION

With hallux rigidus, loss of motion in the first MP joint and difficulty pushing off with the great toe are common. Patients with midfoot arthritis have tenderness and often a dorsal bump on palpation of the midfoot. Patients with talonavicular or talocalcaneal arthritis may show a loss of inversion and eversion of the hindfoot compared with the opposite foot; however, ankle motion is relatively normal. Patients with ankle arthritis have swelling, loss of ankle motion, and often walk with the leg externally rotated.

### DIAGNOSTIC TESTS

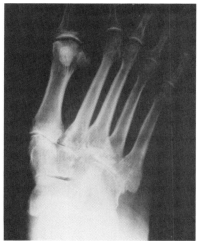

**Figure 2**
Primary degenerative arthritis of the midfoot with involvement of all columns.

*Reproduced with permission from Beaman DN, Saltzman CL, Arthritis of the midfoot, in Mizel MS, Miller RA, Scioli (eds) OKU Foot and Ankle 2. Rosemont, IL, American Academy of Orthopaedic Surgeons, 1998, p 294.*

Weight-bearing radiographs reveal the typical sign of degenerative or traumatic arthritis, including osteophytes (spurs) and joint space narrowing. The first MP joint usually shows dorsal osteophytes protruding from the metatarsal head. In midfoot arthritis, joint space narrowing is especially evident at the second tarsometatarsal joint (**Figure 2**). Talonavicular arthritis is best viewed on an AP radiograph of the foot. With talocalcaneal arthritis, the lateral view of the foot reveals loss of the normal talocalcaneal joint space. Ankle arthritis usually causes loss of joint space, which can be seen on both AP (**Figure 3**) and lateral ankle views.

CT can be helpful when the extent of arthritis is uncertain, especially in the midfoot, where the bony anatomy is sometimes difficult to view on plain radiographs.

## DIFFERENTIAL DIAGNOSIS

Charcot arthropathy (history of diabetes, swelling that is disproportionate to symptoms)

Gout (redness and swelling)

Tendinitis (normal radiograph)

## ADVERSE OUTCOMES OF THE DISEASE

Pain and difficulty with ambulation are common with untreated foot and ankle arthritis.

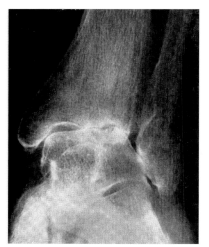

**Figure 3**
AP view of ankle showing loss of joint space and ankle arthritis.

## Treatment

Initial therapy consists of shoe modifications, orthotic inserts, and NSAIDs.

A stiff-soled shoe with a rocker bottom will help relieve symptoms in patients with hallux rigidus.

Midfoot arthritis can be temporized with a rigid custom orthotic insert or a steel shank inserted into the sole of the shoe. Patients with refractory symptoms will benefit from a surgical midfoot fusion.

Talonavicular and subtalar arthritis can be temporized with a medial longitudinal arch support or the more rigid UCBL (University of California Biomechanics Laboratory) orthoses. Corticosteroid injections and NSAIDs can be helpful. Predictable pain relief can be obtained with subtalar arthrodesis. Ankle motion is retained after a subtalar fusion.

Ankle arthritis is treated initially with a custom-molded ankle-foot orthosis (AFO) and NSAIDs. Injection of a corticosteroid also may be beneficial (see Ankle Joint Injection, pp 429-430). In mild to moderate cases, debridement of the joint may defer the need for fusion. Ankle arthrodesis will benefit patients with refractory symptoms. Function is surprisingly good after an ankle fusion because midfoot dorsiflexion and plantar flexion increase. Total ankle replacement remains an investigational technique.

## Adverse outcomes of treatment

Infection, nonunion, and persistent pain can occur after foot and ankle fusions.

## Referral decisions/Red flags

Acute onset of pain with no patient history of trauma should raise suspicion of a stress fracture. Persistent and disabling pain needs further evaluation. Chronic symptoms can be relieved by surgical fusion.

# PROCEDURE

## ANKLE JOINT INJECTION

### MATERIALS

Sterile gloves

Bactericidal skin preparation solution

Two 3-mL syringes

One 22-gauge needle

3 mL of 1% lidocaine

1 mL of 40 mg/mL corticosteroid preparation without epinephrine

Sterile adhesive dressing

### STEP 1

Wear protective gloves at all times during this procedure and use sterile technique.

### STEP 2

Cleanse the skin with a bactericidal skin preparation.

### STEP 3

Palpate the soft spot over the ankle joint just medial to the anterior tibial tendon (**Figure 1**). Use a 3-mL syringe with a 22-gauge needle, and inject 2 mL of the 1% lidocaine anesthetic into the subcutaneous tissue of the soft spot.

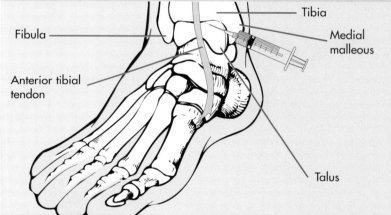

**Figure 1**
Proper location for injection.

Fibula • Anterior tibial tendon • Tibia • Medial malleous • Talus

### STEP 4

Advance the needle into the joint by directing the needle slightly laterally and superiorly. Inject 1 mL of 1% lidocaine anesthetic. If the needle is in the joint, injection of the fluid should meet no resistance. Leave the needle in place and exchange the syringe.

### STEP 5

Inject 1 mL of 40 mg/mL corticosteroid preparation. Injection of the fluid should meet no resistance. Withdraw the needle.

### STEP 6

Dress the puncture wound with sterile adhesive dressing.

# ANKLE JOINT INJECTION (CONTINUED)

## ADVERSE OUTCOMES

Injury to the distal branch of the saphenous nerve is possible. Slow atrophy at the site of the injection is possible secondary to subcutaneous steroid deposition.

## AFTERCARE/PATIENT INSTRUCTIONS

Remind the patient that one third of patients may experience a flare-up of symptoms with increased joint pain for 1 to 2 days. NSAIDs or analgesics may be given during this period. Ice may be helpful for the first 24 hours.

# BUNIONETTE

ICD-9 Code
727.1
Bunion

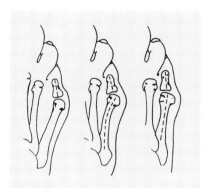

**Figure 1**
Angles measured in the assessment of a bunionette deformity.

*Reproduced with permission from Coughlin MJ: The bunionette deformity: Etiology and treatment, in Gould JS (ed): Operative Foot Surgery. Philadelphia, PA, WB Saunders, 1994, p 54.*

## SYNONYM

Tailor's bunion

## DEFINITION

A bunionette, sometimes referred to as a tailor's bunion, is a deformity of the fifth metatarsophalangeal (MP) joint that is analogous to a bunion (hallux valgus) deformity of the great toe. A bunionette is characterized by prominence of the lateral aspect of the fifth metatarsal head and medial deviation of the small toe (**Figure 1**). A bunionette is associated with frequent wearing of tight, narrow, pointed-toe shoes.

## CLINICAL SYMPTOMS

Patients report pain and problems finding comfortable shoes.

## TESTS

### PHYSICAL EXAMINATION

Deformity is evident on physical examination. An overlying hard corn is frequently present.

### DIAGNOSTIC TESTS

Weight-bearing AP radiographs will show medial deviation of the fifth proximal phalanx and lateral deviation of the fifth metatarsal shaft and/or a prominence on the lateral aspect of the fifth metatarsal head. The joint usually is normal.

## DIFFERENTIAL DIAGNOSIS

Cavovarus foot deformity (leading to excessive weight bearing and pain over the fifth metatarsal)

Inflammatory arthropathy (rheumatoid arthritis, leading to deviation of the small toe)

## ADVERSE OUTCOMES OF THE DISEASE

The most common problem is persistent pain aggravated by shoe wear. Patients also can have associated hard and soft corns, with possible ulceration and infection.

## TREATMENT

Patients should be advised to select proper shoes with a soft upper and a roomy toe box. A shoe repair shop can stretch the shoe over the bunionette. A modified metatarsal pad also can help shift pressure off the fifth metatarsal head. The pad is cut lengthwise on a diagonal, then applied to the lateral aspect of the toe box, just proximal to the bunionette prominence (see Application of a Metatarsal Pad, p 433). A medial longitudinal arch support can help a patient who has a flexible flatfoot. This orthotic device rotates the forefoot slightly, which decreases direct pressure over the bunionette prominence.

With continued symptoms, surgical excision of the bunionette or realignment osteotomy of the fifth metatarsal may be required.

## ADVERSE OUTCOMES OF TREATMENT

Persistent pain despite metatarsal pad application is possible. Surgical risks include persistent pain, infection, incomplete correction, and neuroma formation from injury to the cutaneous nerves in the surgical field.

## REFERRAL DECISIONS/RED FLAGS

Failure of nonoperative treatment indicates the need for further evaluation.

# PROCEDURE

## APPLICATION OF A METATARSAL PAD

### MATERIALS

Felt, silicone, or gel metatarsal pad

Temporary marker (lipstick, eyeliner)

### STEP 1

Ask the patient to mark the painful spot on the bottom of the foot with a material that transfers easily, such as lipstick or eyeliner (**Figure 1**). The mark should be approximately 0.5 cm square.

### STEP 2

Instruct the patient to stand in a shoe, without socks, to transfer the mark to the inside of the shoe.

### STEP 3

Place a metatarsal pad into the shoe just proximal to (toward the heel), not directly under, the mark (**Figure 2**). This ensures that the painful area is suspended by the proximally placed pad.

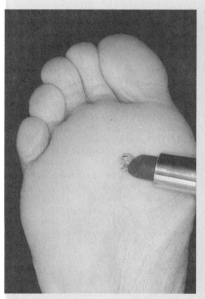

**Figure 1**
Marking the painful area.

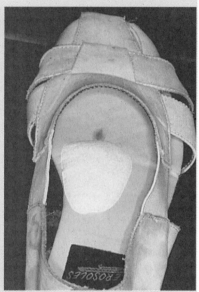

**Figure 2**
Placing the metatarsal pad.

Prefabricated, off-the-shelf felt or gel pads are easy to use, inexpensive, and effective, and they come in different sizes to accommodate different-sized lesions and feet.

### AFTERCARE/PATIENT INSTRUCTIONS

If the pad is effective, a custom-made orthotic can be fabricated that can be transferred from shoe to shoe.

# CHRONIC LATERAL ANKLE PAIN

### ICD-9 Codes
715.17
  Osteoarthritis, localized, primary, foot and ankle
718.87
  Ankle/foot instability
719.47
  Pain in joint; foot and ankle
726.79
  Peroneal tenosynovitis
727.06
  Tenosynovitis and synovitis of foot and ankle

## DEFINITION

Chronic pain on the lateral aspect of the ankle is a common complaint that often follows an inversion injury. However, other conditions may cause chronic lateral ankle pain and should be considered in the differential diagnosis.

## CLINICAL SYMPTOMS

Patients typically report pain on the lateral aspect of the ankle. Episodes of giving way and repeated sprains are typically associated with instability. Between sprains, however, the patient will have periods that are symptom-free. Patients with a bone, cartilage, or tendon lesion often report constant, dull pain over the involved area.

## TESTS

### PHYSICAL EXAMINATION

Identifying focal tenderness using one finger is the key element of the examination and can often identify the source of the problem. Identify any area of swelling. Range of motion should be assessed for both the ankle and subtalar joints. Assess laxity of the ankle and subtalar joints. Test sensation of the sural and superficial peroneal nerves.

Lidocaine injections can be very helpful in differentiating the source of a patient's symptoms. An intra-articular injection of 5 mL of 1% lidocaine into the ankle joint, for example, should provide transient pain relief in a patient with anterolateral impingement syndrome. Other common areas for differential injection include the subtalar joint and peroneal sheath.

### DIAGNOSTIC TESTS

AP, lateral, and mortise radiographs of the ankle joint are obtained for suspected ankle pathology. AP, lateral, and oblique radiographs of the foot are obtained for suspected foot pathology. If ankle or subtalar joint laxity is suspected, stress radiographs (varus and anterior) are helpful and should often include comparison stress views of the opposite, uninjured side. If the radiographs are normal, and occult bony pathology is suspected, a technetium 99m bone scan, limited to AP and lateral views of both feet and ankles, will identify the lesion. Although not specific, the bone scan is very sensitive and will detect most bony lesions, including occult fractures, arthritic changes, and tumors. If the bone scan is abnormal and an occult fracture is suspected, CT with thin cuts through the area in question should be diagnostic. If a stress fracture or tendon injury is suspected (eg, tenosynovitis, a partial tear, or rupture of a tendon), MRI is appropriate. In these cases, the radiologist should be directed to the specific area of the tendon in question.

# DIFFERENTIAL DIAGNOSIS

## ANTEROLATERAL IMPINGEMENT SYNDROME

Anterolateral impingement of the talus with inversion (lateral gutter syndrome) occurs after an inversion ankle sprain. The borders of the lateral gutter of the ankle include the talus medially, fibula laterally, and tibia superiorly, bordered by the anterior/inferior tibiofibular ligament. Following a sprain, chronic scar tissue in the lateral gutter causes the anterolateral impingement. This condition is common in athletes who often report pain and tenderness along the anterolateral aspect of the ankle. The pain is absent at rest and present with activities. These patients usually do not report buckling or giving way, or show any signs of instability. Examination reveals tenderness and swelling along the anterior talofibular ligament and lateral gutter. Radiographs, MRI, technetium 99m bone scan, and CT scan appear normal, so this condition is often overlooked. An intra-articular injection of lidocaine will provide transient pain relief. Initial treatment should include an anti-inflammatory medication, physical therapy, and a possible steroid injection. Arthroscopic debridement of the lateral gutter provides definitive treatment.

## CHRONIC ANKLE/SUBTALAR INSTABILITY

Following an inversion sprain, chronic instability of the ankle and /or subtalar joint may develop. These patients report frequent turning and generalized weakness in the ankle and an inability to return to full sports or daily activities. The cause can be inadequate rehabilitation or inadequate healing, with subsequent attenuation of one or more ligaments. After a moderate to severe inversion injury, a patient will often lose proprioception, range of motion, and muscle strength. A mild contracture of the Achilles tendon also can develop. Six weeks of physical therapy, directed specifically at increasing proprioception and range of motion, will often benefit these patients. The use of an ankle brace during sports activities also can be of significant benefit. If symptoms persist, further evaluation is required. Anterior drawer and inversion stress tests should be assessed. Stress radiographs and diagnostic injections can be helpful. Reconstruction of the ligaments or checkrein tenodesis transfers are the two types of operative management.

## NERVE INJURY

Injury by direct blow, stretch, entrapment, or even transection of the superficial peroneal or sural nerves can be a cause of chronic lateral ankle pain. Repetitive stretching or nerve compression typically causes symptoms over the site of a fascial band or bony ridge. Patients report diffuse dull, achy pain on the lateral aspect of the ankle, and burning, tingling, or radiating pain in the nerve distribution. Plantar flexion and inversion of the ankle and foot will often aggravate the symptoms. Focal tenderness and radiating paresthesias with percussion over the site of nerve injury (Tinel sign) is diagnostic. A more generalized neurologic examination should include an evaluation of the L4, L5, and S1 nerve roots to rule out a proximal nerve lesion. Electromyography and nerve conduction velocity studies often are not helpful in the diagnosis of superficial peroneal or sural nerve lesions. Many of these injuries will resolve spontaneously but some require operative intervention.

## OCCULT BONY PATHOLOGY

Routine radiographs identify most fractures in the foot and ankle, but osteochondral lesions of the talus, avulsion fractures of the calcaneus, lateral process fractures of the talus, and stress fractures of the fibula may not be obvious. A bone scan is an excellent initial study if these injuries are suspected. Once diagnosed, an occult bony lesion often can be treated with 4 to 6 weeks of immobilization. For persistent symptoms, excision of a loose bone fragment, arthroscopic debridement of an osteochondral lesion, or possible surgical fusion of an arthritic joint may be required.

## PERONEAL TENOSYNOVITIS/PERONEAL TENDON SUBLUXATION

A common cause of chronic lateral ankle pain is tenosynovitis from a tear or subluxation of one of the peroneal tendons. The peroneus brevis is most commonly affected by a tear, usually just posterior to the tip of the fibula. Patients report chronic retromalleolar swelling, pain, and tenderness. Recurrent subluxation of the peroneal tendons over the lateral ridge of the fibula also may be associated with this condition. MRI is helpful in the evaluation of peroneal pathology. A simple tenosynovitis may be treated with cast immobilization for 4 to 6 weeks. However, a tear or chronic subluxation of the tendon usually requires operative treatment.

## SUBTALAR JOINT ARTHRITIS

Early arthritis of the subtalar joint may be difficult to identify. These patients present with chronic lateral ankle pain that is aggravated by standing and walking activities, particularly on uneven terrain. Examination reveals limited inversion and eversion. Special radiographic views and/or differential injections may be required to confirm early arthritis in this joint.

## SUBTALAR JOINT SYNOVITIS/SINUS TARSI SYNDROME

Similar to anterolateral impingement syndrome, this condition can be characterized by a chronic synovitis of the subtalar joint, often following an inversion injury. Examination reveals focal pain over the lateral entrance to the sinus tarsi, which is the lateral entrance to the subtalar joint. Patients often have slight restriction and discomfort with passive subtalar motion. Diagnostic studies usually are normal, although MRI may detect chronic inflammation within the subtalar joint. The treatment is similar to lateral gutter syndrome. Surgical debridement of the subtalar joint will often be curative.

# Corns and Calluses

| ICD-9 Code |
| --- |
| 700 |
| Corns and calluses |

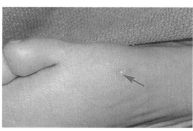

**Figure 1**
Clinical appearance of a seed callus beneath the fifth metatarsal head.

*Adapted with permission from Donley BG, Gates NT: Interdigital corns, in Myerson MS (ed): Foot and Ankle Clinics: Lesser Toe Deformities. Philadelphia, PA, WB Saunders, 1998, vol 3, no 2, p 296.*

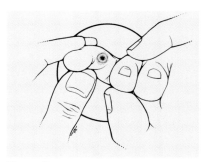

**Figure 2**
Soft interdigital corn on the medial aspect of small toe.

*Adapted with permission from Donley BG, Gates NT: Interdigital corns, in Myerson MS (ed): Foot and Ankle Clinics: Lesser Toe Deformities. Philadelphia, PA, WB Saunders, 1998, vol 3, no 2, p 296.*

## Synonyms

Clavus
Callosity
Heloma durum
Heloma molle

## Definition

Callus is a hyperkeratotic lesion of the skin that forms in response to excessive pressure over a bony prominence. When the callus forms on a toe, it is called a corn. When it forms elsewhere (as under a metatarsal head), it is called a callus. A persistent callus on the sole of the forefoot also is referred to as intractable plantar keratosis (**Figure 1**).

A callus usually occurs beneath the metatarsal heads and is associated with metatarsalgia, a general term for pain overlying one or several of the metatarsal heads. Pain can be caused by the callus itself or by some other manifestation of chronic pressure overload of the metatarsal head, such as synovitis of the joint, attritional tearing of the metatarsophalangeal ligaments, or claw toe deformity. Pressure overload also may be secondary to a cavus foot or wearing high-heeled shoes.

Corns usually occur from inappropriately tight shoe wear, with subsequent development of toe deformities (hammer toe, bunionette, claw toe). Hard corns (heloma durum) occur over bony prominences, whereas soft corns (heloma molle) develop between the toes in the web space (**Figure 2**). Periungual corns are small but painful lesions that occur at the edge of a nail, often in association with a mallet toe or improper shoe fit.

## Clinical symptoms

Patients with corns and calluses typically report pain with walking or wearing shoes.

## Tests

### Physical examination

The pared surface of a callus has a uniform waxy appearance. Warts and calluses generally can be distinguished by palpation. Warts generally are tender when pinched from side to side, whereas corns and calluses are tender with direct pressure. Plantar warts usually do not develop over a bony prominence. Corns occur over or between the toes.

When tenderness exists over the dorsal surface of the MP joint, perform the drawer test to assess joint instability.

## DIAGNOSTIC TESTS

None

## DIFFERENTIAL DIAGNOSIS

Foreign body (history of penetrating wound)

Morton neuroma (perineural fibrosis occurring between the third and fourth metatarsal heads or second and third metatarsal heads, no callus)

Plantar warts (virus lesions occurring on non–weight-bearing areas, may have a nearby satellite lesion, and pared surface has multiple tiny points of hemorrhage near the base)

Synovitis of the MP joint (tenderness over the dorsal MP joint, no plantar callus, painful drawer test)

## ADVERSE OUTCOMES OF THE DISEASE

Persistent pain or ulceration of the skin can develop. Metatarsalgia, when caused by ligament tears or MP synovitis, can result in gradual subluxation of the joint and deformity of the toe.

## TREATMENT

Paring and pressure relief are the principal treatment of corns (see Trimming a Corn or Callus, pp 440-441). Paring involves shaving the lesion layer by layer with a scalpel after the skin is prepared with alcohol or iodine. The goal is to remove enough of the avascular keratin to restore a more normal contour to the skin without drawing blood. This can be accomplished using a #15 blade, without anesthetic, when performed gradually and with care. Paring also provides excellent short-term pain relief. Patients then should be instructed in self-care, using a pumice stone or callus file to regularly debride these lesions after soaking the foot or after a shower.

Treatment of metatarsalgia includes use of a metatarsal pad (see Application of a Metatarsal Pad, pp 433-434), trimming the callus/corn, and correction of associated problems, such as improper shoe fit and claw toe deformities. Pressure is relieved by wearing roomier shoes, using commercially available silicone cushions, or inserting small foam donut pads or metatarsal pads to shift pressure from the lesion. For soft corns, a small amount of lamb's wool or a silicone spacer between the toes can wick away moisture and help cushion the area.

When nonoperative measures fail, surgical treatment to remove the underlying bony prominences is indicated. With soft corns, syndactylization (creating a partial webbing of the involved toes) may be required.

## ADVERSE OUTCOMES OF TREATMENT

Infection and bleeding can occur from excessively deep paring. Paring a soft corn can be especially difficult because of its awkward location in the web space. Medicated keratolytic corn pads often cause maceration and can result in infection; therefore, these pads are probably best avoided.

## Referral decisions/Red flags

Failure to respond to nonoperative treatment, presence of ulceration, and/or infection are indications for further evaluation of hyperkeratotic lesions. Deformity or persistent metatarsalgia also requires further evaluation.

# PROCEDURE

## TRIMMING A CORN OR CALLUS

### MATERIALS

Sterile gloves

Scalpel with #15 or #17 blade

### STEP 1

Wear protective gloves at all times during the procedure, and use excellent lighting and sterile technique.

### STEP 2

Anesthesia is not required to trim a corn or callus; however, prior to the procedure, the patient should soak the foot in water for several minutes to soften the skin.

### STEP 3

Place the blade tangential to the lesion to shave the excess skin (**Figure 1**). Bleeding should not occur.

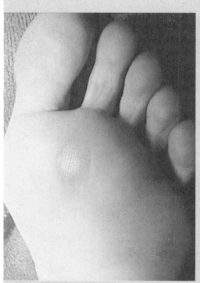 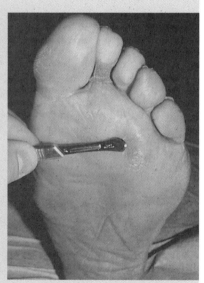

**Figure 1**
Trimming a callus A, A diffuse callus. B, Placement of the blade.

### STEP 4

Take special care with a corn on the toe because the skin is thin and can be fragile. Shell out several millimeters of the hard central core of a plantar callus with the sharp tip of the blade.

# TRIMMING A CORN OR CALLUS (CONTINUED)

## ADVERSE OUTCOMES

Paring down a corn or callus too deeply may expose subcutaneous tissue. If bleeding occurs, the corn or callus has been trimmed too deeply. A wart tends to bleed because of its hypervascularity.

## AFTERCARE/PATIENT INSTRUCTIONS

Instruct the patient to continue to pare down the lesion daily after a shower or bath with a pumice stone or nail file.

# THE DIABETIC FOOT

**ICD-9 Code**

**713.5**
Arthropathy associated with neuro-logic disorders

## SYNONYMS

Charcot arthropathy
Neuropathic foot

## DEFINITION

Diabetes is a group of metabolic disorders characterized by high blood glucose levels. The four major categories are type 1 (insulin-dependent diabetes mellitus), type 2 (non–insulin-dependent diabetes mellitus), gestational diabetes mellitus, and diabetes secondary to other conditions. Types 1 and 2 are the most common forms, with approximately 5% to 10% of all cases of diabetes identified as type 1 and 85% to 90% as type 2.

Diabetic foot problems are a major health problem in the United States and are a common cause of hospitalization and amputation. Patients present with skin ulceration, infection, and/or Charcot arthropathy. The primary etiology is peripheral nerve impairment that results in loss of protective sensation, autonomic dysfunction, and/or motor impairment. With inadequate sensory feedback, skin breakdown results from unperceived repetitive trauma. Vascular insufficiency also may contribute to foot problems in patients with diabetes.

Patients with autonomic dysfunction have dry, scaly, and cracking skin, a condition that predisposes the skin to ulceration.

Motor neuropathy leads to weakness of the intrinsic muscles of the foot, claw toe deformities, subluxation or dislocation of the metatarsophalangeal (MP) joints, abnormal plantar positioning of the metatarsal heads, increased pressure on the sole of the foot, skin breakdown, ulcers, deep infections, and osteomyelitis. Extrinsic forces, such as tight shoes, can contribute to skin breakdown.

Charcot arthropathy results from the disturbance of normal pain and proprioceptive sensation. The result is progressive disruption of joint stability and severe bony deformities.

## CLINICAL SYMPTOMS

Patients may have no symptoms or they may report foot pain at night, characterized as burning and tingling secondary to neuritic involvement. With abnormal areas of pressure, skin breakdown follows, leading to a painless ulcer. Deep infections and osteomyelitis may subsequently develop, usually with a sudden increase in swelling, redness, and drainage and sometimes pain.

Patients with Charcot arthropathy have noticeable swelling, warmth, and redness (**Figure 1**), even though pain is only mild or absent. Charcot arthropathy may be misdiagnosed as cellulitis, osteomyelitis, or gout.

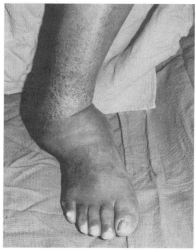

**Figure 1**
Severe deformity from Charcot breakdown of the ankle joint.

*Reproduced with permission from Harrelson JM: The diabetic foot: Charcot arthropathy, in Heckman JD (ed): Instructional Course Lectures 42. Park Ridge, IL, American Academy of Orthopaedic Surgeons, 1993, p 144.*

# TESTS

## PHYSICAL EXAMINATION

A thorough evaluation of the feet is an essential component of the examination of patients with diabetes. A significant number of amputations can be avoided simply by preventive measures and early treatment of skin lesions. Light touch should be tested. Protective foot care and wearing well-cushioned shoes is particularly necessary in patients who cannot feel a 10-g, 5.07-diameter, nylon filament applied to the plantar aspect of the foot.

Diabetic ulcers are insensate and can be easily inspected and probed to determine depth and size. If bone can be probed, osteomyelitis is likely to be present.

Examination of a Charcot joint reveals a hot, red, swollen foot with intact skin. Pulses usually are strong in patients with Charcot arthropathy. A Charcot foot elevated above the heart for 1 minute will lose its redness, whereas a foot affected by cellulitis, soft-tissue abscess, and/or osteomyelitis will not.

## DIAGNOSTIC TESTS

Plain radiographs are necessary to help rule out osteomyelitis and Charcot arthropathy (**Figure 2**). Vascular studies are appropriate when pulses are absent or when the patient has a nonhealing ulcer. MRI can help confirm a deep abscess or osteomyelitis but usually is not necessary. Combined technetium-iridium bone scans have been used in difficult cases to differentiate Charcot arthropathy from osteomyelitis.

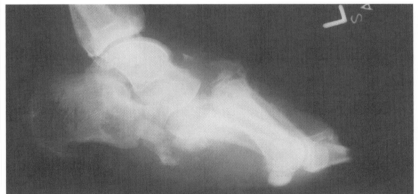

**Figure 2**
Lateral radiograph showing Charcot degeneration of the midfoot.

*Reproduced with permission from Harrelson JM: The diabetic foot: Charcot arthropathy, in Heckman JD (ed): Instructional Course Lectures 42. Park Ridge, IL, American Academy of Orthopaedic Surgeons, 1993, p 144.*

# DIFFERENTIAL DIAGNOSIS

Cellulitis (soft-tissue infection, most likely associated with skin breakdown)

Gout (painful lesion, increased serum uric acid)

Osteomyelitis (usually beneath an open skin ulcer)

Other neuropathies (Charcot-Marie-Tooth disease, alcoholic neuropathy, spinal cord neuropathy)

## ADVERSE OUTCOMES OF THE DISEASE

Skin ulceration, Charcot joint, chronic osteomyelitis, and gangrene all occur in the diabetic foot. Amputation may be necessary.

## TREATMENT

The goal of treatment is patient education and prevention (see Care of Diabetic Feet, pp 445-447). Good control of serum glucose is paramount. Any neuropathy that has occurred is irreversible. When a problem exists, aggressive treatment is needed to avoid a more serious and debilitating situation. The appearance of a callus is the first phase of a diabetic ulcer and signals the need for adaptive shoe wear (cushioned shoes and soft, molded insoles) and close follow-up.

Treatment of a diabetic ulcer requires removing the pressure causing the ulcer, allowing the ulcer to heal, and prescribing optimal shoe wear to prevent recurrence. Accommodative shoe wear, an orthotic device, and total contact casting can be used for superficial ulcerations. For deeper ulcerations, these measures are often inadequate, and surgery may be required. An associated equinus contracture should be corrected by serial casting or percutaneous heel cord lengthening.

Treatment of a deep infection must be aggressive and prompt. The infection is often polymicrobial. Skin swab cultures are inaccurate. Bone biopsy provides more definitive cultures to direct antibiotic therapy. Any abscess should be considered an emergency and drained surgically. Osteomyelitis can be treated surgically with debridement of the affected bone. Digit or ray (toe plus metatarsal) amputation is often needed to eradicate osteomyelitis of the toes or metatarsal heads.

In the initial stage of a Charcot joint, the foot and ankle need to be unweighted and stabilized, usually with a cast. After the acute swelling and erythema have subsided, the patient can begin bearing weight with continued use of a cast or customized, clamshell short leg brace. The patient must be advised that the period of immobilization can be lengthy, often up to 12 months, and that a permanent brace might be required for ambulation. When Charcot arthropathy is properly recognized and treated, acceptable limb salvage can be achieved. Occasionally, surgical reconstruction by arthrodesis is needed for severe deformity that cannot be treated with bracing.

## ADVERSE OUTCOMES OF TREATMENT

The adverse outcomes of treatment are the same as those for diabetes and, in addition, include surgical complications of infection, ischemia, and death.

## REFERRAL DECISIONS/RED FLAGS

Unexplained pain in a diabetic foot, sudden onset of swelling and pain, and nonhealing ulcerations all signal the need for further evaluation.

## ACKNOWLEDGMENT

Information regarding the sensory testing nylon filament was provided by the Filament Project, 5445 Point Clair Road, Caryville, LA 70721.

# PROCEDURE

## CARE OF DIABETIC FEET

### CARE OF THE FEET

1. Never walk barefoot; always wear shoes or slippers.

2. Wash feet daily with mild soap and water.

   - Always test the water temperature with your hands or elbows before putting your feet in the water.
   - After washing, pat your feet dry; do not rub vigorously.
   - Use only one thickness of towel to dry your feet, especially between the toes.
   - Use a skin moisturizing lotion to prevent skin from getting dry and cracked; however, do not use these lotions between the toes.

3. Inspect your feet daily for puncture wounds, bruises, pressure areas and redness, and blisters.

   - Puncture wounds—Have you stepped on any nails, glass, or tacks?
   - Bruises—Feel for swelling.
   - Pressure areas and redness—Check the six major locations for pressure on the bottom of the foot:
     a. Tip of the big toe
     b. Base of the little toe
     c. Base of the middle toes
     d. Heel
     e. Outside edge of foot
     f. Across the ball of the foot (metatarsal heads)
   - Blisters—Check the six major locations on the bottom of the foot for blisters, plus the tops of the toes and the back of the heel. *Never* pop a blister!

4. Seek treatment by a physician for any foot injuries or open wounds.

5. Do not use Lysol disinfectant, iodine, cresol, carbolic acid, kerosene, or other irritating antiseptic solutions to treat cuts or abrasions on your feet. These products will damage soft tissue.

6. Do not use sharp instruments, drugstore medications, or corn plasters on your feet. Always seek the advice of your physician for any condition that needs such care.

7. Protect your feet.
   - Wear loose bed socks while sleeping.
   - Avoid frostbite by wearing warm socks and shoes during cold weather.
   - Do not use a heating pad on your feet.
   - Do not place your feet on radiators, furnaces, furnace grills, or hot water pipes.

SECTION 7 | FOOT AND ANKLE

# CARE OF DIABETIC FEET (CONTINUED)

4st.

- Do not hold your feet in front of the fireplace, circulators, or heaters.
- Do not use a hair dryer on your feet.

8. Place thin pieces of cotton or lamb's wool between your toes if there is maceration of the skin between your toes or if your toes overlap.

9. Do not sit cross-legged; it can decrease circulation to your feet.

10. Take care of your toenails in the following manner:
    - Soak or bathe feet before trimming nails.
    - Make sure that you trim your nails under good lighting.
    - Trim toenails straight across.
    - Never trim toenails into the corner.
    - If toenails are thick, see your physician and use a nail file or emery board for trimming.
    - Consult your physician when there are any signs of an ingrown toenail. Do not treat an ingrown toenail with drugstore medications; however, you can place a thin piece of cotton or waxed dental floss under the toenail. (See Ingrown Toenail, pp 468-469)

## SOCKS AND STOCKINGS

1. Wear clean, dry socks daily. Make certain that there are no holes or wrinkles in your socks or stockings.

2. Wear thin, white, cotton socks in the summer; they are more absorbent and porous. Change them if your feet sweat excessively.

3. Wear square-toe socks; they will not squeeze your toes.

4. Wear pantyhose or stockings with a garter belt. It is important that you do not wear or use the following:
   - Elastic-top socks or stockings, or knee-high stockings
   - Circular elastic garters
   - String tied around the tops of stockings
   - Stockings that are rolled or knotted at the top

## SHOEWEAR

1. Always wear proper shoes. Check the following components daily to ensure that your shoes fit properly and will not damage your feet:
   - Shoe width—Make sure that the shoes are wide and deep enough to give the joints of your toes breathing room. Shoes that are too narrow will cause pressure bruises and blisters on the inside and outside edges of your foot at the base of the toes.

SECTION 7 | FOOT AND ANKLE

77

ESSENTIALS OF MUSCULOSKELETAL CARE | AMERICAN ACADEMY OF ORTHOPAEDIC SURGEONS

# CARE OF DIABETIC FEET (CONTINUED)

- Shoe length—Shoes that are too short will cause pressure and blisters on the tops of your toes.

- Back of shoe—Looseness at the heel will cause blisters at your heels.

- Bottom of heel—Make sure there are no nails. The presence of holes indicates that there are nails in the heels.

- Sole—Make sure that the sole is not broken. A break in the sole will allow nails or other sharp objects to puncture the skin.

2. Be careful about the type of new shoes you purchase. Use the following guidelines when you look for new shoes:

   - Buy new shoes in the evening to allow for swelling in your feet.

   - Inspect your feet once an hour for the first few days. Look for red areas, bruises, and blisters.

   - Do not wear your new shoes for more than a half day for the first few days.

   - The following components in shoes are desirable:
     a. Laces or adjustable closure
     b. Soft leather tops (to allow feet to breathe; they mold to the feet)
     c. Crepe soles (to provide a good cushion for walking)

   - Avoid the following components in shoes:
     a. Elastic across the tops of the shoes
     b. Pointed-toe styles (they constrict the toes)
     c. High heels
     d. Shoes made of plastic (retain moisture and do not allow the feet "to breathe")

3. Put your shoes on properly.
   - Inspect the inside of each shoe before putting it on. Make sure to remove any small stones or debris. Be certain that the inside of the shoe is smooth.
   - Loosen the laces before putting on or taking off your shoes. Make sure that the tongue is flat, with no wrinkles.
   - Be certain that you do not tie your laces either too tightly or too loosely.

# FRACTURE OF THE ANKLE

ICD-9 Code

824.8
Fracture of ankle; unspecified,
closed

## DEFINITION

Ankle fractures may injure the lateral malleolus (distal fibula), the medial malleolus, the posterior lip of the tibia (posterior malleolus), the collateral ligamentous structures, and/or the talar dome. Stable fractures involve only one side of the joint (eg, a fracture of the distal fibula without injury to the medial deltoid ligament) (**Figure 1**). Unstable ankle fractures involve both sides of the ankle joint and may be bimalleolar or trimalleolar. Bimalleolar injuries are either fractures of the lateral and medial malleolus, or a fracture of the distal fibula with disruption of the deltoid ligament. Trimalleolar injuries include a fracture of the posterior malleolus. Posterior dislocation of the ankle also may be present with a trimalleolar fracture. This injury is described as a trimalleolar fracture-dislocation (**Figure 2**).

Stable injuries can be treated symptomatically, but an unstable injury is vulnerable for displacement and subsequent posttraumatic arthritis.

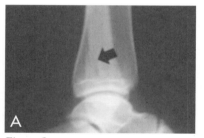 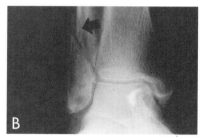

**Figure 1**
Stable fractures of the ankle. A, Nondisplaced fracture of the lateral malleolus. B, Minimally displaced fracture of the lateral malleolus.

## CLINICAL SYMPTOMS

Patients usually report acute pain following trauma. The etiologies are as varied as the circumstances, but usually some element of rotation or twisting has occurred.

## TESTS

### PHYSICAL EXAMINATION

Swelling medially, laterally, and/or posteriorly accompanies most ankle fractures. Marked tenderness is evident at the fracture site. A palpable gap may be apparent on the medial side. External rotation or lateral displacement of the foot from the tibia may be present as well.

A fracture of the distal fibula (lateral malleolus) with tenderness over the medial deltoid ligament is presumed to be an unstable bimalleolar injury.

Palpate the proximal fibula for tenderness because this, coupled with swelling of the medial ankle, can indicate a Maisonneuve fracture, which is an

**Figure 2**
Displaced trimalleolar ankle fracture that requires immediate reduction.

*Reproduced with permission from Grantham SA: Trimalleolar ankle fractures and open ankle fractures, in Greene WB (ed): Instructional Course Lectures XXXIX. Park Ridge, IL, American Academy of Orthopaedic Surgeons, 1990, pp 105-111.*

unstable external rotation injury that includes fracture of the proximal fibula, a tear of the medial deltoid ligament, and a disruption of the tibiofibular syndesmotic ligaments.

Assess circulatory status and posterior tibial, superficial peroneal and deep peroneal nerve function distal to the fracture. Lacerations should be assessed for association with an open fracture.

## DIAGNOSTIC TESTS

AP, lateral, and mortise (15° internally rotated AP) radiographs will reveal most fractures. The relationships of the tibia, fibula, and talus are clearest in the mortise view (**Figure 3**). AP and lateral views should include the proximal fibula and tibia when there is tenderness in that area.

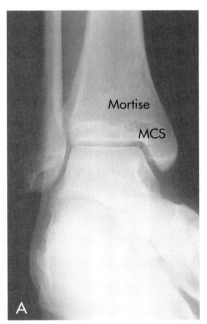 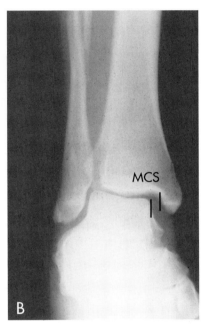

**Figure 3**
A, 15° internal rotation mortise view of the ankle (MCS=medial clear space). B, Lateral fibular fracture with deltoid disruption and widening of the MCS.

*Reproduced with permission from Stiehl JB: Ankle fractures with diastasis, in Greene WB (ed): Instructional Course Lectures XXXIX. Park Ridge, IL, American Academy of Orthopaedic Surgeons, 1990, pp 95–103.*

Minimally displaced fractures may not appear on initial radiographs; therefore, radiographs should be repeated in 10 to 14 days when such a fracture is suspected.

With a rotational injury, a shear or osteochondral fracture of the lateral articular surface of the talus can occur. This is best seen on the mortise view (**Figure 4**). CT may be required for evaluation of complex fractures.

## DIFFERENTIAL DIAGNOSIS

Ankle sprain (inversion injury, lateral tenderness, normal radiographs)

Charcot arthropathy (diffuse swelling, erythema, minimal tenderness)

Fracture of the base of the fifth metatarsal (focal tenderness)

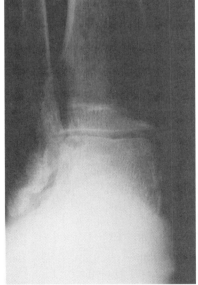

**Figure 4**
Lateral talar dome fracture.

Maisonneuve fracture (widening of syndesmosis, tenderness over the proximal fibula)

Osteochondral fracture of the talar dome, lateral process of the talus, or anterior process of the calcaneus (focal tenderness over the fracture site)

## ADVERSE OUTCOMES OF THE DISEASE

Posttraumatic arthritis, instability, deformity, complex regional pain syndrome, nerve injury, and compartment syndrome are possible.

## TREATMENT

Stable fractures of the distal fibula can be treated with a weight-bearing cast or brace for 4 to 6 weeks. Unstable but nondisplaced fractures require a non-weight-bearing short or long leg cast and more prolonged immobilization. Unstable, displaced fractures require either closed or open reduction. In most cases, open reduction provides better restoration of joint function. Osteochondral fragments should be removed. Concomitant dislocation should be reduced as soon as possible to relieve pressure on the skin and neurovascular structures. Open fractures require immediate surgical debridement.

## ADVERSE OUTCOMES OF TREATMENT

Infection, nonunion, malunion, posttraumatic arthritis, and complex regional pain syndrome can occur.

## REFERRAL DECISIONS/RED FLAGS

Patients with an unstable fracture or osteochondral fragments need further evaluation. All open fractures or open joint injuries require immediate evaluation.

# FRACTURES OF THE CALCANEUS AND TALUS

## ICD-9 Codes
825.0
    Fracture of calcaneus, closed
825.20
    Fracture of talus

## SYNONYMS

Heel fracture

Aviator's fracture (talus)

## DEFINITION

The two bones of the hindfoot, the talus and calcaneus, usually are fractured as a result of severe trauma, such as a motor vehicle accident or fall from a height. However, these two fractures seldom occur together. Most fractures of the talus and calcaneus involve the articular surface and are serious injuries.

## CLINICAL SYMPTOMS

Patients often report acute pain and inability to bear weight.

## TESTS

### PHYSICAL EXAMINATION

Examination reveals swelling and tenderness. Assess function of the superficial peroneal, deep peroneal, sural, medial and lateral plantar nerves distal to the fracture. With swelling, the pulses might not be palpable. Check capillary refill of the toes.

Compartment syndrome is difficult to evaluate with calcaneal and talar injuries; however, notable swelling in the area of the arch is suggestive of a plantar compartment syndrome.

Falls that fracture the calcaneus or talus also may cause a bending force and compression fracture of the lumbar spine. Palpate the spine for tenderness.

### DIAGNOSTIC TESTS

AP and lateral radiographs of the hindfoot are indicated, along with AP and mortise views of the ankle (**Figure 1**). AP and lateral views of the spine should be obtained if there is spinal tenderness. CT may be necessary if further evaluation is needed.

## DIFFERENTIAL DIAGNOSIS

Ankle fracture (ankle swelling or deformity; evident on radiograph)

Associated lumbar spine fracture (pain and tenderness in the lower back)

Medial or lateral ankle ligament injury (swelling and tenderness over involved ligaments)

Talocalcaneal dislocation (deformity of the hindfoot)

SECTION 7 | FOOT AND ANKLE

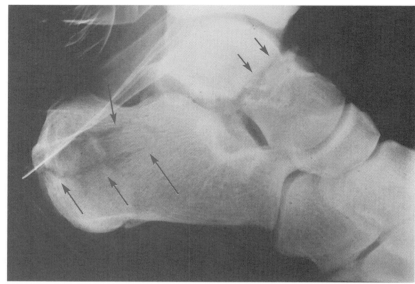

**Figure 1**
Fracture of the talus and calcaneus (arrows).

*Reproduced with permission from Levine AM (ed): Orthopaedic Knowledge Update: Trauma. Rosemont, IL, American Academy of Orthopaedic Surgeons, 1996, pp 191-209.*

## ADVERSE OUTCOMES OF THE DISEASE

The adverse outcomes of either type of fracture are potentially severe and disabling, and treatment is difficult. Fractures of the talus often interrupt the blood supply to the body of the talus and can lead to osteonecrosis. Chronic pain, posttraumatic arthritis, osteonecrosis of the talus, tarsal tunnel syndrome, complex regional pain syndrome, or plantar compartment syndrome can result from either a calcaneal or talar fracture.

## TREATMENT

Immediate treatment consists of splinting with a well-padded posterior splint from the toe to the upper calf. The extremity should be elevated above the level of the heart and ice applied for 20 minutes every 1 to 2 hours.

Many of these fractures require surgical reduction and fixation to minimize later complications.

## ADVERSE OUTCOMES OF TREATMENT

Posttraumatic degenerative arthritis frequently occurs after both of these injuries. Nonunion, postoperative infection, and complex regional pain syndrome also are possible.

## REFERRAL DECISIONS/RED FLAGS

Patients with fractures of the calcaneus or talus or a dislocation of the talocalcaneal joint need further evaluation immediately upon diagnosis.

# FRACTURE OF THE METATARSALS

ICD-9 Code
825.25
Fracture of other tarsal and
metatarsal bones, closed;
metatarsal bones(s)

## SYNONYM
Forefoot fracture

## DEFINITION
Fractures of the metatarsal bones usually heal with nonoperative treatment; however, a zone 2 fracture of the proximal diaphysis of the fifth metatarsal (classic Jones fracture) requires more extensive immobilization, and a zone 3 fracture of this bone (**Figure 1**) can result in nonunion or delayed union.

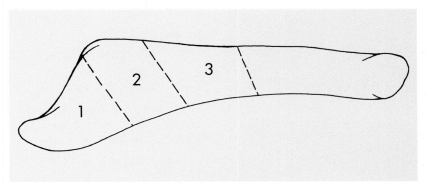

**Figure 1**
The three anatomic zones at the base of the fifth metatarsal: zone 1 includes the articular surface of the fifth metatarsocuboid joint; zone 2 encompasses the articulation of the proximal fourth and fifth metatarsals; zone 3 extends 1.5 cm distal to zone 2.

*Reproduced with permission from Dameron TB, Jr, Fractures of the proximal fifth metatarsal: Selecting the best treatment option. J Amer Acad Orthop Surg 1995;2:110-114.*

## CLINICAL SYMPTOMS
Pain on weight bearing and swelling are common. Stress fractures usually occur after a sudden increase in activity, such as a new training regimen (increase in intensity or distance), change in running surface, or even prolonged walking.

## TESTS
### PHYSICAL EXAMINATION
Examination reveals swelling, ecchymosis, and tenderness over the fractured metatarsal.

### DIAGNOSTIC TESTS
AP, lateral, and oblique radiographs of the foot should demonstrate the fracture.

SECTION 7 | FOOT AND ANKLE

## DIFFERENTIAL DIAGNOSIS

Lisfranc dislocation or sprain (tarsometatarsal joint)

Lisfranc fracture (tarsometatarsal joint)

Metatarsalgia (plantar pain and tenderness over the metatarsal head)

Morton neuroma (plantar pain and tenderness between the metatarsal heads)

## ADVERSE OUTCOMES OF THE DISEASE

Both malunion and nonunion are possible; however, nonunion is uncommon except in association with a fracture in zone 2 or 3 of the proximal fifth metatarsal. Malunion of a metatarsal shaft or neck fracture can result in metatarsalgia with a plantar callus. Compartment syndrome can develop after severe trauma or multiple metatarsal fractures.

## TREATMENT

Treatment of nondisplaced metatarsal neck and shaft fractures includes the use of a short leg cast, fracture brace, or wooden-soled shoe. The device that requires the minimum amount of immobilization while providing adequate comfort should be selected. Weight bearing is permitted as tolerated. In most cases, radiographs should be repeated after 1 week to identify any displacement, then at 6 weeks to confirm healing. Tenderness at the fracture site will diminish as the fracture heals. A fracture of the first metatarsal is often the result of a high-impact injury and may require surgery (**Figure 2**).

Multiple metatarsal fractures and fractures with more than 4 mm of displacement or an apical angulation of more than 10° (seen in the lateral view) may require either closed or open reduction to reestablish a physiologic weight-bearing position of the metatarsal head.

Fractures of the proximal fifth metatarsal may be easy or difficult to manage. Avulsion fractures of the base of the fifth metatarsal (zone 1) or proximal metaphyseal fractures (zone 2) do well with nonoperative treatment. Immobilization with an air stirrup, wooden-soled shoes, or fracture brace is continued until symptoms subside. Acute fractures in zone 2 are more difficult to treat. Most cases will heal with cast immobilization, but treatment of these injuries should start with non-weight-bearing ambulation in a short leg cast for 6 to 8 weeks. Some patients, such as athletes, are better treated by early internal fixation. Fractures in zone 3 often resemble a stress fracture with prodromal symptoms suddenly exacerbated by an inversion injury. These need operative intervention to avoid problems of nonunion or delayed union.

## ADVERSE OUTCOMES OF TREATMENT

Malunion with painful plantar callosities under the metatarsal heads or dorsal corns caused by friction over a prominent metatarsal head can occur.

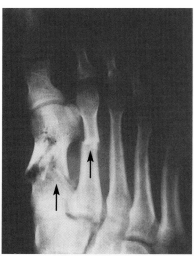

**Figure 2**
Radiograph showing fractures of the first (arrow, left) and second (arrow, right) metatarsals.

*Reproduced with permission from Shereff MJ: Fractures of the forefoot, in Greene WB (ed): Instructional Course Lectures XXXIX. Park Ridge, IL, American Academy of Orthopaedic Surgeons, 1990, p 135.*

## Referral decisions/Red flags

Multiple metatarsal fractures, a metatarsal fracture with more than 4 mm of displacement or more than 10° of angulation, possible compartment syndrome, and/or proximal fifth metatarsal fracture in zones 2 or 3 are all indications for further evaluation. Displaced or comminuted fractures of the first metatarsal also indicate the need for further evaluation. Open fractures require immediate surgical intervention.

# FRACTURE-DISLOCATION OF THE MIDFOOT

ICD-9 Code

838.03
Closed dislocation, tarsometatarsal joint

## SYNONYM

Lisfranc fracture-dislocation

## DEFINITION

Fracture-dislocations of the midfoot, commonly called Lisfranc fracture-dislocations, are easy-to-miss, traumatic disruptions of the tarsometatarsal joints. Injury to these joints can occur as a result of significant trauma or from an indirect mechanism, as may occur in athletics or as a result of tripping. The critical injury involves the second tarsometatarsal joint. The second metatarsal "keys" into a slot in the cuneiforms and is the stabilizing apex for the other tarsometatarsal joints.

## CLINICAL SYMPTOMS

Patients often report a sprain. Pain is localized to the dorsum of the midfoot. The swelling may be relatively mild.

## TESTS

### PHYSICAL EXAMINATION

This injury is easily missed and sometimes misdiagnosed as a foot or ankle sprain. Examination reveals maximum tenderness and swelling over the tarsometatarsal joint rather than the ankle ligaments. During examination, stabilize the hindfoot (calcaneus) with one hand and rotate and/or abduct the forefoot with the other hand (**Figure 1**). This maneuver produces severe pain with a Lisfranc injury but only minimal pain with an ankle sprain.

### DIAGNOSTIC TESTS

AP, lateral, and oblique radiographs of the foot should be obtained. Spontaneous reduction after complete dislocation may occur. Subtle injuries may be more apparent on weight-bearing radiographs. Look for the normal colinearity of the medial aspect of the middle cuneiform with the medial aspect of the second metatarsal on the AP radiograph (**Figure 2**). The oblique view should show similar colinearity of the medial aspect of the fourth metatarsal and the medial aspect of the cuboid. Comparison views of the uninjured foot can be helpful.

When the AP radiograph shows that the second metatarsal base has shifted laterally, even by only a few millimeters, a Lisfranc fracture-dislocation has occurred (**Figure 3**). A small avulsion fracture between the base of the first and second metatarsals indicates disruption of the ligament connecting the base of the second metatarsal and medial cuneiform (Lisfranc ligament) and instability of the tarsometatarsal joints.

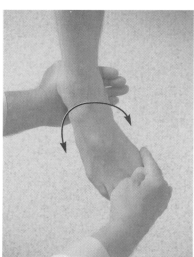

**Figure 1**
Stabilize the hindfoot with one hand and rotate and/or abduct the forefoot with the other.

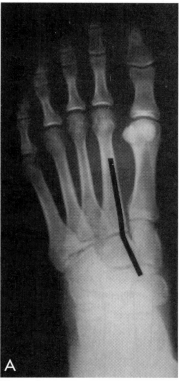
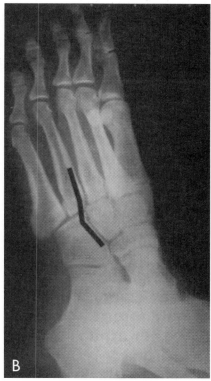

**Figure 2**
The normal radiographic relationship of the metatarsals and cuneiforms. A, AP view. Note the consistent relationship at the second metatarsal and the middle cuneiform. B, Oblique view. Note unbroken line at the medial fourth metatarsal base and medial cuboid.

*Reproduced with permission from Lutter LD, Mizel MS, Pfeffer GP (eds): Orthopaedic Knowledge Update: Foot and Ankle. Rosemont, IL, American Academy of Orthopaedic Surgeons, 1994, p 261.*

When radiographs are normal but physical examination suggests injury to the tarsometatarsal joints, stress radiographs of the midfoot under local anesthetic or sedation may be indicated. If confusion still exists, CT or MRI is helpful in confirming the diagnosis.

## DIFFERENTIAL DIAGNOSIS

Ankle fracture (bony tenderness over the malleolus)

Ankle sprain (focal tenderness over the lateral ankle ligament)

Metatarsal fracture (focal tenderness over the metatarsal)

Navicular fracture (focal tenderness over the navicular)

Midfoot arthritis (chronic pain and tenderness, no recent history of trauma)

## ADVERSE OUTCOMES OF THE DISEASE

Adverse outcomes include midfoot instability, deformity, and arthritis. Compartment syndrome with subsequent ischemic contracture, claw toes, and sensory impairment also can occur.

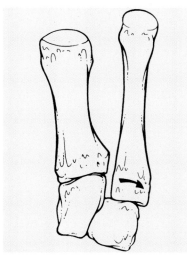

**Figure 3**
Lisfranc fragment, with lateral shift of the second metatarsal.

*Reproduced with permission from Alexander IJ (ed): The Foot: Examination and Diagnosis. New York, NY, Churchill Livingstone, 1990, p 131.*

## TREATMENT

Nondisplaced injuries are treated by 6 to 8 weeks of non–weight-bearing cast immobilization, followed by use of a rigid arch support for 3 months. A fracture or fracture-dislocation with any displacement requires surgical stabilization.

## ADVERSE OUTCOMES OF TREATMENT

Due to injury of the articular cartilage, traumatic arthritis may develop even after appropriate cast immobilization or surgical treatment.

## REFERRAL DECISIONS/RED FLAGS

Because these injuries are frequently missed, they warrant a low threshold for further evaluation and diagnostic testing. Even a minimally displaced fracture-dislocation requires surgical reduction. Any possibility of compartment syndrome requires immediate surgical evaluation.

# FRACTURES OF THE PHALANGES

ICD-9 Code
826.0
    Fracture of one or more phalanges
    of foot; closed

## SYNONYM

Broken toe

## DEFINITION

Phalangeal fracture, commonly known as a broken toe, usually involves the proximal phalanx and is caused by direct trauma. They rarely result in major disability. The fifth, or little, toe is the most commonly affected.

## CLINICAL SYMPTOMS

Patients have pain, swelling, or ecchymosis.

## TESTS

### PHYSICAL EXAMINATION

Examination may reveal deformity of the toe, but local bony tenderness, swelling, and ecchymosis are often the only principal findings.

### DIAGNOSTIC TESTS

AP radiographs usually confirm the diagnosis.

## DIFFERENTIAL DIAGNOSIS

Freiberg infraction (osteonecrosis of the metatarsal head)

Ingrown toenail/paronychia (inflammation of the fold of tissue around the toenail)

Metatarsalgia (plantar tenderness over the metatarsal head)

Metatarsophalangeal synovitis (tenderness over the metatarsophalangeal [MP] joint)

## ADVERSE OUTCOMES OF THE DISEASE

Permanent deformity is an uncommon possibility.

## TREATMENT

Phalangeal fractures are treated by buddy taping the fractured toe to an adjacent toe, usually the toe medial to the fractured one. A gauze pad can be placed between the toes to absorb moisture and prevent maceration of the skin from sweating. The tape and gauze should be changed as often as needed.

Closed reduction under a digital block or open reduction and pinning is rarely necessary but should be considered for markedly angulated fractures or fractures involving the articular surface of the MP joints of all toes or interphalangeal joint of the great toe.

## ADVERSE OUTCOMES OF TREATMENT
Chronic swelling and deformity of the toe are possible.

## REFERRAL DECISIONS/RED FLAGS
Patients with an open fracture or a displaced intra-articular fracture (especially at the MP joint) need further evaluation.

# PROCEDURE

## DIGITAL ANESTHETIC BLOCK (FOOT)

### MATERIALS

Sterile gloves

Bactericidal skin preparation solution

Ethyl chloride spray

10-mL syringe

18-gauge needle

25-gauge, 1½" needle

10 mL of 1% lidocaine or 0.5% bupivacaine, both *without* epinephrine

Adhesive dressing

### STEP 1

Wear protective gloves at all times during the procedure and use sterile technique.

### STEP 2

Use the 18-gauge needle to draw 10 mL of the local anesthetic into the syringe, then switch to the 25-gauge needle to preserve sterility.

### STEP 3

Cleanse the dorsal surface of the foot with bactericidal solution on either side of the metatarsal heads.

### STEP 4

Freeze the dorsal skin with ethyl chloride spray.

### STEP 5

Insert the 25-gauge needle into the soft-tissue space on either side of the metatarsal head until it just begins to tent the plantar skin (**Figure 1**). Remember that the sensory nerves travel along the plantar side of the metatarsal.

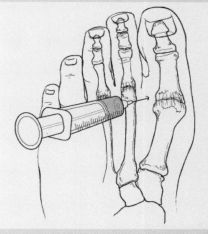

**Figure 1**
Insert the needle on either side of the metatarsal head.

## STEP 6

Withdraw the needle approximately 1 cm or until the tip rests at the level of the plantar aspect of the metatarsal head.

## STEP 7

Inject 3 mL of anesthetic, then an additional 2 mL while the needle is withdrawn. Make certain that some of the anesthetic is deposited subcutaneously around the dorsal sensory nerves.

## STEP 8

Repeat the procedure on the other side of the metatarsal of the toe that is to be anesthetized. Within 1 to 2 minutes, the involved toe should become numb.

## STEP 9

Dress the puncture wound with a sterile adhesive dressing.

## ADVERSE OUTCOMES

Although rare, infection is possible. Necrosis of a digit is possible if epinephrine is used in the anesthetic solution.

## AFTERCARE/PATIENT INSTRUCTIONS

Advise the patient that a collection of fluid on the plantar aspect of the foot may appear but that the fluid will dissipate within several hours after the block.

# HALLUX RIGIDUS

ICD-9 Code
735.2
    Hallux rigidus

## SYNONYMS

Hallux limitus

Great toe arthritis

## DEFINITION

Hallux rigidus is degenerative arthritis of the metatarsophalangeal (MP) joint of the great toe and the most common site of arthritis in the foot. The principal symptoms are pain and stiffness, especially as the toe moves into dorsiflexion. Hallux rigidus is the second most common malady of the great toe and affects approximately 2% of the population between the ages of 30 and 60 years.

## CLINICAL SYMPTOMS

Patients have pain in the great toe joint with activity, especially in the toe-off phase of gait as the MP joint goes into extension. The osteophytes that develop on the dorsum of the toe can become red and irritated with shoe wear (**Figure 1**). The dorsal sensory nerves of the great toe can be irritated by the associated swelling.

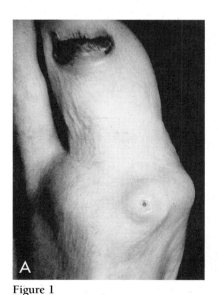 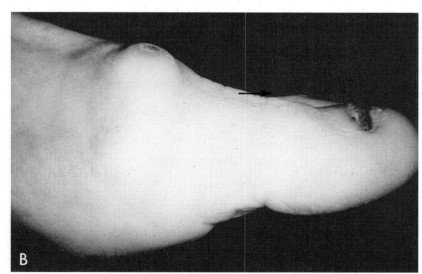

**Figure 1**
A, Top view of dorsal prominence from underlying bony osteophyte. B, Lateral view of same (arrow).

*Reproduced with permission from Mann RA: Hallux rigidus, in Greene WB (ed): Instructional Course Lectures XXXIX. Park Ridge, IL, American Academy of Orthopaedic Surgeons, 1990, pp 15-21.*

# TESTS

## PHYSICAL EXAMINATION

Stiffness of the great toe with loss of extension at the MP joint is the hallmark. Osteoarthritic spurs develop primarily on the dorsal portion of the first metatarsal head (**Figure 2**). The toe is in normal alignment.

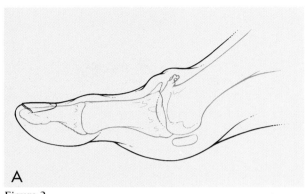

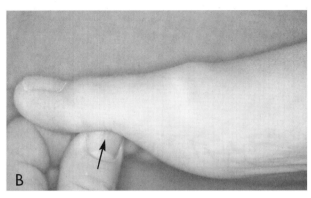

**Figure 2**
A, Hallux rigidus osteophytes. B, Loss of extension (arrow) is the hallmark.

*Reproduced with permission from Alexander IJ: The Foot: Examination and Diagnosis. New York, NY, Churchill Livingstone, 1990, p 65.*

## DIAGNOSTIC TESTS

AP and lateral radiographs show narrowing of the MP joint of the great toe and osteophytes, predominantly on the dorsal and lateral aspects of the great toe (**Figure 3**).

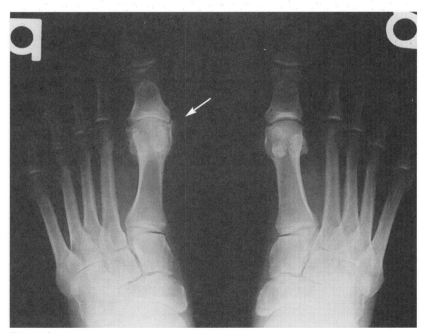

**Figure 3**
Standing AP radiograph of the feet. *Left,* foot with advanced arthritic changes (arrow). *Right,* foot with small medial and lateral spurs.

## DIFFERENTIAL DIAGNOSIS

Gout (recurrent episode of erythema and swelling, positive clinical history)

Hallux valgus (bunion and valgus angulation of the great toe)

Turf toe (history of injury, pain on the plantar aspect of MP joint accentuated by extension of the toe)

## ADVERSE OUTCOMES OF THE DISEASE

Pain aggravated by walking is common.

## TREATMENT

Nonoperative treatment consists of wearing a shoe with a large toe box to decrease pressure on the toe. A stiff-soled shoe modified with a steel shank or rocker bottom limits dorsiflexion of the great toe and decreases pain caused by motion in the arthritic joint. Patients should be advised to avoid wearing high-heeled shoes. NSAIDs, ice, and contrast baths also can help decrease inflammation and control symptoms for a short period of time (see Contrast Baths, p 425).

Surgical treatment consists of either excision of the dorsal osteophytes or fusion of the joint (arthrodesis). Resection of the joint may be indicated in some patients. An artificial joint implant is not recommended.

## ADVERSE OUTCOMES OF TREATMENT

NSAIDs can cause gastric, renal, or hepatic complications. No adverse outcomes associated with treatment have been found to occur, other than the usual surgical complications.

## REFERRAL DECISIONS/RED FLAGS

Failure of nonoperative treatment is an indication for further evaluation.

# HALLUX VALGUS

ICD-9 Code
735.0
  Hallux valgus (acquired)

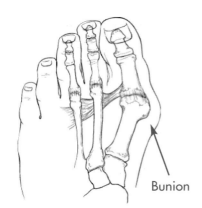

**Figure 1**
Anatomy of a hallux valgus.

Bunion

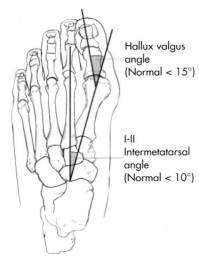

Hallux valgus angle
(Normal < 15°)

I-II Intermetatarsal angle
(Normal < 10°)

**Figure 2**
Measure the angle shown above from the patient's standing AP radiograph.

*Adapted with permission from Pedowitz W: Bunion deformity, in Pfeffer G, Frey C (eds): Current Practice in Foot and Ankle Surgery. New York, NY, McGraw Hill, 1993, pp 219–242.*

## SYNONYMS

Bunion

Metatarsus primus varus

## DEFINITION

Hallux valgus is lateral deviation of the great toe at the metatarsophalangeal (MP) joint that can lead to a painful prominence of the medial aspect of the first metatarsal head (bunion) (**Figure 1**). The female-to-male ratio of symptomatic hallux valgus is approximately 10:1.

## CLINICAL SYMPTOMS

Pain and swelling, aggravated by shoe wear, are the principal complaints.

## TESTS

### PHYSICAL EXAMINATION

A hypertrophic bursa is evident over the medial eminence of the first metatarsal. The great toe is pronated (rotated inward) with subsequent callus on its medial aspect. Irritation of the medial plantar sensory nerve can cause numbness or tingling over the medial aspect of the great toe. Assess the valgus angulation at the MP joint (Normal valgus at the MP joint is < 15°). Measure range of motion at the MP joint. Most patients with hallux valgus have relatively normal MP motion (extension 60° to 70° and flexion 30°). Evaluate the lesser toes for associated deformities. A second toe that overrides the laterally deviated great toe is a frequent problem. Other lesser toe problems include corns, calluses, hammer toes, and bunionette (a bunion-like prominence on the lateral side of the fifth MP joint).

## DIAGNOSTIC TESTS

The severity of a bunion deformity is graded by measuring forefoot angles on weight-bearing AP radiographs of the foot. The normal hallux valgus angle is < 15°, and a normal intermetatarsal (IM) angle is < 10° (**Figure 2**). Radiographs also are used to assess lateral subluxation of the sesamoids, the shape of the metatarsal head, degenerative changes in the MP joint, valgus at the interphalangeal (IP) joint, and lesser toe abnormalities. A weight-bearing lateral radiograph of the foot is less helpful but is important for evaluating any lesser toe subluxation or arthritic changes of the great toe MP joint.

## DIFFERENTIAL DIAGNOSIS

Gout (articular and periarticular inflammation and tenderness)

Hallux extensus (cock-up toe, or extension of the great toe)

Hallux interphalangeus (lateral deviation of the great toe at the IP joint)

Hallux rigidus (osteoarthritis of the first MP joint)

Hallux varus (medial deviation of the great toe at the MP joint)

Inflammatory arthropathy (rheumatoid arthritis leading to deviation of the great toe)

## ADVERSE OUTCOMES OF THE DISEASE

Chronic pain is a primary symptom and requires alterations in activity and shoe modifications (greater shoe width and minimal heel height).

## TREATMENT

The initial treatment is patient education and shoe wear modifications. These modalities usually are sufficient for mild to moderate deformities. Shoes should have adequate width at the forefront and should be constructed of soft uppers, with no thick stitching over the medial eminence. An orthotist or a shoe repair professional can stretch the shoe directly over the bunion. High heels place undue pressure on the forefoot and bunion prominence and should be avoided. Physical therapy, splints, and bracing are not helpful, although occasionally a medial longitudinal arch support can decrease pressure on a bunion of a patient with a pronated flatfoot.

No treatment is needed for asymptomatic hallux valgus, even if the deformity continues to progress. For patients who have continued disability despite nonoperative treatment, several well-established surgical procedures are available. Indications for different procedures are based on the severity of the hallux valgus, the IM angle, and joint congruity. Joint replacement is rarely indicated because of the high complication rate.

## ADVERSE OUTCOMES OF TREATMENT

Surgical treatment can result in recurrence, undercorrection, overcorrection (hallux varus), decreased function, stiffness, pain, malunion or nonunion of an osteotomy, and transfer lesions (metatarsalgia).

## REFERRAL DECISIONS/RED FLAGS

Persistent pain despite shoe modifications indicates the need for further evaluation. Patients with persistent pain may benefit from surgical correction.

SECTION 7 | FOOT AND ANKLE

# INGROWN TOENAIL

ICD-9 Code
703.0
Diseases of nail; ingrowing nail

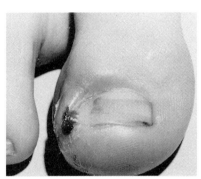

**Figure 1**
Ingrown toenail.

*Reproduced with permission from Lutter LD, Mizel MS, Pfeffer GB (eds): Orthopaedic Knowledge Update: Foot and Ankle. Rosemont, IL, American Academy of Orthopaedic Surgeons, 1994, p 54.*

## SYNONYMS
Paronychia
Infected toenail
Onychocryptosis

## DEFINITION
With an ingrown toenail, the distal margin of the nail grows into the adjacent skin causing irritation, inflammation, and possibly secondary bacterial or fungal infection. The condition is virtually limited to the great toe. Ingrown toenails are associated with improper trimming of the toe nail, tight shoes, hereditary predisposition, subungual pathology, congenital incurved nail, thickened nail, direct trauma, or any combination of these factors (**Figure 1**).

With improper trimming, the toenail is cut in a curved fashion similar to trimming fingernails. This allows the sharp edge of the nail to grow into the more prominent skin margins (nail fold) found at the end of toenails. Properly trimmed toenails are cut straight across to keep the lateral margin of the toenail beyond the nail fold. Some people have toenails that have a naturally incurved shape. Ingrown toenails may occur in these patients even with proper trimming techniques. Soft-tissue hypertrophy over a normal nail plate secondary to trauma or tight shoes also may cause an ingrown toe nail. Skin breakthrough creates a portal of entry for a secondary bacterial or fungal infection.

## CLINICAL SYMPTOMS
Stage I (inflammation) is characterized by induration, swelling, and tenderness along the nail fold. In stage II (abscess), the patient has purulent or serous drainage, increased tenderness, and increased erythema. In stage III (granulation), granulation tissue grows onto the nail plate, inhibiting drainage. This stage is less painful than stage II.

## TESTS
### PHYSICAL EXAMINATION
The diagnosis is clinical; visual inspection is the basis for staging the condition.

### DIAGNOSTIC TESTS
Radiographs may be obtained of stage II and stage III ingrown toenails to rule out a subungual exostosis and osteomyelitis.

## DIFFERENTIAL DIAGNOSIS

Felon (deep abscess on the plantar aspect of the toe)

Onychomycosis (fungal infection of the nail)

Osteomyelitis (bone infection with changes on radiograph)

Paronychia (superficial abscess on the base of the toenail)

Subungual exostosis (osteochondroma beneath the nail)

## ADVERSE OUTCOMES OF THE DISEASE

Progressive pain, paronychia, felon, nail plate deformity, and osteomyelitis are all possible. Hematogenous seeding of other organs may occur but is very uncommon.

## TREATMENT

Stage I: Warm soaks, proper nail trimming, accommodative shoe wear, and clean socks are all necessary. With a blunt instrument, insert cotton or waxed dental floss beneath the nail to lift the edge of the nail from its embedded position. Exchange packing daily until the nail has grown out sufficiently. Nonconstrictive shoes or sandals prevent extrinsic irritation of the inflamed skin.

Stage II: Initial treatment should include foot soaks along with broad-spectrum oral antibiotics (cephalosporin). Partial excision of the nail under digital block should be performed when the patient has severe pain, when there is a risk of secondary infection to a prosthetic joint, or when a course of oral antibiotics fails to treat associated infection (see Digital Anesthetic Block [Foot], pp 461-462). Partial nail excision is preferred (see Nail Plate Avulsion, pp 470-472). Complete nail excision increases the risk of upward deformation of the nail bed (clubbing). An avulsed nail requires 3 to 4 months to regrow.

Stage III: Partial or complete nail plate excision with or without ablation of the germinal matrix of the nail is indicated.

## ADVERSE OUTCOMES OF TREATMENT

Adverse outcomes include recurrence (50% to 70% with excision alone), nail plate deformity, upturned nail or clubbed nail after complete nail plate excision, and poor cosmesis.

## REFERRAL DECISIONS/RED FLAGS

Failure of nonoperative treatment or the presence of stage III disease is an indication for further evaluation.

# PROCEDURE

## NAIL PLATE AVULSION

### MATERIALS

Sterile gloves

Bactericidal skin preparation solution

¼" Penrose drain or a strip cut from a rubber glove (optional)

Materials to administer a digital block (see Digital Anesthetic Block [Foot])

Strong small scissors or anvil nail cutter

Small hemostat

Nonadherent sterile gauze

Sterile dressing material

### ANATOMY

A recurrent ingrown toenail or paronychial infection makes it necessary to remove a portion of the nail plate, usually in the great toe. The lateral or medial margins of the nail, or both, may be involved.

Removal of the entire nail plate is described below. Partial removal involves undermining the lateral or medial third of the nail, vertically cutting the nail with strong small scissors or an anvil nail cutter at the junction of the lateral or medial third, and avulsing the small segment adjacent to the nail fold.

### STEP 1

Wear protective gloves at all times during the procedure and use sterile technique.

### STEP 2

Cleanse the toe with a bactericidal solution.

### STEP 3

Follow the steps in the procedure titled Digital Anesthetic Block (Foot) to administer a digital block.

### STEP 4

Wrap a ¼" strip of rubber around the base of the toe to act as a tourniquet and control bleeding (optional).

### STEP 5

Using a small scissors or hemostat, elevate the nail plate from the underlying nail bed (Figure 1).

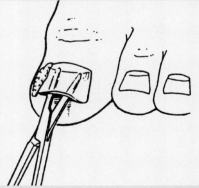

**Figure 1**
Elevate the nail plate from the nail bed.

# NAIL PLATE AVULSION (CONTINUED)

## STEP 6

Separate the proximal cuticle (nail fold) from the nail plate.

## STEP 7

Grasp the free portion of the nail plate with a hemostat and avulse it (**Figure 2**), then palpate the nail bed to ensure that no spikes of nail tissue remain.

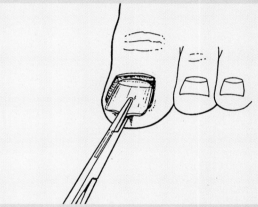

**Figure 2**
Avulse the nail plate.

## STEP 8

If a tourniquet was used, remove it and apply compression to stop local bleeding.

## STEP 9

Apply nonadherent sterile gauze over the exposed nail bed and wrap the entire toe with a sterile dressing.

## ADVERSE OUTCOMES

Because of recurrence of ingrown toenails after nail plate avulsions, permanent ablation of the nail matrix may be required.

## PERMANENT ABLATION

This procedure may be necessary and can be performed by curettage and/or phenol ablation of the nail matrix.

# Nail Plate Avulsion (continued)

## Aftercare/Patient Instructions

Instruct the patient to remove the dressing and gauze in 48 hours and replace them with an adhesive strip. Also instruct the patient to pack a wisp of cotton from a cotton ball or waxed dental floss under the advancing edge of the newly growing nail over the next few months to prevent the edge of the nail from digging into the exposed soft tissue.

# MALODOROUS FEET

ICD-9 Code
780.8
Hyperhidrosis

## SYNONYM

Sweaty feet syndrome

## DEFINITION

Sweat, the main offender, is a secretion of the eccrine glands of the skin. The thick skin of the soles can contain as many as 3,000 eccrine glands per square inch. Fluid intake, aspirin, other medications, and emotional stress all can increase sweating. The temperature inside shoes can easily reach 102°F. Poor hygiene, increased moisture, and heat cause the normally occurring bacteria to proliferate and produce isovaleric acid, the substance associated with foot odor.

Some people are born with a genetic defect that causes excessive sweating, or hyperhidrosis. In most people, environmental conditions and emotional stress trigger severe sweat production.

## ADVERSE OUTCOMES OF THE DISEASE

Smelly feet are a troubling problem that can result in social embarrassment, poor acceptance in the work environment, and accelerated damage to footwear. Some people become so used to their odor (osmic adaptation) that they are unaware of its presence.

## TREATMENT

Initial treatment should focus on reducing local sweating and inhibiting the growth of bacteria. Frequent foot washing and dusting the feet with absorbent powder is helpful.

Shoes and socks should be changed at least once a day. Shoes that "breathe" should be worn; leather breathes, but plastic does not. Shoes should be allowed to air out for 24 hours after use, and shoes permeated with odor should be discarded.

Soaking the feet in strong black tea for 30 minutes a day for a week can help. The tannic acid in the tea kills the bacteria and closes the pores, keeping feet dry longer. Use two tea bags per pint of water; boil for 15 minutes; add 2 quarts of cool water; then soak the feet in the cool solution. A solution of 1 part vinegar and 2 parts water also can be tried.

Persistent foot odor can indicate a low-grade infection, as can occur with athlete's foot, or a severe case of hereditary sweating. Bacterial or fungal infections are best managed with medicated creams or oral medication. Proper foot hygiene (washing, frequent shoe and sock changes) also is essential to help cure these infections.

Severe hereditary hyperhidrosis requires medical management to suppress sweating and the growth of bacteria. At bedtime, apply a topical solution of 20% aluminum chloride hexahydrate and wrap the feet in kitchen plastic wrap. This procedure should be followed for two consecutive nights, then repeated every 3 to 7 nights until sweating is reduced. Aluminum chloride hexahydrate is available in 10% solutions for those sensitive to the stronger preparation.

High-voltage current delivered through a tap-water bath (iontophoresis) can decrease sweat production. Fifteen-minute treatments are repeated two or three times a week until sweating is reduced. Maintenance therapy requires repeat treatments at 3- to 4-week intervals. This therapy is effective but requires special equipment and trained personnel.

Surgical sympathectomy (excision of the nerve that controls sweating) can have dramatic results but may produce unpleasant side effects.

## ADVERSE OUTCOMES OF TREATMENT
Side effects of sympathectomy are possible.

## REFERRAL DECISIONS/RED FLAGS
Symptoms of bacterial or fungal infection or of hyperhidrosis are indications for further evaluation.

# METATARSALGIA

ICD-9 Code

726.70
Enthesopathy of ankle and tarsus,
unspecified

## SYNONYM
Forefoot pain

## DEFINITION
Metatarsalgia is a general term indicating forefoot pain localized under one or more of the lesser metatarsals. Abnormal metatarsal length with alteration of weight-bearing forces can be a cause of metatarsalgia. Toe deformities such as claw or hammer toe can lead to metatarsalgia by causing displacement of the plantar fat pad and loss of cushioning under the metatarsal heads. Callus formation occurs, and this thickened skin can be a major component of the patient's symptoms. A persistent callus on the sole of the foot is called intractable plantar keratosis.

## CLINICAL SYMPTOMS
Activity-related pain is localized to the plantar aspect of the forefoot directly over the metatarsal heads. The patient may complain about the diffuse callus formation.

## TESTS
### PHYSICAL EXAMINATION
Observe the alignment of the toes. Evaluate swelling, range of motion, and stability of the metatarsophalangeal (MP) joints. Palpate for swelling or masses along the plantar and dorsal aspects of the metatarsals as well as adjacent interspaces. Note the extent of any callus and whether it is discrete or diffuse. A discrete callus is tender with direct pressure. Evaluate digital nerve function.

### DIAGNOSTIC TESTS
Standing AP and lateral radiographs of the foot should be obtained to assess metatarsal and toe alignment.

## DIFFERENTIAL DIAGNOSIS
Claw toe-related pain (plantar displacement of the metatarsal heads and fat pad)

Metatarsal stress fracture (localized tenderness and radiographic findings)

Interdigital neuroma (numbness in the involved web space)

Intractable plantar keratosis (persistent callus on sole of foot)

Forefoot mass (ganglion or other tumor)

MP synovitis (swelling of the joint, dorsal tenderness)

Plantar wart (tender with circumferential pressure)

## Adverse Outcomes of the Disease

Progressive pain and difficulty walking

## Treatment

Accommodative shoes, a metatarsal pad (see Application of a Metatarsal Pad, p 433) or an orthotic device is the key to treatment. A thickened callus can be shaved (see Corns and Calluses, pp 437-439). Nonoperative treatment usually is successful, but if these measures fail, surgery to realign the toes and/or metatarsal head can be considered. Removal of the metatarsal head should be avoided.

## Adverse Outcomes of Treatment

Inadequate pain relief, delayed union, nonunion, and transfer lesions (stress with resultant pain transferred to the adjacent metatarsal) are possible complications of surgical treatment.

## Referral Decisions/Red Flags

Symptoms that persist despite nonoperative care indicate the need for further evaluation.

# MORTON NEUROMA

ICD-9 Code
355.6
Mononeuritis of lower limb; lesion
of plantar nerve

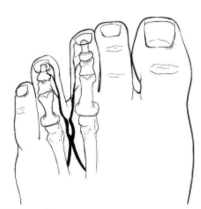

**Figure 1**
Interdigital neuroma between the
metatarsal heads.

*Adapted with permission from McElvenny RT: The etiology
and surgical treatment of intractable pain about the fourth
metatarsophalangeal joint (Morton's toe). J Bone Joint Surg
1943;25A:675-679.*

## SYNONYMS

Plantar neuroma
Interdigital neuroma

## DEFINITION

Morton neuroma, also referred as plantar interdigital neuroma, is not a true neuroma but rather a perineural fibrosis of the common digital nerve as it passes between the metatarsal heads. The fibrosis is secondary to repetitive irritation of the nerve. The condition is most common between the third and fourth toes (third web space) (**Figure 1**). Morton neuroma occurs less frequently in the second web space (between the second and third toes) and rarely in either the first or fourth intermetatarsal space. The simultaneous occurrence of two neuromas is extremely uncommon. Morton neuroma has a female-to-male ratio of 5:1, probably related to compression of the nerve by tight shoe wear.

## CLINICAL SYMPTOMS

Plantar pain in the forefoot is the most common presenting symptom. Dysesthesias into the affected two toes or burning plantar pain that is aggravated by activity also is common. Occasionally, patients report numbness in the adjacent toes of the involved web space. Night pain is rare. Many patients state that they feel as though they are "walking on a marble" or that there is "a wrinkle in my socks." Relief often is obtained by removing the shoe and rubbing the ball of the foot. Symptoms are aggravated by wearing high-heeled or tight, restrictive shoes.

## TESTS

### PHYSICAL EXAMINATION

Isolated pain on the plantar aspect of the web space is consistent with an intermetatarsal neuroma. Apply direct plantar pressure to the interspace with one hand and then squeeze the metatarsals together with the other hand. Morton neuroma is indicated by increased tenderness and pain radiating to the toes.

Inspect the plantar surface for calluses, then palpate dorsally along metatarsal shafts and plantarly over the metatarsal heads to evaluate for stress fractures or metatarsalgia, respectively. Evaluate sensory function of the digital nerves. Stress each tarsometatarsal joint by grasping the midfoot with one hand and moving each metatarsal in a dorsoplantar direction to rule out midfoot arthritis. Similarly, grasp the metatarsal shaft and, while keeping the toe parallel to the metatarsal, try to displace the digit dorsally, then plantarly. Pain or excess motion with this maneuver indicates synovitis or inflammation of the metatarsophalangeal (MP) joint.

## DIAGNOSTIC TESTS

Radiographs are normal in patients with Morton neuroma. MRI and ultrasound can detect a neuroma but are unreliable and their use is not commonly indicated.

## DIFFERENTIAL DIAGNOSIS

Hammer toe (flexion deformity of the proximal interphalangeal joint)

Metatarsalgia (plantar tenderness over the metatarsal head)

Metatarsophalangeal synovitis (tenderness and swelling directly over the MP joint)

Stress fracture (dorsal metatarsal tenderness)

## ADVERSE OUTCOMES OF THE DISEASE

Chronic, intermittent pain and the need for shoe and activity modifications are possible.

## TREATMENT

Patients should be advised to wear a low-heeled, soft-soled shoe with a wide toe box. Pain relief also can be obtained using metatarsal pads to spread the metatarsal heads and take pressure off the nerve.

Locate the neuroma on the plantar aspect of the foot in the soft tissue between the involved metatarsal heads. Ask the patient to mark the painful spot on the bottom of the foot with a material that transfers easily, such as lipstick or eyeliner. Instruct the patient to stand, without socks, in a shoe to transfer the mark to the inside of the shoe. Place the pad into the shoe directly over the mark. This ensures that the metatarsal heads are kept apart and away from the neuroma when the patient is bearing weight. Note that this placement differs from the placement of a pad for metatarsalgia. Felt or gel pads are inexpensive, effective, and come in different sizes to accommodate different sized shoes and feet of different sizes. Advise the patient that, if the pad is effective, a more permanent orthotic can be fabricated that can be transferred from shoe to shoe.

A mixture of 1 to 2 mL of lidocaine without epinephrine and 1 mL (10 mg/mL) of corticosteroid injected just proximal to the metatarsal heads can be both diagnostic and therapeutic (see Morton Neuroma Injection, pp 480-481). Multiple injections should be avoided.

If symptoms persist or recur, surgical excision of the neuroma or division of the transverse metatarsal ligament is indicated.

## ADVERSE OUTCOMES OF TREATMENT

Symptoms can persist or recur after nonoperative treatment. Symptoms can recur or become worse after surgical excision of the neuroma if a painful stump of nerve develops.

## REFERRAL DECISIONS/RED FLAGS

Persistent pain despite shoe or insert modifications or injection of cortico-steroid indicates the need for further evaluation.

# PROCEDURE

## MORTON NEUROMA INJECTION

### MATERIALS

Sterile gloves

Bactericidal skin preparation solution

Ethyl chloride spray

3-mL syringe

18-gauge needle

25-gauge, 1-to-1½" needle

1 mL of 10 mg/mL corticosteroid preparation

2 mL of 1% lidocaine or 0.5% bupivacaine, both *without* epinephrine

Adhesive dressing

### STEP 1

Wear protective gloves at all times during the procedure and use sterile technique.

### STEP 2

Use the 18-gauge needle to draw 1 mL of the 10 mg/mL corticosteroid preparation and 2 mL of the local anesthetic into the syringe, then switch to the 25-gauge needle to preserve sterility.

### STEP 3

Cleanse the dorsal skin between the metatarsal heads with bactericidal solution.

### STEP 4

Freeze the dorsal skin with ethyl chloride spray.

### STEP 5

Place the needle in line with the metatarsophalangeal joint, which is approximately 1 to 2 cm proximal to the web of the toe (**Figure 1**).

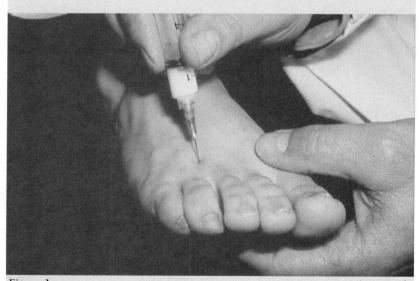

**Figure 1**
Proper location for injection for Morton neuroma.

# Morton Neuroma Injection (continued)

## Step 6

Insert the needle into the plantar aspect of the foot so that the tip gently tents the skin. Withdraw the needle approximately 1 cm so that the tip is where the neuroma is found, at the level of the plantar metatarsophalangeal joint.

## Step 7

Inject the corticosteroid-anesthetic mixture around the neuroma, taking care not to inject into the plantar fat pad.

# NAIL FUNGUS INFECTION

**ICD-9 Code**
110.1
    Dermatophytosis, of nail

## SYNONYMS
Dermatophytic onychomycosis
Tinea ungulum

## DEFINITION
Fungal infection of the nail (onychomycosis) occurs four times more frequently in the toes compared to the fingers. *Trichophyton rubrum* and *T mentagrophytes* cause 90% of the infections. Approximately 50% of patients are older than age 70 years. The problem may be primarily cosmetic, or the nail may become so hypertrophic that it interferes with shoe wear and is painful.

## CLINICAL SYMPTOMS
Patients report discoloration, thickening, and difficulty in trimming the nails.

## TESTS
### PHYSICAL EXAMINATION
Thickening and chalky yellow or white discoloration of the nail is observed (Figure 1).

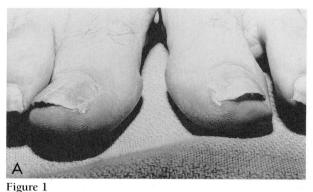
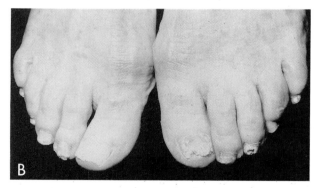

**Figure 1**
A, Early form of fungal infection. The hyponychium is affected, followed by the nail bed and plate. B, All three layers of the nail plate are infected. Treatment will require an oral antifungal agent.

*Reproduced with permission from Chou LB: Skin and nail disorders, in Mizel MS, Miller RA, Scioli MW (eds): Orthopaedic Knowledge Update Foot and Ankle 2, American Academy of Orthopaedic Surgeons, Rosemont, IL 1998, p 34.*

### DIAGNOSTIC TESTS
Diagnosis is made by microscopic examination of nail scrapings and potassium hydroxide slide preparation.

### DIFFERENTIAL DIAGNOSIS
Onychogryphosis (severe nail deformity, curling at the edge of the nail)

Repetitive trauma (ridges and cracking of the nail with thickening)

## ADVERSE OUTCOMES OF THE DISEASE

A thickened nail can make shoe wear difficult.

## TREATMENT

Treatment options include observation with periodic trimming of the thickened nail, removal of the nail, and/or medications. Topical medications are less effective than oral agents because topical medications cannot penetrate the thickened nail. Recently developed oral agents such as itraconazole, fluconazole, ketoconazole, and terbinafine have been shown to be effective in the treatment of onychomycosis. For example, itraconazole 200 mg per day given continuously or as a pulse dose (200 mg twice daily for 1 week per month for 3 consecutive months) has been reported to achieve a mycologic cure of 64% at 12 months, with 88% of patients showing marked improvement.

## ADVERSE OUTCOMES OF TREATMENT

Oral therapy is costly and can elevate hepatic enzyme levels. These levels should be tested periodically (especially in patients with a history of hepatic dysfunction). Rare cases of hepatobiliary dysfunction have been reported.

## REFERRAL DECISIONS/RED FLAGS

None

# ORTHOTIC DEVICES

## DEFINITION

Proper shoe fit, shoe modifications, inserts, pads, and orthoses can significantly relieve common foot complaints. An orthosis can support an area of collapse, cushion an area of pressure, accommodate fixed deformity, limit motion, equalize limb length, and reduce shear of the foot in the shoe. The appropriate use of shoe orthoses, commonly referred to as "orthotics," depends on an adequate physical examination and a basic understanding of foot alignment and functions.

## FOOT TYPES AND FUNCTIONS

During gait, the normal foot changes from a supple, shock-absorbing structure to a rigid lever for push-off. At heel strike, the foot is supple, allowing shock absorption and accommodations to uneven ground. During midstance, the foot is converted to a rigid lever that supports full body weight while allowing continued progression of the limb (roll over).

A cavus (highly arched) foot is rigid, cannot unlock during early stance, and lacks shock absorption. A pes planus (flatfoot) foot is extremely supple and often does not effectively supinate to form a rigid lever for push-off.

Many types of simple orthotic devices can be dispensed directly from the physician's office or are available at drugstores, sporting goods stores, and shoe stores. Custom orthoses are used for more complex problems or after off-the-shelf devices fail (**Figure 1**).

## TYPES OF ORTHOTIC DEVICES

### PADS/INSERTS

1. Full-contact insert (full length): A prefabricated rubber or silicone insert that reduces shock by absorbing normal and shear forces.

2. Full-contact orthosis: An orthosis that is molded to the shape of the patient's foot. These are often posted (ie, bringing the ground up to the foot) to improve foot alignment and biomechanics, accommodate a deformity, and/or cushion the foot.

3. Soft orthosis: An orthosis that is used primarily for cushioning but offers little control of foot motion.

4. Semirigid orthosis: The most common type of orthosis; it provides reasonable strength and durability and is made to help control alignment of the foot during gait.

5. Rigid orthosis: An orthosis that offers maximum durability and support but requires a precise fit because it provides little flexibility.

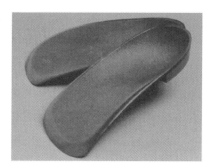

**Figure 1**
Custom orthoses.

*Reproduced with permission from Prolab, San Francisco, CA.*

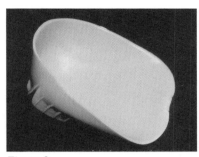

**Figure 2**
Heel insert.

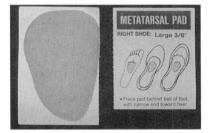

**Figure 3**
Metatarsal pad.

*Reproduced with permission from Hapad, Inc, Bethel Park, PA.*

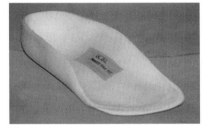

**Figure 4**
UCBL orthosis.

6. Heel insert (eg, felt, foam, gel, rubber, or silicone): Prefabricated, shock-absorbing device available over the counter (**Figure 2**).

7. Heel wedge: A device that is tapered to support varus or valgus hindfoot.

8. Scaphoid pad (arch cookie): A medial longitudinal arch pad that provides support for a flatfoot.

9. Metatarsal pad: A pad that is fixed to an insert or the bottom of the shoe (**Figure 3**).

10. Toe crest: An insert that elevates a toe to relieve pressure at the tip (for mallet toe).

11. Toe separator: A pad that is placed between toes to decrease friction. It is used for calluses and corns.

12. UCBL (University of California Biomechanics Laboratory) orthoses: A type of full-contact orthosis that stabilizes the hindfoot by using medial and lateral vertical supports. Used for midfoot plantar fasciitis or a moderate pes planovalgus foot (**Figure 4**).

## SHOES/MODIFICATIONS

1. Extra-depth shoe: A shoe with increased depth that accommodates forefoot problems, such as a hammer toe, and allows room for inserts.

2. Shoe lift: A device that partially or fully corrects limb length discrepancy. Typically, a ¼" lift can be accommodated inside the shoe. Any elevation up to ½" needs to be added to the outside of the shoe.

3. Metatarsal bar: An internal or external transverse bar that unloads the forefoot (for metatarsalgia).

4. Rocker bottom sole: Contouring sole of shoe to simulate the roll over phase of gait and therefore reduce forces on the plantar surface of the foot during walking.

5. Solid Ankle Cushion Heel (SACH): Soft material that replaces the posterior portion of the shoe's heel to reduce shock at heel strike.

6. Running shoes: Shoes that are designed for shock absorbency. Typically, 50% of shock absorbency is lost at 300 to 500 miles. Running shoes should be replaced at least every 6 months.

7. Shoe fit: Measure the foot by tracing the width of the forefoot while standing barefoot. The forefoot width of the shoe should be approximately ½" wider that this measurement.

8. Thomas heel: Medial extension of the heel to support flatfoot.

# APPLICATION OF ORTHOTIC DEVICES

Table 1 lists the type of orthotic therapy needed for specific foot conditions.

## Table 1
### Recommended Orthotic Treatment for Specific Diagnoses

| Diagnosis | Orthotic therapy |
| --- | --- |
| Bunions and/or bunionettes | Wide toe box, stretch shoes, soft seamless uppers, "bunion shield" type pad |
| Cavus foot (rigid) | Soft orthotic cushions to distribute pressures evenly |
| Flatfoot (adult) | Asymptomatic: No special orthotic or shoe treatment indicated<br>Symptomatic: Semirigid insert or longitudinal arch pad, medial heel wedge, extended heel counter |
| Flatfoot (child) | No special orthotic or shoe treatment indicated. Normal in infancy, with more than 97% correcting spontaneously |
| Hallux rigidus | Full-length prefabricated stiff insert, Morton extension inlay, or rocker bottom sole |
| Hammer toe or claw toe | Accommodative shoe wear, toe crest |
| Metatarsalgia | Wide shoes, metatarsal pads, or metatarsal bars |
| Morton neuroma | Wide toe box, metatarsal pad with neuroma positioning |
| Neuropathic ulceration | Full-contact cushioned orthosis, extra-depth or custom shoes, rocker bottom sole to unload forefoot |
| Plantar fasciitis | Prefabricated heel insert (silicone, rubber, or felt) |
| Runner's painful knee | Sport orthotic inlay: Full-length, soft, prefabricated (decreases pronation and stress) |

# PLANTAR FASCIITIS

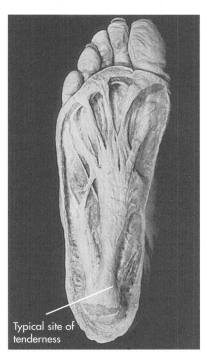

Typical site of tenderness

**Figure 1**
Plantar fascia with digital extension to toes.

## SYNONYMS

Heel spur
Heel pain syndrome
Plantar heel pain

## DEFINITION

The plantar fascia arises from the medial tuberosity of the calcaneus and extends to the proximal phalanges of the toes (**Figure 1**). The plantar fascia provides support to the foot and as the toes extend during the stance phase of gait, the plantar fascia is tightened by a windlass mechanism, resulting in elevation of the longitudinal arch, inversion of the hindfoot, and a resultant external rotation of the leg.

Plantar fasciitis is the most common cause of heel pain in adults. The etiology is probably a degenerative tear of part of the fascial origin from the calcaneus, followed by tendinosis-type reaction. Chronic degenerative changes in the fibers of the plantar fascia are the predominant histologic finding. Plantar fasciitis affects women twice as often as men and is more common in overweight persons. It is not associated with a particular foot type.

## CLINICAL SYMPTOMS

Onset of symptoms is usually insidious and not related to a fall or twisting injury. Patients report focal pain and tenderness directly over the medial calcaneal tuberosity and 1 to 2 cm distally along the plantar fascia. The pain is often most severe on awakening or when rising from a resting position because the first few steps stretch the plantar fascia. Prolonged standing and walking also increases the pain. Sitting typically relieves symptoms.

## TESTS

### PHYSICAL EXAMINATION

Examination reveals tenderness directly over the plantar medial calcaneal tuberosity and 1 to 2 cm distally along the plantar fascia. Often considerable pressure must be applied to this area during the examination to reproduce weight-bearing stress and the patient's symptoms. Patients may have tightness in the Achilles tendon. Passive dorsiflexion of the toes (windlass mechanism) may cause increased pain.

### DIAGNOSTIC TESTS

Radiographs are not necessary as part of the initial evaluation if the patient's history and examination are consistent with a diagnosis of plantar fasciitis. Standing lateral radiographs should be obtained before an injection of corticosteroid or for patients who continue to have symptoms after 6 to 8 weeks of nonoperative treatment. Standing lateral radiographs also may be indicated for patients with systemic symptoms or pain at rest.

A heel spur (osteophyte) develops in the origin of the flexor brevis muscle just superior to the plantar fascia in approximately 50% of patients (**Figure 2**). However, the spur is not a source of pain and is present in 20% of similar-age adults who do not have plantar fasciitis.

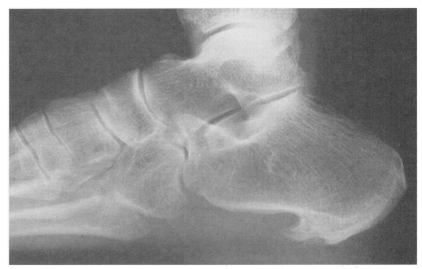

**Figure 2**
Radiographic appearance of a plantar heel spur.

Although not necessary for diagnosis, a bone scan will show increased uptake at the medial calcaneal tuberosity. MRI, which also is not necessary for diagnosis or treatment, will show thickening of the origin of the plantar fascia, as well as marrow edema in the calcaneal tuberosity.

## DIFFERENTIAL DIAGNOSIS

Acute traumatic rupture of the plantar fascia (ecchymosis, tenderness, swelling over the proximal plantar fascia)

Calcaneal stress fracture (rare, tenderness with medial and lateral pressure of the calcaneus)

Calcaneal tumor (rare, pain at rest, night pain)

Fat pad atrophy/contusion (tenderness over an abnormally prominent calcaneal tuberosity)

Sciatica (radicular symptoms)

Seronegative spondyloarthropathy (typically bilateral enthesitis of the plantar fascia, other sites of enthesitis and arthralgic joints involved)

Tarsal tunnel syndrome (paresthesias and numbness on the plantar aspect of the foot)

## ADVERSE OUTCOMES OF THE DISEASE

Patients can experience chronic heel pain and a significant alteration in daily activities. Altered gait may aggravate forefoot, knee, hip, or back problems.

## TREATMENT

Over 95% of patients with plantar fasciitis can be managed satisfactorily with nonoperative treatment. Patients should be informed that it commonly takes 6 to 12 months for symptoms to resolve. Avid walkers and joggers need counseling concerning alternative exercise regimens, such as use of a stationary bike.

Initial treatment should include an orthotic device, such as a silicone, rubber, or felt heel pad (**Figure 4**), along with a home program of stretching exercises. To stretch the Achilles tendon, the patient should lean forward against a wall, keeping one knee straight with the heel on the ground while bending the other knee (**Figure 5**). This maneuver can be done with either one or both legs, depending on whether one or both heels are painful. As the patient bends forward, he or she should feel the calf muscles stretch. The stretch should be held for 10 seconds. Patients should repeat this exercise several times each day.

For the plantar fascia stretching exercise, the patient should be instructed to lean forward over a table, chair, or countertop, spread the feet apart with one foot in front of the other, flex the knees, and squat down slowly. The heels must be kept on the ground as long as possible during the squat. As the patient squats, he or she should feel the heel cord and plantar fascia stretch as the heels finally start to lift from the ground. The patient should stretch and hold for 10 seconds, then relax and straighten. Patients should repeat this exercise several times each day.

Some studies suggest that a night splint should be used as part of initial treatment. The night splint holds the ankle and foot in slight extension, which maintains the Achilles tendon and plantar fascia in a stretched position during sleep.

Contrast baths, ice, NSAIDs, and/or shoes with shock-absorbing soles also can be used to decrease inflammation in the painful heel (see Contrast Baths, p 425).

If symptoms are unchanged after 8 weeks, injection of corticosteroid into the heel may be indicated (see Injection for Plantar Fasciitis, pp 491-492). A formal physical therapy consultation may be necessary to help direct the patient's continued stretching program.

If symptoms persist, the use of a nonremovable cast or custom orthotic device should be considered. Surgical treatment typically consists of partial release of the plantar fascia.

## ADVERSE OUTCOMES OF TREATMENT

NSAIDs can cause gastric, renal, or hepatic complications. Fat pad necrosis or rupture of the plantar fascia can develop from improper injection of corticosteroids. Surgical treatment may not improve symptoms and also can cause complete disruption of the plantar fascia.

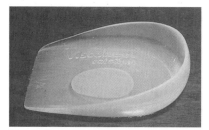

**Figure 3**
Heel pad.

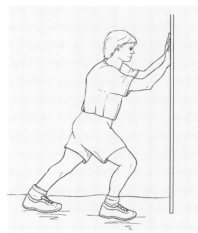

**Figure 4**
Achilles stretching exercise.

*Adapted with permission from the American Orthopaedic Foot and Ankle Society, Seattle, WA.*

SECTION 7 | FOOT AND ANKLE

## Referral decisions/Red flags

Patients whose symptoms do not respond to nonoperative treatment need further evaluation. Surgical release should be considered only after 6 to 12 months of intense nonoperative management.

# PROCEDURE

## INJECTION FOR PLANTAR FASCIITIS

### MATERIALS

Sterile gloves

Bactericidal skin preparation solution

Ethyl chloride spray

Lateral radiograph of the heel

5-mL syringe

18-gauge needle

21-gauge 1-to-1½" needle

Mixture of 1 mL of 10 to 40 mg/mL of corticosteroid preparation and 4 mL of 1% lidocaine, without epinephrine

Adhesive dressing

### STEP 1

Wear protective gloves at all times during the procedure and use sterile technique.

### STEP 2

Use the 18-gauge needle to draw 1 mL of 40 mg/mL corticosteroid preparation and 4 mL of the local anesthetic into the syringe, then switch to the 21-gauge needle to preserve sterility.

### STEP 3

Prepare the medial aspect of the heel.

### STEP 4

Spray ethyl chloride onto the medial heel to freeze the skin.

### STEP 5

Measure the soft-tissue thickness beneath the calcaneus directly on the radiograph.

### STEP 6

Using the measurement from the radiograph as a guide, palpate the calcaneus medially where it begins to curve upward. Insert the 21-gauge needle into this area, which is approximately 2 cm from the plantar surface of the foot (Figure 1).

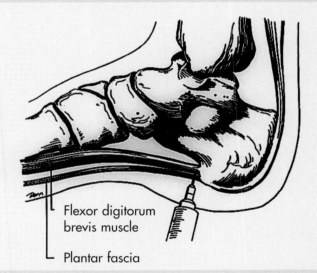

Flexor digitorum brevis muscle

Plantar fascia

**Figure 1**
Proper location for injection.

# INJECTION FOR PLANTAR FASCIITIS (CONTINUED)

## STEP 7

Advance the needle down to the calcaneus until it hits the bone. Walk the tip of the needle distally along the bone to the plantar surface of the calcaneus. The needle should be immediately superior (deep) to the plantar fascia.

## STEP 8

Advance the needle to its hilt and inject 3 mL of the anesthetic-corticosteroid mixture. Inject the remaining 2 mL of the preparation while withdrawing the needle 2 cm, then withdraw the needle completely. Make certain that you do not inject the anesthetic-corticosteroid preparation into the medial subcutaneous tissue or the fat pad of the heel that is superficial to the plantar fascia.

## STEP 9

Dress the puncture wound with a sterile adhesive bandage.

## ADVERSE OUTCOMES

Injection of a corticosteroid into the superficial fat pad can cause fat necrosis, with loss of cushioning of the plantar heel. The injection may cause rupture of the plantar fascia.

## AFTERCARE/PATIENT INSTRUCTIONS

Advise the patient that transient numbness of the heel can occur. Also explain that heel pain could return in a few hours when the anesthetic agent wears off and that the corticosteroid might take a few weeks to have an effect on the symptoms.

# POSTERIOR HEEL PAIN

ICD-9 Code
726.71
    Achilles bursitis or tendinitis

## SYNONYMS

Haglund syndrome
Insertional Achilles tendinitis
Pump bump

## DEFINITION

Pain in the posterior heel around the insertion of the Achilles tendon can originate from one or more of the following structures: the insertion of the
Achilles tendon into the calcaneus (insertional Achilles tendinitis); the retrocalcaneal bursa (retrocalcaneal bursitis); a prominent process of the calcaneus
impinging on the Achilles tendon (Haglund syndrome); or inflammation of
the bursa between the skin and the Achilles tendon (pump bump). The exact
etiology may be confusing because frequently one or more of these areas are
involved at the same time (**Figure 1**).

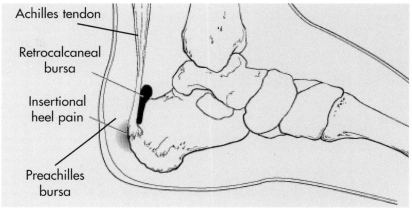

**Figure 1**
Sites of posterior heel pain.

## CLINICAL SYMPTOMS

Patients with a prominent process of the calcaneus initially develop a bursa
that is irritated by shoe wear and causes a pump bump (**Figure 2**). In later
years, insertional tendinitis with calcification and degenerative tears of the
Achilles tendon are most often seen. Start-up pain as well as pain after activity is common, as is a limp. Shoe wear can be difficult because of the direct
pressure on the posterior heel prominence.

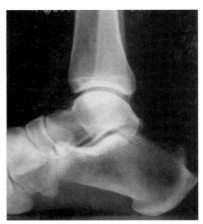

**Figure 2**
Prominent superior process of calcaneus with calcification of tendon.

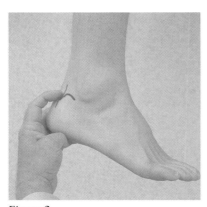

**Figure 3**
Palpate on either side of the Achilles tendon insertion.

# TESTS

## *PHYSICAL EXAMINATION*

Examination reveals swelling and tenderness at the posterior heel. The prominence is usually larger on the lateral side of the heel. A superficial bursa (pump bump) that is soft can be present and inflamed by shoe wear.

The Achilles tendon may be diffusely thickened and inflamed. Retrocalcaneal bursitis can cause pain anterior to the Achilles tendon that is increased by squeezing the bursa from side to side and just anterior to the Achilles tendon. (**Figure 3**).

## *DIAGNOSTIC TESTS*

Lateral radiographs of the heel may show calcification of the Achilles tendon and spur formation. A prominent posterosuperior process of the calcaneus also might be apparent.

# DIFFERENTIAL DIAGNOSIS

Achilles tendon avulsion (palpable defect in the tendon, positive Thompson test)

Os trigonum syndrome (posterolateral pain increased with forced dorsiflexion)

Plantar fasciitis (pain below the calcaneus)

Stress fracture of the calcaneus (midcalcaneal bony tenderness)

# ADVERSE OUTCOMES OF THE DISEASE

Difficulty with shoe wear and sports activities is possible, as is chronic pain and limping.

# TREATMENT

A heel lift or open-back shoes will minimize pressure on the inflamed area. Ice massage and contrast baths will decrease inflammation (see Contrast Baths, p 425). Achilles tendon stretching exercises should be used if an equinus contracture is present. Casting for 4 to 6 weeks may alleviate symptoms. Surgical intervention will remove the prominent bone and diseased tendon.

# ADVERSE OUTCOMES OF TREATMENT

Surgical removal of bone and debridement of the Achilles tendon can predispose to rupture.

# REFERRAL DECISIONS/RED FLAGS

Recalcitrant pain or failure to respond to nonoperative management indicates the need for further evaluation.

# PLANTAR WARTS

ICD-9 Code
078.19
Viral warts, unspecified; other specified viral warts

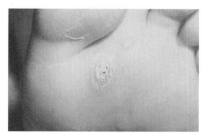

**Figure 1**
Clinical appearance of a plantar wart.

*Reproduced with permission from California Pacific Medical Center, San Francisco, CA.*

## SYNONYM

Verruca vulgaris

## DEFINITION

Plantar warts are hyperkeratotic lesions caused by a papillomavirus that develops on the sole of the foot. The peak incidence is in the second decade and is more commonly observed in athletic youngsters.

## CLINICAL SYMPTOMS

Patients have painful, slightly raised lesions on the sole of the foot. These lesions may occur in clusters known as "mosaic warts."

## TESTS

### PHYSICAL EXAMINATION

Warts usually appear on non–weight-bearing areas on the sole of the foot. Normal papillary lines of the skin (fingerprint pattern) cease at the margin of the lesion (**Figure 1**). The lesions usually are very tender if pinched side to side, a finding not observed with a corn or callus. By contrast, a corn is tender with direct pressure. A plantar wart can occur anywhere on the sole, whereas a callus is associated with a bony prominence. Superficial paring of a wart with a scalpel reveals punctate hemorrhage and a fibrillated texture. A callus is avascular and on paring has a uniform texture that resembles yellow candle wax.

### DIAGNOSTIC TESTS

When doubt exists, histopathologic examination of a specimen confirms the diagnosis. However, this type of testing is seldom necessary, given the characteristic gross appearance after superficial paring.

## DIFFERENTIAL DIAGNOSIS

Callus (hyperkeratotic lesion that forms in response to a bony prominence)

Foreign body (correlates with history and examination)

Plantar fibromatosis (fibroblastic reaction in plantar fascia)

## ADVERSE OUTCOMES OF THE DISEASE

Plantar warts are often persistent; they can spread to other areas of the foot, grow larger, and leave scars on the sole of the foot.

## TREATMENT

Most lesions resolve spontaneously within 5 to 6 months, so aggressive treatment should be reserved for unusually large, painful, or persistent lesions.

Initial treatment commonly includes superficial paring, followed by the use of a keratolytic agent, such as salicylic acid in liquid or salve form. The lesion should then be covered with occlusive tape to ensure that the medication stays within the desired area and debrides the necrotic layers of tissue upon removal of the tape. Medication should be applied twice daily for 1 month.

Warts that are resistant to initial treatment will sometimes respond to intralesional injection of approximately 1 mL of local anesthetic with epinephrine. Electrocautery, cryotherapy with liquid nitrogen, laser ablation, or curettage may be performed under local anesthetic. Care should be taken to avoid causing necrosis of the deep dermis, which can produce intractable, painful scarring on the sole of the foot. In curettage, for example, the subcutaneous fat should not be visible when the procedure is finished. Intralesional injections of bleomycin and radiation therapy also have been described for severe, recalcitrant lesions, but these options are best performed by specialists with experience in their use.

## ADVERSE OUTCOMES OF TREATMENT

Secondary infection can occur after treatment. Intractable scarring from excessively deep ablation is also a significant risk.

## REFERRAL DECISIONS/RED FLAGS

Persistent or recurring warts warrant further evaluation.

# POSTERIOR TIBIAL TENDON DYSFUNCTION

## SYNONYMS

Acquired flatfoot
Posterior tibial tendon rupture
Posterior tibial tendon insufficiency

## DEFINITION

The posterior tibial tendon is one of the main supporting structures of the medial ankle and arch. Posterior tibial tendon dysfunction is the primary cause of medial ankle pain in the middle-aged patient. Demographically, the classic presentation is an overweight woman who is older than age 55 years. Steroid injections, diabetes, hypertension, and/or previous injury to the foot are other risk factors. The posterior tibial tendon is thickened and shows degenerative changes. As a result, the posterior tibialis muscle is ineffective and its function of supporting the medial longitudinal arch is lost. As a result, a flatfoot develops. Initially the foot is flexible, but over time the deformity becomes fixed and the hindfoot joints develop arthritic changes.

## CLINICAL SYMPTOMS

Pain and swelling on the medial aspect of the ankle are the most common complaints. Usually patients state that they have lost the arch and that the ankle rolls in. The onset of symptoms is insidious, and there is usually no history of trauma. Although pain and tenderness initially is along the medial aspect of the foot, lateral pain ultimately develops as the collapsed flatfoot abuts the fibula during gait.

## TESTS

### PHYSICAL EXAMINATION

Both feet should be examined from the knee down with the patient standing. Examination shows swelling and tenderness posterior and inferior to the medial malleolus, along the course of the posterior tibial tendon. The medial arch is decreased or completely flattened. The heel shows increased valgus and with advanced changes the forefoot is in abduction. When viewed from behind, the affected foot will show "too many toes" because of the forefoot abduction and hindfoot valgus (**Figure 1**).

Posterior tibial strength is decreased on both manual muscle testing as well as functional maneuvers. Normally a patient with both hands placed on a wall can perform a toe rise on one leg, and during this maneuver, the posterior tibial tendon will pull the heel into inversion. Patients with dysfunction or rupture of the posterior tibial tendon cannot perform a complete heel rise on

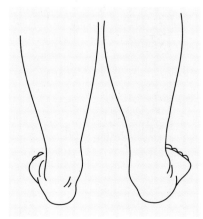

**Figure 1**
"Too many toes" sign

SECTION 7 | FOOT AND ANKLE

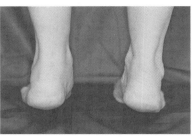

**Figure 2**
The left heel does not rotate inward (varus) when the patient stands on her toes.

one leg, and when this test is performed while standing on both legs, normal inversion of the heel does not occur (**Figure 2**).

## DIAGNOSTIC TESTS

Standing AP and lateral radiographs of the foot reveal a flatfoot, with alignment changes at the talonavicular and other joints. MRI of the posterior tibial tendon may be useful in equivocal situations.

## DIFFERENTIAL DIAGNOSIS

Congenital pes planus (bilateral, present since childhood)

Lisfranc fracture-dislocation (history of trauma, pain in the midfoot)

Medial ankle laxity (rare, abnormal ankle radiographs)

Medial malleolus stress fracture (focal bony tenderness)

Tarsal coalition (fixed deformity, onset as adolescent or young adult)

## ADVERSE OUTCOMES OF THE DISEASE

A progressive, painful flatfoot with gait disturbance is common. A severe flatfoot makes shoe wear or even bracing difficult.

## TREATMENT

Tenosynovitis of the tendon without a flatfoot should be treated with a short leg cast or cast brace for 4 weeks, NSAIDs, and activity limitation. After the cast is removed, a molded ankle-foot orthosis may be used as the tendinitis resolves. An injection of corticosteroid may weaken the already pathologic tendon and is not recommended. When nonoperative treatment fails, surgical debridement of the tendon may be indicated.

Once a flexible flatfoot starts to develop, the use of a medial heel wedge, a medial longitudinal arch support, or a molded ankle-foot orthosis can help. A UCBL (University of California Biomechanics Laboratory) orthotic insert can be effective. Often surgery is required. If the deformity is relatively mild, then a tendon transfer, often combined with realignment osteotomy and/or ligament reconstructive procedures, can be done. However, once a rigid flatfoot develops, stabilization of the hindfoot by arthrodesis is the better alternative.

## ADVERSE OUTCOMES OF TREATMENT

Tendon transfer surgery may fail, requiring an arthrodesis of the hindfoot.

## REFERRAL DECISIONS/RED FLAGS

Patients with unexplained medial ankle pain require further evaluation because a medial ankle sprain rarely occurs. Patients with a recent onset of flatfoot deformity also require further evaluation.

# RHEUMATOID FOOT AND ANKLE

ICD-9 Code
714.0
Rheumatoid arthritis

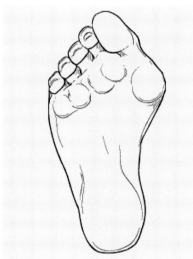

**Figure 1**
Metatarsalgia develops as the fat pad is pulled distally and the metatarsal heads become more prominent.

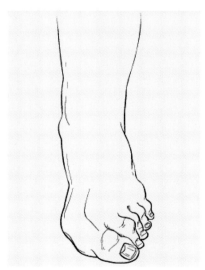

**Figure 2**
Hallux valgus and lesser toe deformities are associated with rheumatoid arthritis.

## DEFINITION

Ninety per cent of patients with rheumatoid arthritis are estimated to have symptoms that are related to the foot or ankle. Longevity of the disease correlates with the presence and severity of symptoms. Ninety percent of patients report symptoms in the forefoot and midfoot, and 67% report symptoms in the ankle and hindfoot. Chronic synovitis leads to stretching of the capsule and ligaments of the joints with subsequent malalignment of the joints, and ultimately to bony deformities such as hallux valgus, claw toes with subluxated or dislocated metatarsophalangeal (MP) joints, and end-stage arthritis of the ankle or subtalar joint.

## CLINICAL SYMPTOMS

Patients present with loss of motion and pain on weight bearing.

Metatarsalgia commonly occurs with subluxation/dislocation of the lesser toe MP joints, claw toes, and distal migration of the fat pad (**Figure 1**). Severe hallux valgus often accompanies lesser toe deformities (**Figure 2**).

In the hindfoot, tenosynovitis of the posterior tibial tendon can produce medial ankle pain and swelling. Early arthritis of the talonavicular or subtalar joint also is common and typically occurs before ankle involvement.

The ankle is usually one of the last joints to be involved in rheumatoid arthritis.

## TESTS

### PHYSICAL EXAMINATION

Metatarsophalangeal synovitis, with focal pain and swelling over the MP joints, may be the presenting complaint in patients with rheumatoid arthritis. Bilateral symptoms, multiple joint involvement, and the presence of nodules should lead to clinical suspicion of rheumatoid arthritis.

### DIAGNOSTIC TESTS

Laboratory tests reveal an elevated erythrocyte sedimentation rate and positive rheumatoid factor. Radiographs reveal soft-tissue swelling, osteopenia, subchondral erosions, and malalignment. Lateral drift occurs at the MP joints and at the talonavicular joint (**Figure 3**).

## DIFFERENTIAL DIAGNOSIS

Posterior tibial tendon dysfunction (swelling and tenderness over the posterior tibial tendon)

Seronegative spondyloarthropathies (enthesitis such as plantar fasciitis or Achilles tendinitis)

Traumatic arthritis (history of preceding trauma)

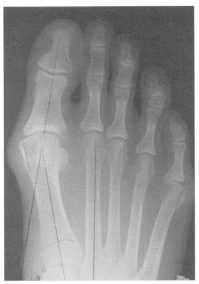

**Figure 3**
AP radiograph of foot showing severe hallux valgus and dislocated metatarsophalangeal joints.

## ADVERSE OUTCOMES OF THE DISEASE

Pain, progressive deformity, and metatarsalgia with plantar ulcerations are common if the condition remains untreated.

## TREATMENT

Medical management can improve symptoms and slow the progression of disease. Disease-modifying agents (such as methotrexate) have been shown to decrease synovitis and slow progression of the disease. Corticosteroid injections can be helpful for inflamed joints and significant tenosynovitis.

An extra-depth accommodative shoe with a molded insole and metatarsal bar often relieves metatarsalgia. A UCBL (University of California Biomechanics Laboratory) orthosis can provide significant pain relief for a patient who has a flexible hindfoot deformity. A molded ankle-foot orthosis can be used for more extensive disease involvement.

The most reliable surgery for forefoot deformity involves fusion of the first MP joint with metatarsal head resections. Implant arthroplasty of the great toe is rarely indicated.

Tenosynovectomy is only a temporizing procedure and is rarely indicated. Most patients with severe arthritis of the hindfoot joints require triple arthrodesis (talocalcaneal, talonavicular, and calcaneocuboid joints). Patients still have dorsiflexion and plantar flexion through the ankle joint after a triple arthrodesis.

Significant ankle arthritis may require arthrodesis. Patients with rheumatoid arthritis who have severe ankle destruction often have subtalar joint involvement. Injections into the joints can help determine which is more symptomatic. When both joints are involved, a pantalar (tibiotalocalcaneal) fusion should be performed. Total ankle replacements in patients with rheumatoid arthritis remains investigational.

## ADVERSE OUTCOMES OF TREATMENT

Foot deformities can progress even with optimal medical management.

## REFERRAL DECISION/RED FLAGS

Persistent pain despite medical management signals the need for further evaluation.

# SESAMOIDITIS

ICD-9 Code
733.99
  Sesamoiditis

## SYNONYM
Dancer's toe

## DEFINITION
The sesamoid bones are embedded in the flexor hallucis brevis tendon beneath the first metatarsal head (plantar surface). Sesamoid disorders include inflammation, fracture, and arthritis. Sesamoiditis occurs from repeated stress of the sesamoid and the subsequent inflammation. Fractures of the sesamoid may be acute or stress related.

## CLINICAL SYMPTOMS
Pain under the first metatarsal head is noted, with or without swelling and ecchymosis (**Figure 1**). The usual stresses involve dancing or running, but sesamoiditis also can be caused by trauma from falls or more commonly by forced dorsiflexion of the great toe with acute onset of pain.

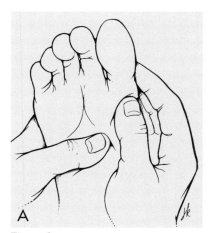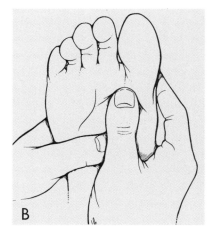

**Figure 1**
A, Location of the medial sesamoid. B, Location of the lateral sesamoid.
*Reproduced with permission from Alexander IJ: The Foot: Examination and Diagnosis. New York, NY, Churchill Livingstone, 1990, p 65.*

## TESTS

### PHYSICAL EXAMINATION
With both sesamoiditis and sesamoid fractures, examination reveals focal tenderness at the sesamoid bone directly beneath the metatarsal head. The tender spot will move with the sesamoid as the great toe is flexed and extended. Dorsiflexion of the toe is painful.

## DIAGNOSTIC TESTS

AP, lateral, and axial radiographs of the sesamoid bones are indicated. An oblique view of the sesamoid also may be helpful in visualizing a fracture line. Bipartite or multipartite sesamoid bones are common, occurring in 25% of the population. These normal variants have smooth margins and should not be confused with fractured sesamoids that have sharp margins. Comparison views of the opposite foot or a bone scan may be helpful.

## DIFFERENTIAL DIAGNOSIS

Hallux rigidus (limited dorsiflexion, dorsal spur, dorsal tenderness)

Hallux valgus (pain medially, lateral deviation of the great toe)

Metatarsalgia (tenderness over the plantar aspect of a lesser metatarsal)

Neuroma (pain and tenderness over the medial sensory nerve)

## ADVERSE OUTCOMES OF THE DISEASE

Without treatment, the patient may have pain and a limp. Nonunion may occur following an acute fracture.

## TREATMENT

An acute sesamoid fracture is best treated with a stiff-soled shoe or a removable short leg fracture brace. Patients may change to a stiff-soled shoe with a wide toe box as symptoms permit, usually about 4 weeks after the injury. A J-shaped (dancer's) pad can help relieve pressure under the first metatarsal head once the fracture has healed and the patient begins to ambulate in everyday shoes.

Patients with sesamoiditis should be advised to avoid wearing high-heeled shoes. For more severe symptoms, taping the great toe in plantar flexion, using sesamoid pads, or wearing a removable short leg fracture brace for 4 to 6 weeks can relieve pressure on the sesamoids and decrease inflammation. If these measures fail, excision of the sesamoid may be required.

## ADVERSE OUTCOMES OF TREATMENT

Hallux valgus or varus is rare but can develop following removal of a sesamoid.

## REFERRAL DECISIONS/RED FLAGS

Persistent pain is an indication for further evaluation.

# SHOE WEAR

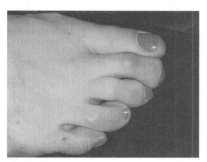

**Figure 1**
The foot takes the shape of the shoe, not vice versa.

Shoes protect and cushion the feet and in many cases serve a cosmetic purpose. Improperly fitted or improperly manufactured shoes are the cause of many foot deformities. Women who consistently wear high-heeled shoes with a narrow toe box have an increased incidence of bunions, hammer toes, corns, and—ultimately—foot surgery (**Figure 1**). Foot size increases with age, and many adult men and women continue to buy the same size shoe without having their foot measured. Patients need instruction about proper fitting shoes.

## SHOE DESIGN AND LASTING TECHNIQUES

Shoes are designed in seven basic styles: pump, Oxford, sandal, mule, boot, clog, and moccasin. Fashionable shoes come in variations of these styles, although the design of some fashionable footwear can indicate that little regard has been shown for proper shoe function.

The last is the three-dimensional form (either straight or curved) on which the base of the shoe is made. The shape of the toe box, instep, and curve of the shoe is determined by the last. The straighter the last, the straighter the shoe and the more medial support the shoe can provide.

Common methods of lasting include slip lasting, board (or flat) lasting, and combination lasting. A slip-lasted shoe is constructed by sewing together the upper, like a moccasin, then gluing it into the sole. This method makes a lightweight, flexible shoe with no tortional rigidity.

With board-lasting or flat-lasting techniques, the upper is fastened to the insoles with tacks or staples. This construction makes a stable but less flexible shoe.

Combination lasting uses more than one technique for the same shoe. Shoes made in this way are typically board-lasted in the rear for stability and slip-lasted in the forefoot for flexibility.

## SHOE ANATOMY

### OUTER SOLE

The outer sole makes contact with the ground and usually is attached to the midsole (**Figure 2**). Most athletic shoes have outer soles made of hard carbon rubber or blown rubber compounds. The outer sole provides pivot points and can be designed with a herring bone pattern, suction cups, radial edges, or asymmetric studs. These design patterns enhance stability and traction.

### MIDSOLE AND WEDGE

The midsole and the heel wedge are located between the inner and the outer sole and are attached to both. These components provide cushioning, shock absorption, lift, and control.

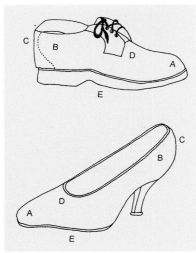

**Figure 2**
Anatomy of the shoe. A, Toe box; B, Quarter; C, Counter; D, Vamp; E, Outsole. The insole is hidden inside the shoe and provides the surface on which the foot rests.

*Reproduced with permission from Yodlowski ML, Femino JE: Shoes and orthoses, in Mizel MS, Miller RA, Scioli MW (eds): Orthopaedic Knowledge Update Foot and Ankle 2, American Academy of Orthopaedic Surgeons, Rosemont, IL 1998, pp 55-64.*

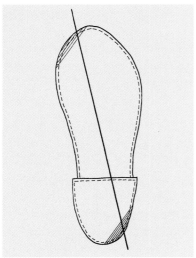

**Figure 3**
Normal wear pattern.

*Reproduced with permission from Yodlowski ML, Femino JE: Shoes and orthoses, in Mizel MS, Miller RA, Scioli MW (eds): Orthopaedic Knowledge Update Foot and Ankle 2, American Academy of Orthopaedic Surgeons, Rosemont, IL 1998, pp 55-64.*

## HEEL COUNTER

The heel counter is a firm cup built into the rear of the shoe that holds the heel in position and helps control excessive foot motion.

## TOE BOX

The toe box may include a stiff material inserted between the lining and outer surface in the toe area to prevent collapse and protect the toes.

## TONGUE

The tongue is designed primarily to protect the dorsum of the foot from dirt, moisture, and pressure.

## SOCK LINERS, ARCH SUPPORTS, AND INSERTS

The sock liner covers the insole and provides comfort and appearance. This liner acts primarily as a buffer zone between the shoe and the foot. Arch supports, heel cups, and other types of padding provide additional support, cushioning, and motion control.

## WELT

The welt is a strip of leather or other material that joins the upper with the outer sole.

## SHOE ANALYSIS AND FIT

Whenever patients have a foot or ankle complaint, evaluation of their shoes should be an integral part of the examination. Wear patterns are generally predictable, with the normal wear pattern on the outer sole slightly medial at the toe and lateral at the heel (**Figure 3**). Abnormalities in the wear pattern indicate problems with alignment and gait. A tracing of the weight-bearing foot should be compared to a tracing of the shoe (**Figure 4**).

Although proper fitting of shoes is not an exact science, relying on a number of easy-to-follow guidelines can help. Shoes always should be fit to the weight-bearing foot at the end of the day, when feet are at their largest. Shoes cannot be stretched to the shape of the foot. The upper should not wrinkle with flexion, and the foot should not bulge over the welt. The end of the longest toe of the larger foot should be within $^3/_8$" to $^1/_2$" of the end of the toe box. The forefoot should not be crowded, and the toes should easily extend. The shoe should provide a relatively snug grip at the counter above the heel. High heels should be avoided because this style exerts excessive pressure on the front of the foot. Above all else, shoes should be comfortable from the moment they are tried on.

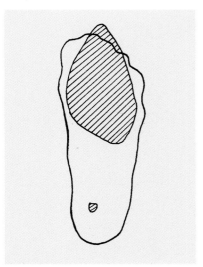

**Figure 4**
There is often a large mismatch between the contour of a patient's foot (solid line) and the shoe they are wearing (shaded area). Note the compression of the forefoot and the very small contact area of the high heel. Such a tracing can often disclose the cause of a patient's foot pain.

*Reproduced with permission from Yodlowski ML, Femino JE: Shoes and orthoses, in Mizel MS, Miller RA, Scioli MW (eds): Orthopaedic Knowledge Update Foot and Ankle 2, American Academy of Orthopaedic Surgeons, Rosemont, IL 1998, pp 55-64.*

## ADVERSE OUTCOMES FROM POOR SHOE FIT

Bunion, hammer toes, neuromas, corns and calluses, and ingrown toenails are all possible.

# SOFT-TISSUE MASSES OF THE FOOT AND ANKLE

ICD-9 Codes

727.43
    Ganglion and cyst of synovium,
    tendon, and bursa, unspecified
728.71
    Plantar fascial fibromatosis

## SYNONYMS

Plantar fibromas
Nodular fasciitis
Mucoid cyst
Fibromatosis
Ledderhose disease

## DEFINITION

Ganglia and plantar fibromas are the most common soft-tissue tumors in the foot and ankle. Other lesions are not included in this chapter.

A ganglion is a cystic tumor that contains gelatinous fluid and arises from a joint capsule or tendon sheath. Ganglia of the foot or ankle usually are small, 2- to 3-cm masses that arise on the top or side of the foot.

A plantar fibroma is a benign thickening of the plantar fascia that can vary in size from 1 to 6 cm. Plantar fibromas may evolve to plantar fibromatosis (nodular fasciitis of the plantar fascia), a condition that is similar histologically to Dupuytren disease of the palmar fascia. Compared to Dupuytren disease, plantar fibromatosis is less likely to cause severe deformities of the toes or feet.

## CLINICAL SYMPTOMS

A ganglion cyst typically is a painless, soft nodule but may cause problems with aching, nerve compression, or shoe wear. A plantar fibroma is a firm mass on the bottom of the foot that may be painful and is more likely to interfere with shoe wear.

## TESTS

### PHYSICAL EXAMINATION

A ganglion cyst is a discrete mass that is usually movable with side-to-side pressure. A plantar fibroma can be focal or can have multiple, discrete masses that are hard (rubbery) and are part of the plantar fascial band.

### DIAGNOSTIC TESTS

Plain radiographs are typically normal. Aspiration of a ganglion with an 18-gauge needle will return a straw-colored, gelatinous material. Sophisticated diagnostic imaging generally is not necessary for either a ganglion cyst or a plantar fibroma.

## DIFFERENTIAL DIAGNOSIS

Giant cell tumor of the tendon sheath (solid mass, inability to aspirate soft core)

Lipoma (subcutaneous fatty deposit)

Malignant sarcoma (synovial sarcoma, fibrosarcoma)

Neurofibroma (often tubular along the course of the nerve)

## ADVERSE OUTCOMES OF THE DISEASE

Patients may report persistent discomfort and difficulty with shoe wear. Malignant degeneration of a plantar fibroma is possible, but the risk is small.

## TREATMENT

The wall of the ganglion can be pierced three or four times with an 18-gauge needle to release the gelatinous core and promote complete collapse of the cyst. Care should be taken to avoid an overlying sensory nerve. If the ganglion recurs and continues to be symptomatic, it should be excised. The efficacy of corticosteroid injection into a ganglion has not been proven.

A plantar fibroma is best treated with shoe modifications and an orthotic device. Surgical excision is indicated in patients with significant persistent symptoms or if the fibroma has increased significantly in size.

## ADVERSE OUTCOMES OF TREATMENT

Surgical excision of a plantar fibroma should be avoided, if possible, because of the high rate of recurrence and potential for a painful plantar surgical scar.

## REFERRAL DECISIONS/RED FLAGS

If the diagnosis of the mass is not clear based on anatomy, examination, radiographs, and aspiration, further evaluation is needed to rule out other etiologies. Recurrence of a ganglion following aspiration usually requires surgical excision.

# STRESS FRACTURES OF THE FOOT AND ANKLE

SECTION 7 | FOOT AND ANKLE

ICD-9 Codes
824
　Fracture of ankle
825.2
　Fracture of tarsal and metatarsal
　bones

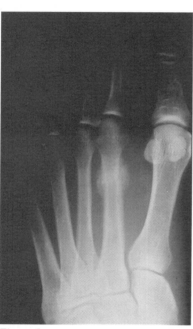

**Figure 1**
AP radiograph showing a healed stress
fracture of the second metatarsal.

## SYNONYMS
March fracture
Insufficiency fracture

## DEFINITION
A stress fracture is caused by repetitive overloading. The bone fails when the fatigue process exceeds the reparative process. Stress fractures often result from an increased level of activity or after beginning a different type of activity, such as military training or initiating walking for exercise. Conditions that weaken the bone predispose patients to stress fractures; therefore, these injuries are sometimes referred to as insufficiency fractures. Young, athletic women are at risk because of the triad of amenorrhea, osteopenia, and overexercise. Older women are at risk because of osteoporosis.

The metatarsals are the most common site of a stress fracture site (especially the second metatarsal), but these fractures also can be seen in other bones of the foot and ankle including the navicular, calcaneus, and fibula (**Figures 1-3**). Theoretically, any bone exposed to repetitive stress can sustain a stress fracture.

## CLINICAL SYMPTOMS
Patients present with the insidious onset of pain and swelling. The pain increases with weight-bearing activity and is relieved by rest. Metatarsal fractures will present with a diffusely swollen dorsal forefoot, whereas fibula fractures produce a swollen lateral ankle. Some patients report hearing a crack or pop as the incomplete stress fracture became a complete break.

## TESTS
### PHYSICAL EXAMINATION
Localized point tenderness and concomitant swelling directly over the fracture site are the most reliable physical signs. Ecchymosis occasionally is observed.

### DIAGNOSTIC TESTS
Early radiographs (less than 2 weeks from onset of symptoms) are usually normal, but after 3 to 4 weeks, radiographs show healing callus at the fracture site. A bone scan is more sensitive than a radiograph and can be positive by 5 days (**Figure 4**). MRI can confirm the diagnosis but is not routinely used.

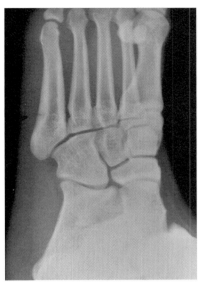

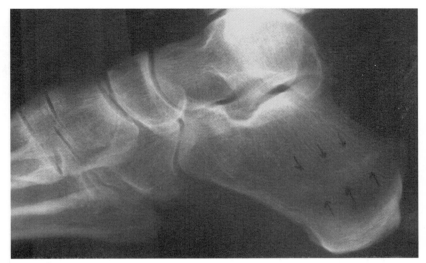

**Figure 3**
Calcaneal stress fracture seen as density (between arrows).

**Figure 2**
Stress fracture of the fifth metatarsal.

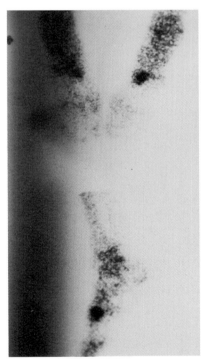

**Figure 4**
Stress fracture.

## DIFFERENTIAL DIAGNOSIS

Gout (redness, erythema)

Metabolic bone disorders (multiple stress fractures)

Morton neuroma (pain and tenderness in the intermetatarsal space)

Neoplasm (pain at night or at rest)

Synovitis of the second metatarsophalangeal joint (swelling and tenderness of the joint)

## ADVERSE OUTCOMES OF THE DISEASE

Chronic stress fractures may require prolonged immobilization to heal. Displacement of fractures with continued unprotected activity can lead to malunion or nonunion that requires surgical procedures. This is more likely with fifth metatarsal (Jones fracture) and navicular stress fractures.

## TREATMENT

Treatment for most patients is based on reduced activity and protective footwear. For metatarsal stress fractures, a stiff-soled shoe, wooden-soled postoperative sandal, or removable short leg fracture brace shoe will be sufficient. Most patients with calcaneal and fibula fractures will benefit from 2 to 4 weeks of immobilization in a short leg walking cast. Because of the high rate of nonunion, navicular and fifth metatarsal fractures both should be casted, and the patient should use crutches and avoid bearing weight on the involved limb. Internal fixation is often a better alternative for a stress fracture of the fifth metatarsal.

## Adverse outcomes of treatment

Metatarsal stress fractures can displace in the sagittal plane and lead to a painful callus. NSAIDs may retard osteogenesis and should be avoided during fracture healing.

## Referral decisions/Red flags

Navicular, fifth metatarsal, and all fibula stress fractures require further evaluation early after diagnosis. Failure to heal by 4 to 6 weeks or recurrent fractures suggest the need for a metabolic work-up.

# Tarsal Tunnel Syndrome

**ICD-9 Code**
355.5
Tarsal tunnel syndrome

## Synonym
Posterior tibial nerve entrapment

## Definition
Tarsal tunnel syndrome describes the symptom complex associated with compression neuropathy of the posterior tibial nerve or its branches posterior to the medial malleolus (**Figure 1**). Although an analogy to carpal tunnel syndrome of the upper extremity has been suggested, the only real similarity is the name. In contrast with carpal tunnel syndrome, tarsal tunnel syndrome is much less common, its symptoms are more vague and intermittent, and its diagnosis more difficult. Numerous causes of tarsal tunnel syndrome have been reported including compression from a ganglion or bony lesion, but most cases are of unknown etiology.

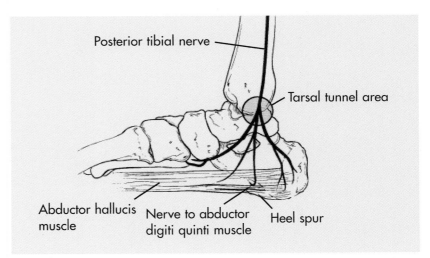

**Figure 1**
Anatomy of the tarsal tunnel.

## Clinical symptoms
Most patients complain of diffuse, poorly localized pain along the medial ankle. Paresthesias (tingling) or dysthesias (burning) along the medial ankle and into the arch are a common component of the symptom complex. The pain is often worse after walking and also can occur at night.

## Tests
### Physical examination
The physical examination reveals tenderness over the tarsal tunnel just posterior to the medial malleolus (**Figure 2**). Percussion over the posterior tibial

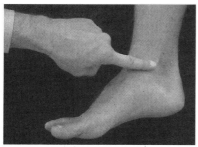

**Figure 2**
Tenderness over the tarsal tunnel just posterior to the medial malleolus is indicative of tarsal tunnel syndrome.

nerve (Tinel sign) should reproduce the symptoms. Decreased sensation in the distribution of the posterior tibial nerve on the plantar aspect of the foot also can be present.

### DIAGNOSTIC TESTS

Radiographs of the foot and ankle are necessary to rule out bony pathology, but the radiographs are usually normal. MRI can be useful for determining an etiology such as a ganglion, but the MRI usually is normal. Electrodiagnostic testing may identify tibial nerve entrapment; however, a positive or negative test does not always correlate with intraoperative findings or clinical outcomes.

### DIFFERENTIAL DIAGNOSIS

Complex regional pain syndrome (discoloration of foot, skin and temperature changes)

Diabetic neuropathy (history of diabetes, bilateral loss of nerve function in a stocking distribution)

Herniated lumbar disk (leg and thigh pain)

Peripheral neuropathy (stocking distribution)

Posterior tibial dysfunction (pain associated with pes planus)

### ADVERSE OUTCOMES OF THE DISEASE

Persistent pain and numbness are possible, and severe numbness can lead to plantar ulcers. Complex regional pain syndrome also can develop.

### TREATMENT

For patients with flatfeet and significant pronation, an orthotic device used to support the medial arch and decrease stretch along the tibial nerve may alleviate symptoms. Review of the surgical results shows a lower success rate for tarsal tunnel release compared with that for carpal tunnel release.

### ADVERSE OUTCOMES OF TREATMENT

Symptoms may not resolve completely if permanent nerve damage has occurred. Surgical nerve release can lead to increased scarring and increased symptoms. The results of revision tarsal tunnel surgery are extremely poor, especially when an adequate decompression of the nerve was performed during the initial procedure.

### REFERRAL DECISIONS/RED FLAGS

Further evaluation is needed for patients who have one or more of the following conditions: severe or progressive symptoms; loss of motor strength, which can indicate a herniated disk; or severe pain to light touch, which can indicate complex regional pain syndrome.

# TOE DEFORMITIES

ICD-9 Codes
734.8
    Claw toe (acquired)
735.4
    Hammer toe (acquired)
735.8
    Other acquired deformities of toe

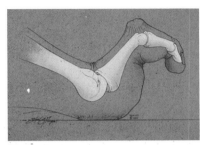

**Figure 1**
Clinical appearance of a claw toe.

## DEFINITION

Deformities of the lesser toes are categorized as three types: hammer toes, claw toes, and mallet toes. These deformities are most commonly caused by constrictive, improperly fitting shoes. They also are caused by an imbalance of the intrinsic (arising from the foot) and extrinsic (arising from the leg) muscles.

A claw toe has fixed extension of the metatarsophalangeal (MP) joint and flexion of the proximal interphalangeal (PIP) joint (**Figure 1**). A flexion contracture of the distal interphalangeal (DIP) joint may be present as well. Claw toes usually affect all of the lesser toes of the foot and often are secondary to a neurologic disorder such as Charcot-Marie-Tooth disease, or an inflammatory arthritis such as rheumatoid arthritis. Patients with diabetes who have a peripheral neuropathy commonly develop claw toes.

A hammer toe has a flexion deformity of the PIP joint with no significant deformity of the DIP or MP joints (**Figure 2**). The flexion deformity of the PIP joint may cause some passive extension of the MP joint when the patient is standing, but the MP joint is in neutral alignment when the foot is examined in a non–weight-bearing position.

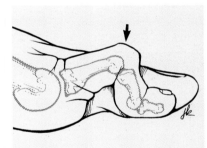 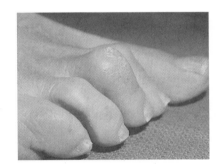

**Figure 2**
Clinical appearance of a hammer toe.

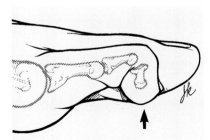

**Figure 3**
Clinical appearance of a mallet toe.

A mallet toe has a flexion deformity at the DIP joint with relatively normal alignment of the PIP and MP joints (**Figure 3**). Hammer toes and mallet toes can be isolated to a single toe due to improper shoe wear. The second toe is most commonly affected.

## CLINICAL SYMPTOMS

Pain, deformity, and difficulty with shoe wear are the common complaints of patients with lesser toe deformities. A corn can develop on the dorsum of the PIP joint or tip of the toe. These calluses are painful and can become infected. In patients with hyperextension of the MP joint, the metatarsal head is displaced plantarly with resultant increased pressure, callus, and pain on the plantar side of the forefoot.

## TESTS

### PHYSICAL EXAMINATION

Examine the patient in both standing and sitting positions. Note alignment, the presence of corns, and flexibility and stability of the MP, PIP, and DIP joints. Evaluate alignment and mobility of the ankle and hindfoot joints. Look for a cavus foot associated with neurologic disorders. Evaluate sensory and motor function of the foot and lower extremities.

### DIAGNOSTIC TESTS

Radiographs are helpful only in planning surgery and to rule out osteomyelitis when ulceration of the toe has occurred. Neurologic work-up may be indicated in patients with claw toes and a high arch.

## DIFFERENTIAL DIAGNOSIS

Neurologic or rheumatologic disorder (claw toes)

## ADVERSE OUTCOMES OF THE DISEASE

Without treatment, patients have difficulty with shoe wear, and persistent painful corns and calluses. Ulceration can lead to infection and possible osteomyelitis.

## TREATMENT

Shoe modification with soft, roomy toe boxes to accommodate these deformities is the mainstay of treatment. A shoe repair shop can help by stretching shoes to accommodate single hammer and mallet toe deformities. Commercially available running and walking shoes often provide enough depth to accommodate most deformities. Shoes with heels higher than 2¼" should be avoided. Over-the-counter, protective cushions are helpful when corns develop.

Passive stretching of the toes can keep the toes flexible and prevent a fixed deformity.

Commercially available straps to hold the toes in place can provide symptomatic relief (**Figure 4**). In addition, the patient can tape the toe into flexion at the MP joint. With a narrow strip of tape, begin on the plantar aspect of the foot under the metatarsal head, looping over the dorsum of the proximal phalanx and crossing back to the starting point while holding the toe flexed at the MP joint.

Surgical correction may be necessary for fixed deformities. The goals of surgery are not cosmesis, but alignment of the toes to comfortably accommodate footwear. Postoperatively, the toes tend to sit flat but do not have normal range of motion and tend to swell for several months.

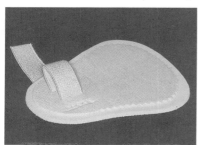

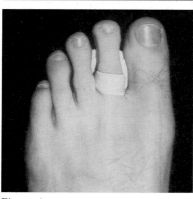

**Figure 4**
Type of splint used for a claw toe.

## Adverse outcomes of treatment

Continued pain, corns, and recurrent deformity are possible.

## Referral decisions/Red flags

Failure of nonoperative treatment or persistent ulceration requires further evaluation. Patients with vascular insufficiency are poor candidates for surgical treatment.

# TURF TOE

**ICD-9 Code**
845.12
Sprains and strains of ankle and
foot; metatarsophalangeal (joint)

## SYNONYM

First metatarsophalangeal joint sprain

## DEFINITION

Turf toe is a sprain of the first metatarsophalangeal (MP) joint that most commonly occurs with hyperextension but can occur with any forced range of motion. The term "turf toe" was coined because the incidence of these injuries increased with the use of artificial turf on athletic playing fields. Turf toe injuries can have significant morbidity, and in some studies account for more missed playing time than ankle sprains.

## CLINICAL SYMPTOMS

Patients usually report swelling, tenderness, and limited motion of the first MP joint. A grade 1 sprain is a stretch injury of the capsule, with the athlete usually able to participate in sports with mild symptoms. A grade 2 sprain is a partial tear of the plantar ligamentous complex of the MP joint. These patients have moderate swelling, ecchymosis, and decreased range of motion. A grade 3 sprain is a complete tear of the MP ligamentous complex. Marked swelling, bruising, and limited motion occur with grade 3 injuries. The patient can neither compete athletically nor walk normally.

## TESTS

### PHYSICAL EXAMINATION

Assess the degree of swelling, ecchymosis, range of motion, and gait.

### DIAGNOSTIC TESTS

Radiographs are useful to detect associated avulsion fractures, evaluate joint congruity, and rule out preexisting arthritic changes. When the diagnosis is in question, a bone scan or MRI can help exclude other possibilities such as sesamoid or metatarsal fractures.

## DIFFERENTIAL DIAGNOSIS

Hallux rigidus (arthritis of the first MP joint)

Sesamoid stress fracture (focal pain over the sesamoid)

## ADVERSE OUTCOMES OF THE DISEASE

Instability and arthritis (hallux rigidus) of the first MP joint can develop. Symptomatic loose bodies and osteochondritic lesions can occur.

## TREATMENT

Nonoperative treatment with rest, ice, compression, and elevation usually is sufficient. Early range of motion is started as symptoms allow. Grade 3 injuries require protected weight bearing or immobilization for 1 to 2 weeks, with a 4- to- 6-week period of rest from athletics. Taping, orthotic devices, or a rocker bottom sole to restrict MP motion may decrease symptoms. Surgical intervention is seldom necessary except in the case of displaced intra-articular or avulsion fractures.

## ADVERSE OUTCOMES OF TREATMENT

Delayed return to sports activities, hallux rigidus, and acquired hallux varus or valgus can occur.

## REFERRAL DECISIONS/RED FLAGS

Intra-articular fractures can require open reduction or excision. Urgent surgical intervention is necessary for an irreducible dislocation. Osteochondral lesions or loose bodies also require further evaluation.

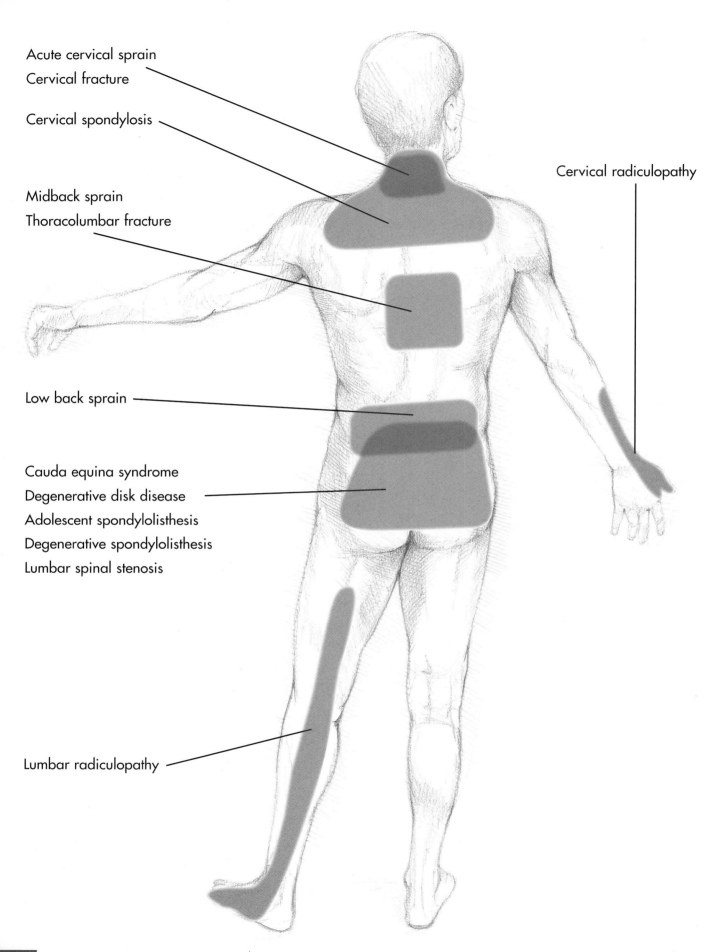

Acute cervical sprain
Cervical fracture

Cervical spondylosis

Cervical radiculopathy

Midback sprain
Thoracolumbar fracture

Low back sprain

Cauda equina syndrome
Degenerative disk disease
Adolescent spondylolisthesis
Degenerative spondylolisthesis
Lumbar spinal stenosis

Lumbar radiculopathy

# SPINE

**Section Editor**
Robert K. Snider, MD
Orthopaedic Surgeon
Billings, Montana

Darrel S. Brodke, MD
Assistant Professor
Department of Orthopedics
University of Utah Health Sciences Center
Salt Lake City, Utah

Jeffrey S. Fischgrund, MD
Attending Spine Surgeon
Department of Orthopaedics
William Beaumont Hospital
Royal Oak, Michigan

Harry N. Herkowitz, MD
Chairman
Department of Orthopaedics
William Beaumont Hospital
Royal Oak, Michigan

Alan M. Levine, MD
Director, Alvin and Lois Lapidus Cancer Institute
Head, Division of Orthopedic Oncology at
Sinai Hospital
Clinical Professor
Orthopaedic Surgery and Oncology
University of Maryland School of Medicine
Baltimore, Maryland

James T. Lovitt, MD
Billings, Montana

Gregory S. McDowell, MD
Co-Director, Northern Rockies Regional Spine Injury
Center
Orthopaedic Surgeons PSC
St. Vincent Hospital and Health Center
Billings, Montana

Peter V. Teal, MD
Billings, Montana

# SPINE—AN OVERVIEW

Common degenerative disorders of the spine do not cause loss of life or limb, but they do alter function and comfort and often threaten employment or recreational activities. Low back pain affects 60% to 80% of the adult population at some time; therefore, it may be less a disease than a natural attendant of aging (Table 1). Patients between the ages of 30 and 50 years find chronic back pain particularly frustrating as these years coincide with peak economic, social, and family demands. Most episodes of back and neck pain resolve within a few weeks with little residual effect, but back pain is significant because it is often a patient's first illness that substantially interferes with their function. Patients with persistent pain are often dissatisfied with treatment programs because of the recurring nature of their problem.

## Table 1
### Common Spinal Conditions by Age Group

| Age group | Common conditions |
| --- | --- |
| Younger than 10 years | Intervertebral diskitis, myelomeningocele, osteoblastoma, leukemia, congenital kyphosis, and scoliosis |
| 11-19 years | Spondylolisthesis, kyphosis (Scheuermanns disease) |
| 20-29 years | Disk injuries (central disk protrusion, disk sprain), spondylolisthesis, spinal fracture |
| 30-39 years | Cervical and lumbar disk herniation or degeneration |
| 40-49 years | Cervical and lumbar disk herniation or degeneration, spondylolisthesis with radicular pain |
| 50-59 years | Disk degeneration, herniated disk, metastatic tumors |
| 60 years | Spinal stenosis, disk degeneration, herniated disk, spinal instability, metastatic tumors |

For most back problems, it is important to perform a thorough medical history and establish a diagnosis (Table 2). Nonoperative treatment should be provided before further intervention is considered. During this time, patients should continue working, although job modifications may be needed. Ultimately, some patients may need to change jobs, a move that can have significant economic and psychologic consequences. In addition, litigation following vehicular injury and workers' compensation issues often clouds the treatment process with concerns of causation and aggravation. Educating patients about their spinal problems and the impact these problems have on their lives is a challenge that demands patience and concern.

## Table 2
### Common Presentation of Spinal Problems

| Problem | Associated signs and symptoms | Possible diagnosis |
| --- | --- | --- |
| Neck pain | Paravertebral discomfort relieved with rest and aggravated with activity | Acute neck sprain |
| | Limited motion or morning stiffness | Cervical spondylosis |
| Neck and arm pain | A younger patient with an abnormal upper extremity neurologic examination | Cervical radiculopathy due to herniated nucleus pulposus |
| | An older patient with limited motion and pain on extension | Cervical radiculopathy due to cervical spondylosis |
| | Urinary dysfunction with global sensory changes, weakness, and an abnormal gait | Cervical myelopathy secondary to cervical spondylosis or trauma |
| | Shoulder pain and a positive impingement sign | Shoulder pathology |
| | Tinel sign and nondermatomal distribution of symptoms | Peripheral nerve entrapment |
| Back pain | Paravertebral discomfort relieved with rest and aggravated with activity | Acute low back sprain |
| | Limited motion or stiffness | Degenerative disk disease, ankylosing spondylitis |
| | Unrelenting night pain and weight loss | Tumor |
| | Fevers, chills, and sweats | Infection or intervertebral disk infection |
| Back and leg pain | A younger patient with an abnormal lower extremity neurologic examination | Lumbar radiculopathy due to herniated nucleus pulposus |
| | An older patient with poor walking tolerance and a stooped gait | Spinal stenosis |
| | Tenderness over the lateral hip and discomfort at night | Trochanteric bursitis |

The most significant adverse outcomes of spinal disease are myelopathy or paralysis. These problems may develop in association with trauma, tumors, spinal stenosis, a cauda equina syndrome, sudden progression of spondylolisthesis, or a lumbar radiculopathy.

The most serious etiology of back pain is a malignant tumor, most of which are metastatic, and some of which cause bony collapse and paralysis. The tumors that most commonly metastasize to bone are prostate, breast, lung, renal, adrenal, and thyroid.

## TYPE OF PAIN

Night pain that interrupts or prevents sleep, along with fever and weight loss, may indicate a malignancy or infection. Acute, posttraumatic pain may indicate an associated fracture. Low back pain is distinctly uncommon in children and always warrants evaluation.

# LOCATION OF PAIN

## NECK PAIN
Pain located in the neck, trapezial, and interscapular areas most commonly occurs in association with degeneration of the intervertebral disk. Pain from an acute cervical sprain (whiplash) is usually self-limiting.

## NECK AND RADICULAR ARM PAIN
When accompanied by referred pain into the arm, neck pain may be the result of an entrapment of a cervical nerve root by a herniated disk or bony spur. For screening diagnostic information, see **Figure 1**. Many patients with a herniated cervical disk are more comfortable when they place the hand of the symptomatic arm on their head, since this position reduces the tension on the nerve. In contrast, patients with intrinsic shoulder problems feel more comfortable with their arms at their sides. With peripheral nerve entrapment syndromes, such as carpal tunnel syndrome, patients may report arm pain and a lesser degree of neck pain.

## LOW BACK PAIN
Low back pain typically occurs in the midline at about the L4 or L5 level. Many patients indicate that this pain radiates to the sacroiliac or buttock areas. Back problems that affect patients between the ages of 20 and 30 years are often related to sprains of the soft-tissue structures of the back, including the ligamentous support portion of the intervertebral disk, the annulus fibrosus. The annulus may weaken with repeated small tears, leading to degenerative disk disease in later years. Young adults with spondylolisthesis may have recalcitrant back pain and may have to change jobs. With seronegative spondyloarthropathies (such as ankylosing spondylitis), patients often have back pain with morning stiffness that lasts longer than 30 minutes.

With aging and degeneration of the intervertebral disk, associated arthritis may develop in the facet joints and contribute to the chronic back pain often seen after age 40 years. Back pain associated with spinal stenosis may be aggravated by spinal extension (standing or walking upright or sleeping supine). Diffuse idiopathic skeletal hyperostosis (DISH) often becomes symptomatic after age 50 years and primarily affects men.

Extra-spinal causes of back pain include pancreatitis, kidney stones, pelvic infections, and tumors or cysts of the reproductive tract.

## BACK AND RADICULAR LEG PAIN
Unilateral leg pain is common with herniation of an intervertebral disk, usually at the L4-5 or L5-S1 vertebral levels. This pain is typically worse with sit-

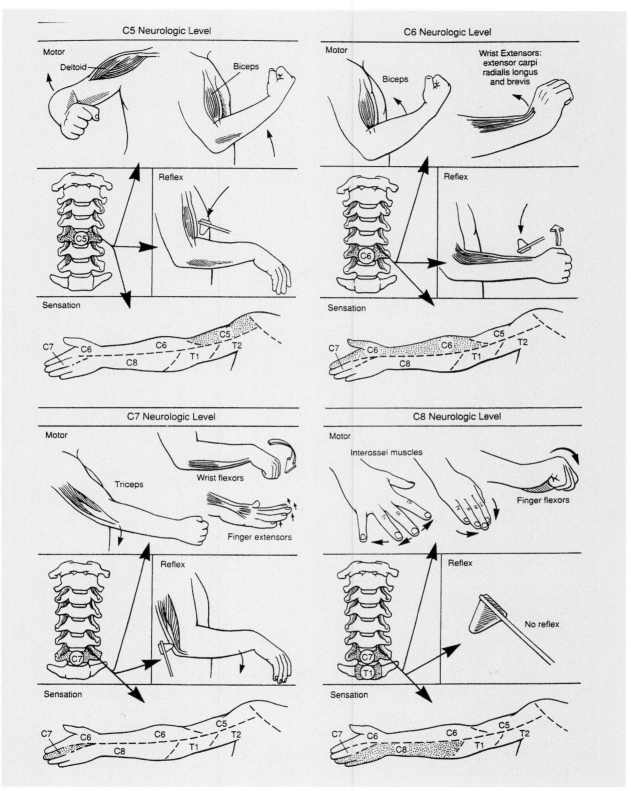

**Figure 1**
Neurologic evaluation of the upper extremity (C5-6, C6-7).

*Reproduced with permission from Klein JD, Garfin SR: History and physical examination, in Weinstein JN, Rydevik BL, Somtag VKH (eds): Essentials of the Spine. New York, NY, Raven Press, 1995, pp 71–95.*

ting and is associated with sciatic tension signs (straight-leg raising test, flip sign) as well as altered sensation, motor strength, and reflexes in the lower extremity (**Figure 2**). Trochanteric bursitis in women mimics sciatica, and the two problems may coexist. Lumbar disk herniation uncommonly occurs at a more proximal level. In this situation, radicular symptoms are in a different location and femoral nerve stretch signs are positive.

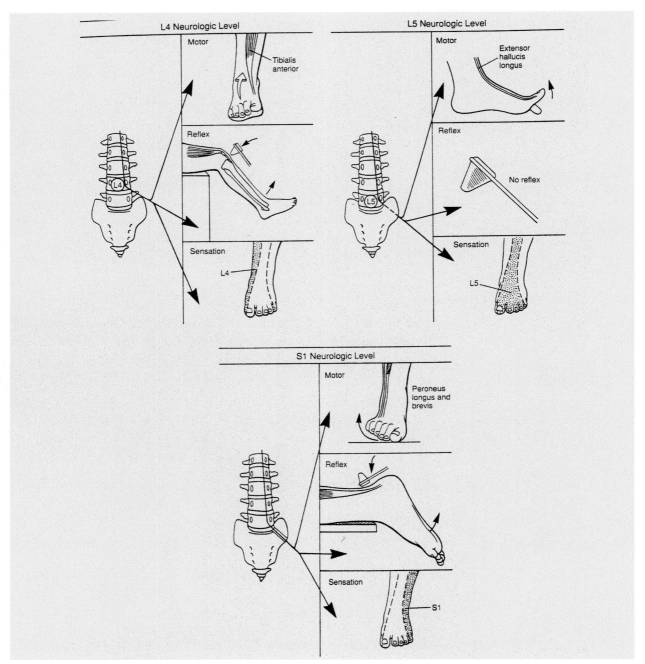

**Figure 2**
Neurologic evaluation of the lower extremity (L4-5).

*Reproduced with permission from Klein JD, Garfin SR: History and physical examination, in Weinstein JN, Rydevik BL, Somtag VKH (eds): Essentials of the Spine. New York, NY, Raven Press, 1995, pp 71–95.*

Bilateral leg pain may indicate spinal stenosis, a large central disk rupture with cauda equina syndrome, or spondylolisthesis, especially after the age of 40 years. Exercise-induced leg pain (unilateral or bilateral) may signify spinal stenosis. Spinal stenosis is typically more severe at the L3-4 and L4-5 interspaces.

Extra-spinal causes of nerve root entrapment or irritation include hip disease, pyriformis syndrome, ovarian cysts, and retroperitoneal lesions.

# Deformity

Kyphosis is best seen from the side with the patient bending forward. Scoliosis is associated with rotation of the spinal column that is more obvious when the patient bends forward. Scoliosis is usually idiopathic, but patients should be evaluated for other causes such as neurofibromatosis or spinal cord lesions. Spondylolisthesis usually occurs at the lumbosacral joint and is accompanied by tight hamstring muscles (inability to toe-touch). Onset of a spinal deformity in adulthood suggests spinal instability, osteoporosis, or a tumor. These conditions may be accompanied by compromise of the spinal nerve roots.

# Trauma

All spinal trauma must be evaluated radiographically. Some bony injuries are subtle, especially in the cervical spine, and the potential consequences of misdiagnosis can be devastating. Spinal fractures are often accompanied by other life-threatening visceral, head, or skeletal injuries. For various reasons some spinal injuries may be missed initially in the multiply injured patient even after an appropriate work-up. Special imaging of the spine should be left to the discrimination of the consultant to avoid unnecessary reduplication of these expensive tests.

# Gender

Women have an increased incidence of the following spinal conditions: scoliosis in adolescence, metastatic breast cancer and trochanteric bursitis in later adulthood, and osteoporosis with vertebral body fractures and increased kyphosis after menopause.

Men have an increased incidence of the following spinal conditions: kyphosis in adolescence, ankylosing spondylitis in adulthood, multiple myeloma and DISH in later adulthood, and metastatic carcinomas from the prostate and lung.

In conclusion, spinal problems may be associated with radicular pain into a limb and may have serious etiologies. Most, however, are related to degenerative changes associated with aging or growth.

# PHYSICAL EXAMINATION
# SPINE

## Inspection/Palpation

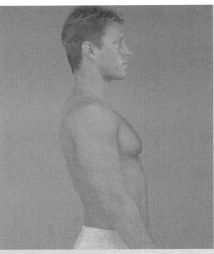

### Lateral view

With the patient standing, inspect for deviations in normal cervical lordosis, thoracic kyphosis, and lumbar lordosis. Loss of cervical lordosis or lumbar lordosis occurs with painful conditions such as acute sprains, fractures, infectious or neoplastic processes.

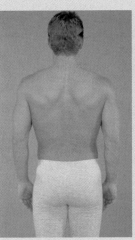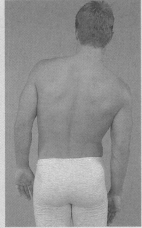

### Posterior view

Inspect the spine for normal, straight alignment (left). Moderate to severe scoliosis will be obvious. Also inspect for muscle atrophy. A lumbar list might be present in association with a herniated disk or other condition in which the patient will lean to one side to alleviate nerve root compression (right).

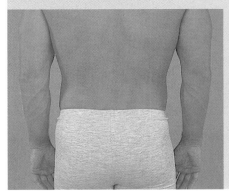

### Pelvic tilt

Observe the patient standing with the feet together and the knees straight. Inspect or palpate the top of the iliac crests. A pelvis that is not level usually indicates limb-length inequality, but it may be secondary to curvature of the spine.

# Inspection/Palpation

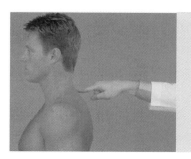

### Spinous process

Palpate the spinous processes to define the alignment of the spine. C7 (shown in figure) is the most prominent cervical spinous process. The top of the thyroid cartilage is at the level of the C4 vertebral body, and the cricoid cartilage is parallel to the C6 vertebral body. Lumbar landmarks include the top of the posterior iliac crest, usually at the same level as the L4 vertebral body, and the posterior superior iliac spine, indicated by the dimples of Venus, at the same level as the S2 vertebral body.

# Range of Motion–Cervical Spine

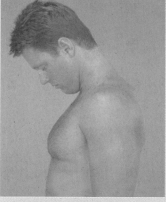

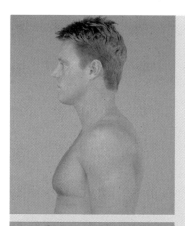

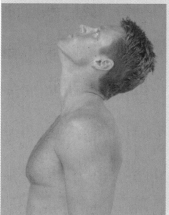

### Flexion and extension: Zero Starting Position

The Zero Starting Position is with the neck aligned with the trunk (top). Stabilize the trunk so that motion does not occur in the thoracic spine. Assess flexion with forward bending of the cervical spine (center) and extension with posterior inclination (bottom). Flexion and extension are typically estimated visually in degrees; however, limited flexion can also be measured as the distance the chin lacks in touching the sternum.

# Range of Motion–Cervical Spine

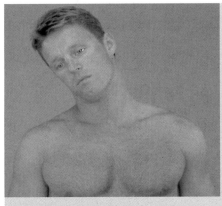

## Lateral bend

The Zero Starting Position is with the nose vertical and in line with the axis of the trunk. Stabilize the trunk so that motion occurs only at the neck. Right lateral bend is with the head inclined toward the right, and left lateral bend is the opposite direction. The degree of motion is the angle between the vertical axis and midaxis of the face.

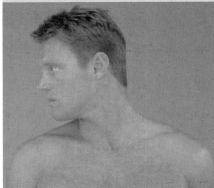

## Rotation

The Zero Starting Position is the same as that for lateral bend. Rotation is estimated in degrees. To measure rotation with the neck in maximum flexion is primarily an estimate of upper cervical vertebral rotation.

# Range of Motion–Lumbar Spine

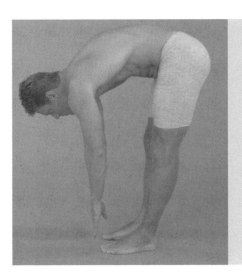

## Flexion-extension, visual estimation

The Zero Starting Position is with the patient standing with the hips and knees straight and the trunk in line with the lower extremities. The feet should be comfortably apart to facilitate movement of the spine, and the arms should hang in a relaxed, extended position. With the spine at maximum flexion, measure the distance between the fingertips and the floor. If at maximum flexion the fingertips are more than 10 cm from the floor, there is an increased association with lumbar radiculopathy or nonorganic pathology. The former is more likely with a positive flip sign.

# Range of Motion–Lumbar Spine

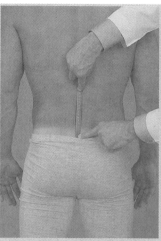
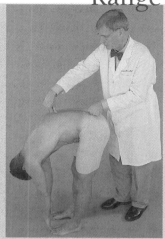

### Flexion, simplified skin distraction

This test uses principles previously described with the modified Schober test, but the landmarks for the simplified skin distraction test provide more precise measurements of lumbar spine motion.

With the patient in the Zero Starting Position, measure a 15-cm span, starting distally on a line with the posterior superior iliac spines (dimples of Venus) (left). Ask the patient to bend to a position of maximum flexion, and then measure the distance between these end points again (right). The degree of lumbar flexion is the distance between these points on maximum flexion minus 15 cm. Normal lumbar flexion is 5 to 7 cm of skin distraction.

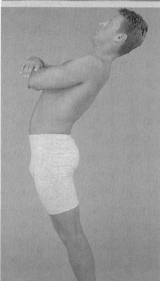

### Extension, simplified skin distraction

Lumbar extension can be estimated visually or quantified by the skin distraction technique. Mark a 15-cm span as described previously. Ask the patient to place the spine in maximum extension, and then measure the distance between the end points. The degree of extension is the distance measured in maximum extension minus 15 cm.

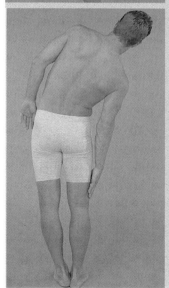

### Lateral bending, tape measure method

Use of a tape measure to evaluate lateral bend quantifies the degree of restricted motion and correlates with disability. Mark the thigh at the tip of the long finger with the patient in the Zero Starting Position and with the spine positioned in lateral maximum bend. Record the distance between the two positions (normal range is 15 to 30 cm).

# Muscle Testing–Cervical Spine

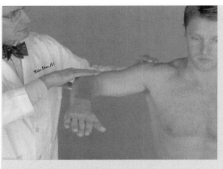

## C5–Deltoid muscle

With the patient seated, abduct the shoulder to 90°. Push down on the arm to resist activity of the deltoid. A ratchety, giving way motion is a nonorganic sign. True weakness is uniform.

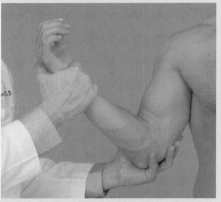

## C5–Biceps

With the patient seated, ask the patient to flex the elbow in a supinated position as you apply resistance. The biceps also is innervated by C6, but if C5 is intact, biceps strength should be at least grade 3. Test C5 sensation by assessing light touch on the lateral aspect of the arm.

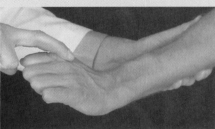

## C6–Radial wrist extensors

Flex the patient's fingers to eliminate wrist extension activity by the finger extensor muscles, then ask the patient to extend the wrist in a radial direction as you apply resistance. Test C6 sensation by assessing light touch on the volar aspect of the thumb.

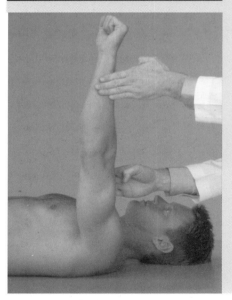

## C7–Triceps

With the patient supine and the shoulder flexed approximately 90°, ask the patient to extend the elbow as you apply resistance.

# Muscle Testing–Cervical Spine

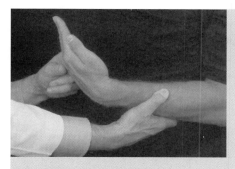

### C7–Flexor carpi radialis

With the patient seated, place the fingers in extension to eliminate wrist flexor activity by the finger flexor muscles, and then ask the patient to flex the wrist in a radial direction as you apply resistance. Test C7 sensation by assessing light touch on the volar aspect of the long finger.

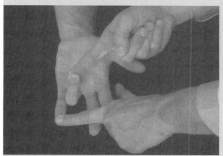

### C8–Flexor digitorum sublimus to ring finger

Stabilize the long, index, and little fingers in extension and ask the patient to flex the fingers as you apply resistance. Test C8 sensation by assessing light touch on the volar aspect of the little finger.

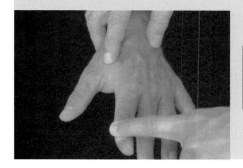

### T1–First dorsal interossei

Ask the patient to abduct the index finger as you apply resistance. Palpate the muscle belly of the first dorsal interossei to confirm activity of the muscle. Test T1 sensation by assessing light touch on the medial aspect of the arm proximal to the elbow.

# Muscle Testing–Lumbar Spine

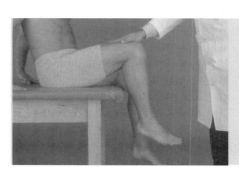

### L1–Hip flexors

With the patient seated, ask the patient to flex the hip as you apply resistance. Check light touch on the proximal and anterior aspects of the thigh to test sensation.

# Muscle Testing–Lumbar Spine

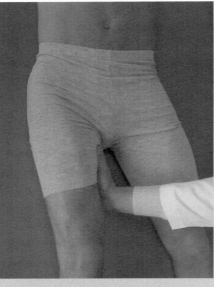

### L2–Hip adductors

With the patient supine, ask the patient to adduct the thigh as you apply resistance. The hip adductors are also innervated by L3 and L4, but if L2 is intact, the hip adductors are at least grade 3. Check light touch at the middle portion of the anterior aspect of the thigh to test L2 sensation.

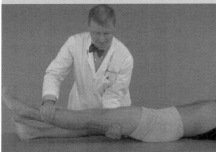

### L3–Quadriceps

With the patient supine, ask the patient to extend the knee as you apply resistance. Check light touch just below the patella to test L3 sensation.

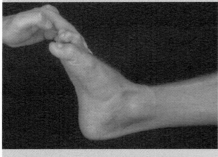

### L4–Anterior tibialis

With the patient seated, have the patient flex the toes to eliminate dorsiflexor activity by the toe extensor muscles. Ask the patient to dorsiflex the ankle in an inverted position as you apply resistance. Check light touch just above the medial malleolus to test L4 sensation.

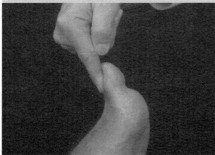

### L5–Extensor hallucis longus

With the patient supine or seated, stabilize the foot in a neutral position with one hand and ask the patient to extend the great toe as you apply resistance. Check light touch in the first web space to test L5 sensation.

# Muscle Testing–Lumbar Spine

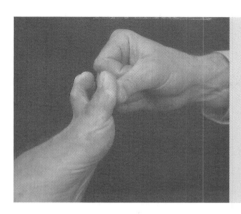

## S1–Flexor hallucis longus

With the patient supine or seated, stabilize the foot in a neutral position with one hand and ask the patient to flex the great toe as you apply resistance. Check light touch on the lateral border of the foot to test S1 sensation.

# Special Tests

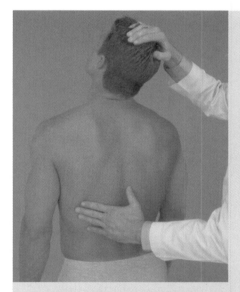

## Spurling test

Ask the patient to extend the neck while tilting the head to the side. This maneuver narrows the neural foramen and will increase or reproduce radicular arm pain associated with cervical disk herniations or cervical spondylosis.

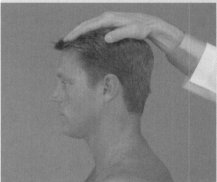

## Axial loading

With the patient standing, push down on the patient's head; this maneuver may provoke neck pain in some patients with disk pathology, but increased low back pain from this maneuver is usually a nonorganic finding.

Special Tests

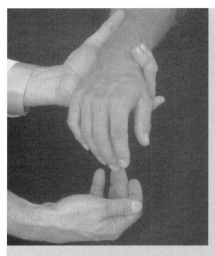

### Hoffmann reflex

With the patient seated and the patient's relaxed hand cradled in yours, flick the long finger nail and look for index finger and thumb flexion as a sign of long-tract spinal cord involvement in the neck.

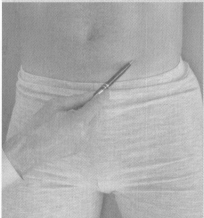

### Superficial abdominal reflex

With the patient supine, stroke lightly toward the umbilicus. The normal reflex is movement of the umbilicus toward the stimulated side. Absence of this motion may suggest spinal cord pathology in the cervical or thoracic region. Perform the test in the upper and lower quadrants on on both sides.

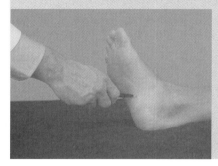

### Babinski sign

With the patient supine, stroke lightly upward on the plantar surface of the foot and look for great toe extension (withdrawal response) and fanning of the lesser toes as a sign of long-tract spinal cord involvement. Also called flexor plantar response.

# Special Tests

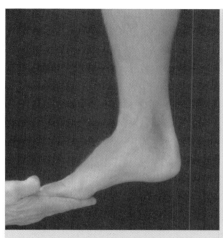

### Ankle clonus

With the patient seated, dorsiflex the ankle suddenly and observe for rhythmic beating (clonus), noting the duration of and the number of "beats." This is another sign of long-tract spinal cord involvement.

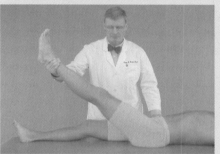

### Straight-leg raising

This test places the L5 and S1 nerve roots and the sciatic nerve under tension. With the patient supine and relaxed, elevate the leg until either the knee begins to bend or the patient reports severe pain in the buttock or back. Record the degree of elevation at which pain occurs. Next, dorsiflex the ankle to determine whether this motion increases pain (further stretch of the L5 and S1 nerve roots). Plantar flexion of the ankle relieves sciatic tension. Increased back pain with this maneuver is probably nonorganic.

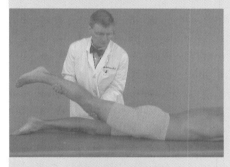

### Reverse straight-leg raising

The reverse straight-leg raising test is a traditional way to place the L1–4 nerve roots under tension. With the patient prone, lift the hip into extension while keeping the knee straight. Increased pain suggests compression of the upper lumbar nerve roots.

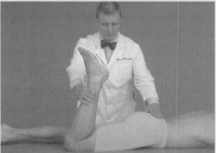

### Prone rectus femoris test

This test also places the L1–4 nerve roots under tension. With the patient prone, maintain the hip in a neutral position while flexing the knee. Increased pain suggests compression of the upper lumbar nerve roots.

# Special Tests

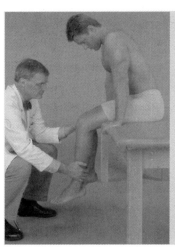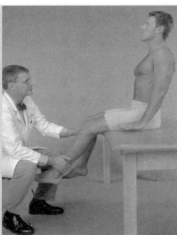

## Flip sign

With the patient seated and hands resting on the edge of the table, examine the patient's reflexes, test toe extensor strength, and then knee extensor strength (left). Next, distract the patient by asking whether he or she has knee problems (focusing the patient's attention on the knee and away from the back), then lift the foot and extend the knee (right). Measure the degree of knee flexion reached when back pain occurs. Patients with sciatic tension will immediately flip back in acute pain and may hit the wall. The flip sign correlates with straight-leg raising pain under 45° of elevation.

# CAUDA EQUINA SYNDROME

## ICD-9 Code

**344.60**
Cauda equina syndrome, without mention of neurogenic bladder

## DEFINITION

The distal end of the spinal cord, the conus medullaris, terminates at the L1-2 level. Below this, the spinal canal is filled with the L2-S4 nerve roots, known as the cauda equina. Compression of roots distal to the conus causes paralysis without spasticity.

The cauda equina syndrome results from a relatively sudden reduction in the volume of the lumbar spinal canal that causes compression and paralysis of multiple nerve roots. The sacral roots that control bladder and anal function are midline and are particularly vulnerable. Causes include central disk herniations, epidural abscess, epidural hematoma, and fracture or other trauma. Onset can be immediate with a fracture or can occur over a few hours or days with other conditions. Cauda equina syndrome usually requires emergency surgery to relieve nerve root compression and stop progression of neurologic loss. Even with prompt recognition and immediate decompression, recovery of neurologic function is often incomplete.

## CLINICAL SYMPTOMS

Radicular pain and numbness typically involve both legs; however, symptoms are often more severe in one extremity (**Figure 1**). Lower extremity pain may diminish as paralysis progresses. Leg weakness can manifest as stumbling, difficulty rising from a chair, or foot drop. Patients often report difficulty voiding or loss of urinary and anal sphincter control.

Patients may have a history of preexisting spinal stenosis with a sudden increase in symptoms, or the history may reveal sudden onset of pain following lifting, or recent spine surgery with the subsequent onset of fever, chills, and increased back and leg pain.

## TESTS

### PHYSICAL EXAMINATION

Watch the patient walk. Inability to rise from a chair without the assistance of armrests (quadriceps and/or hip extensor weakness) and inability to walk on the heels or toes (ankle dorsiflexor and plantar flexor weakness) suggest multiple nerve root dysfunction. Evaluate motor and sensory function of the lumbosacral nerve roots, including anal sphincter tone and/or perianal numbness. Patients seen in the emergency department for acute back pain may receive an injection of narcotics that causes acute urinary retention and confounds the diagnosis of cauda equina syndrome.

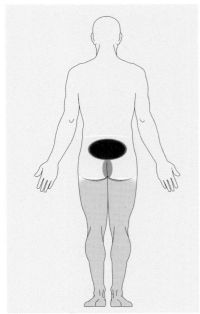

**Figure 1**
Pain diagram for cauda equina syndrome.

## DIAGNOSTIC TESTS

AP and lateral radiographs of the lumbar spine are important to identify structural problems such as a fracture and spondylolisthesis. A CBC and erythrocyte sedimentation rate can confirm a suspected infection.

## DIFFERENTIAL DIAGNOSIS

Guillain-Barré syndrome (intact sensation possible, normal MRI)

Herniated disk (unilateral radicular symptoms and motor weakness, normal rectal tone and perianal sensation)

Metastatic tumor (lymphoma or leukemia, abnormal blood studies, pathologic fracture)

Multiple sclerosis (no history of trauma, patchy numbness, diplopia, facial and/or upper extremity numbness)

Spinal cord tumor (positive Babinski sign, patchy numbness above L2, spasticity)

## ADVERSE OUTCOMES OF THE DISEASE

Permanent paralysis and loss of sphincter function (urinary and anal) are possible. The danger is relating bladder symptoms to age-related conditions of female cystocele or male prostatism without considering sphincter paralysis.

## TREATMENT

Cauda equina syndrome is a surgical emergency. Immediate decompression is almost always necessary once the anatomic lesion is defined.

## ADVERSE OUTCOMES OF TREATMENT

Wound infection and postoperative hematoma are possible.

## REFERRAL DECISIONS/RED FLAGS

Any unexplained neurologic deficit, loss of normal bowel or bladder function, increasing pain not controlled by simple analgesics, or decreasing pain in the face of increasing neurologic deficit are cause of concern.

# CERVICAL RADICULOPATHY

ICD-9 Codes

722.0
Displacement of cervical intervertebral disk without myelopathy
723.4
Other disorders of cervical region,
brachial neuritis or radiculitis

## SYNONYM

Herniated cervical disk

## DEFINITION

Cervical radiculopathy is referred neurogenic pain in the distribution of a cervical nerve root or roots, with or without associated numbness, weakness, or loss of reflexes. The usual cause in young adults (< 40 years of age) is herniation of a cervical disk, which entraps the root as it enters the foramen. In older patients, a combination of foraminal narrowing due to vertical settling of the disk space and arthritic involvement of the facet and uncovertebral joint is the most common cause of lateral nerve root entrapment.

## CLINICAL SYMPTOMS

Neck pain and radicular pain with associated numbness and paresthesias in the upper extremity in the distribution of the involved root are common (**Figure 1**). Muscle spasms or fasciculations in the involved myotomes sometimes occur. Other symptoms may include weakness, lack of coordination, changes in handwriting, diminished grip strength, dropping objects from their hand, and difficulty with fine manipulative tasks. Occipital headaches and pain radiating into the paraspinal and scapular regions also may occur.

Symptoms indicative of cervical myelopathy, such as trunk or leg dysfunction, gait disturbances, bowel or bladder changes, and signs of upper motor neuron involvement, occur more commonly with stenosis of the cervical spinal canal.

Patients may state that they can relieve the pain by placing their hands on top of their head, as this decreases tension on the involved nerve root.

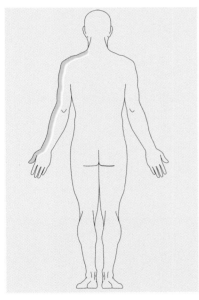

**Figure 1**
Typical pain diagram for a patient with cervical radiculopathy.

## TESTS

### PHYSICAL EXAMINATION

Cervical lordosis may be reduced and the range of neck motion may be mildly restricted. Extension and axial rotation (Spurling test) will often cause pain in the arm or shoulder. Assess motor and sensory function of the C5-T1 nerve roots as well as upper extremity reflexes and other upper motor neuron signs. Careful examination for signs of shoulder pathology, vascular disturbances, and peripheral nerve entrapment also is necessary. A complete neurologic examination should be performed (**Table 1**).

Signs of upper motor neuron involvement can suggest spinal cord compression.

## Table 1
### Clinical Features of Common Cervical Syndromes

| Disk | Pain | Sensory change | Motor weakness atrophy | Reflex change |
|---|---|---|---|---|
| C4-5 (C5 root) | Base of neck, shoulder, anterolateral aspect of arm | Numbness in deltoid region | Deltoid, biceps | Biceps |
| C5-6 (C6 root) | Neck, shoulder, medial border of scapula, lateral aspect of arm, radial aspect of forearm | Dorsolateral aspect of thumb and index finger | Biceps, wrist extensors pollicus longus | Biceps, brachioradialis |
| C6-7 (C7 root) | Neck, shoulder, medial border of scapula, lateral aspect of arm, dorsum of forearm | Index, long fingers, dorsum of hand | Triceps and/or finger extensors | Triceps |

## DIAGNOSTIC TESTS

Plain radiographs may identify regions of spondylosis or degenerative involvement of the disk and the facet. MRI or CT with intrathecal contrast confirms the diagnosis and can help in resolving a diagnostic dilemma (**Figures 2 and 3**), but these are not necessary in routine care. Electromyography and nerve conduction velocity studies help in some instances to identify the location of neurologic dysfunction but are used primarily in preoperative planning.

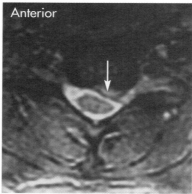

**Figure 2**
Axial MRI image of a cervical disk herniation in a younger patient.

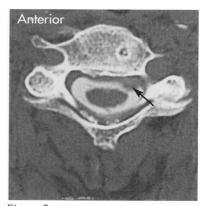

**Figure 3**
Axial CT scan with intrathecal contrast of a cervical disk herniation in a younger patient.

## DIFFERENTIAL DIAGNOSIS

Adhesive capsulitis (restricted passive and active motion of the shoulder)

Demyelinating conditions (varying symptoms, intensity, and location)

Myocardial ischemia (abnormal ECG or stress tests)

Peripheral nerve entrapment (Phalen test, Tinel test at elbow or wrist)

Rotator cuff disease (painful wince with active shoulder abduction and circumduction movements)

Thoracic outlet syndrome (positive EAST maneuver)

## ADVERSE OUTCOMES OF THE DISEASE

Muscle paralysis, weakness, or chronic pain syndromes can develop, or the condition may progress to a myelopathy with cord involvement, although the latter is rare.

## TREATMENT

Spontaneous resolution of all or most symptoms occurs within 6 to 12 weeks in most patients. With radicular pain, a short course of oral steroids and adequate non-narcotic pain medication is indicated. Avoid the use of oral narcotics to prevent narcotic addiction in patients in whom chronic pain syndromes develop. Cervical traction and physical therapy are helpful in the first 2 to 4 weeks. Manipulation of the cervical spine is contraindicated in patients with osteoporosis, restricted motion, rheumatoid arthritis, advanced age, carotid or vertebral atherosclerosis, or tumors, or in children, in patients on anticoagulants, or in patients with associated radiculopathy or myelopathy.

## ADVERSE OUTCOMES OF TREATMENT

Quadriparesis, herniation of an intervertebral disk, stroke, or vertebral fracture can follow manipulation of the cervical spine.

## REFERRAL DECISIONS/RED FLAGS

Failure of nonoperative treatment, atrophy, motor weakness, or signs of myelopathy may require surgical evaluation. Patients with any signs that suggest a demyelinating condition, infection, or tumor require further evaluation. Radicular symptoms with intolerable pain require early specialty evaluation.

# CERVICAL SPONDYLOSIS

## ICD-9 Codes

721.0
  Cervical spondylosis without myelopathy
721.1
  Cervical spondylosis with myelopathy
723.0
  Spinal stenosis in cervical region

## SYNONYMS

Degenerative disk disease of the cervical spine
Cervical arthritis

## DEFINITION

Cervical spondylosis is the nomenclature for degenerative disk disease in the cervical spine. This condition is produced by ingrowth of bony spurs, buckling or protrusion of the ligamentum flavum, and/or by herniation of disk material. The result is narrowing of the neural foramen and possible stenosis of the cervical spinal canal. Cervical spondylosis can cause neck pain, cervical radiculopathy, and/or cervical myelopathy.

## CLINICAL SYMPTOMS

The most common symptoms are stiffness and chronic neck pain that is worse with upright activity. Some patients report grinding or popping in the cervical region with motion. Paraspinous muscle spasm may occur, as may headaches that seem to originate somewhere in the neck. Increased irritability, fatigue, sleep disturbances, and impaired work tolerance also may develop. Radicular symptoms and pain may occur in the upper extremities with lateral recess stenosis and nerve root entrapment (Figure 1).

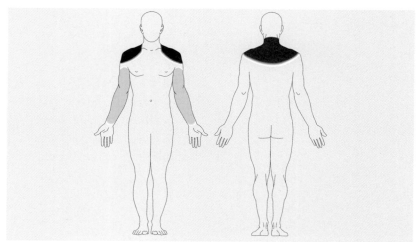

**Figure 1**
Typical pain diagram for a patient with cervical spondylosis.

Narrowing of the spinal canal and resultant myelopathy are more common in older men. Typical symptoms of cervical myelopathy include sensory abnormalities in the upper extremities and motor weakness and spasticity in the lower extremities. Gait and urinary function are often abnormal as well.

Loss of vibration and position sense (posterior column deficits) are more common in the feet than in the upper extremities. A concomitant radiculopathy in the upper extremity may obscure the diagnosis of cervical myelopathy.

## TESTS

### PHYSICAL EXAMINATION

Examination may reveal tender spots along the lateral neck or along the spinous processes posteriorly. Motion may be limited or cause pain. Assess sensory and motor function of the upper (C5-T1) and lower (L1-S1) nerve roots. Evaluate gait as well as bowel and bladder function. With myelopathy, flexion may produce electric shocks that travel down the spine, arms, or legs. A Hoffmann reflex, clonus, hyperreflexia, and Babinski sign (an extensor toe response) are possible, as are gait disturbances and global weakness.

Patients with radiculopathy may have signs that mimic a herniated cervical disk, including abnormal reflexes and motor and sensory function. The Spurling test is frequently positive.

### DIAGNOSTIC TESTS

AP and lateral radiographs are necessary (**Figure 2**). Findings on the lateral view include sclerosis in the intervertebral disk area with osteophytes (bone spurs) projecting anteriorly. Osteophytes also may project from the posterior portion of the vertebral body into the spinal canal, producing stenosis of the cervical canal (**Figure 3**). Anterior subluxation of one vertebra onto the vertebra below increases the probability of cervical stenosis and associated neurologic findings. Degenerative findings are most common at the C5-6 and C6-7 disk spaces.

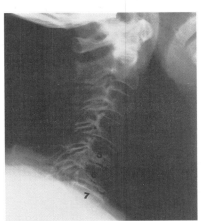

**Figure 2**
Lateral radiograph of an older patient with advanced cervical spondylosis.

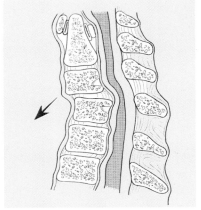

**Figure 3**
Degenerative disk changes and degenerative subluxations causing canal stenosis.

*Adapted with permission from Bohlmann HH: Cervical spondylosis with moderate to severe myelopathy. Spine 1977;2:151-162.*

## DIFFERENTIAL DIAGNOSIS

Metastatic tumor (night pain that prevents sleep)

Soft cervical disk herniation (generally seen in younger patients)

Spinal cord tumor (myelopathy)

Syringomyelia (loss of superficial abdominal reflexes, insensitivity to pain)

Vertebral subluxation (in rheumatoid arthritis or following acute trauma)

## ADVERSE OUTCOMES OF THE DISEASE

Chronic pain, myelopathy, or mixed myeloradiculopathy are possible. Note that these sequelae of cervical spondylosis occur more commonly when the condition is advanced.

## TREATMENT

Supportive treatment and reassurance may be adequate, but symptoms may last several months or become chronic. NSAIDs or other non-narcotic pain medication will often be adequate. Amitriptyline may be useful. Avoid prescribing narcotic analgesics. Patients also may benefit from a cervical pillow or cervical roll and physical therapy.

Surgery decompression and fusion may be necessary for patients with intractable pain, progressive neurologic findings, or symptoms of cervical myelopathy and spinal cord compression.

## ADVERSE OUTCOMES OF TREATMENT

NSAIDs may cause gastric, renal, or hepatic complications. Sedation from tricyclics and adverse reactions with monoamine oxidase inhibitors are possible. Narcotic addiction is also possible. Monoparesis or loss of specific nerve root function may occur, and although uncommon, quadriparesis or quadriplegia is also possible.

## REFERRAL DECISIONS/RED FLAGS

Intractable neck pain that is not responsive to treatment, neurologic symptoms that affect either the upper or lower extremities, lack of coordination, and radicular symptoms related to neck motion all indicate the need for further evaluation.

# CERVICAL SPRAIN

ICD-9 Code
847.0
  Sprains and strains of other and
  unspecified parts of back, neck

## SYNONYM
Neck strain

## DEFINITION

Cervical sprain is a common condition that is usually self-limiting. By strict definition, an acute cervical sprain is a muscle injury in the neck. However, because the deep location of the soft-tissue structures in the neck do not permit differentiation of what is injured by either physical examination or sophisticated imaging modalities, this term also is used to describe ligamentous injuries of the facet joints or intervertebral disks. Whatever soft-tissue structures have been injured, the diagnostic and treatment protocols are similar (eg, rule out unstable injuries and neurologic dysfunction and then provide symptomatic treatment).

A whiplash mechanism (acceleration-deceleration of the neck with rapid flexion-extension) is common in motor vehicle accidents. These injuries may cause prolonged disability despite no apparent instability. The cause is probably a combination of relatively severe ligamentous/muscle injury combined with nonorganic overlay.

## CLINICAL SYMPTOMS

The pain may follow an incident of significant trauma or may be spontaneous in onset. Nonradicular, nonfocal neck pain is most common, noted anywhere from the base of the skull to the cervicothoracic junction. Pain is often worse with motion and may be accompanied by paraspinal spasm and discomfort in the region of the trapezius muscle (**Figure 1**). Occipital headaches are common in the early phase and can persist for months. Pain following trauma often persists longer than sprains of spontaneous onset. Patients may report increased irritability, fatigue, sleep disturbances, and difficulty concentrating. Work tolerance may be impaired.

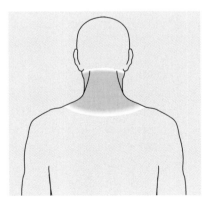

**Figure 1**
Typical pain diagram for a patient with an acute cervical examination.

## TESTS

### PHYSICAL EXAMINATION

Examination reveals areas of tenderness in the paraspinous muscles, spinous processes, interspinous ligaments, or medial border of the scapula. Limited motion is common, involving either rotation, lateral bending, and/or flexion and extension. Pain is often noted at the extremes of motions. The neurologic examination is normal, and usually there is no visible deformity in the neck.

### DIAGNOSTIC TESTS

AP, lateral, and odontoid radiographs are necessary if the patient has a history of trauma, or associated neurologic deficit, or if the patient is elderly. All seven cervical vertebrae must be seen. Anterior displacement of the pharyngeal air shadow indicates soft-tissue swelling and possible disruption of the intervertebral disk or anterior longitudinal ligament and requires further evaluation. The width of the prevertebral soft tissue at the level of C3 should not exceed 7 mm in normal adults. The normal lordotic curve may be straightened or reversed with muscle spasm, but this finding also is noted in approximately 10% of normal adults. Preexisting degenerative changes may be noted and are most commonly age related and most frequent at C5-6 or C6-7.

If the patient has severe pain, the screening radiographs, along with flexion-extension lateral views, should be examined for signs of instability that include more than 3.5-mm translation of a vertebral body and/or more than 11° of angulation of adjacent vertebrae.

## DIFFERENTIAL DIAGNOSIS

Cervical disk herniation (neurologic abnormality and radicular pain)

Cervical spine tumor or infection (night pain, weight loss, history, fever, chills, sweats)

Dislocation or subluxation of the spine (evident on radiographs)

Inflammatory conditions of the cervical spine (rheumatoid arthritis with abnormal radiographs)

Sociogenic/malingering/secondary gain (inconsistent or exaggerated findings)

Spinal fracture (abnormal radiograph)

## ADVERSE OUTCOMES OF THE DISEASE

Symptoms completely resolve in most patients within the first 4 to 6 weeks. Resolution typically is delayed with whiplash, but most symptoms resolve within 6 to 12 months with few residual complaints.

Patients with subtle disk disruptions and injuries superimposed on existing degenerative conditions of the joints and disks of the cervical spine can have intractable pain. In some instances, radiculopathy due to lateral nerve root entrapment or myelopathy due to central spinal stenosis can develop.

## TREATMENT

Providing the patient with reassurance about anticipated improvement is an important first step. Acute care involves 1 or 2 weeks with a soft cervical collar, appropriate pain medications, and/or short-term NSAIDs. Muscle relaxants can help if the patient has spasm. Commercially available cervical pillows help with sleep.

Massage, cervical traction, and ultrasound may help, especially with severe pain in the first 4 weeks. Avoid narcotic medications after the first week or two. Amitriptyline is often of value if symptoms persist.

Manipulation of the cervical spine is contraindicated in patients with osteoporosis, restricted motion, rheumatoid arthritis, carotid or vertebral atherosclerosis, or tumors. Manipulation is also contraindicated in the elderly, in children, and in patients on anticoagulants or with associated radiculopathy or myelopathy.

Aerobic activities, such as walking, should be started as soon as possible. Add isometric exercises as the patient's comfort improves, preferably in the first 2 weeks. Encourage an early return to normal activities and work.

## ADVERSE OUTCOMES OF TREATMENT

NSAIDs can cause gastric, renal, or hepatic complications. If the patient's condition fails to improve, reactive depression can develop. Chronic pain syndrome and drug dependence are also possible if treatment fails. Manipulation can result in herniation of an intervertebral disk or fracture or fracture-dislocation of a vertebra.

## REFERRAL DECISIONS/RED FLAGS

Pain refractory to treatment, nerve root deficit, myelopathy, or a diagnostic dilemma indicate the need for further evaluation.

# FRACTURE OF THE CERVICAL SPINE

ICD-9 Code

805.0
Fracture of vertebral column without mention of spinal cord injury, cervical, closed

## DEFINITION

Cervical spine fractures and ligamentous injuries are commonly the result of high-energy trauma, such as a motor vehicle accident, fall from a height, or a diving accident. These fractures must be suspected and either identified or ruled out in all trauma patients who report neck pain. In addition, the history and examination of unconscious or intoxicated patients are compromised, and such patients involved in an accident require radiographs to rule out cervical spine injuries.

## CLINICAL SYMPTOMS

Severe neck pain, paraspinous muscle spasm, and/or point tenderness are the most common presenting symptoms. Pain that radiates into the shoulder or arm with associated numbness or tingling suggests nerve root impingement. Global sensory or motor deficits suggest spinal cord injury. In patients with multiple trauma, other injuries may be so painful as to distract the patient. Therefore, in these patients, the absence of neck pain on initial examination does not "clear" or eliminate the possibility of a cervical spine injury.

## TESTS

### PHYSICAL EXAMINATION

Inspect for swelling and contusions. Palpate for tenderness and paraspinal spasm. A gap or a step-off between spinous processes suggests malalignment. Evaluate motor and sensory function of the upper and lower extremity nerve roots as well as the sensory status of the thoracic dermatomes. Perianal sensation, sphincter tone, and bulbocavernosus reflex also should be assessed in any patient with a neurologic deficit.

### DIAGNOSTIC TESTS

AP, lateral, and odontoid views are standard. Injuries at the upper and lower portions of the cervical spine are most commonly missed. The lateral radiograph must include the occiput superiorly and the top of T1 inferiorly. Occasionally, a swimmer's view is required to visualize the cervicothoracic junction.

The lateral radiograph should be evaluated for anterior soft-tissue swelling, height of the vertebral body, and alignment of the vertebral bodies, facet joints, and spinous processes. The odontoid view should be checked for odontoid fracture (often subtle), C1 lateral mass widening, and occipital condyle position. The AP radiograph can show subtle malalignment of the spinous processes; this finding indicates rotational malalignment secondary to facet fracture or dislocation.

If no fracture is seen, the radiographs should be carefully evaluated for other signs of instability, including more than 3.5 mm translation of a vertebral body or more than 11° of angulation of adjacent vertebral bodies. Flexion-extension lateral views should be obtained only after a three-view series has been cleared. Note that flexion-extension radiographs may not detect ligamentous instability if paraspinal spasm is still present. Therefore, in the acute situation, other studies may be required to rule out a fracture or significant ligamentous injury.

## DIFFERENTIAL DIAGNOSIS

Acute disk herniation (normal radiographs with or without neurologic deficit)

Cervical sprain (normal radiographs with muscle pain/tenderness)

High thoracic fracture (evident on swimmer's view or thoracic radiographs)

## ADVERSE OUTCOMES OF THE DISEASE

Severe injury may result in complete or incomplete quadriplegia. Nerve compression with radiculopathy may also occur. Chronic neck pain and fatigue may result from deformity or associated muscle injury.

## TREATMENT

The cervical spine must be immobilized during extrication and transport of all patients who sustain high-energy trauma or who have suspected neck injuries. Immediate IV steroids (methylprednisolone 30 mg/kg bolus followed by a continuous drip of 5.4 mg/kg/h for 23 hours) should be considered for patients who have sustained a spinal cord injury.

Patients whose initial radiographs and neurologic examination are normal but who have persistent pain should wear a cervical collar for 7 to 10 days. Repeat the examination, and obtain three-view cervical spine radiographs if symptoms persist. If these radiographs are normal, flexion-extension lateral radiographs should be obtained. If these are normal, then the patient may start a neck stretching and strengthening physical therapy program with scapular stabilization.

## ADVERSE OUTCOMES OF TREATMENT

As with adverse outcomes of the disease, complete or incomplete quadriplegia, radiculopathy, or chronic pain can result from the treatment.

## REFERRAL DECISIONS/RED FLAGS

Patients with a fracture, dislocation, subluxation, instability, or neurologic deficit require further evaluation. A high index of suspicion for occult injury should be maintained in patients who are intoxicated, uncooperative, or unconscious.

# FRACTURE OF THE THORACIC AND LUMBAR SPINE

**ICD-9 Codes**

805.2
Fracture of the vertebral column without mention of spinal cord injury, dorsal (thoracic), closed

805.4
Fracture of the vertebral column without mention of spinal cord injury, lumbar, closed

## DEFINITION

Fractures of the thoracic or lumbar spine generally occur as a result of high-energy trauma such as motor vehicle accidents or falls from a height. They also can occur following minimal trauma in patients who have diminished bone strength from osteoporosis, tumors, infections, or a long-term history of steroid use.

The fracture pattern usually determines fracture stability and likelihood of neural injury. Simple compression fractures involving only the anterior half of the vertebral body are generally stable, as are some burst fractures (compression fractures extending to the posterior third of the vertebral body). Flexion-distraction injuries that disrupt anterior and posterior bone and ligamentous structures are highly unstable.

## CLINICAL SYMPTOMS

Moderate to severe back pain related to a traumatic event is the most common presenting symptom. The pain is exacerbated by motion. Numbness, tingling, weakness, or bowel and bladder dysfunction suggest nerve root or spinal cord injury.

## TESTS

### PHYSICAL EXAMINATION

Inspect the trunk, chest, and abdomen for swelling and ecchymosis. Tenderness to palpation or light percussion occurs at the level of injury. A step-off (forward shift) or gap between spinous processes with swelling, and hematoma formation are the hallmark signs of an unstable flexion-distraction or burst fracture. Evaluate motor and sensory function of all nerve roots distal to the injury. Diffuse numbness, weakness, loss of reflexes, ankle clonus, or a positive Babinski sign indicates spinal cord injury. Examination of perianal sensation, sphincter function, and the bulbocavernosus reflex are particularly important with an associated spinal cord injury. Evaluate the abdomen and chest for possible associated injuries.

### DIAGNOSTIC TESTS

AP and lateral radiographs of the thoracic and lumbar spine are indicated. When a spine fracture is identified, the radiograph should be scrutinized for adjacent or nonadjacent fractures, as well. Oblique views can supplement the standard examination, if needed.

In the lateral view, compression and burst fractures show loss of height of the anterior wall of the vertebral body and resultant kyphotic deformity (**Figure 1**). Unstable flexion-distraction injuries show widening of the space between adjacent spinous processes in the lateral view. The AP view may

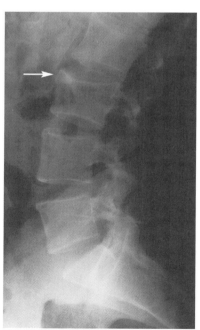

**Figure 1**
Lateral radiograph showing a minimal compression fracture of the lumbar spine.

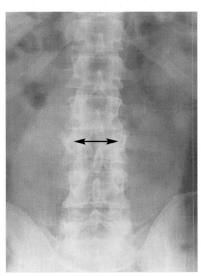

**Figure 2**
AP radiograph showing a burst fracture of the lumbar spine with widening of the interpedicular distance (arrows).

reveal transverse process fractures or widening of the interpedicular distance with an unstable burst (**Figure 2**). Rotation of one vertebral body in relation to the one below indicates instability. Any injury other than a simple compression fracture requires additional imaging studies.

## DIFFERENTIAL DIAGNOSIS

Herniated lumbar disk (no fracture, able to walk, single nerve root)

Thoracic or lumbar muscle strain (no neurologic findings or fractures)

Visceral injuries (abnormal abdominal examination and radiographs, ultrasound, or CT scan)

## ADVERSE OUTCOMES OF THE DISEASE

Loss of nerve or spinal cord function, persistent painful instability or deformity, and impaired function are serious sequelae of some spinal injuries.

## TREATMENT

Preventing neurologic damage, restoring stability, and restoring normal function are the goals of treatment. Initial extrication, transportation, and evaluation in the emergency department require the use of spinal precautions, including a spine board and log rolling. If radiographs reveal no fracture or instability and no neurologic deficits are present, these precautions may be lifted.

Isolated transverse process fractures do not affect stability but can indicate injury to adjacent visceral organs. A thoracolumbar corset can be used for symptom control.

Simple compression fractures with wedging of less than 20° and no posterior vertebral or posterior element involvement can be managed with a hyperextension brace for 12 weeks, to be worn during sitting and standing activities. Pain management may require short-term oral narcotics. Emphasize walking but restrict bending, stooping, twisting, and lifting more than 20 lb. Encourage the patient to return to work as quickly as possible, with job modifications as needed. Exercises to strengthen spinal extensor muscles can supplement walking after the brace is removed.

Other injuries usually require more aggressive treatment. Patients with a spinal cord injury should be started on steroids immediately. Unstable burst fractures, flexion-distraction injuries, and fracture-dislocations are usually treated by internal fixation and spinal fusion.

## ADVERSE OUTCOMES OF TREATMENT

Progressive collapse with kyphotic deformity can occur, resulting in chronic pain and/or neurologic compromise. Chronic muscle pain can also develop if the trunk muscles are not adequately strengthened after immobilization is discontinued.

## REFERRAL DECISIONS/RED FLAGS

Any neurologic deficit is a sign of significant injury and requires further evaluation. Burst fractures, flexion-distraction injuries (or any injury to the posterior column of the spine), fractures with vertebral rotation, and fracture-dislocations all require further evaluation and treatment.

# Low Back Sprain

ICD-9 Codes
847.2
    Sprains and strains of other and
    unspecified parts of back, lumbar
847.1
    Sprains and strains of other and
    unspecified parts of back, thoracic

## SYNONYMS

Low back pain
Pulled low back
Lumbar sprain

## DEFINITION

Low back pain is the most frequent cause of lost work time and disability in adults younger than age 45 years. Most symptoms, however, are of limited duration, with 85% of patients demonstrating significant improvement and returning to work within 1 month. The 4% of patients whose symptoms persist longer than 6 months generate 85% to 90% of the costs to society for treating low back pain.

By strict definition, a low back sprain is an injury to the paravertebral spinal muscles. However, the term also is used to describe ligamentous injuries of the facet joints or anulus fibrosus. In the latter condition, the disk does not herniate into the spinal canal, but substances can leak from the nucleus pulposus that induce inflammation and cause irritation of the lumbosacral nerve roots. Due to the deep location of the lumbar soft tissues, localizing an injury to a specific structure is difficult, if not impossible. Furthermore, in this area, whatever muscle or ligamentous structures have been injured, the treatment protocols are similar.

Repeated lifting and twisting or operating vibrating equipment most often precipitates a back sprain. Other risk factors include poor fitness, poor work satisfaction, smoking, and hypochondriasis. Recurrent episodes are separated by many months or years; more frequent recurrences suggest degenerative disk disease.

## CLINICAL SYMPTOMS

Patients report the acute onset of low back pain, often following a lifting episode. The lifting may be a trivial event, such as leaning over to pick up a piece of paper. The pain often radiates into the buttocks and posterior thighs (**Figure 1**). Patients may have difficulty standing erect and may need to change position frequently for comfort. This condition often first occurs in the young adult years. When this condition is a patient's first major episode of pain, he or she may show signs of nonorganic behavior, such as exaggerated responses, generalized hypersensitivity to light touch, or facial grimacing.

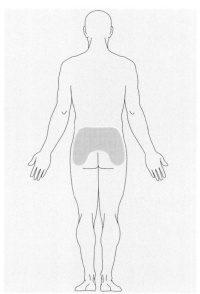

**Figure 1**
Typical pain diagram for a patient with low back sprain.

# TESTS

## PHYSICAL EXAMINATION

Examination reveals diffuse tenderness in the low back or sacroiliac region. Range of motion of the lumbar spine, particularly flexion, is typically reduced and elicits pain. The degree of lumbar flexion and the ease with which the patient can extend the spine are good parameters by which to evaluate progress. The motor and sensory function of the lumbosacral nerve roots and lower extremity reflexes are normal.

## DIAGNOSTIC TESTS

Plain radiographs usually are not helpful for patients with acute low back strain, as they typically show changes appropriate for their age. In adolescents and young adults, there is little or no disk space narrowing, whereas in adults older than age 30 years, there is variable disk space narrowing and/or spurs.

For patients with atypical symptoms, such as pain at rest or at night or a history of significant trauma, AP and lateral radiographs are necessary. These views help to identify or rule out infection, bone tumor (visualize up to T10), fracture, or spondylolisthesis.

# DIFFERENTIAL DIAGNOSIS

Ankylosing spondylitis (family history, morning stiffness, limited mobility of the lumbar spine)

Drug-seeking behavior (exaggerated symptoms, inconsistent and nonphysiologic examination)

Extraspinal causes (ovarian cyst, nephrolithiasis, pancreatitis, ulcer disease)

Fracture of the vertebral body (major trauma or minimal trauma with osteoporosis)

Herniated nucleus pulposus or ruptured disk (unilateral radicular pain symptoms that extend below the knee and are equal to or greater than the back pain)

Infection (fever, chills, sweats, elevated erythrocyte sedimentation rate)

Myeloma (night sweats, men older than age 50 years)

# ADVERSE OUTCOMES OF THE DISEASE

Functional impairment is the primary disability. This can be of great significance for any patient whose normal activities are strenuous and whose general health is otherwise excellent, but young adults, in particular, have difficulty accepting a condition that can impair function for several weeks.

## Treatment

Treatment focuses on relieving symptoms, with a short period of bed rest (1 to 2 days) and NSAIDs or other non-narcotic pain medications (7 to 14 days). Muscle relaxants may be helpful in the first 3 to 5 days, but narcotic analgesics and sedatives should be avoided. Couple medications with reassurance. Once the acute pain has diminished, emphasize aerobic conditioning and strengthening regimens. The goal is to assist the patient in returning to normal activity within 4 weeks.

## Adverse outcomes of treatment

NSAIDs can cause gastric, renal, or hepatic complications. Although rare, manipulation may result in herniation of the intervertebral disk.

## Referral decisions/Red flags

Neurologic abnormalities, unresponsive pain syndromes, or an unusual cause for the pain indicates the need for further evaluation.

# LUMBAR DEGENERATIVE DISK DISEASE AND CHRONIC LOW BACK PAIN

ICD-9 Codes

722.52
Degeneration of thoracic or lumbar intervertebral disk, lumbar, or lumbosacral disk
724.2
Low back pain

## DEFINITION

Degeneration of the intervertebral disk is a physiologic event of aging modified by such factors as injury, repetitive trauma, infection, heredity, and tobacco use. As the hydrophilic properties of the nucleus pulposus degrade, the disk loses height and formerly tight ligaments become loose. Motions such as sliding and twisting create tears in the anulus fibrosus. Osteoarthritis and chronic low back pain develop.

Chronic low back pain is a condition in which symptoms have persisted for more than 3 months. Symptoms usually present between the third and sixth decades. Symptoms are typically recurrent and episodic, but in some patients can be unremitting. Degenerative disk disease and chronic low back pain can interfere with the patient's vocation and ability to lead an active life; therefore, improvement in functional and occupational disability is most important.

## CLINICAL SYMPTOMS

Low back pain that radiates to one or both buttocks is the hallmark symptom (**Figure 1**). The pain is often described as "mechanical" in that it is aggravated by activities such as bending, lifting, stooping, or twisting. Patients may report stiffness or have a history of intermittent sciatica (ie, pain radiating down the back of the leg), but discomfort in the back is the predominant symptom. The pain is typically relieved with lying down or a night's rest; however, some patients can be troubled with nighttime awakenings.

While depression usually is not the cause of chronic low back pain, it can complicate treatment and therefore this possibility should be evaluated.

## TESTS

### PHYSICAL EXAMINATION

Lumbar and sacroiliac tenderness is a common finding. Patients also can exhibit a side or forward list from muscle spasm. Motor and sensory function of the lower extremity nerve roots as well as the lower extremity reflexes is normal. Straight-leg raising and spinal motion may be mildly restricted. While not characteristic, nonorganic findings, such as widespread sensitivity to light touch, nonanatomic localization of symptoms, inappropriate grimacing, inconsistent actions, and exaggerated pain behaviors may be seen with this condition.

### DIAGNOSTIC TESTS

AP and lateral radiographs often show age-appropriate changes, such as anterior osteophytes and reduced height of the intervertebral disks on the lateral

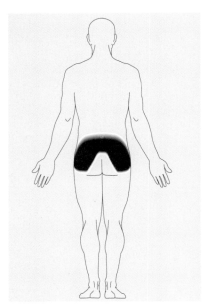

**Figure 1**
Typical pain diagram for a patient with lumbar degenerative disk disease.

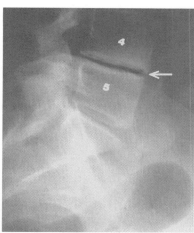

**Figure 2**
Lateral radiograph showing marked degenerative changes affecting the disk between L4 and L5.

view. Often there is a "vacuum sign" with apparent air (nitrogen) in the disk space (**Figure 2**).

## DIFFERENTIAL DIAGNOSIS

Depression (abnormal Beck Depression Inventory[1], sleep disturbance)

Drug-seeking behavior (inappropriate physical findings)

Extraspinal causes (ovarian cyst, nephrolithiasis, pancreatitis, abdominal aortic aneurysm, ulcer disease)

Illness behavior (multiple surgeries, multiple illnesses)

Inflammatory arthritides (morning stiffness for more than 30 minutes, positive HLA-B27, elevated erythrocyte sedimentation rate)

Intervertebral disk infection or vertebral osteomyelitis (history of excruciating pain, fever, history of IV drug use, recent infection)

Metastatic tumors, myeloma, lymphoma (pathologic fractures, severe night pain, weight loss, fatigue)

Osteoporosis with compression fractures (female gender, previous fracture)

Spinal tuberculosis (lower socioeconomic groups, history of AIDS)

Workplace dissatisfaction (discontent with boss, job)

## ADVERSE OUTCOMES OF THE DISEASE

Patients with more severe symptoms can have limited vocational and avocational activities, recreation, and sleep disturbances. Mood, sexuality, and concentration can be adversely affected. Deconditioning can be the result of reduced activities, making both symptoms and any occupational dysfunction worse.

## TREATMENT

This condition can be considered a chronic pain management problem. Intermittent use of NSAIDs or other non-narcotic pain medications should be recommended. Antidepressants can be suggested, if appropriate, and reassurance is appropriate after ruling out the more serious causes of back pain. Weight reduction, physical activity, and exercise 30 minutes daily (walking, swimming, or biking, with lumbar flexion and/or extension exercises) are also important. These patients should not smoke.

## ADVERSE OUTCOMES OF TREATMENT

NSAIDs can cause gastric, renal, or hepatic complications. Do not label patients "disabled." Suggest a modified work schedule and more recreational activities that improve general conditioning. Narcotic abuse or dependency can be a problem for patients who resort to narcotic analgesics.

## REFERRAL DECISIONS/RED FLAGS

Further evaluation is needed for patients who have fever, chills, unexplained weight loss, a history of cancer, significant nighttime pain, or a history of pain for more than 6 to 12 months. Other indications for additional evaluation include the presence of pathologic fractures, obvious deformity, saddle anesthesia, loss of major motor function, bowel or bladder dysfunction, abdominal pain, or visceral dysfunction.

## REFERENCE

1. Beck AT, et al: Assessment of depression: The depression inventory. *Mod Probl Pharmacopsychiatry* 1974;7:151-169.

# LUMBAR HERNIATED DISK

ICD-9 Codes

722.10
Displacement of thoracic or lumbar intervertebral disk without myelopathy

724.4
Thoracic or lumbosacral neuritis or radiculitis, unspecified (Radicular syndrome of lower limb)

## SYNONYMS

Sciatica

Lumbar radiculopathy

Neurogenic leg pain

## DEFINITION

The intervertebral disk is composed of the nucleus pulposus, a gel-like material that cushions axial compression, and the anulus fibrosus, a specialized ligamentous structure surrounding the nucleus pulposus that helps to stabilize the spine while it performs lifting and bending activities. These activities, however, also increase pressure on the nucleus pulposus. Through weaker parts of the anulus fibrosus, eg, posterolateral component, the nucleus pulposus may bulge or herniate into the lumbar canal. The resultant herniated disk syndrome (commonly called sciatica) causes pain and/or numbness and/or weakness in one or both lower extremities. In part, the pain results from direct mechanical compression of the nerve root and in part from chemical irritation of the nerve root by substances in the nucleus pulposus.

Disk herniation most commonly occurs at the L4-5 or L5-S1 levels with subsequent irritation of the L5 or S1 nerve root. Herniations at more proximal intervertebral levels constitute only 5% of all lumbar disk herniations.

Herniated lumbar disk affects about 2% of the population, but only 10% to 25% of those patients have symptoms that persist longer than 6 weeks. Because less than 10% have significant symptoms after 3 months, only a limited number of patients require surgical treatment.

## CLINICAL SYMPTOMS

The onset of symptoms is often abrupt, but may be insidious. Unilateral radicular leg pain is frequently accompanied by low back pain. Some patients report preexisting back pain that disappears when the leg pain begins, signaling the herniation.

The pain is often severe and is exaggerated by sitting, walking, standing, coughing, and sneezing. Typically, the pain radiates from the buttock down the posterior or posterolateral leg to the ankle or foot (**Figure 1**). Patients have a difficult time finding a position of comfort. Usually, lying on their back with a pillow under the knees or lying on their side in a fetal position provides some relief.

Upper or midlumbar radiculopathy (L1 to L4 nerve root compression) refers pain to the anterior aspect of the thigh and often does not radiate below the knee.

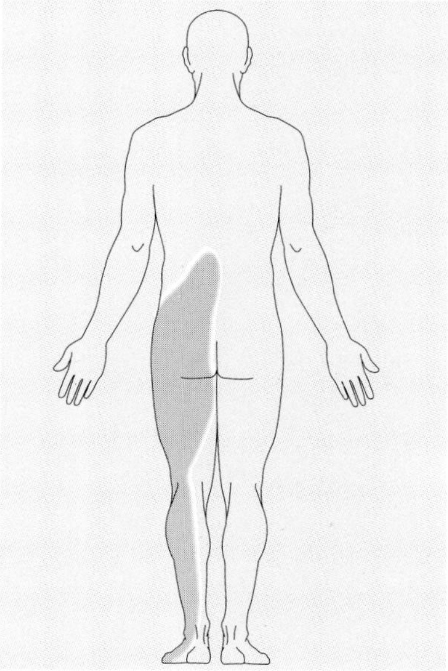

**Figure 1**
Pain diagram of patient with lumbar radiculopathy.

SECTION 8 | SPINE

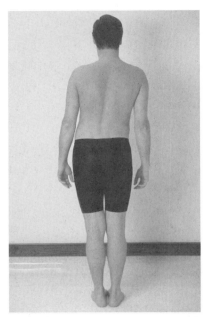

**Figure 2**
Trunk shift, or "list," to right.

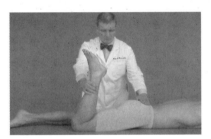

**Figure 3**
Prone rectus femoris test.

# TESTS

## PHYSICAL EXAMINATION

With the patient standing, look for a list (trunk shifts to one side) (**Figure 2**). With the patient sitting, observe for pain and spinal extension (leaning back) when the leg is raised (flip sign), as these signs are highly reliable for a herniated disk, especially when coupled with back pain reproduced with supine straight-leg raising limited to less than 45° of leg elevation. Patients with lumbar radiculopathy are often tender in the sciatic notch, and lumbar motion may be restricted in flexion and/or extension.

Evaluate motor and sensory function of the lumbosacral nerve roots as well as the deep tendon reflexes. With the patient supine, evaluate straight-leg raising on the involved and uninvolved limbs. This test places the L5 and S1 nerve roots on stretch. Ipsilateral restriction of straight-leg raising is common with a variety of lumbar spine problems, but a positive crossed straight-leg raising test (pain in the involved leg or buttock that occurs when lifting the uninvolved leg) is highly specific for lumbar nerve root entrapment. To put the upper lumbar nerve roots on stretch, perform a reverse straight-leg raising test. With the patient prone, either extend the hip or do the prone rectus femoris test (**Figure 3**).

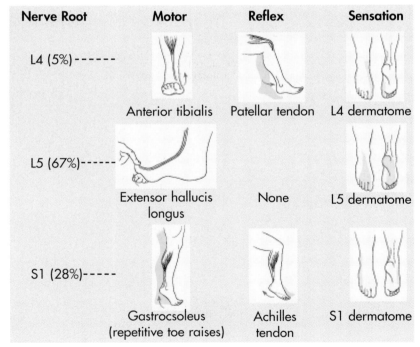

| Nerve Root | Motor | Reflex | Sensation |
|---|---|---|---|
| L4 (5%) | Anterior tibialis | Patellar tendon | L4 dermatome |
| L5 (67%) | Extensor hallucis longus | None | L5 dermatome |
| S1 (28%) | Gastrocsoleus (repetitive toe raises) | Achilles tendon | S1 dermatome |

**Figure 4**
Typical motor, sensory, and reflex findings with common lumbar radiculopathies.

*Adapted with permission from Kasser JR (ed): Orthopaedic Knowledge Update 5. Rosemont, IL, American Academy of Orthopaedic Surgeons, 1996, pp 609–624.*

Classic findings include the following (**Figure 4**):
- L3-4 disk (L4 nerve root) can produce weakness in the anterior tibialis, numbness in the shin, thigh pain, and an asymmetric knee reflex. About 5% of disk ruptures occur at this level.

- L4-5 disk (L5 nerve root) can produce weakness in the great toe extensor, numbness on the top of the foot and first web space, and posterolateral thigh and calf pain.
- L5-S1 disk (S1 nerve root) can produce weakness in the great toe flexor as well as gastrocsoleus with inability to sustain tiptoe walking, numbness in the lateral foot, posterior calf pain and ache, and an asymmetric ankle reflex.

## DIAGNOSTIC TESTS

Plain radiographs usually demonstrate age-appropriate changes. MRI can be useful if there is a diagnostic dilemma or as a part of preoperative planning (**Figure 5**) but is otherwise not necessary unless there are progressive neurologic changes or intolerable pain.

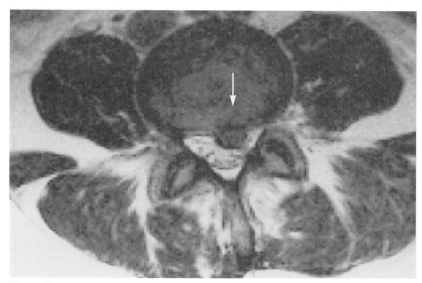

**Figure 5**
Preoperative axial MRI scan showing herniated lumbar disk (arrow).

## DIFFERENTIAL DIAGNOSIS

Cauda equina syndrome (perianal numbness, urinary overflow incontinence or retention, reduced anal sphincter tone, bilateral involvement)

Demyelinating conditions (clonus)

Extraspinal nerve entrapment (abdominal or pelvic mass)

Hip or knee arthritis (decreased internal rotation of hip, knee deformity or effusion)

Lateral femoral cutaneous nerve entrapment (sensory only, lateral thigh)

Spinal stenosis (older population)

Thoracic cord compression (clonus, spasticity, high sensory pattern, abdominal reflexes)

Trochanteric bursitis (no tension signs, pain down lateral thigh and leg, exquisite tenderness over the trochanter)

Vascular insufficiency (absent posterior tibial pulse, claudication, trophic changes)

## ADVERSE OUTCOMES OF THE DISEASE

Cauda equina syndrome with permanent motor loss, urinary incontinence, and sensory numbness can develop. Specific root deficit, with permanent dysesthesia, pain, or weakness may occur.

## TREATMENT

NSAIDs should be used in the acute phase, along with 1 to 3 days of bed rest. Muscle relaxants and/or narcotic medications may be helpful in the acute phase but typically should not be prescribed for longer than 7 to 10 days. Patients should limit sitting, prolonged standing, or walking and take frequent rests. Patients also should be reassured that most disk herniations resolve without residual problems.

Many ruptures with a significant inflammatory component will improve within 3 to 6 weeks. If not, specialty evaluation should be considered.

A short course of oral steroids (5 days) or an epidural injection may reduce leg pain within the first 2 weeks after herniation. However, recent studies indicate that epidural steroids do not change the natural history of the syndrome or significantly alter pain that has persisted for more than 2 weeks.

## ADVERSE OUTCOMES OF TREATMENT

NSAIDs can cause gastric, renal, or hepatic complications. Progression of neurologic deficit, or persistent numbness and weakness can occur despite treatment.

## REFERRAL DECISIONS/RED FLAGS

Patients with any of the following conditions need further evaluation: cauda equina syndrome; urinary retention; perianal numbness; motor loss; severe single nerve root paralysis; progressive neurologic deficit; radicular symptoms that persist for more than 6 weeks; intractable leg pain; or recurrent episodes of sciatica that interfere with the patient's life activities.

# LUMBAR SPINAL STENOSIS

ICD-9 Code

724.02
    Spinal stenosis other than cervical,
    lumbar region

## SYNONYM

Neurogenic claudication

## DEFINITION

Lumbar spinal stenosis is narrowing of one or more levels of the lumbar spinal canal and subsequent compression of the nerve roots. Anatomically, lumbar stenosis may affect as many as 30% of the population over age 60 years, yet only a portion of these individuals have symptoms. At this age, spinal stenosis is typically degenerative in origin; however, patients with achondroplasia or other conditions causing a congenitally small spinal canal may experience symptoms in their 20s or 30s.

In order of descending likelihood, L4-5, L3-4, and L1-2 are the levels most commonly involved. At L5-S1, the stenosis usually is not central but foraminal, involving the same root (L5) as central canal stenosis at the L4-5 level.

## CLINICAL SYMPTOMS

The stenosis typically is anatomically severe before symptoms occur. Onset of symptoms may be indolent or follow a lifting incident or minor trauma. A common pattern of presentation is neurogenic claudication causing radicular complaints (with or without associated back pain) in one or both legs. Neurogenic claudication differs from vascular claudication, but these conditions can coexist (Table 1). With neurogenic claudication, symptoms progress from a proximal to distal direction. Walking or prolonged standing causes fatigue and weakness in the legs (Figure 1). Pain with vascular claudication stops when the patient stops walking, but neurogenic claudication does not immediately subside when walking stops.

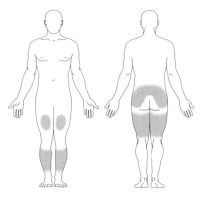

**Figure 1**
Typical pain diagram for a patient with spinal stenosis.

## Table 1
### Comparison of Vascular to Neurogenic Claudication

| Evaluation | Vascular | Neurogenic |
|---|---|---|
| Claudication distance | Fixed | Variable |
| Relief of pain | Standing | Sitting-flexed |
| Walk up hill | Pain | No pain |
| Bicycle ride | Pain | No pain |
| Type of pain | Cramp, tightness | Numbness, ache, sharp |
| Pulses | Absent | Present |
| Bruit | Present | Absent |
| Skin | Loss of hair, shiny | Normal |
| Atrophy | Rarely | Occasional |
| Weakness | Rarely | Occasional |
| Back pain | Uncommon | Common |
| Limitations of spinal movement | Uncommon | Common |

*Reproduced with permission from Herkowitz HN, Spinal stenosis: clinical evaluation, in Eilert RE (ed), Instructional Course Lectures XLI. Rosemont, IL, American Academy of Orthopaedic Surgeons, 1992, p 184.*

Extension of the spine narrows the spinal canal; flexion increases canal diameter. Therefore, patients may obtain short-term relief by leaning forward (stooping); grocery shopping is often completed by leaning on the carts. Relief after sitting varies depending on the degree of neural compression. Patients who sleep on their backs (with the spine extended) might awaken after a few hours with back and leg pain.

Lumbosacral pain at presentation is less common and is associated with walking or standing. A vague aching in the legs or leg weakness also is possible.

Spondylolisthesis (degenerative or spondylolytic), vascular insufficiency, and osteoarthritis of the hips are often associated with spinal stenosis. Obesity may be a predisposing factor.

## TESTS

### PHYSICAL EXAMINATION

Muscle weakness in the legs is often subtle, so it is best elicited by examination after walking on a treadmill. Proprioception can be impaired, resulting in a mildly positive Romberg test. Sensory changes are segmental if present but can involve more than one spinal level. Reflexes can be diminished. The posterior tibial pulse is normal unless the patient has concomitant vascular disease. Some patients will have a lumbar scoliosis. With bowel or bladder symptoms, sphincter tone can be decreased. Since many of these patients have concomitant prostate disease or stress incontinence, genitourinary evaluation is necessary to differentiate these processes.

### DIAGNOSTIC TESTS

AP and lateral radiographs (including up to T10 in the lateral view) can show spondylolisthesis or significant narrowing of the intervertebral disk (**Figure 2**). Some patients are osteopenic, as well. Radiographs can show evidence of an old burst fracture of the vertebral body.

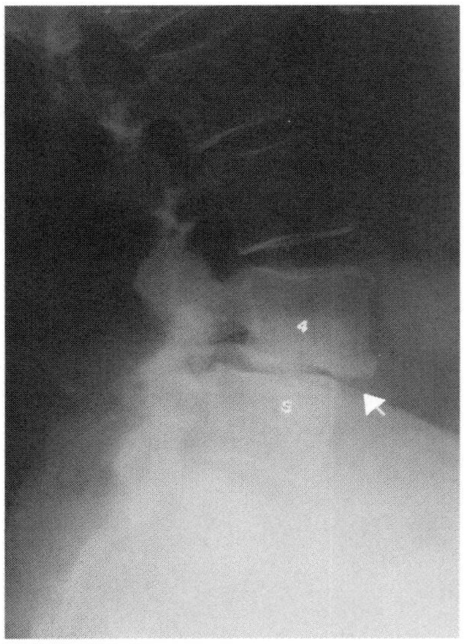

## DIFFERENTIAL DIAGNOSIS

Abdominal aortic aneurysm (palpable pulsatile mass)

Arterial insufficiency (distance to claudication constant, recovery after rest, absent or diminished pulses)

Diabetes mellitus (abnormal glucose metabolism, nonsegmental numbness, skin changes)

Folic acid or vitamin $B_{12}$ deficiency (confirmed by laboratory tests, anemia)

Infection (fever, elevated erythrocyte sedimentation rate, intervertebral disk narrowed)

Tumor (patchy neurologic deficit, bone destruction, severe night pain)

## ADVERSE OUTCOMES OF THE DISEASE

The rate of progression varies widely, from none to rapid. Many patients tolerate this condition well and never develop any neurologic deficit. However, pain and limited function can become severe and lead to a secondary depres-

**Figure 2**
Lateral radiograph of a patient with degenerative spondylolisthesis at L4 on L5 (arrow).

sion. Standing erect may become impossible, forcing the patient to adopt a stooped posture. Claudication can develop after walking only a few feet. Cauda equina syndrome develops in some patients, with loss of bowel and bladder function.

## TREATMENT

An exercise or physical therapy program that focuses on flexing the spine is recommended. Flexion of the spine increases intraspinal volume. Bicycling is one exercise that is done with the spine in flexion. Improving abdominal muscle tone lifts the pelvis anteriorly and flexes the lumbar spine; however, reduction of intra-abdominal fat is crucial to meet this objective. Lumbar flexion exercises (on all fours, arching the back, or in the fetal position) increase spinal canal volume. Exercises that extend the spine (swayback) should be avoided.

Intermittent use of NSAIDs can help. Long-term use of narcotics is reserved for patients with severe symptoms who are not surgical candidates. Folic acid or vitamin $B_{12}$ supplementation can be used empirically or following testing.

## ADVERSE OUTCOMES OF TREATMENT

Neural damage during decompression is possible. Prolonged use of NSAIDs can cause renal failure, hepatotoxicity, and gastrointestinal ulcer disease. The chronic use of narcotics is associated with its own set of problems when these drugs are used inappropriately.

## REFERRAL DECISIONS/RED FLAGS

Any neurologic deficit, gait disturbance, or bowel and bladder dysfunction should be evaluated further. Since these changes may not be reversed following surgery, the goal of treatment is to prevent progression. If nonoperative treatment is ineffective, specialty consultation is indicated. Night pain that disturbs sleep usually is an indication of advanced disease for which further evaluation is indicated.

# METASTATIC DISEASE

ICD-9 Codes
198.5
　　Secondary malignant neoplasm of
　　other specified site, bone and
　　bone marrow
733.13
　　Pathologic fracture, vertebrae

## SYNONYM

Pathologic fracture

## DEFINITION

Malignant tumors involving the spine can be either primary (rare) or metastatic (common). Metastatic disease to the vertebrae occurs at some time in the clinical course in approximately 50% of all patients who have solid tumors. The highest prevalence is with carcinoma of the breast, lung, prostate, colon, thyroid, and kidney.

Osseous involvement of the vertebrae is much more common than involvement of the spinal cord or dura. The most likely etiology is hematogenous spread, depositing neoplastic cells in the vertebral body through the Batson plexus (a unique venous plexus of the spine characterized by collateral connections to the inferior vena cava and a general lack of valves).

Metastatic disease may become clinically evident by one of several different presentations: 1) as an incidental finding in asymptomatic patients; 2) in patients with known primary tumors who are being evaluated for possible metastatic disease by bone scan, MRI, or CT; 3) as localized spinal pain; or 4) as neurologic findings in patients with or without previous history of a primary tumor.

## CLINICAL SYMPTOMS

Pain is the most common presenting symptom. The pain often is first noted following trivial trauma, is typically constant, and progressively worsens as the days or weeks pass. Weight-bearing activities (standing, sitting) aggravate the pain, whereas lying down typically relieves it. Pain that prevents sleep and persists through the night is highly suspicious for a neoplasm.

With compression of the nerve roots, the pain associated with cervical or lumbar tumors also has a radicular component to the extremities. Similar nerve root entrapment by tumors in the thoracic spine cause a band-like distribution of pain around the chest. When the compression involves a nerve root, radicular symptoms and associated sensory loss and/or motor weakness are restricted to a single extremity. With more generalized sensory and motor dysfunction, cervical or thoracic cord compression or cauda equina syndrome should be suspected, especially if the patient reports difficulty walking or bowel or bladder dysfunction. Patients may report that the sensation diminishes progressively from the affected level distally.

The rate of disease progression and neurologic dysfunction can be slow, evolving over weeks or months, or more rapid in aggressive tumors. Progression can be more difficult to identify in patients taking high dosages of pain medication for metastatic disease elsewhere. Acute onset of quadriplegia or paraplegia can occur (infrequently) with rapid enlargement of a soft-tissue tumor mass or following a pathologic fracture that compresses the spinal cord.

## TESTS

### PHYSICAL EXAMINATION

An area of tenderness to palpation and/or percussion along the spinous processes is common. Tumors in the posterior elements (lamina, spinous process) may be palpable. A patient with a vertebral body collapse can develop increased kyphosis at the level of fracture. Assess motor and sensory function of all nerve roots distal to the lesion. Check deep tendon and other appropriate spinal cord reflexes.

If the primary tumor has not been previously diagnosed, the patient will need a complete evaluation with particular emphasis on the thyroid, breasts, chest, kidney, and prostate.

### DIAGNOSTIC TESTS

Initial radiographic evaluation requires high-quality AP and lateral radiographs. Cervical spine radiographs should also include odontoid views and show all vertebrae from the occiput to T1. Lumbar spine radiographs should include the bodies of T10 to the tip of the coccyx, with a spot lateral view of the lumbosacral junction, if needed for clarity. A radiopaque marker placed to the side of the area of percussion tenderness helps focus the area of concern. The lateral view may show collapse with loss of height of the vertebral body or areas of bony destruction with lytic or blastic lesions in the vertebral body. The AP view may show loss of the integrity of the pedicles, often the first radiologic sign of tumor involvement.

A technetium Tc 99m bone scan is the best screening study to identify widespread metastatic disease because it evaluates the spine as well as other axial (pelvis) and appendicular (extremity) bones.

## DIFFERENTIAL DIAGNOSIS

Degenerative arthritis (fracture rare, bone dense)

Infection (loss of disk space, sclerosis)

Multiple myeloma (men older than age 50 years, fracture from trivial trauma)

Osteoporotic fracture (generalized osteopenia, pedicles intact)

Traumatic fracture (normal bone, widening of bone in AP and lateral views)

## ADVERSE OUTCOMES OF THE DISEASE

Involvement of one area of the spine with metastatic disease does not usually change the overall survival rate, but spinal deformity and/or intractable pain pose considerable problems in patient care. Spinal involvement with neurologic deficit compromises quality of life and may shorten life with complications of paraplegia. Quadriplegia and paraplegia are the most serious sequelae of pathologic fracture.

## TREATMENT

Treatment of spinal tumors is based on the degree of bony involvement, the type of symptoms, and patient preference. Chemotherapy, hormonal therapy, or radiation is appropriate for asymptomatic tumors detected during evaluation for metastatic disease. Radiation therapy is appropriate for painful metastases without serious deformity or neural compression. Alternative methods are considered in tumors that are insensitive to radiation (renal cell carcinoma). With pain and neurologic deficit, the most effective way to improve neural function and overall function is surgical decompression, generally with adjunctive postoperative radiation therapy. Surgical intervention results in improved neurologic function in approximately 85% of patients.

## ADVERSE OUTCOMES OF TREATMENT

Neurologic deterioration persists in some patients, despite adequate decompression, because of recurrent tumor or tumor involvement in the vascular supply to the spinal cord. Surgical wound complications are more common if the surgery follows radiation therapy or if the patient is taking oral steroids.

## REFERRAL DECISIONS/RED FLAGS

Patients with known prior malignancies and spinal symptoms or patients with intractable pain require specialty evaluation, as do patients in whom trivial trauma produces a spinal fracture even in the presence of osteoporosis.

# Scoliosis in Adults

ICD-9 Codes

737.30
  Scoliosis (and kyphoscoliosis), idiopathic
737.43
  Curvature of spine associated with other conditions, scoliosis

## Definition

Scoliosis is a lateral curvature of the spine. In adults, the condition is classified as either a deformity that developed during childhood or a deformity that developed after skeletal maturity, usually secondary to degenerative disk disease and/or degenerative spondylolisthesis. Changes that occur with aging, such as osteoporosis, degenerative disk disease, spinal stenosis, and degenerative spondylolisthesis, can contribute to and/or confound the symptoms and progression of either condition.

## Clinical symptoms

The most common presenting symptom is pain localized to the midthoracic, thoracolumbar, midlumbar, or lower lumbar region. The most common overlapping syndrome is degenerative disk disease, which also causes lower lumbar pain. Neurologic dysfunction and radicular pain are most commonly associated with compression of the L4 or L5 nerve root due to asymmetric hypertrophy of the facet joints, asymmetric disk degeneration, and mild rotatory subluxation.

Another presenting symptom is curve progression. These patients report that the "hump" on their back is getting bigger, that they are leaning to the side more, or that they are losing height. Patients older than age 60 years more commonly report these problems.

Cardiopulmonary decompensation rarely is evident in adult-onset scoliosis. Symptoms related to pulmonary compromise are associated with severe neuromuscular curves.

## Tests

### Physical examination

The entire spine should be inspected and palpated with the patient standing. The relative height of the shoulders and iliac wings should be noted, as should any asymmetry at the waist. Decompensation is evaluated by measuring the distance a plumb line from C7 deviates to the right or left of the gluteal cleft. Forward bending also exaggerates the asymmetry of the posterior rib cage and thoracolumbar junction. Pain to palpation may be present in the area of the iliolumbar ligaments and sacroiliac joint and usually is related to degenerative disk disease. Neurologic examination should include evaluation of reflexes as well as motor and sensory function of the lumbosacral nerve roots.

### Diagnostic tests

Standing posteroanterior and lateral radiographs should be obtained on a 36" cassette, with spot views obtained of the specific painful areas. Electromyography is rarely indicated but can be helpful to distinguish radiculopathy from neuropathy in patients with diabetes mellitus.

## Differential diagnosis

Congenital scoliosis (vertebral body abnormality, childhood or adolescent presentation)

Degenerative disk disease with asymmetric disk space collapse (normal vertebral shape, sharp curve over few segments)

Degenerative spondylolisthesis with accompanying lateral listhesis and disk degeneration (forward or backward slip of vertebral body)

Neuromuscular scoliosis (neurologic abnormalities and weakness)

Severe disk herniation with sciatic scoliosis and radiculopathy (unilateral neurologic signs, normal vertebral contour)

Vertebral osteomyelitis (fever, severe local pain, lysis of bone in vertebral body, narrowing of disk)

Traumatic or pathologic vertebral fracture (wedge-shaped vertebral body, history of trauma)

## Adverse outcomes of the disease

Increased pain and deformity with diminished functional activity are possible. With increased cosmetic deformity, patients may become less social.

## Treatment

Many patients can be managed nonoperatively with intermittent NSAIDs and exercise, eg, walking, lumbar flexion exercises. Severe pain requires stabilization (fusion) and possible decompression of spinal stenosis.

## Adverse outcomes of treatment

NSAIDs may cause gastric, renal, or hepatic complications. Complications of operative management may include increased pain, increased deformity, infection, pseudarthrosis, instrumentation failure, or paralysis. The postoperative complication rate is much higher in adults than in adolescents.

## Referral decisions/Red flags

Progressive neurologic deterioration requires emergency management. Patients who report that they cannot walk more than two blocks because of pain, respiratory dysfunction, or weakness require specialty evaluation. Any change in the deformity requires further evaluation as well.

# SPINAL ORTHOTICS

## CERVICAL

### SOFT CERVICAL COLLAR

This foam-covered orthosis is appropriate for short-term use in cervical sprains or intermittent use to alleviate pain in patients with cervical spondylosis. The common error is to select a soft cervical collar that is too big, thus thrusting the neck into extension. A collar that positions the neck in approximately 10° of flexion maximizes the space for the nerve roots as they pass through the vertebral foramen. Patients should be on an isometric exercise program to avoid loss of intrinsic muscle support.

### PHILADELPHIA COLLAR

This molded polystyrene brace provides better control of cervical rotation and is preferred for transport and initial immobilization of patients with suspected cervical fractures. Some patients prefer this support to the cervical collar in the treatment of acute sprains; however, unless rotational control is necessary (C1-2 injury), most people prefer the greater comfort of a soft cervical collar.

### RIGID CERVICAL ORTHOTICS

A hard cervical collar limits flexion and extension better than a soft cervical collar. Greater restriction of neck motion is obtained by a brace that extends from the neck to the midthoracic spine. For example, the Miami J orthosis (Jerome Medical, Moorsetown, NJ) is basically a Philadelphia collar that has a rigid plastic component extending to the middle of the chest. As such, it greatly restricts rotation that primarily occurs in the upper cervical spine as well as the flexion and extension and lateral bending that occurs to a greater degree in the lower cervical spine.

### HALO BRACE

This brace provides superior immobilization of the cervical spine. The halo portion is rigidly secured to the head by four screws inserted into the outer table of the skull. Bars connect the halo portion to a plastic vest that surrounds the chest. Virtually no cervical spinal motion occurs in a patient wearing this brace.

## THORACIC

### THORACOLUMBOSACRAL CORSET

A standard lumbosacral corset with a proximal extension provides adequate support for patients with osteoporosis or acute thoracic sprains involving the lower thoracic spine. Some corsets are equipped with metal stays or plastic inserts that are bent to conform to the patient's spine. Women may reject this brace because of irritation under their breasts; the orthotist may need to modify the brace to ensure patient compliance.

### JEWETT OR OTHER SIMILAR THREE-POINT ORTHOSIS

The basic principle of this type of orthotic is three-point fixation, with pressure over the sternum and pubis anteriorly and over the midspine posteriorly. Most are aluminum and bendable to fit the patient. These braces limit flexion and extension of the thoracic spine but provide limited rotational control. Due to their limited contact areas and light weight, patient tolerance usually is good. This type of orthosis is useful for patients with thoracic sprains or simple compression fractures.

### TOTAL-CONTACT THORACOLUMBAR ORTHOSIS

These braces are either prefabricated modules that are fitted based on measurements of the torso or made from a plaster mold of the patient's torso. The latter provides better total contact and rotational control but is more expensive. These braces usually are constructed of hard plastic anterior and posterior clamshells lined with a soft material that attach together on the sides. These braces are used primarily as definitive treatment in patients with stable burst fractures of the thoracolumbar spine or as a postoperative aid following spinal fusion.

## LUMBAR

### ELASTIC BELTS

These braces do not limit lumbar spine motion and probably do not prevent injury. With a mild lumbar strain, they may provide some proprioception and abdominal support.

### LUMBOSACRAL CORSET

The standard lumbosacral corset can be worn with or without internal stays of metal or plastic. These devices limit motion to a limited degree and are most useful for an adjunct to pain control following a lumbar sprain or acute disk. The time period of bracing should be short and accompanied by an exercise program once the acute pain has subsided.

### RIGID ORTHOTICS

See the descriptions for the three-point and total-contact orthoses.

# SPONDYLOLISTHESIS: DEGENERATIVE

ICD-9 Code
738.4
    Acquired spondylolisthesis

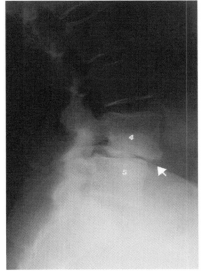

**Figure 1**
Lateral radiograph of a patient with degenerative spondylolisthesis at L4 on L5 (arrow).

## DEFINITION

Degenerative spondylolisthesis is forward slippage of a lumbar vertebral body that is caused by degeneration and alterations in the facet joints in conjunction with degenerative changes in the intervertebral disk. By definition, the lamina and pars interarticularis are intact. This condition occurs most frequently between the fourth and fifth vertebral bodies, is more common in women older than age 40 years, and has an increased incidence in black women.

Retrolisthesis is posterior slippage of a lumbar vertebral body. This condition also develops secondary to degenerative changes.

## CLINICAL SYMPTOMS

Back pain that is aggravated by bending, lifting, or twisting activities is common. Narrowing of the lateral recesses can cause a radiculopathy. Narrowing of the central canal can cause neurogenic claudication or other symptoms of spinal stenosis.

## TESTS

### PHYSICAL EXAMINATION

Inspect and palpate the spine for any curvature, loss of lordosis, or step-off of the spinous processes. Evaluate motor and sensory function of the L1-S4 nerve roots. Diminished knee and/or ankle reflexes are often present; however, these findings are common in the older population. While motor examination is usually normal, strength testing after walking may reveal weakness in toe or heel walking or in great toe dorsiflexion strength. There may be a palpable step-off when palpating the spinous processes.

### DIAGNOSTIC TESTS

AP and lateral radiographs are adequate. The lateral view will show slippage of one vertebra onto another, usually with the superior vertebra displaced several millimeters relative to the one below (**Figure 1**). The involved disk space frequently shows degeneration and narrowing.

## DIFFERENTIAL DIAGNOSIS

Iatrogenic instability (following diskectomy or decompression)

Pathologic fracture (from tumor)

Posttraumatic instability (history of fracture)

Spondylolisthesis (pars defect, as a residual of adolescent spondylolisthesis)

## ADVERSE OUTCOMES OF THE DISEASE

Disabling back pain or functional neurologic impairment associated with spinal canal stenosis or radiculopathy is possible.

## TREATMENT

Flexion exercises, stretching exercises, occasional corset wear, and intermittent use of NSAIDs may be of benefit. Most patients require lifestyle changes, including avoiding repetitive bending, heavy lifting, and trunk twisting. Severe pain that does not respond to nonoperative management requires further evaluation (eg, MRI) and consideration of surgical decompression and/or stabilization.

## ADVERSE OUTCOMES OF TREATMENT

NSAIDs may cause gastric, renal, or hepatic complications and may interact with other medications.

## REFERRAL DECISIONS/RED FLAGS

Patients with symptoms of spinal stenosis (neurogenic claudication) after walking two blocks or less require further evaluation. Patients with cauda equina syndrome (perianal numbness and/or bowel or bladder impairment) require immediate evaluation.

# Spondylolisthesis: Isthmic

**ICD-9 Code**
738.4
  Acquired spondylolisthesis

## Definition

Spondylolisthesis occurs when one vertebral body slips in relation to the one below. In children this usually occurs between L5 and S1. A defect develops at the junction of the lamina with the pedicle (pars interarticularis), leaving the posterior element without a bony connection to the anterior element. Most likely this condition is a fatigue fracture that developed in the preadolescent years and failed to heal. If the defect only is present, the patient has spondylolysis. When the vertebral body slides forward, producing the "slip" or "listhesis," the condition is called spondylolisthesis. Patients who participate in activities that place severe stress on this area, such as gymnastics and football, have a higher incidence of this condition.

## Clinical symptoms

This condition may be asymptomatic or minimally symptomatic; however, adolescent and adult patients may develop back pain that radiates posteriorly to or below the knees and is worse with standing (**Figure 1**). Frequently, they experience spasms in the hamstring muscles manifested by the inability to bend forward and have very limited straight-leg raising. True nerve compression symptoms are rare.

## Tests

### Physical examination

Examination may reveal diminished lumbar lordosis and flattening of the buttocks. Palpate the spinous processes. With significant spondylolisthesis, a "step-off" is noted with the spinous process of the slipped vertebra that is "left behind" being more prominent than the one above.

Hamstring spasm is manifested by marked limitation in the ability to bend forward or passive straight-leg raise with the patient supine. Neurologic deficits are rare.

### Diagnostic tests

With forward slippage (spondylolisthesis) lateral radiographs demonstrate forward translation of L5 relative to S1 (expressed as a percentage of the AP width of the vertebral body) (**Figure 2**). A defect in the pars interarticularis is evident on the oblique views (an absent neck in the "Scotty dog") (**Figure 3**). This is the only radiographic abnormality if the condition is limited to a spondylolysis.

Increasing slippage can be evaluated with radiographs taken at 6-month intervals (or sooner if symptoms increase) until growth is complete.

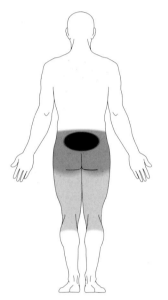

**Figure 1**
Typical pain diagram for a patient with isthmic spondylolisthesis.

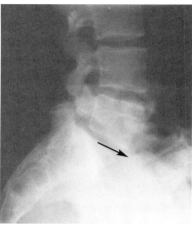

**Figure 2**
Lateral radiograph of a grade 2 to 3 spondylolisthesis at the lumbosacral junction (arrow).

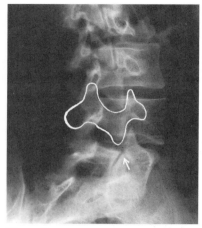

**Figure 3**
Oblique radiograph shows a normal "Scotty dog" appearance to the lamina (outlined area). In the vertebra below, the neck of the Scotty dog is broken (see arrow) and is the site of the pars interarticularis defect of spondylolisthesis.

## DIFFERENTIAL DIAGNOSIS

Intervertebral disk injury (no "step-off" or slip, and no defect seen on plain radiograph)

Intervertebral diskitis (elevated erythrocyte sedimentation rate and fever)

Osteoid osteoma (night pain, abnormal bone scan, pain relieved with aspirin)

Spinal cord tumor (sensory findings, upper motor neuron signs)

## ADVERSE OUTCOMES OF THE DISEASE

Progressive or complete slip of the vertebral body, chronic back pain and disability, neurologic paralysis of the lower lumbar nerve roots, or bowel and bladder involvement (cauda equina syndrome) are possible.

## TREATMENT

Strengthening and flexibility exercises and observation with periodic radiographs (a standing spot lateral view usually is adequate) are indicated until growth is nearly complete. Activities that may aggravate the condition, such as gymnastics or football line play, should be discontinued. A custom-fitted thoracolumbosacral orthosis may control pain but probably will not decrease slippage.

## ADVERSE OUTCOMES OF TREATMENT

Despite treatment, unrecognized progression of the forward slip can develop.

## REFERRAL DECISIONS/RED FLAGS

Patients with significant pain and/or obvious slippage need further evaluation.

## Section Editor
### Walter B. Greene, MD
Chairman and J. Vernon Luck, Jr,
Distinguished Professor
Department of Orthopaedic Surgery
University of Missouri School of Medicine
Columbia, Missouri

David D. Aronsson, MD
Professor
Department of Orthopaedics and
Rehabilitation
Department of Pediatrics
University of Vermont College of Medicine
Burlington, Vermont

Robert M. Bernstein, MD
Assistant Chief of Staff
Shriners Hospitals for Children—
Los Angeles
Los Angeles, California

R. Dale Blasier, MD
Professor of Orthopaedic Surgery and
Pediatrics
Division of Pediatric Orthopaedics
University of Arkansas for Medical Sciences
Little Rock, Arkansas

Robert M. Campbell, Jr, MD
Associate Professor
Department of Orthopaedics
University of Texas Health Science Center
San Antonio, Texas

Jon R. Davids, MD
Director, Motion Analysis Laboratory
Orthopaedic Department
Shriners Hospitals for Children—Greenville
Greenville, South Carolina

Frederick R. Dietz, MD
Professor
Department of Orthopaedic Surgery
University of Iowa College of Medicine
Iowa City, Iowa

James C. Drennan, MD
Professor
Department of Orthopaedics and
Rehabilitation
University of New Mexico School of
Medicine
Albuquerque, New Mexico

Marybeth Ezaki, MD
Associate Professor
Department of Orthopaedic Surgery
University of Texas Southwestern Medical
School
Texas Scottish Rite Hospital for Children
Dallas, Texas

Keith R. Gabriel, MD
Assistant Chief of Staff
Shriners Hospitals for Children—
Twin Cities
Minneapolis, Minnesota

Gaia Georgopoulos, MD
Associate Professor
Department of Orthopaedic Surgery
University of Colorado Health Sciences
Center
Denver, Colorado

M. Mark Hoffer, MD
Lowman Professor
Orthopedic Hospital
Los Angeles, California

Walter W. Huurman, MD
Professor
Orthopaedic Surgery and Pediatrics
Department of Orthopaedic Surgery and
Rehabilitation
University of Nebraska Medical Center
Omaha, Nebraska

Kosmas J. Kayes, MD
Assistant Professor, Pediatric Orthopedics
Department of Orthopaedic Surgery
Indiana University School of Medicine
Indianapolis, Indiana

Vincent S. Mosca, MD
Associate Professor and Chief of Pediatric
Orthopedics
University of Washington School of
Medicine
Director, Department of Orthopedics
Children's Hospital and Regional Medical
Center
Seattle, Washington

Prasit Nimityongskul, MD
Professor and Interim Chair
Department of Orthopaedic Surgery
University of South Alabama College of
Medicine
Mobile, Alabama

Brad W. Olney, MD
Clinical Professor
Section of Orthopaedics
University of Kansas Medical School—
Wichita
Wichita, Kansas

William L. Oppenheim, MD
Professor and Head, Pediatric Orthopedics
Department of Orthopaedic Surgery
UCLA Medical Center
Los Angeles, California

Hamlet A. Peterson, MD, MS
Emeritus Professor of Orthopedic Surgery
Mayo Medical School
Division of Pediatric Orthopaedic Surgery
Mayo Clinic
Rochester, Minnesota

William A. Phillips, MD
Professor, Orthopaedics and Pediatrics
Chief, Pediatric Orthopaedics and Scoliosis
Baylor College of Medicine
Texas Children's Hospital
Houston, Texas

Peter D. Pizzutillo, MD
Director
Department of Orthopaedic Surgery
St. Christopher's Hospital for Children
Philadelphia, Pennsylvania

Thomas L. Schmidt, MD
Chief and Professor
Pediatric Orthopaedic Surgery
The Children's Mercy Hospital
Kansas City, Missouri

Perry L. Schoenecker, MD
Chief of Staff
Shriners Hospitals for Children—St. Louis
Professor of Orthopedic Surgery
Washington University School of Medicine
Acting Chairman of Orthopedic Surgery
St. Louis Children's Hospital
St. Louis, Missouri

Kit M. Song, MD
Associate Director
Department of Orthopedics
Children's Hospital and Regional Medical
Center
Seattle, Washington

# PEDIATRIC ORTHOPAEDICS

George Sotiropoulos, MD
Department of Child Health
University of Missouri—Columbia
Hospitals and Clinics
Columbia, Missouri

L.T. Staheli, MD
Professor Emeritus
Department of Orthopedics
University of Washington School of
Medicine
Seattle, Washington

J. Andy Sullivan, MD
Professor and Don H. O'Donoghue
Professor and Chair
Department of Orthopaedic Surgery
Children's Hospital of Oklahoma
Oklahoma City, Oklahoma

Michael D. Sussman, MD
Former Chief of Staff
Shriners Hospitals for Children—Portland
Portland, Oregon

George H. Thompson, MD
Director, Pediatric Orthopaedics
Rainbow Babies and Children's Hospital
Department of Orthopaedics
Case Western Reserve University School of
Medicine
Cleveland, Ohio

Jeffrey D. Thomson, MD
Director
Department of Orthopaedic Surgery
Connecticut Children's Medical Center
Hartford, Connecticut

Stuart L. Weinstein, MD
Ignacio V. Ponseti Chair and Professor of
Orthopaedic Surgery
Department of Orthopaedic Surgery
University of Iowa College of Medicine
Iowa City, Iowa

# PEDIATRIC ORTHOPAEDICS—AN OVERVIEW

The oft-quoted statement "Children are not just small adults," is particularly germane for pediatric disorders of the musculoskeletal system. Fractures, soft-tissue injuries, neurologic disorders, and infections have unique features and different considerations in children. Furthermore, the effect of growth must always be considered as it may be a positive or negative factor in the treatment of these disorders. For that reason, *Essentials of Musculoskeletal Care* includes this separate section on pediatric orthopaedics.

## AGE AND GENDER

Because degenerative joint disease takes years to develop, pain from a skeletal deformity is uncommon during childhood. Therefore, understanding the natural history of these conditions is critical to knowing whether treatment is needed. Some "deformities" in children are normal for the age. For example, genu varum or bowlegs is normal at birth, but by the time a child reaches age 3 years, normal alignment is a "knock-knee" or relatively large amount of genu valgum.

Considering age and gender can be helpful when evaluating children. For example, a boy between the ages of 4 and 8 years who has proximal thigh pain and a limp most likely has Legg-Calvé-Perthes disease. Similar symptoms in adolescent boys suggest a slipped capital femoral epiphysis. Female infants are more likely to have hip dysplasia, whereas clubfoot is more common in male infants. Adolescent girls are more likely to have scoliosis, but kyphosis of the spine is more common in adolescent boys.

## GROWTH

Growth, with its associated remodeling potential, may be a tremendous ally in treatment. This is particularly true in the newborn period, when simply splinting a very dysplastic hip for a few months will result in a normal joint that functions well for a lifetime. Certain angular deformities in pediatric fractures also may completely remodel. This allows greater latitude in closed management of fractures in children.

Growth, however, may exacerbate pediatric disorders. Fractures that damage the physis or growth plate may cause progressive angulation or shortening of the limb. Progressive angulation also may occur from asymmetric compression on one side of the physis. As a result, growth from that side of the physis is inhibited and an angular deformity develops. Examples include progressive bowleg deformity in infantile tibia vara (occurring in obese children who start walking at an early age) and rickets (weakening of the bony structure at the growth plate).

# NEUROMUSCULAR DISORDERS

Bones grow and muscles have to "catch up." Many pediatric neuromuscular disorders such as cerebral palsy, myelomeningocele, and muscular dystrophy cause muscle weakness and muscle imbalance (greater weakness on one side of the joint). Muscle imbalance plus growth results in contracture of the muscle and possible bony deformity. For example, in a child with cerebral palsy, the hip adductor and flexor muscles are often more spastic and therefore stronger than the opposing hip abductors and extensors. With growth, this muscle imbalance may cause progressive contracture of the adductors and flexors, as well as dysplasia of the femur and acetabulum, and subluxation or dislocation of the hip.

# VARIABLES IN SOFT-TISSUE INJURIES

As children grow, their coordination and psyche also are developing. As a result, competitive sports require adaptation of the game to the age and size of the child. Overuse injuries in the adult primarily manifest themselves as either microscopic tears or complete rupture of the musculotendinous junction or within the substance of the tendon. In children, the bone-tendon junction is the weak link. The result is different types of overuse syndromes. For example, Osgood-Schlatter disease results from microscopic avulsion fractures at the insertion of the patellar tendon during adolescence when the child is relatively big and active and when the relatively weak secondary ossification center of the proximal tibia is developing.

# VARIABLES IN INFECTION AND ARTHRITIS

The higher incidence of hematogenous osteomyelitis in children is related to the unique anatomy of metaphyseal circulation in children. Hematogenous septic arthritis also is more common in children. Chronic arthritides such as juvenile rheumatoid arthritis also are different in children. The etiology of this difference is less clear but may be related to a developing immune system causing a different response to triggering agents.

# PHYSICAL EXAMINATION
# PEDIATRIC ORTHOPAEDICS

## Inspection/Palpation

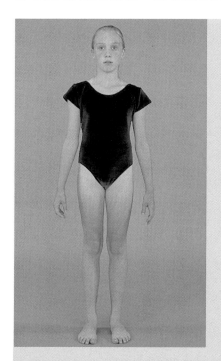

### Anterior view

With the patient standing, inspect alignment of the legs for knock-knee (genu valgum), bowleg (genu varum), internal femoral torsion (patellae point toward one another), external femoral torsion (patellae face away from each other and not straight ahead), and limb-length inequality (pelvis not level). Also, look for increased angulation at the elbow or extreme shoulder height asymmetry. Look for asymmetry in the angle formed by the humerus and forearm (elbow carrying angle). Unilateral deformity may indicate an acute injury or deformity from a congenital or traumatic growth disturbance.

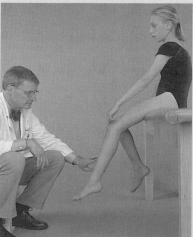

### Palpation

A young child may not be able to verbalize the site of his or her pain. Initiate palpation by touching an area that is probably not involved. Palpate from this area to the region of suspected involvement. Even though the child may be apprehensive and crying, a change in discomfort can be identified as the tender area is palpated.

# Range of Motion

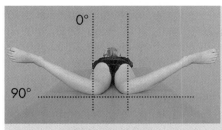

### Hip internal rotation

Measure internal rotation with the hip in extension for a more accurate reflection of femoral torsion. With the patient prone, flex the knees to 90° to the Zero Starting Position and rotate the legs outward. This maneuver positions the hip into internal rotation. With restricted unilateral motion, one hip will stop moving and the other will continue to move. With increased femoral anteversion, internal rotation will exceed external rotation by 30° or more.

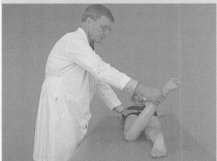

### Hip external rotation

With the child prone and knees together, rotate the legs inward while stabilizing the pelvis. This maneuver positions the hip into external rotation. Compare the two sides. Rotation of the hips is typically symmetric.

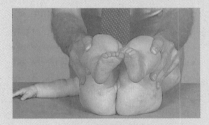

### Hip abduction–infants

Assess hip abduction in neonates and infants with the hips flexed as children this age have some degree of normal hip flexion contracture. Thigh lengths should be equal. Abduct the child's legs. Abduction in children this age should be symmetric and should exceed 50° to 60°. Limited abduction suggests developmental dislocation of the hip.

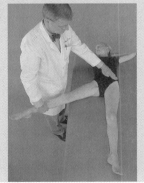

### Hip abduction–older children

Assess hip abduction with the hip in extension and the pelvis level. Place one finger on the contralateral anterior superior iliac spine. This hand will sense when the pelvis starts to tilt (limit of hip abduction). Abduct the hip until the pelvis starts to tilt and estimate the degree of movement.

# Special Tests

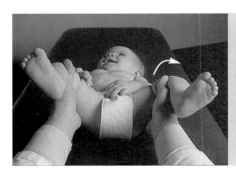

### Barlow sign

The Barlow sign dislocates an unstable neonatal hip. Stabilize the pelvis by placing one hand on the pelvis (symphysis pubis). Place your other hand with the long finger over the greater trochanter and the thumb on the medial thigh. Flex and then adduct the hip. If the hip is located but unstable, the femoral head will dislocate with a clunk or with a sensation of slippage as the leg is adducted. This test should be performed with very little force.

# Special Tests

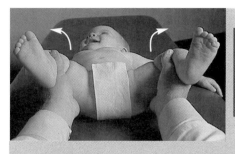

### Ortolani "reduction" sign

The Ortolani sign reduces a dislocated hip in a neonate or young infant. Flex the hips to 90°. Place your long finger over the greater trochanter and your thumb over the inner thigh. Abduct both hips, pushing the femoral head into the acetabulum with your long finger. A positive test is a clunk or sensation of reduction as the femoral head slips over the rim of the acetabulum and relocates.

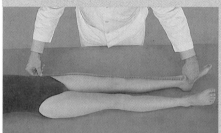

### Limb-length discrepancy

Measure with a tape measure from anterior superior iliac spine to the prominence of the medial malleolus. Alternatively, different-sized wooden blocks can be placed under the short leg while the patient is standing. When the iliac crests are level, the thickness of the blocks indicates the amount of limb-length discrepancy.

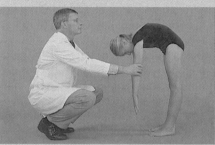

### Scoliosis, forward bending

The vertebral body rotates with scoliosis, pulling the transverse process and ribs posteriorly on the convex side. The resulting posterior prominence is more apparent with the forward bending test. Ask the patient to bend forward with the knees straight and with both arms hanging free, as you stand first behind and then in front of the patient. Inspect along the spine. A prominence on forward bending indicates scoliosis. Measure the amount of rotational prominence with a scoliometer.

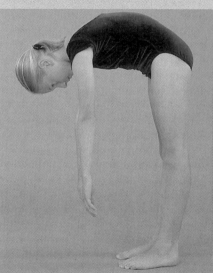

### Kyphosis

Examine the thoracic spine from the side. Look for excessive round back in the thoracic spine. Ask the patient to bend forward with arms hanging free. If the patient is not able to touch the toes, the reason may be tight hamstrings secondary to Scheuermann kyphosis or spondylolisthesis in the lower lumbar spine.

# ANTERIOR KNEE PAIN

ICD-9 Codes
717.9
Pathologic plica
732.4
Osgood-Schlatter disease
Sinding-Larsen-Johannson syndrome
732.7
Osteochondritis dissecans
736.6
Bipartite patella
Patellofemoral dysfunction

## DEFINITION

Pain about the anterior aspect of the knee is common in adolescents; however, a definite cause is not always identifiable. Idiopathic pain may be secondary to a subclinical disruption (strain) of the developing musculoskeletal structures, as these are under increased stress from the growth spurt and exuberant adolescent activities. This is particularly true at secondary ossification centers that, at this age, are the weak link to repetitive movement and muscular contraction.

## CLINICAL SYMPTOMS

Patients typically report a history of indolent onset of peripatellar pain that is activity related. Swelling and giving way usually are absent, but if reported, these symptoms are mild, vague, and inconclusive. If the patient reports more definitive symptoms of instability, then problems such as patellar subluxation or a torn meniscus are more likely.

## TESTS

### PHYSICAL EXAMINATION

Hip rotation should be assessed to exclude the possibility of slipped capital femoral epiphysis.

Ask the patient to place one finger on the spot that hurts the most. Adolescents with anterior knee pain often will report that they cannot identify an exact spot but will state that "it hurts all over." With encouragement, however, many will be able to localize the area of most severe pain and this can be an aid in diagnosis. Examine the knee for effusion, any restricted motion, ligamentous stability, abnormal patellar tracking, and other signs of patellar instability, as shown in the physical examination in the Knee section.

### DIAGNOSTIC TESTS

Screening radiographs include AP and lateral views of the knee. Specific views are listed within the description of the differential diagnosis. Special imaging studies such as CT with the knee extended and flexed 20° or a kinematic MRI may be required for patients who have persistent pain.

## DIFFERENTIAL DIAGNOSIS

### PATELLOFEMORAL DYSFUNCTION

Patellofemoral dysfunction is common and ranges from subtle maltracking of the patella as the knee moves from extension to flexion to episodes of recurrent dislocation. Chondromalacia of the patella is an adverse outcome.

With mild patellofemoral dysfunction, the history is poorly localized knee pain that is aggravated by stair climbing, jumping, or even prolonged sitting.

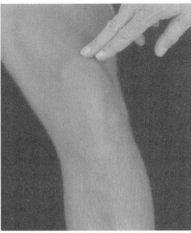

**Figure 1**
To perform the apprehension test by displacing the patella laterally with the knee extended. Flex the knee. This maneuver may cause pain on apprehension as the patella subluxates or dislocates over the lateral femoral condyle.

Maltracking of the patella may be evident as the knee moves from full extension to 30° of flexion, but abnormalities are often subtle. The patella apprehension sign may be present with more overt instability (**Figure 1**). Patella compression may cause pain but is often nonspecific. Much of the physical examination entails ruling out other causes of knee pain. If patellofemoral dysfunction is suspected, a tangential view of the patella should be included.

Patellofemoral dysfunction usually responds to nonoperative therapy that is based on strengthening the quadriceps muscle while avoiding or minimizing stress across the patellofemoral joint. Closed chain kinetic exercises (eg, step downs and partial squats) keep the foot in contact with the ground and diminish patellofemoral contact forces. A stretching program is indicated for any patient with hamstring, rectus femoris, or iliotibial band tightness. Recalcitrant cases require operative treatment to realign the quadriceps mechanism.

### SINDING-LARSEN-JOHANSSON SYNDROME

Sinding-Larsen-Johansson syndrome is jumper's knee (patella tendinitis) that occurs during childhood. Patients typically are boys between 9 and 12 years old who report activity-related pain localized to the inferior pole of the patella. The pathophysiology of this syndrome is microscopic tears or an avulsion injury at the junction of the inferior pole of the patella and the patella tendon. The prognosis of Sinding-Larsen-Johansson syndrome is uniformly good because as the patella grows, progressive ossification envelopes and thus anchors the area of heterotopic ossification. By contrast, the older adolescent or adult with jumper's knee may have continued symptoms that ultimately require operative intervention.

The examination is normal except for the localized tenderness at the inferior pole of the patella. Radiographs may show small areas of heterotopic ossification at the inferior pole. Treatment is activity modifications. Complete resolution of symptoms is universal but may take several months.

A similar overuse process may occur at the superior pole of the patella. This condition, quadriceps tendinitis, is not as common as Sinding-Larsen-Johansson syndrome because the triangular shape of the patella concentrates muscular contraction forces at the inferior pole. Except for a difference in location, the history, examination, treatment, and expected results of quadriceps tendinitis in children are similar to those of Sinding-Larsen-Johansson syndrome.

### BIPARTITE PATELLA

A bipartite patella is a separate ossification center of the superior lateral corner of the patella, typically seen as an incidental finding on radiographs (**Figure 2**). However, a bipartite patella may become a source of anterior knee pain.

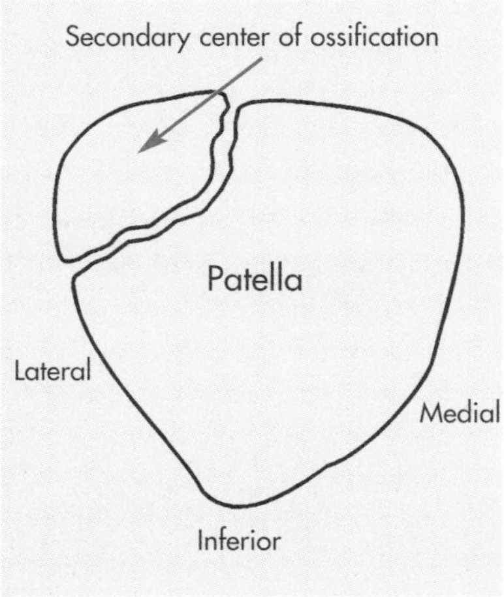

In the acute situation, the patient presents after a fall or injury with tenderness and swelling localized to the superolateral corner of the patella. This most likely results from strain of the fibrous attachments of the ossification center. Treatment is based on the history and degree of tenderness. Short-term immobilization for 3 to 4 weeks with a removable brace usually is sufficient.

Secondary center of ossification

Patella

Lateral

Medial

Inferior

**Figure 2**
The separate ossification center seen in bipartite patella.

In chronic cases, patients report pain after running and jumping activities. Activity modifications may resolve the symptoms, but some cases are recalcitrant to nonoperative therapy and require excision of the superolateral fragment with reattachment of the quadriceps tendon.

## PATHOLOGIC PLICA

A plica is a normal fold in the synovium that may become thickened and fibrotic as a result of a direct blow or repetitive stress. The medial patella plica is most likely to be affected. The patient typically presents with anteromedial knee pain and, with further questioning, reports a history of popping, snapping, or pseudolocking. Examination reveals a clicking sensation as the knee flexes in a 40° to 60° arc. With the knee flexed 60°, the tender plica is brought into a prominent position and may be palpated medial to the patella.

Nonoperative therapy is often successful and includes activity modifications and NSAIDs. Arthroscopic excision is appropriate for patients with persistent symptoms.

## OSTEOCHONDRITIS DISSECANS

In the knee, osteochondritis dissecans (OCD) most likely results from repetitive stress that causes osteonecrosis of the underlying bone and, ultimately, a subchondral stress fracture. The most common location is the medial femoral condyle. These lesions may heal or, with continued stress, the dissection may progress to cause a fissure or separation in the articular cartilage. Ultimately, continued stress may result in a loose body as the lesion becomes completely separated from surrounding bone, commonly known as a loose body in the joint.

The onset of most cases is during childhood. Symptoms, however, may not begin until either the late adolescent or adult years. When OCD presents during early adolescence, the articular cartilage may have buckled, but frequently it has not separated. Making the diagnosis is important because during the growing years OCD has the potential to heal.

A typical history is pain and stiffness after running and sports activities. Occasionally, the child will note swelling of the knee with activity. The examination may be unremarkable or may demonstrate mild effusion or quadriceps atrophy. Radiographs are necessary to make a diagnosis. In addition to AP and lateral views, a tunnel view is helpful in outlining lesions in the posterolateral aspect of the medial femoral condyle (**Figure 3**).

The prognosis depends on the size of the lesion and the age of the child. Lesions less than 1 cm in diameter do well, while those greater than 2 cm have a poor prognosis for healing with nonoperative management. Younger children have greater potential to repair osteonecrotic bone before the lesion starts separating. After the distal femoral physis closes, the lesion is very unlikely to heal.

Nonoperative management involves activity modifications so that symptoms do not occur. Parents particularly need to be advised that the patient will not be able to participate in sports for 3 to 12 months. Activity modifications should continue just as long after operative treatment. Successful nonopera-

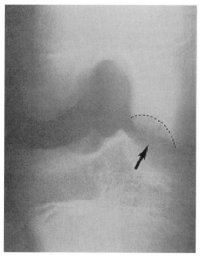

**Figure 3**
Tunnel view of the knee showing osteochondritis dissecans (arrow).

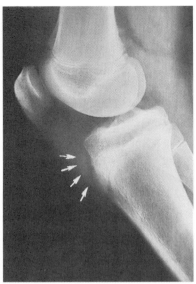

**Figure 4**
Symptomatic tibial tubercle ossicle (arrows) in a 13-year-old boy.

tive management results in a normal knee, whereas the long-term results after operative treatment are less predictable.

The indications for operative treatment include a loose body, an unstable lesion, or persistent symptoms despite compliant nonoperative care.

## OSGOOD-SCHLATTER DISEASE

Osgood-Schlatter disease (or condition) results from repetitive injury and small avulsion injuries at the patellar tendon insertion into the secondary ossification center of the tibial tuberosity. Onset of this disorder during early adolescence coincides with development of this secondary ossification center. Overuse explains the increased incidence in children who are active in sports.

Examination reveals tenderness and swelling at the tibial tuberosity. Radiographs may be normal or demonstrate heterotopic ossification anterior to the tibial tuberosity (**Figure 4**).

Treatment consists of activity modifications to permit healing of the microscopic avulsion fractures. For severe or recalcitrant symptoms, short-term immobilization for 4 to 8 weeks may be beneficial.

Detailed information about Osgood-Schlatter disease is provided on pp 684-685.

# BACK PAIN

ICD-9 Codes
724.1
    Pain in thoracic spine
724.2
    Low back pain

## SYNONYM
Backache

## DEFINITION
Pain in the thoracic or lumbar spine is not as common in children, but compared with that in adults, is more often due to organic causes (sometimes serious) when present for more than a few weeks.

## CLINICAL SYMPTOMS
The nature of onset, as well as the location, character, and radiation of the pain should be determined. Back pain accompanied by neurologic signs and symptoms (eg, radicular pain, muscle weakness, gait abnormalities, sensory changes, bowel and bladder dysfunction) or systemic symptoms (eg, fever, malaise, and weight loss) suggest an organic cause. Night pain often signals a more serious problem.

## TESTS

### PHYSICAL EXAMINATION
Examine the spine with special emphasis on identifying deformities, loss of motion, muscle spasm, and areas of tenderness. Assess gait, motor and sensory function of all appropriate nerve roots, straight leg and reverse straight leg raising tests, deep tendon reflexes, and pathologic reflexes (Babinski sign). Test superficial abdominal reflexes by lightly stroking the skin in a diagonal direction toward the umbilicus. Perform the test in all four quadrants. A normal reflex is deviation of the umbilicus toward the side of the test in all four quadrants. Asymmetric abdominal reflexes may be the only finding in a child with syringomyelia or other spinal cord pathology; however, this reflex may be absent or asymmetric in healthy children.

Abnormal neurologic findings may be a late manifestation of a tumor. Therefore, a normal neurologic examination does not eliminate serious problems.

### DIAGNOSTIC TESTS
The extent of the evaluation depends on the duration and degree of symptoms as well as the results of the physical examination. No laboratory or radiographic studies are necessary if the examination is normal and symptoms are mild and of limited duration.

For symptoms in the thoracic and lumbar regions, standing AP and lateral radiographs of the entire spine provide more information because these views permit standardized measurement of deformity. Oblique views may be helpful for patients who have symptoms in the lumbar spine.

AP, lateral, oblique, and open-mouth odontoid views of the cervical spine are indicated for patients with neck pain. Flexion-extension lateral views of the cervical spine also may be necessary.

The need for additional imaging studies (eg, bone scan, MRI, CT) depends on the suspected etiology. The need for and sequencing of these tests depends on the differential diagnosis.

## DIFFERENTIAL DIAGNOSIS

Differential diagnosis of pediatric back pain is shown in Table 1. Muscle strain is the most common cause of thoracic and lumbar pain in children. Scheuermann disease may present with pain in the thoracic and thoracolumbar regions, while spondylolysis and spondylolisthesis are common causes of pain in the lumbar and lumbosacral regions. Idiopathic scoliosis rarely

## Table 1
### Differential Diagnosis of Back Pain in Children

| Etiology | Condition |
| --- | --- |
| Congenital | Congenital spine anomalies<br>Diastematomyelia |
| Developmental | Scoliosis<br>Kyphosis (Scheuermann disease) |
| Traumatic | Upper cervical spine instability<br>Occult fractures<br>Pathologic fractures<br>Muscle strain<br>Spondylolysis and spondylolisthesis<br>Herniated disk<br>Slipped vertebral apophysis |
| Infectious | Diskitis<br>Vertebral osteomyelitis<br>Tuberculosis |
| Systemic | Chronic infection<br>Storage diseases<br>Juvenile osteoporosis |
| Juvenile arthritis | Ankylosing spondylitis<br>Juvenile rheumatoid arthritis |
| Neoplastic | |
| Benign | Osteoid osteoma<br>Osteoblastoma<br>Aneurysmal bone cyst<br>Langerhan cell histiocytosis |
| Malignant | Spinal cord tumor<br>Neuroblastoma<br>Leukemia<br>Osteogenic sarcoma<br>Metastatic disease |
| Psychogenic | |

causes pain in children, but scoliosis associated with syringomyelia, tethered spinal cord, or neoplasms may present as back pain.

## ADVERSE OUTCOMES OF THE DISEASE

When back pain has an organic cause, failure to diagnose may result in progression of the condition. In certain conditions, such as instability of the upper cervical spine, tumors, or infections, failure to diagnose may ultimately result in spinal cord or peripheral nerve injury.

## TREATMENT

Treatment of back pain in children is diagnosis specific. Because of the extensive differential diagnoses, it is not possible to discuss all aspects of treatment here.

If there are no ominous symptoms or neurologic abnormalities, then observation with activity modifications and mild analgesics is appropriate initially. More extensive studies will be necessary if the pain does not improve within 1 to 2 months, if the pain progresses, or if new symptoms and findings develop.

## ADVERSE OUTCOMES OF TREATMENT

Adverse outcomes of treatment are also diagnosis specific. The principal adverse outcome is lack of improvement or worsening of symptoms despite treatment. This indicates failure to recognize an underlying organic cause for the pain.

## REFERRAL DECISIONS/RED FLAGS

The following factors suggest a serious underlying etiology: 1) persistent or increasing pain; 2) pain accompanied by systemic symptoms such as fever, malaise, or weight loss; 3) neurologic symptoms or findings; 4) bowel or bladder dysfunction; 5) onset of symptoms at a young age, especially 4 years of age or younger (possible tumor); and 6) a painful thoracic scoliosis. If these findings occur, further evaluation is necessary.

# ELBOW PAIN

ICD-9 Code
719.42
    Pain in joint, upper arm

## FRACTURES
Supracondylar humerus
Lateral condyle humerus
Medial condyle humerus
Medial epicondyle humerus
Radial head
Olecranon
Occult fractures

## SOFT-TISSUE INJURIES
Dislocation
Hemarthrosis
Sprain
Subluxation of the radial head (nursemaid's elbow)

## INFECTION

## CHRONIC PAIN
Traction apophysitis of the elbow
Panner disease
Osteochondritis of the capitellum
Tumors

## DEFINITION
Elbow pain in children is most often caused by an acute or chronic injury to bone or soft tissues. Excessive throwing and the subsequent valgus stress cause most chronic elbow pain in children. The focus of this chapter is on soft-tissue injuries. Fractures are discussed in a separate chapter.

## CLINICAL SYMPTOMS
Patients with acute conditions report pain, tenderness, swelling, and most often a history of falling on an outstretched arm. For those with chronic pain, the common history is aching pain over the involved area that is activity related.

## TESTS
### PHYSICAL EXAMINATION
For patients with acute conditions, evaluate the status of the median, ulnar, and radial nerves distal to the injury. Assess radial and ulnar pulses as well. With obvious deformity, position or splint for comfort and proceed with

radiographs. In other children, attempt to find the site of maximum tenderness and perform a gentle evaluation of elbow motion.

For children with chronic pain, assess the point of maximum tenderness. Mild swelling and limited motion may be present. Palpate for a mass to exclude an atypical tumor. Palpate the ulnar nerve while moving the elbow to rule out a subluxating ulnar nerve.

## DIAGNOSTIC TESTS

AP and lateral radiographs of the elbow should be obtained for all acute injuries. A fracture or dislocation may be obvious or subtle. The radial head should be directed towards the capitellum on both views. Comparison views are helpful with subtle injuries.

With chronic pain, AP and lateral radiographs may be normal or may show an avulsion fracture, or fragmentation and heterotopic ossification of the medial epicondyle (Little Leaguer elbow), or fragmentation and irregularity of the capitellum.

## DIFFERENTIAL DIAGNOSIS

### OCCULT FRACTURES

A posterior fat pad sign is associated with occult fractures in children. Overlying the distal humerus are an anterior and posterior fat pad. These structures are within the elbow joint capsule. In a normal elbow, the anterior fat pad can be seen on a lateral radiograph, but the posterior fat pad usually is not seen. Any process that causes an elbow effusion will elevate the anterior and posterior fat pads and make both structures visible (**Figure 1**). In children who have a positive posterior fat pad sign and no evidence of fracture on initial radiographs, the incidence of a subsequent bony injury being demonstrated ranges from 6% to 76%. The greater incidence is noted in studies that include repeat AP, lateral, and oblique radiographs obtained 2 to 3 weeks after the injury.

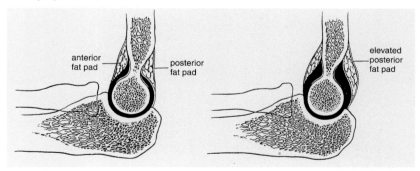

**Figure 1**
Normal anterior and posterior fat pads (left) and anterior and posterior fat pads elevated from an effusion (right).

*Reproduced with permission from Skaggs DL, Mirzayan R: The posterior fat pad sign in association with occult fracture of the elbow in children. J Bone Joint Surg, 1999;81A:1429-1433.*

A child with a posterior fat pad sign and no apparent fracture on initial radiographs or signs of septic arthritis should be assumed to have an occult, nondisplaced fracture. A posterior long arm splint or a long arm cast should be used for 2 to 3 weeks. Bony injuries that demonstrate only a posterior fat pad sign at initial evaluation are mild, nondisplaced fractures. If no tenderness is noted at the 2- to 3-week evaluation, immobilization can be discontinued. In this situation, there is no evidence that repeat radiographs alter treatment.

### DISLOCATION

Dislocation of the elbow is typically posterior. Associated injuries such as fracture of the medial epicondyle or other fractures can occur. The medial epicondyle fracture can be displaced and incarcerated in the joint. Closed reduction usually is successful.

### HEMARTHROSIS

An elbow hemarthrosis is a diagnosis of exclusion. Examination demonstrates swelling of the joint, and radiographs typically show a posterior fat pad sign. Aspiration of the joint is diagnostic and will decrease discomfort.

### SPRAINS

Elbow sprains are uncommon in children because the bone is the weak link. Short-term immobilization is appropriate.

### SUBLUXATION OF THE RADIAL HEAD

This condition, also called a pulled elbow or nursemaid's elbow, is the most common elbow injury in children younger than age 5 years. This injury is associated with increased ligamentous laxity. The mechanism of injury is a pull on the forearm when the elbow is extended and the forearm pronated. The annular ligament, which wraps around the neck of the radius, slips proximally and becomes interposed between the radius and ulna.

Immediately after the injury, the child will cry, but the initial pain quickly subsides. Thereafter, the child is reluctant to use the arm but otherwise does not appear to be in great distress. The extremity is held by the side with the elbow slightly flexed and the forearm pronated. Tenderness over the radial head and resistance on attempted supination of the forearm are the only consistent findings. Radiographs are normal.

To reduce the subluxation, place your thumb over the radial head and supinate the forearm. If this maneuver fails to produce the snap of reduction, then flex the elbow. Resistance may be perceived just before reaching full flexion. As the elbow is pushed through that resistance, the annular ligament will slip back into normal position and a snap will be perceived as the radial head reduces. If the reduction is successful, the child will begin to use the extremity normally in a few minutes. The exception is the child who presents 1 to 2 days after injury. At this time, swelling of the annular ligament may both obscure the snap that signals a successful reduction and also prevent immediate resumption of normal function. However, if the elbow has full flexion and supination, the radial head has been reduced. Immobilization is probably not necessary, as parents report that slings are quickly discarded.

### INFECTION

Infection as a cause of acute elbow pain is relatively uncommon. For example, in one study of pediatric infections, the elbow accounted for only 12% of septic arthritis. These conditions, however, should be considered when evaluating a child with elbow pain. The possibility of infection is more likely with an acute onset of pain, no history of injury, and an elevated temperature.

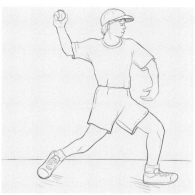

**Figure 2**
Throwing athletes impose valgus stress on the elbow.

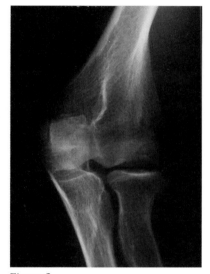

**Figure 3**
AP radiograph demonstrating radiolucency typical to osteochondritis dissecans of the capitellum.

*Reproduced with permission from Peterson RK, Savoie FH III, Field LD: Osteochondritis dissecans of the elbow, in Zuckerman JD (ed), Instructional Course Lectures 48, American Academy of Orthopaedic Surgeons, Rosemont, IL, 1999, pp 393-398.*

## CHRONIC PAIN

These injuries may affect either the medial (tension) or lateral (compression) side of the humerus. Medial injuries can be acute (avulsion fracture of the medial epicondyle) or gradual in onset (traction apophysitis of the medial epicondyle, better known as Little Leaguer elbow) (**Figure 2**). Lateral involvement is secondary to osteonecrosis of the capitellum. When children younger than age 10 years are affected, the condition typically is called Panner disease and has a good prognosis.

Chronic injuries generally are self-limited. Resting the arm, with no throwing for 3 to 6 weeks, is indicated followed by rehabilitation to restore elbow motion and upper extremity strength. Osteonecrosis of the capitellum in adolescents, called osteochondritis dissecans or OCD, has a more guarded prognosis (**Figure 3**). This condition can result in an osteochondral loose body, which causes a locking or catching sensation, and is more likely to cause residual symptoms and consideration of operative treatment. Intra-articular loose bodies secondary to osteochondritis dissecans should be removed operatively if they are causing pain and/or intermittent locking of the joint.

Tumors, although very uncommon about the elbow in children, are more likely with chronic pain, no history of injury, pain at rest, night pain, and pain that is getting worse.

# FOOT AND ANKLE PAIN

| ICD-9 Codes |
| --- |
| 682.7 |
|   Abscess, foot |
| 732.5 |
|   Calcaneal apophysitis |
|   Accessory navicular |
|   Freiberg infraction |
|   Osteochondral lesion of talus |
|   Os trigonum |
| 733.49 |
|   Osteonecrosis of navicular |
| 754.61 |
|   Tarsal coalition |
| 755.66 |
|   Hallux valgus |
| E920.9 |
|   Nail puncture wound |

## DEFINITION

Foot and ankle pain in a child generally is caused by specific clinical conditions; however, trauma, infection, and tumors are potential causes as well.

## CLINICAL SYMPTOMS

A history of a significant injury combined with localized findings generally suggests some type of trauma. However, children have numerous minor injuries to the lower extremities, and parents might attribute symptoms to a particular injury or episode when, in fact, the actual condition has nothing to do with trauma. Furthermore, injuries in younger children may occur away from the parents or others, and young children are typically unable to give an exact account of how the injury occurred.

Determining whether the problem is acute or chronic also provides information about its etiology. A recent onset of symptoms generally is associated with traumatic or infectious conditions.

Questions about systemic symptoms such as malaise, swelling, and fever are important with either acute-onset conditions or chronic symptoms. Fever and swelling are more likely to suggest infectious or possibly malignant conditions.

## TESTS

### PHYSICAL EXAMINATION

Infections in the foot usually have a history of direct penetrating injuries such as a nail puncture wound. If the incident occurred within the preceding 24 to 72 hours, the diagnosis is most likely a soft-tissue cellulitis or abscess.

Physical examination can often localize the area of tenderness to a specific anatomic site. This step is extremely helpful in arriving at the correct diagnosis. Older children can often point with one finger to the spot that hurts the most, which helps localize the anatomic site and greatly narrows the differential diagnosis.

The foot should be examined for areas of swelling, erythema, or ecchymosis. Ecchymosis is generally a sign of traumatic injury, whereas erythema suggests an inflammatory or infectious process. The ankle and subtalar joints should be evaluated for range of motion and tenderness on range of motion. Decreased inversion and eversion can suggest a tarsal coalition, while painful range of motion of the joint can indicate an inflammatory or infectious process.

### DIAGNOSTIC TESTS

Radiographs are needed when a fracture or chronic process is suspected. Physical examination should be used to determine whether the problem is in the foot or ankle. If the problem is localized to the foot, AP, lateral, and oblique views of the foot are taken. AP and lateral views of the ankle can be ordered if the ankle is the area of concern. If findings on the radiographs could be a normal variant, comparison views of the opposite foot can be taken.

More sophisticated imaging studies are sometimes necessary. A bone scan can be helpful if a stress fracture or infectious process is suspected. CT is generally best for benign bony lesions, while MRI provides better information on soft-tissue lesions and malignant processes.

# Differential diagnosis

## Hindfoot

### Calcaneal apophysitis

Calcaneal apophysitis is characterized by pain in the posterior aspect of the heel that occurs after play and sports activities and most commonly affects active, prepubertal children. Tenderness at the posterior aspect of the calcaneus is common. Radiographs typically are not needed. Short-term activity modifications or restriction is indicated. Detailed information about calcaneal apophysitis is provided on pp 604-605.

### Os trigonum

The os trigonum is an accessory ossicle of the posterior talus that usually is a normal anatomic variant. However, this secondary center of ossification may become symptomatic in older adolescents and adults, particularly those who participate in ballet or soccer. Patients commonly report posterior ankle pain that is activity related. Pain also develops secondary to posterior impingement of the os trigonum between the talus and tibia during plantar flexion. Surgical excision may be required.

### Osteochondral lesion of the talus

This lesion typically affects adolescents, particularly athletes. The pain is exacerbated by activity and is localized to the ankle region. Radiographs of the ankle usually confirm the diagnosis, although MRI may be necessary in some cases.

### Tarsal coalition

Tarsal coalition is the most common cause of rigid flatfeet in children. Symptoms typically develop during the second decade. The onset of pain generally is insidious but can be associated with an injury or change in activity. Hindfoot motion is markedly restricted, and spasm of the peroneal muscles can be elicited by quickly inverting the foot. Talocalcaneal bars are difficult to see on routine radiographs; therefore, CT is necessary to confirm the diagnosis. Treatment depends on the presentation of symptoms. Detailed information about tarsal coalition is provided on pp 714-716.

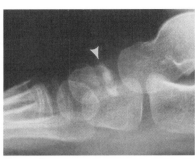

**Figure 1**
Lateral radiograph of the foot showing a shattered, fragmented navicular (arrow).

*Reproduced with permission from Kasser JR (ed): Orthopaedic Knowledge Update 5. Rosemont, IL, American Academy of Orthopaedic Surgeons, 1996, pp 503–514.*

# MIDFOOT

## OSTEONECROSIS OF THE NAVICULAR

This condition, sometimes called Köhler disease, primarily affects children (usually boys) ages 4 to 8 years. Patients limp, turn out their foot while walking, and may report pain in the medial arch. Radiographs show a dense, fragmented, thin navicular (**Figure 1**). A short leg walking cast for 4 to 8 weeks relieves pain, improves walking (less pain), and may speed resolution of the osteonecrosis. However, the eventual outcome is good whether casting or activity modifications are chosen.

## ACCESSORY NAVICULAR

Accessory navicular is an anatomic variant in which a secondary center of ossification forms at the medial aspect of the navicular and may become symptomatic during adolescence. Patients report pain and swelling on the medial side of the foot. Activity or shoe wear may exacerbate the pain. Radiographs may be necessary, depending on the presentation and history of symptoms. Treatment generally is limited to short-term activity restrictions or shoe modifications. However, a walking cast or even operative treatment may be necessary, depending on the symptoms and history. Detailed information about accessory navicular is provided on pp 602-603.

# FOREFOOT

## FREIBERG INFRACTION

Freiberg infraction is osteonecrosis involving the head of the second metatarsal, most likely a result of trauma, and typically affects adolescents. The pain is exacerbated by activity. Examination reveals tenderness under the second metatarsal head, sometimes swelling on the dorsal aspect of the metatarsal head and pain at the extremes of dorsiflexion and plantar flexion. Radiographs usually show evidence of the condition within 2 to 3 weeks of the onset of symptoms (**Figure 2**). Treatment options include activity modifications, a metatarsal pad, or short-term casting. Occasionally, operative treatment is required to remove loose bodies or to realign the metatarsal head.

## HALLUX VALGUS

Hallux valgus may develop during adolescence. At this age, most patients are asymptomatic, but some may report pain. Treatment principles are similar to those for adults. Detailed information about hallux valgus is presented on pp 466-467.

# OTHER FOOT PROBLEMS

## ENTHESITIS

Enthesitis is characterized by pain and inflammation at a bone-tendon insertion but is uncommon in children. Disorders such as Achilles tendinitis or plantar fasciitis may be the presenting symptoms of a seronegative spondyloarthropathy.

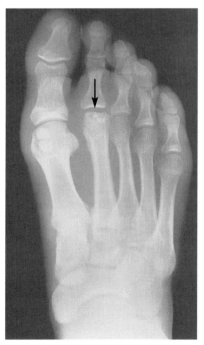

**Figure 2**
Radiograph showing Freiberg infraction. Note flattening and fragmentation at the head of the second metatarsal (arrow).

## INFECTION

Infection in the foot usually is secondary to a direct penetrating injury, such as a nail puncture wound. If symptoms develop within 24 to 72 hours after the injury, the cellulitis or abscess usually is secondary to a *Staphylococcus aureus* infection. If swelling and erythema develop several days after the injury, the infection usually is a septic arthritis or osteomyelitis secondary to *Pseudomonas aeruginosa* that requires surgical debridement.

## SPRAINS, STRAINS, AND FRACTURES

Sprains, strains, and fractures of the foot and ankle occur but are relatively uncommon until late adolescence. Most of these injuries in children can be managed by nonoperative modalities. In a child who has a history of an inversion injury and tenderness over the distal fibular physis, the most likely diagnosis is a nondisplaced fracture of the physis. This injury is best treated with a cast.

## TUMORS

Tumors in the foot and ankle are uncommon at all ages. The most common benign bony tumor in children is a unicameral or aneurysmal bone cyst involving the calcaneus. Osteoid osteoma affecting the tarsal bones also occurs in children. Ewing sarcoma affecting the tarsal bones or diaphysis of metatarsals is the most common malignant bony lesion involving the foot. The pain, swelling, and radiographic findings in this tumor may mimic osteomyelitis. Of the malignant soft-tissue lesions, synovial cell sarcoma is most common in the foot. Typical symptoms include onset during the second decade of a slowly enlarging mass.

SECTION 9 | PEDIATRIC ORTHOPAEDICS

# GROWING PAIN

ICD-9 Code
729.5
  Pain in limb

## DEFINITION

Growing pain is a condition for which there is no uniform diagnostic consensus. Typically, it is a diagnosis made after more specific pathologic conditions are excluded. Although its true etiology is unknown, growing pain or leg aches are often thought to be the result of overactivity (muscular strain or fatigues). The condition typically occurs in an otherwise healthy, active child. Growing pain is more common in boys, in children with ligamentous laxity, and in 2- to 5-year-old children. Older children, however, also may be affected. The pain or discomfort is commonly localized to the calf but may be perceived in the foot, ankle, knee, or thigh. The problem is often bilateral, but parents may report that one leg seems to hurt more than the other or that one leg hurts some nights while the other leg hurts different nights.

## CLINICAL SYMPTOMS

Leg pain is often described as mild to moderate, intermittent in character, and more noticeable in the evening or at night or following a day of increased activity or sport. Parents generally report using warm or cold compresses, massage, or simple analgesics to relieve the symptoms. Constitutional symptoms such as fever, weight loss, loss of appetite, or malaise are rarely reported.

## TESTS

### PHYSICAL EXAMINATION

Examination of the affected extremity should focus on identifying any masses, inflammation, lymphadenopathy, abnormal joint movement, instability, muscle group atrophy, and any neurologic deficits. With growing pain, the examination is usually normal in all aspects, although the affected extremity can be tender to deep pressure. Flexible flatfeet may be noted, but the gait and pattern of shoe wear is normal.

### DIAGNOSTIC TESTS

Plain radiographs should be considered in children who have a higher intensity of pain or more prolonged symptoms, a history of pain at rest that is not relieved by simple analgesics, or an associated mass. Bone scan, CT, or MRI should be considered if a specific lesion, such as bone or soft-tissue tumor, stress fracture, bone or joint infection, or tarsal coalition, is suspected. Metabolic work-up may be needed if the history and review of systems suggest certain conditions such as leukemia or an endocrinopathy.

## DIFFERENTIAL DIAGNOSIS

Calcaneal apophysitis (heel pain with activity)

Köhler disease (unilateral, pain with activity, foot turned out with walking)

Metabolic/systemic disease (history and review of systems suggestive of leukemia, endocrine disorder, renal osteodystrophy, juvenile chronic arthritis, rheumatic disease)

Subacute osteomyelitis (unilateral, activity-related symptoms)

Trauma (unilateral, toddler's or stress fracture)

Tumor (unilateral, pain more persistent and severe)

## ADVERSE OUTCOMES OF THE DISEASE

Growing pain has a benign and self-limiting course, although the leg aches may occur intermittently for several months. Permanent long-term impairment has not been noted.

## TREATMENT

An explanation of the natural history and expected outcome and perhaps a recommendation about use of simple analgesics usually are sufficient to allay parental fears and to avoid overtreatment. Short-term use of NSAIDs and/or a short period of rest or immobilization before resuming activities, as the level of pain allows, also can be recommended. Operative treatment is not indicated.

## ADVERSE OUTCOMES OF TREATMENT

Overuse of pain medication with subsequent psychological aspects and unnecessary testing are possible.

## REFERRAL DECISIONS/RED FLAGS

Patients with a history of severe, persistent pain along with constitutional symptoms (eg, fever, night sweats, malaise, poor appetite, weight loss) need further evaluation. Findings on physical examination that indicate masses, significant inflammation, lymphadenopathy, circulatory compromise, neuropathy, or myopathy also are a concern. A serious error is to diagnose growing pain or leg aches while overlooking the more specific underlying conditions listed in the differential diagnosis.

# ACCESSORY NAVICULAR

ICD-9 Code
732.5
Juvenile osteochondrosis of foot

## DEFINITION

Accessory navicular is an anatomic variant in which a secondary center of ossification forms in the medial portion of the tarsal navicular bone at the attachment of the posterior tibialis tendon. During adolescence, this may become prominent and symptomatic by virtue of its size, or from repetitive sprains and microfractures at the attachment of the ossicle to the navicular. Symptoms are more common in girls. The disorder is fairly common, with one study observing a 14% incidence of symptoms during adolescence.

## CLINICAL SYMPTOMS

Patients typically report pain and swelling on the medial side of the foot. The pain is exacerbated with activity or with pressure from the overlying shoes. Severe pain is uncommon.

## TESTS

### PHYSICAL EXAMINATION

Tenderness and mild swelling over the medial aspect of the navicular (insertion of the posterior tibialis tendon) is typical. Inversion of the foot against resistance may be painful. A flexible pes planus may be present.

### DIAGNOSTIC TESTS

Radiographs are not necessary with a typical examination and mild symptoms. With persistent or severe symptoms, AP, lateral, and oblique radiographs of the foot will document the disorder and exclude other possibilities. The AP and lateral views should be weight bearing to best demonstrate pes planus or other alignment problems. The oblique view, obtained with the patient supine, often provides the best profile of the accessory ossicle (**Figure 1**). Some patients have a cornuated navicular (shaped like a horn of plenty), resulting from fusion of the accessory ossicle to the navicular.

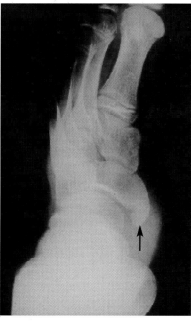

**Figure 1**
Oblique radiograph of the foot demonstrating accessory navicular in a 12-year-old girl.

## DIFFERENTIAL DIAGNOSIS

Flexible pes planovalgus (developmental or acquired)

Posterior tibial tendinitis (swelling in the region of the posterior tibial tendon)

Tarsal coalition (restricted inversion, eversion of the heel)

## ADVERSE OUTCOMES OF THE DISEASE

Patients may experience persistent pain or a limp.

## TREATMENT

Most patients can be treated with short-term restriction of activities and/or shoe modifications to relieve pressure over the prominent navicular (soft material medial to the bump and/or stretching of the shoe). A short period of time in a walking cast may permit healing of the repetitive microfractures and resolution of symptoms. In most cases, the bump is not large and symptoms resolve with cessation of growth. Excision of the prominent portion of the navicular is the treatment of choice for patients with persistent, disabling symptoms.

## ADVERSE OUTCOMES OF TREATMENT

Postoperative infection and a tender medial scar that is irritated by shoe wear are both possible.

## REFERRAL DECISIONS/RED FLAGS

Persistent pain signals the need for further evaluation.

# CALCANEAL APOPHYSITIS

| ICD-9 Code | |
| --- | --- |
| 732.5 | Juvenile osteochondrosis of foot |

## SYNONYM
Sever disease

## DEFINITION
Calcaneal apophysitis most commonly affects active, prepubertal children and is characterized by pain in the posterior aspect of the heel that occurs after play and sports activities. This condition is caused by repetitive stress and microtrauma on the calcaneal apophysis. This weak link is obliterated when the apophysis fuses to the main body of the calcaneus, a process that occurs around age 9 years in girls and age 11 years in boys.

## CLINICAL SYMPTOMS
Patients have posterior heel pain and a limp that is activity related.

## TESTS
### PHYSICAL EXAMINATION
Examination reveals tenderness at the posterior aspect of the calcaneus.

### DIAGNOSTIC TESTS
Radiographs are not diagnostic, and sclerosis at the secondary ossification center is normal (**Figure 1**). With bilateral involvement and a typical history,

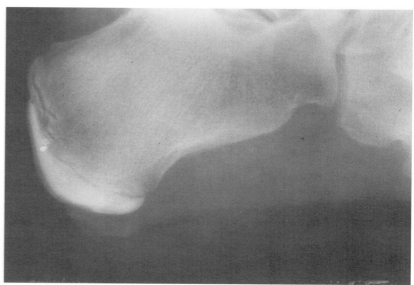

**Figure 1**
Lateral radiograph of the heel in a child (note sclerosis in the secondary ossification center of the calcaneus is normal).

*Reproduced with permission from Wilkins KE: The painful foot in the child, in Bassett FH (ed): Instructional Course Lectures 37. Park Ridge, IL, American Academy of Orthopaedic Surgeons, 1988, pp 77–85.*

radiographs probably are not necessary. With unilateral involvement, a lateral view of the heel is necessary to rule out a unicameral bone cyst.

## DIFFERENTIAL DIAGNOSIS

Achilles tendinitis (can be associated with Reiter syndrome or other seronegative spondyloarthropathies)

Infection (unilateral, elevated erythrocyte sedimentation rate, swelling)

Tumor (unilateral, swelling, night pain)

## ADVERSE OUTCOMES OF THE DISEASE

Pain, a limp, and activity modifications are possible, but there are no long-term sequelae.

## TREATMENT

Treatment includes short-term modification or restriction of the precipitating activity. Shoe modifications using a ¼" heel lift or heel cushion and Achilles tendon stretching can be helpful. Casting is rarely needed but can be used for 4 to 6 weeks if the pain and limp are recalcitrant. Neither surgery nor steroid injection is indicated.

## ADVERSE OUTCOMES OF TREATMENT

There are no long-term sequelae.

## REFERRAL DECISIONS/RED FLAGS

Suspicion of tumor or osteomyelitis indicates the need for further evaluation.

# CAVUS FOOT DEFORMITY

ICD-9 Codes
736.75
    Cavovarus deformity of foot,
    acquired
754.59
    Varus deformities of feet, other
    (Talipes cavovarus)

## SYNONYMS

Pes cavus

High-arched foot

## DEFINITION

Pes cavus is a foot with an abnormally high arch. The forefoot is fixed in equinus relative to the hindfoot. Other terms, such as cavovarus and equinocavovarus, describe additional changes in the hindfoot or ankle.

Children with a cavus foot frequently have an underlying neuromuscular disorder with associated muscle weakness or spasticity. Unless there is a known cause for the cavus foot, children who present with this condition should undergo a thorough diagnostic evaluation. Patients with systemic neuromuscular diseases or idiopathic cavus feet usually have bilateral involvement. Unilateral deformity is associated with localized disorders of the lumbosacral spinal cord.

## CLINICAL SYMPTOMS

Parents often note changes in the arch and toes, difficulty in fitting shoes, or difficulty with repeated ankle sprains. Pain is infrequent during childhood, but with time, painful callosities develop underneath the prominent metatarsal heads. A family history should be obtained because some causes of cavus feet are genetic disorders. Inquire about bowel or bladder symptoms that may be present with spinal cord lesions.

## TESTS

### PHYSICAL EXAMINATION

Inspect the lower extremity to evaluate the alignment of the ankle, heel, midfoot, and toes, and check the plantar aspect of the foot for callosities. A careful neurologic examination of the lower extremities also is necessary. Examine the spine for curvatures, paraspinal spasm, and midline defects such as dimpling or abnormal hairy patches. Examine the upper extremity for weakness of the intrinsic muscles of the hand.

### DIAGNOSTIC TESTS

Standing AP and lateral radiographs of the foot and the entire spine should be obtained. On the spinal radiographs, look for congenital malformations, diastematomyelia, widening of the interpedicular distance, and atypical curve patterns. On the lateral view of a normal foot, a line typically passes through the axis of the talus and first metatarsal. With a cavus foot, dorsal angulation is noted on lines drawn through the axis of the talus and first metatarsal (Figure 1).

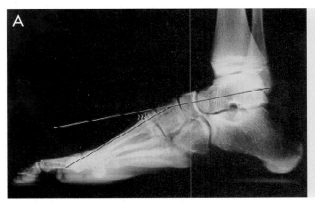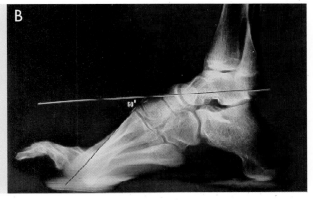

**Figure 1**
A, Radiograph demonstrates a positive angle of Meary caused by cavus foot and associated forefoot equinus. Normally a line passing through the long axis of the talus should go through the first metatarsal. B, In a patient with a more severe deformity, note the claw-toes and the hypertrophy of the cortices of the fifth metatarsal resulting from excessive lateral forefoot weight bearing.

Nerve conduction velocity studies and MRI of the spine may be indicated. Electromyography may distinguish myopathic from neuropathic conditions.

## Differential diagnosis

Charcot-Marie-Tooth disease (peripheral neuropathy with abnormal nerve conduction velocity studies, autosomal dominant most common)

Clubfoot (incomplete correction)

Diastematomyelia (hairy patch on the spine, abnormal spinal radiographs and MRI)

Friedreich ataxia (gait abnormalities, autosomal recessive)

Idiopathic (may be familial, very uncommon, diagnosis of exclusion)

Lipomyelomeningocele (soft-tissue prominence on the lower spine, may be noted only on MRI)

Muscular dystrophy (previous diagnosis)

Myelomeningocele (previous diagnosis)

Poliomyelitis (previous diagnosis)

Spinal cord tether (possible unilateral foot deformity)

Spinal cord tumor (commonly unilateral deformity)

Trauma (residuum of tendon laceration or fracture)

## Adverse outcomes of the disease

Outcome and progression depend on the disease process.

## Treatment

Underlying spinal cord pathology requires operative treatment. Foot deformities may be accommodated in the early stage of the disorder by shoe modifications and arch supports. In children, cavus feet tend to progress, and progressive deformities require operative treatment to correct the deformity and balance muscle forces to maintain the correction. Arthrodesis should not be used primarily but may be helpful as a salvage procedure.

## ADVERSE OUTCOMES OF TREATMENT

With patients who have progressive loss of sensation and proprioception, skin ulcers are more common if the foot remains in an unbalanced position. Charcot arthropathy of the ankle is more likely to occur after a previous triple arthrodesis.

## REFERRAL DECISIONS/RED FLAGS

Further evaluation is recommended upon diagnosis.

# CHILD ABUSE

| ICD-9 Code |
| --- |
| 995.50 |
| Child abuse, unspecified |

## SYNONYMS

Shaken baby syndrome
Nonaccidental trauma
Munchausen syndrome by proxy

## DEFINITION

Approximately 2.4 million reports of child abuse are filed annually in the United States, and 4,000 children die every year as a result of abuse or neglect. Most cases of abuse involve children younger than age 3 years. Firstborn children, premature infants, stepchildren, and handicapped children are at a greater risk. Failure to recognize injuries of child abuse results in a child being returned to the same environment and a 25% risk of serious reinjury and a 5% risk of death.

The critical issue in identifying child abuse is whether the history given by the family adequately explains the child's injuries. Soft-tissue injuries such as bruising, burns, or scars are seen in most patients. Toddlers typically have normal bruises over the chin, the brow, elbows, knees, and shins, but bruises on the back of the head, buttocks, abdomen, legs, arms, cheeks, or genitalia are suspicious for abuse. Fractures also are common in child abuse cases, and these children are more likely to have an additional abdominal injury as a result of blunt trauma.

## THE INVESTIGATIVE INTERVIEW

The guiding principle for the conduct of the interview is to remain objective while calmly and methodically questioning the family. Seldom is a single physical finding conclusive for a diagnosis of child abuse; additional injuries and risk factors in the home must be identified. Other guidelines of the investigative interview include the following:

- interview individual family members in private;

- be attentive, nonjudgmental, and avoid leading questions during the history;

- carefully document the given history of injury verbatim, as well as its source;

- establish a scenario for the injury from each witness, noting carefully any inconsistencies;

- identify who primarily is responsible for feeding and disciplining the child;

- identify all family members and other individuals who have access to the child;

- identify individuals outside the family who have been with the child without family supervision;

- assess for risk factors: boyfriends, stepparents, baby-sitters, and even larger siblings, as these individuals are often abusers;

- note any delay in seeking medical attention for injuries.

When obtaining the social history, inquire about unusual stresses on the family, such as recent loss of a job, separation or divorce, death in the family, housing problems, or inadequate funds for food. Alcohol abuse in the home is a risk factor for child abuse, and maternal cocaine use increases the risk of abuse fivefold.

If family members later change their account of how the injury occurred or any other aspect of the history, do not alter the original account, but date and record the revision as an addendum to the record.

## TESTS

### PHYSICAL EXAMINATION

Carefully conduct a head-to-toe examination to evaluate the child for any suspicious soft-tissue injuries. A thorough examination is important because in most cases of confirmed abuse, there is evidence of prior abuse. Note, in detail, any suspicious soft-tissue injuries. Palpate the face, spine, and upper and lower extremities for tenderness suggestive of fracture. Examine the abdomen for swelling and tenderness. Inspect for physical signs of sexual assault such as bruising or chafing of the genitalia. Physical findings of sexual abuse can be subtle. A physician specializing in sexual abuse may be required to examine the child.

### DIAGNOSTIC TESTS

If the child's mental status is abnormal, evaluate for subdural hematoma and retinal hemorrhage secondary to violent shaking. Check bleeding studies when there is bruising, and order a toxicology screening if there is a history of substance abuse in the family or if there is abnormal mental status. CT of the abdomen is indicated if the head-to-toe examination shows abdominal tenderness or if the results of liver function tests are elevated.

AP and lateral radiographs of all long bones, the hands, feet, spine, and the chest, as well as a skull series, are standard. Do not order a single radiograph or so-called "baby gram." This study does not provide adequate detail and may miss subtle fractures. While there is no predominant fracture pattern seen in child abuse, certain fractures are more suspicious for child abuse than others. Fractures considered highly specific for child abuse include posterior rib fractures, scapula fractures, fractures of the posterior process of the spine, and fractures of the sternum. One type of fracture unique to child abuse is the "corner" or "chip" fracture of the metaphysis that avulses the edge of the metaphysis from the epiphysis because of downward traction or pull on the extremity (**Figure 1**). Spiral fractures are caused by rotational injury, and transverse or oblique fractures are caused by a direct blow. Rib fractures also

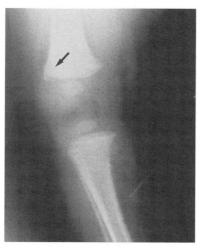

**Figure 1**
AP radiograph of the distal femur with a "corner" or "chip" fracture.

are common and, when healed, may appear only as fusiform thickening of the ribs. A bone scan may be helpful in detecting rib fractures, but it may not show skull fractures or long bone fractures near the epiphyseal growth plates.

Fractures considered to be of moderate specificity for abuse include multiple, especially bilateral, fractures, fractures of different ages, epiphyseal separations, vertebral body fractures, fractures of the fingers, and complex skull fractures. Multiple fractures at various stages of healing without explanation strongly suggest a history of child abuse (**Figure 2**).

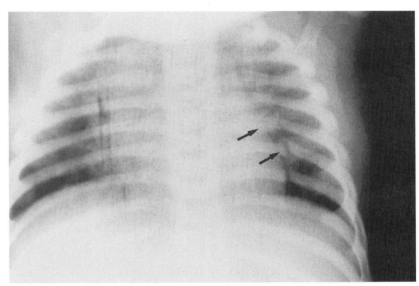

**Figure 2**
Rib fractures at various stages of healing.

The age of fractures can be estimated by their appearance. Seven to 14 days after the injury, new periosteal bone and callus formation can be seen; by 14 to 21 days after the initial injury, there is loss of the definition of the fracture line and maturation of the callus with trabecular formation. More dense callus is seen 21 to 42 days after injury. As the bone remodels to a more normal configuration, fractures older than 6 weeks are distinguished by subtle fusiform sclerotic thickening that is best seen when compared with a normal contralateral bone.

Fractures of low specificity for abuse include clavicle fractures and linear skull fractures. Of note, a vague history of injury or other risk factors for child abuse outweigh fracture specificity in determining child abuse.

It is important to avoid overdiagnosing child abuse. Spiral fractures of the tibia, the so-called "toddler's fracture" can occur in 1- to 3-year-old children as a result of a relatively trivial fall. Spontaneous fractures can occur in diseases such as osteogenesis imperfecta. The presence of osteopenia, a family history of osteogenesis imperfecta, as well as the presence of blue sclera would suggest this disease. Pathologic fractures also are seen in osteomyelitis, tumor, rickets, neuromuscular disease, and other metabolic diseases.

## THE FINAL DIAGNOSIS OF CHILD ABUSE

Once pathologic fractures are excluded, determine whether the child's fracture has been caused by either accidental trauma or inflicted trauma. A diagnosis of accidental trauma can be made when an acute injury is brought promptly to medical attention, has a plausible mechanism of injury, and lacks other risk factors for child abuse. Suspicious injuries must be reported as child abuse.

## REPORTING CHILD ABUSE

In the United States, any physician who reports suspected child abuse in good faith is protected from both civil and criminal liability, but failure to report suspected child abuse exposes the physician to liability. Sexual abuse is a criminal offense and must always be reported. Eliciting help from the hospital's child protection committee is helpful and appropriate. In addition to making notes in the medical record, the physician may be asked to complete a notarized affidavit summarizing findings in the abuse case and stating that the child may be at risk for injury or loss of life if returned to the home environment. The child may then be placed in a foster home until an investigation is completed. The physician must be prepared to defend his or her findings in custodial hearings if the family challenges the actions of child protective services.

# Clubfoot

ICD-9 Code
754.51
Talipes equinovarus

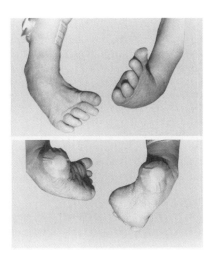

**Figure 1**
Newborn with bilateral congenital clubfoot.

## Synonyms

Congenital clubfoot

Talipes equinovarus

## Definition

Clubfoot, sometimes called talipes equinovarus, is a congenital deformity characterized by four distinct components: plantar flexion (equinus) of the ankle, adduction (varus) of the heel (hindfoot), high arch (cavus) at the midfoot, and adduction of the forefoot (**Figure 1**).

While there are many theories about the causes of clubfoot, none has been proved. Most cases are idiopathic and occur in an otherwise normal infant. Neuromuscular clubfoot is secondary to disorders such as myelomeningocele, arthrogryposis, and congenital constriction band syndrome. Only idiopathic clubfoot is discussed here.

The incidence of clubfoot in boys is twice that in girls. If a family has one child with a clubfoot, the risk in subsequent siblings is 3% to 4%. If one parent and one child in a family have clubfoot, the risk in subsequent children is 25%.

## Clinical symptoms

Infants with clubfoot typically appear as if they could walk on the top or dorsolateral aspect of the foot. In most patients, all four components of a clubfoot are present to some degree, but different aspects of the deformity may be more striking. Plantar flexion (equinus) usually is most severe and is characterized by the foot pointing down, a drawn-up position of the heel, and the inability to pull the calcaneus down when dorsiflexing the foot. The high arch (cavus) may be difficult to see, but with a severe clubfoot, it is indicated by a transverse crease across the sole of the foot. Occasionally, forefoot adduction is relatively severe while the other components appear less severe.

## Tests

### Physical examination

Examination should rule out neuromuscular disorders and determine whether muscle function and sensation are intact. In rare instances, congenital absence of the anterior compartment muscles will occur in association with rigid clubfoot. Absence of muscle function and altered sensation can indicate a spinal cord disorder such as lipomyelomeningocele.

A true idiopathic clubfoot is not fully correctable by passive manipulation. Therefore, a foot that can be placed in a normal position by manipulation is talipes equinovarus caused by intrauterine molding rather than a true club-foot. This problem typically resolves without therapy.

### DIAGNOSTIC TESTS

Radiographs usually are not necessary to confirm the diagnosis or to begin treatment. However, they should be obtained if the diagnosis is unclear or if nonoperative treatment is failing. Standardized stress views provide the most information about the rigidity of deformity and differential diagnosis.

## DIFFERENTIAL DIAGNOSIS

Arthrogryposis (stiffness and weakness of multiple joints of the upper and/or lower extremities)

Congenital constriction band syndrome (partial or circumferential bands of indented skin and underlying tissue, variable distal amputations and deformities including clubfoot)

Distal arthrogryposis (autosomal dominant condition, stiffness of the hands and feet)

## ADVERSE OUTCOMES OF THE DISEASE

When left untreated, children with clubfoot will have a severe disability. Not only are walking and shoe wear severely impaired, but there is the psychological trauma of living with what many perceive as a grotesque deformity.

Even with successful treatment, the affected foot will be smaller and less mobile than a normal foot. The difference is not as obvious with bilateral involvement but is readily apparent with unilateral involvement. The shoe of the affected foot is typically 1 to 1½ sizes smaller than the normal foot. In addition, the calf muscles are smaller in the affected leg and may present a cosmetic problem for which there is no good solution.

## TREATMENT

Manipulation and casting should commence immediately upon diagnosis; with passage of time, the untreated deformity only becomes stiffer and more resistant to nonoperative treatment. Two to 4 months of manipulation and casting are required to correct a clubfoot. The success rate of casting depends on many variables, including the rigidity of the deformity and the experience and skill of the physician. Correction by manipulation usually requires prolonged splinting to minimize the potential for recurrence. Recurrence after casting is most common within the first 2 to 3 years of life, but can happen up to age 5 to 7 years.

Surgery is required when nonoperative treatment fails, usually after 3 to 4 months of treatment. Initial reconstructive procedures range from heel cord lengthening to a complete posterior, medial, and lateral release of the foot. The purpose of surgery is to lengthen or release contracted tendons and ligaments so that the bones can be positioned in normal alignment. Casting is done after surgery to allow healing of the tendon and remodeling of the tarsal bones. Although less common, recurrence also is possible after operative treatment.

Treatment is successful if the foot is in a good weight-bearing position and the child can run and play without pain.

## ADVERSE OUTCOMES OF TREATMENT

Recurrent deformity is more likely to occur if the treatment program did not completely correct the deformity. Overcorrection is possible after surgical release and results in a severe flatfoot with lateral translation of the heel. Flatfoot can also result from casting if the hindfoot varus is not fully corrected before the foot is manipulated into dorsiflexion.

## REFERRAL DECISIONS/RED FLAGS

Immediate diagnosis and specialty evaluation in the first week of life provide the best chance for successful correction by casting and manipulation. Neurologic abnormalities or stiff joints suggest an underlying disorder associated with the clubfoot deformity.

# CONGENITAL DEFORMITIES OF THE LOWER EXTREMITY

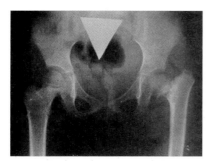

**Figure 1**
Congenital coxa vara in a 5-year-old child.

*Reproduced with permission from Kasser JR (ed): Orthopaedic Knowledge Update 5. Rosemont, IL, American Academy of Orthopaedic Surgeons, 1996, p 353.*

## CONDITIONS

Coxa vara
Congenital dislocation of the knee
Congenital dislocation of the patella
Posteromedial bowing of the tibia
Anterolateral bowing of the tibia
Calcaneovalgus foot
Congenital vertical talus
Congenital short first metatarsal
Congenital curly toe
Polydactyly

## DEFINITION

These conditions are, by definition, present at birth; however, some disorders, such as congenital dislocation of the patella, may not be apparent until the child is older.

## CLINICAL SYMPTOMS

Pain is not present during infancy and early childhood.

## TESTS

### PHYSICAL EXAMINATION

Deviations from normal evoke suspicion. The lower extremities of a newborn have been compressed in the uterus. Therefore, a hip flexion contracture of 40° to 60° and a knee flexion contracture of 20° to 30° are normal in newborns. Likewise, in utero, the ankles and feet are pressed into a dorsiflexed position; therefore, calcaneovalgus posture of the foot is normal.

Disproportionate shortening of the upper and lower extremities or spine suggests a generalized skeletal dysplasia. Other organ systems should be evaluated to rule out other genetic and chromosomal disorders.

### DIAGNOSTIC TESTS

AP and lateral radiographs of the affected extremity are standard.

## COXA VARA

This condition is a relatively uncommon hip disorder characterized by a decrease in the normal neck-shaft angle of the femur (**Figure 1**). The types of coxa vara are congenital, acquired, and developmental. Congenital coxa vara is associated with congenital short femur and proximal femoral focal deficiency. Acquired coxa vara is secondary to metabolic or traumatic conditions.

Developmental coxa vara is an idiopathic condition that develops in early childhood.

The bony deformity alters the mechanics of the hip and causes abductor muscle weakness, a Trendelenburg gait abnormality, and, if unilateral, a limb-length discrepancy. Untreated, the deformity and gait abnormality progress. A realignment osteotomy can improve hip function.

## CONGENITAL DISLOCATION OF THE KNEE

This condition presents as hyperextension of the knee at birth, which ranges from a mild positional deformity that readily responds to short-term splinting to a frank dislocation of the tibia on the femur that is complicated and difficult to treat (**Figure 2**). Associated abnormalities such as hip dislocation or clubfoot are common in patients with true subluxation or dislocation of the knee.

## CONGENITAL DISLOCATION OF THE PATELLA

Congenital dislocation of the patella may not be apparent for several months after birth. Persistent flexion contracture of the knee and external rotation of the leg are suggestive of the diagnosis. The patella may not be palpable in its dislocated lateral position. Ultrasound is helpful in confirming the diagnosis in a younger child whose patella has not started to ossify. Operative treatment is necessary and is more complicated than what is required for adolescents and adults with recurrent dislocation of the patella.

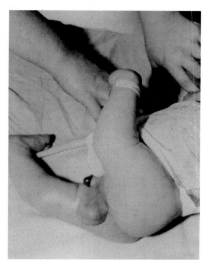

**Figure 2**
Bilateral congenital dislocation of the knees in a newborn. Patient also had associated bilateral dislocated hips and a left clubfoot.

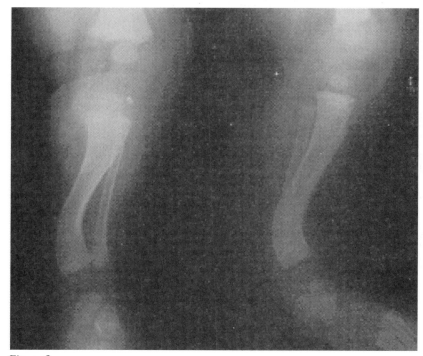

**Figure 3**
Radiograph of infant with congenital posteromedial bow of the tibia.

*Reproduced with permission from Kasser JR (ed): Orthopaedic Knowledge Update 5. Rosemont, IL, American Academy of Orthopaedic Surgeons, 1996, p 441.*

SECTION 9 | PEDIATRIC ORTHOPAEDICS

## POSTEROMEDIAL BOWING OF THE TIBIA

This idiopathic deformity is most obvious and rather striking at birth (**Figure 3**). Posteromedial bowing of the tibia causes the neonate's foot to be in apparent dorsiflexion and valgus, and the deformity initially can be misclassified as a calcaneovalgus foot. The affected limb also is short. The bowing improves with growth, and realignment osteotomy is rarely necessary. A variable degree of limb-length discrepancy persists and typically requires a shoe lift and possibly contralateral epiphysiodesis.

## ANTEROLATERAL BOWING OF THE TIBIA

This condition might or might not be apparent at birth and is often associated with neurofibromatosis (**Figure 4**). Anterolateral bowing of the tibia often progresses to congenital pseudarthrosis of the tibia, a condition that results in an unstable extremity, requires complicated operations and even then has a high failure rate. Infants with anterolateral bowing of the tibia need bracing to prevent, if possible, progression to pseudarthrosis.

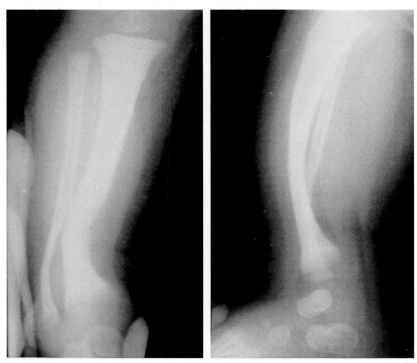

**Figure 4**
AP and lateral radiographs of the tibia showing anterolateral bowing.

## CALCANEOVALGUS FOOT

This condition is common in neonates and is characterized by marked dorsiflexion of the ankle such that the foot may be pressed against the tibia (**Figure 5**). Examination should include an evaluation for deficient activity of the plantar flexors from lipomyelomeningocele or some other neurologic condition. If the child has no neuromuscular disorder, spontaneous correction without sequelae is expected.

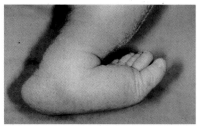

**Figure 5**
Calcaneovalgus foot in a neonate.

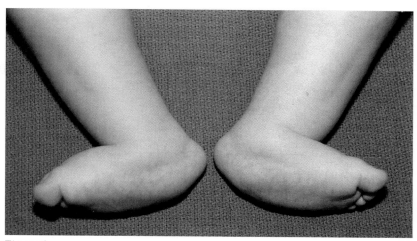

**Figure 6**
Bilateral congenital vertical talus in a 9-month-old infant.

*Reproduced with permission from Kasser JR (ed): Orthopaedic Knowledge Update 5. Rosemont, IL, American Academy of Orthopaedic Surgeons, 1996, p 507.*

## CONGENITAL VERTICAL TALUS

This rigid flatfoot deformity might or might not be recognized at birth (**Figure 6**). The condition may be idiopathic, familial, or associated with a neuromuscular or chromosomal abnormality. Most patients do not respond to serial casting and require operative treatment.

## CONGENITAL SHORT FIRST METATARSAL

Shortening of the great toe is obvious and is often associated with hallux varus. If the great toe is deviated, problems with shoe wear develop. Strapping is ineffective, and operative treatment is required.

## CONGENITAL CURLY TOE

This idiopathic condition is characterized by flexion and medial rotation of the toe. Most children are asymptomatic. Strapping is ineffective. If problems develop with shoe wear, operative treatment of the toe flexors is often successful.

## POLYDACTYLY

The presence of accessory toes often causes trouble with shoe wear (**Figure 7**). Deletion is best performed around 10 months of age, a time when anesthetic problems are less but before the child begins to walk. An earlier consultation often helps the parents understand the treatment and the rationale for timing of surgery.

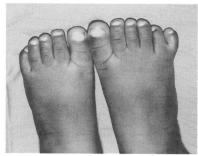

**Figure 7**
Postaxial polydactyly of the right foot.

# CONGENITAL DEFORMITIES OF THE UPPER EXTREMITY

ICD-9 Codes

755.01
    Polydactyly of fingers
755.11
    Syndactyly of fingers without fusion
    of bone
755.50
    Congenital dislocation of the radial
    head
755.53
    Congenital radial-ulnar synostosis

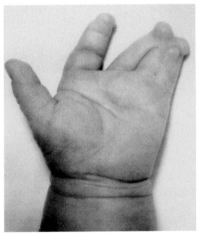

**Figure 1**
Complex syndactyly of the ulnar three-fingers. Note how the long finger is pulled toward the shorter ring and little fingers.

## CONDITIONS

Syndactyly
Polydactyly
Congenital radial-ulnar synostosis
Congenital dislocation of the radial head

## DEFINITION

Congenital deformities are, by definition, present at birth. Syndactyly and polydactyly are obvious; however, congenital dislocation of the radial head and congenital radial-ulnar synostosis usually are not identified until the child is 3 to 10 years of age.

## SYNDACTYLY

Syndactyly is a condition characterized by the lack of normal separation between fingers or toes (**Figure 1**). It can vary from a thin web of skin to a bony fusion (synostosis) between the phalanges. In complete syndactyly, the digits are joined to the tips. In partial syndactyly, there can be increased webbing at the base of the digits or webbing to just short of the tips. Other malformations occur in about 5% of patients.

Because the fingers differ in length, growth may cause progressive deviation of the conjoined fingers. Use of the digits is limited, and cosmesis is an issue for patients. Therefore, children with hand syndactyly should be assessed for operative treatment. In most cases, a skin graft will be needed. The growth differential of syndactyly of the toes is less significant, and function is rarely limited. Therefore, correction of syndactyly of the toes often is not required.

## POLYDACTYLY

Polydactyly is the presence of extra digits in the hand or foot, usually adjacent to the thumb or great toe (preaxial) or lateral to the little finger (postaxial) (**Figure 2**). Extra digits can vary in appearance from a vestigial digit attached by a narrow bridge of skin to a normal-appearing digit with its own metacarpal/metatarsal. Radiographs usually are not needed for diagnostic purposes, only for prognosis and planning operative treatment.

Polydactyly of the hand may not cause functional difficulties, but it is a significant cosmetic deformity. Accessory digits of the foot frequently cause difficulty in shoe wear. Vestigial digits can be ablated by application of a circumferential suture at the base of the skin bridge. Otherwise, removal of extra digits should be delayed until the child is 9 to 10 months of age, a time when

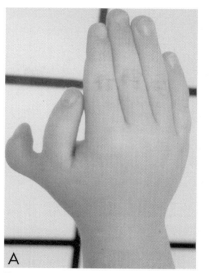
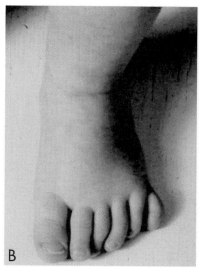

**Figure 2**
A, Polydactyly of the hand expressed as a duplicated thumb. B, Polydactyly of the foot. The widening of the foot presents a problem for shoe fitting.

anesthesia problems are less but before the child will be psychologically affected by the operation. Early consultation often helps the parents understand the treatment. Surgical deletion may be performed earlier if the extra digit interferes with function or if the parents have significant concerns.

## CONGENITAL RADIAL-ULNAR SYNOSTOSIS

In congenital radial-ulnar synostosis, the proximal ends of the radius and ulna fail to separate, resulting in an inability to pronate and supinate the forearm. Children substitute shoulder motion to place the hand in a pronated or supinated position. When the condition is unilateral, there are fewer symptoms because the normal opposite extremity can be used for many activities. This abnormality often is not detected until children are old enough to start using their hands in a purposeful manner.

Limited pronation and supination of the forearm can be readily detected, even during examination of the newborn. Because many young children have lax wrist ligaments, the distal end of the radius and ulna, not the hand, should be grasped and gently pronated and supinated to assess forearm rotation.

After ossification occurs, radiographs demonstrate bony union of the proximal radius and ulna (**Figure 3**).

No treatment is needed if the forearm is in a satisfactory position. Patients with bilateral involvement are more likely to have functional limitations. Surgery to divide the synostosis and restore motion has not been successful in most series. Operative treatment usually is reserved for patients with disability secondary to a forearm positioned in either extreme pronation or supination. Osteotomy to realign the forearm can improve function. This procedure usually is not done until the child is at least age 4 years and may be delayed until the adolescent or adult years if the degree of disability is questionable.

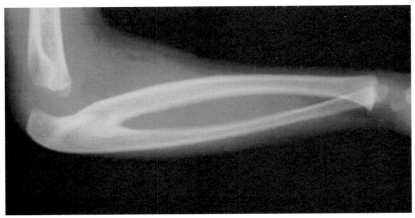

**Figure 3**
Radial-ulnar synostosis. Fusion of the proximal radius and ulna is apparent.

## CONGENITAL DISLOCATION OF THE RADIAL HEAD

Congenital dislocation of the radial head can occur in several directions but most commonly develops posteriorly and typically is bilateral. Elbow deformity and limited motion are the presenting symptoms, but these may not be noticed by the parents for several years. Occasionally, children report pain.

Examination reveals that elbow motion is limited. Rotation is often more limited than flexion and extension. The dislocated radial head often presents as a palpable prominence on the lateral side of the elbow.

Radiographs of the elbow demonstrate the dislocation. The radial head is dome shaped (convex) instead of its normal concave appearance (**Figure 4**).

The deformity and limited elbow motion associated with this condition are often well tolerated. Attempts at open reduction in young children have met with little success. Excision of the radial head after growth is completed can be considered for pain relief but usually does not improve motion.

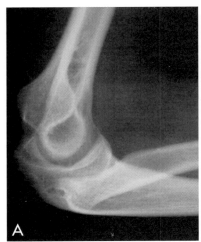
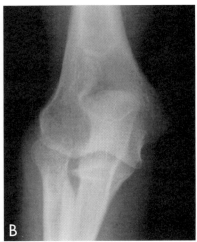

**Figure 4**
Congenital dislocation of the radial head. A, On the lateral view, the radial head is dislocated posteriorly and does not articulate with the humerus. B, On the AP view, the normal concavity of the radial head is lost and replaced by a convexity.

# CONGENITAL DELETIONS OF THE LOWER EXTREMITY

**ICD-9 Codes**
755.34
Proximal femoral focal deficiency
755.36
Tibial hemimelia
755.37
Fibular hemimelia

## CONDITIONS
Fibular hemimelia
Tibial hemimelia
Proximal femoral focal deficiency

## DEFINITION
These disorders are obvious at birth and their appearance can be alarming to parents. Support and counseling by the physician can be critical while the parents are attempting to understand their child's condition. Limb-length discrepancy is the primary functional disability. The discrepancy remains proportional, but the absolute amount increases as the child grows. Many patients will function best with an appropriate amputation. It should be emphasized to the parents that these patients can be quite functional with a prosthesis. Furthermore, many of these patients are otherwise healthy and this also can be emphasized to the parents.

Even though operative treatment usually is not done until the child is 1 year of age or older, early referral to a specialist is helpful. This allows the surgeon time to gain the parents' trust, as the concept of amputation is not easy to accept in a small infant when the absolute discrepancy is small. Providing the parents with an opportunity to meet other affected children at a more advanced stage of growth and development also will be reassuring.

## FIBULAR HEMIMELIA
Fibular hemimelia, sometimes called congenital absence of the fibula, is a sporadic disorder of unknown etiology. It is the most commonly deficient long bone (**Figure 1**). Limb-length discrepancy is universal, ranging from 2 to 16 cm by skeletal maturity.

The deficiency often extends to the lateral border of the foot with associated defects, including absence of the lateral ray(s) of the foot, anomalous bony fusions of the tarsal bones, valgus alignment of the hindfoot, and equinus positioning of the ankle with a ball-and-socket-like ankle joint. Associated milder deformities may occur in the thigh with genu valgum secondary to hypoplasia of the lateral femoral condyle along with mild shortening of the femur.

The goal of treatment is a functional limb. The limb-length discrepancy will increase as the child grows, and the degree of anticipated final discrepancy, in combination with the stability of the hindfoot, will determine the operative treatment. If the anticipated discrepancy is large (8 to 16 cm) and/or the hindfoot is unstable, disarticulation at the ankle and prosthetic fitting is recommended during the first 2 years of life. If the anticipated discrepancy is

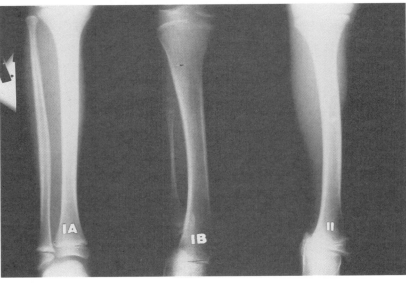

**Figure 1**
Classification of fibular hypoplasia from minimal shortening of the fibula with a ball-and-socket ankle (IA) to complete absence of the fibula (II).

*Reproduced with permission from Kasser JR (ed): Orthopaedic Knowledge Update 5. Rosemont, IL, American Academy of Orthopaedic Surgeons, 1996, pp 437–451.*

small and the hindfoot is stable, other modalities to equalize the leg lengths may be considered.

An adverse outcome of treatment is multiple procedures to maintain a nonfunctional foot and equalize large limb-length discrepancies and then amputating the leg during adolescence. A careful assessment of hindfoot function and anticipated limb-length discrepancy at maturity can help avoid this scenario.

## TIBIAL HEMIMELIA

Tibial hemimelia, also called congenital absence of the tibia, is characterized by partial or complete absence of the tibia (**Figure 2**). This disorder may be sporadic or familial, with most inherited cases secondary to autosomal dominant transmission. Familial cases usually have bilateral involvement and upper extremity deletions. Other disorders that may be associated with tibial hemimelia include congenital heart disease, cleft palate, imperforate anus, hypospadias, hernias, and gonadal malformations.

Involvement of the medial aspect of the foot is common with talipes equinovarus (clubfoot) and absence of medial ray(s). Ironically, tibial hemimelia also can be associated with polydactyly. Shortening of the involved limb is present and, with unilateral involvement, the anticipated discrepancy is typically large (8 to 16 cm). Knee flexion contracture is found when the tibia is totally absent or if the quadriceps is deficient, and the fibula may appear as a bony projection lateral to the lateral femoral condyle.

Treatment is based on function of the quadriceps muscle and the presence or absence of a proximal tibia. If a proximal tibia is present and the quadriceps is functional, disarticulation at the ankle will provide the child with a

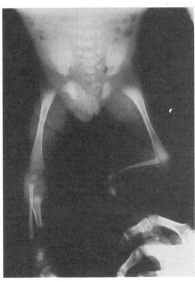

**Figure 2**
Radiograph of an infant with bilateral tibial hemimelia. The patient's right lower limb has incomplete absence of the tibia; on the left, the tibia is completely absent.

good end-bearing stump that can be fit with a below-knee prosthesis. If the proximal tibia or quadriceps muscle is absent, knee disarticulation and fitting with an appropriate prosthesis will provide the best function. In both situations, the limb-length discrepancy can be made up by the length of the prosthesis. Of course the best function occurs when knee function can be salvaged, but even with the knee disarticulation, function is very satisfactory.

## PROXIMAL FEMORAL FOCAL DEFICIENCY

Proximal femoral focal deficiency (PFFD) is an uncommon, sporadic condition of unknown etiology characterized by dysgenesis of the proximal femur with coxa vara and/or pseudarthrosis of the femoral neck. Shortening of the femur is marked, and limb-length discrepancy at maturity ranges from 7 to 25 cm. Associated abnormalities are common and include hip dysplasia, hypoplasia of the lateral femoral condyle, knee instability with absent anterior cruciate ligament, and partial or complete fibular hemimelia. Associated deficiencies in other organ systems are uncommon.

While several classification systems exist, the most simple (and perhaps useful) classification is that by Torode and Gillespie (**Figure 3**). Type A is a congenital short femur, in which the foot lies opposite the midpoint of the contralateral tibia when the limb is gently extended. Overall length discrepancy is less than 20%. In type B, the thigh is very short, with external rotation of the hip and flexion contractures of both the hip and knee, and the foot lies

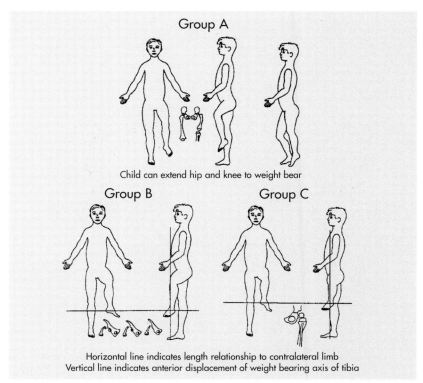

**Figure 3**
Classification of proximal femoral focal deficiency.

*Reproduced with permission from Gillespie R: Classification of congenital abnormalities of the femur, in Herring JA, Birch JG (eds): The Child with a Limb Deficiency. American Academy of Orthopaedic Surgeons, Rosemont, IL, 1998, p 69.*

approximately at the level of the contralateral knee. The overall length discrepancy is about 40%. Type C is characterized by an extremely short femur with pistoning and instability of the hip joint. The foot lies well proximal to the opposite knee.

Patients with type A deformity can be treated with a limb equalization procedure (limb lengthening, contralateral epiphysiodesis, or both). Types B and C usually require some form of amputation and prosthetic fitting because of the expected severe limb-length discrepancy at maturity. Depending on the severity of the hip abnormality, some form of reconstruction also may be necessary. However, in almost all cases, the child will be able to walk, even if the femoral head and acetabulum are completely absent.

# CONGENITAL DELETIONS OF THE UPPER EXTREMITY

ICD-9 Codes

755.21
Transverse deficiency of the forearm
755.26
Radial hemimelia
755.27
Ulnar hemimelia
755.29
Hypoplasia of the thumb

## CONDITIONS

Hypoplasia/Absence of the thumb
Radial hemimelia
Ulnar hemimelia
Transverse deficiency of the forearm

## DEFINITION

These disorders can affect one side of the extremity (eg, hemimelia) or can be a transverse complete deletion. A thorough evaluation is appropriate because some patients will have abnormalities in other organ systems. Deficiency of the thumb, radial hemimelia, ulnar hemimelia, and transverse deficiency of the forearm are most common and are discussed below.

As a general principle, reconstructive surgery usually is not performed before the infant is 6 to 18 months of age; however, early specialty evaluation is helpful to allay anxiety of the parents and grandparents. Furthermore, early consultation allows time for parents to gain an understanding and realistic expectations of the expected function and appearance after operative treatment. Finally, some of these disorders will not benefit from operative treatment, but early discussion concerning principles of prosthetic management will be helpful.

## HYPOPLASIA/ABSENCE OF THE THUMB

The extent of the deficiency is variable. A hypoplastic thumb may be small, unstable, or thin due to deficient development of the thenar musculature. Other disorders are common, including congenital heart disease (Holt-Oram syndrome), craniofacial abnormalities, and vertebral anomalies (VATER association). Fanconi anemia also can develop in later childhood.

If untreated, patients adapt by using the pinch function between the index and long fingers to substitute for the deficient thumb. Patients with unilateral involvement (eg, a normal opposite upper extremity) generally have excellent overall function with minimal impairment.

Operative management is based on the magnitude of the deficiency. Reconstruction is indicated when the hypoplastic thumb is of adequate size and the carpometacarpal joint is stable. Index pollicization (transfer of the index finger to the thumb position, leaving the hand with three fingers) is recommended for more severe deformities.

## RADIAL HEMIMELIA

Radial hemimelia, sometimes called radial club hand, is characterized by radial deviation of the hand, variable presence and stiffness of the thumb, index, and long fingers, variable shortening and bowing of the forearm segment, and variable range of motion at the elbow. Associated disorders include congenital heart disease (Holt-Oram syndrome), craniofacial abnormalities, and vertebral anomalies (VATER association). TAR syndrome (thrombocytopenia with absent radius) also is possible. The unique aspect of TAR syndrome is the presence of an essentially normal thumb. In other syndromes, if the radius is deficient, then the thumb also is hypoplastic or absent.

Operative management is designed to improve the alignment and appearance of the hand relative to the forearm. A centralization procedure ideally is performed between 6 and 18 months of age. Untreated patients can still function surprisingly well. Therefore, operative treatment is contraindicated in patients with short forearms and/or limited elbow motion. These patients do better if the hand remains closer to the midline (eg, radially deviated).

## ULNAR HEMIMELIA

Ulnar deficiencies include a variety of disorders involving either a partial or complete absence of skeletal and soft-tissue elements on the ulnar (postaxial) border of the forearm and hand. Conditions range from hypoplasia of the ulna, in which the ulna is completely present but short, to total aplasia of the ulna, which may be associated with congenital fusion of the radius to the humerus (radiohumeral synostosis). Digital deficiencies are common and variable.

Compared with radial and thumb deletions, ulnar hemimelia is not associated with anomalies of other organ systems. However, patients with ulnar hemimelia are more likely to have disorders elsewhere in the skeletal system, including tibial hemimelia and proximal femoral focal deficiency.

Operative treatment is not commonly indicated for ulnar hemimelia, except for associated digital deformities. Syndactyly release, web space reconstruction, and other procedures, when indicated, can improve hand function.

## TRANSVERSE DEFICIENCY OF THE FOREARM

Transverse deficiency of the forearm, sometimes called congenital below-elbow amputation, is characterized by complete absence of the hand and wrist and a hypoplastic or partially absent forearm. Elbow function is good, even if the radial head is dislocated. This disorder is sporadic, typically unilateral, and generally is not associated with abnormalities in other organ systems, although patients may have congenital constriction band syndrome and other musculoskeletal anomalies.

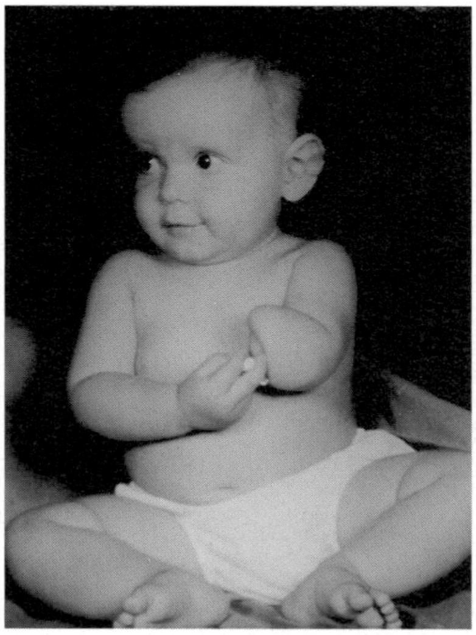

Children with unilateral transverse deficiency of the forearm have minimal functional limitations. Bimanual activities are often performed using the medial aspect of the affected forearm to assist the opposite, uninvolved extremity (**Figure 1**). The principal deficit is cosmetic, which is particularly troublesome during the teenage years.

Operative treatment is rarely necessary. Primitive digital remnants, if present, occasionally are removed for cosmetic reasons.

Prosthetic management is of great interest to families of infants with this condition. The best time to introduce the prosthesis is controversial, though

**Figure 1**
Infant with unilateral transverse deficiency of the forearm already using affected limb to assist the uninvolved extremity.

many centers favor an aggressive "fit when they sit" protocol. This approach is based on the developmental principle that normal bimanual activities begin when an infant is able to sit independently, at about age 6 to 8 months. Others recognize that a prosthesis often impedes an infant's ability to crawl and favor the first fitting after an infant is able to stand and walk independently.

Prosthetic options include the standard body-powered design, consisting of a shoulder harness and a hook terminal device; a myoelectric design, consisting of a mechanical hand that is opened and closed by voluntary forearm muscle activity; and a passive design, consisting of a lightweight, durable, cosmetically appealing, nonmovable hand. The optimal design is based on a number of factors and is best determined on an individual basis.

The principal benefit of prosthetic management is cosmetic, which may be more significant to the parents than the child prior to the teenage years. Function is not consistently improved by any of the prosthetic designs, leading to a high rate of prosthetic rejection.

# DEVELOPMENTAL DYSPLASIA OF THE HIP

ICD-9 Codes

754.30
Congenital dislocation of the hip, unilateral

754.31
Congenital dislocation of the hip, bilateral

## SYNONYMS

Congenital dysplasia of the hip
Congenital dislocation of the hip
Congenital subluxation of the hip

## DEFINITION

Developmental dysplasia of the hip (DDH) encompasses all dysplastic hip disorders, ranging from an in utero rigid dislocation to a typical perinatal hip dislocation to a hip dysplasia that develops during childhood from either extreme ligamentous laxity or from neuromuscular disorders such as cerebral palsy or myelomeningocele. The various nomenclatures previously used (eg, congenital dislocation of the hip, congenital dysplasia of the hip, congenital disease of the hip) were imprecise and confusing because some patients had a hip problem that was neither congenital nor dislocated.

Typical DDH is associated with ligamentous laxity and usually is detectable at birth. Common characteristics include prevalence in the left hip (3:1 ratio), female gender (5:1 ratio), and breech presentation (20% for frank breech presentation). DDH is rarely seen in blacks but is more common in whites of northern European ancestry, American Indians, and families with a history of DDH. Development of torticollis also is associated with DDH.

## CLINICAL SYMPTOMS

Neonates are asymptomatic. Parents often notice a limp, a waddling gait pattern, or a limb-length discrepancy when the infant begins to walk.

## TESTS

### PHYSICAL EXAMINATION

The physical examination is key to the early diagnosis. The examination should be done on a firm surface with the infant relaxed. Hip instability may not be detected if the infant is crying or upset.

Two maneuvers are helpful in detecting hip instability during the neonatal examination (**Figure 1**). The Barlow test should be performed first and is a "sign of exit" as the femoral head dislocates from the socket. To perform this test, flex the infant's hips and knees to 90°, then place your thumb along the medial thigh and the long finger along the lateral axis of the femur. Apply gentle pressure to the knee in a posterior direction while adducting the femur. A positive Barlow test is a "clunk," as the femoral head dislocates from the socket and slides over the posterior lip of the acetabulum.

The Ortolani maneuver is a "sign of relocation" as the femoral head is manipulated back into the acetabulum. To perform this maneuver, flex the

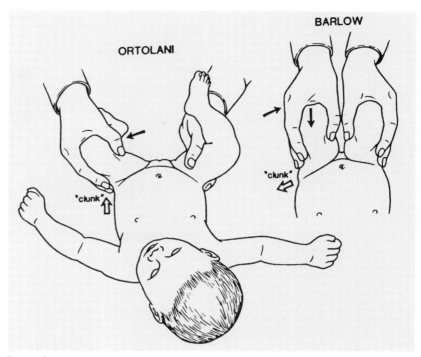

**Figure 1**
Ortolani and Barlow maneuvers.

hips and knees to 90° and position your hands similar to the Barlow maneuver. Abduct the hip while applying gentle pressure from your long finger over the greater trochanter and then pushing the femoral head anteriorly. A positive Ortolani sign is a "clunk" as the femoral head slides over the posterior lip of the acetabulum and into the socket.

In a neonate who has a dislocated hip, the adductors become contracted. As a result, in patients 1 to 3 months of age or older, the hip cannot be relocated by the Ortolani maneuver. The key to diagnosing DDH at this age is recognizing limited hip abduction. In infants, this is most easily detected by flexing the hips and knees to 90° and maximally abducting both hips. Asymmetric abduction suggests unilateral DDH. A unilateral dislocation also is indicated by shortening of the thigh, or a positive Galeazzi sign (unequal knee heights with the hips and knees flexed to 90°). Bilateral DDH is not as obvious. Thigh lengths are equal, and abduction is symmetric. Bilateral DDH is suggested by hip abduction limited to less than 45° to 55°.

## DIAGNOSTIC TESTS

Because a neonate's femoral head is cartilaginous, radiographs of the hip can be difficult to interpret at this time. Radiographs are more accurate in detecting DDH in infants who are 4 to 8 months old. In most neonates, the physical examination is sufficient to make the diagnosis and initiate treatment.

Ultrasound can provide information concerning whether the hip joint is unstable or dislocated and is particularly useful before the femoral head has ossified (**Figure 2**). There is a debate about whether ultrasound screening of newborns should be selective or universal. Currently, most physicians are

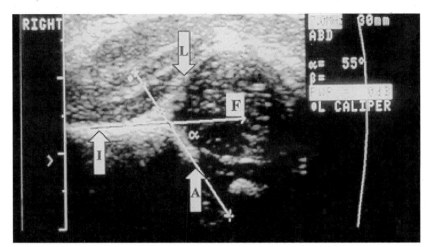

**Figure 2**
Ultrasound of neonatal hip and measurements used to determine unstable hip.

selectively screening infants and recommend an ultrasound only if the infant is at increased risk for DDH or has an equivocal examination.

## DIFFERENTIAL DIAGNOSIS

Cerebral palsy (mild spastic diplegia with tightness of adductors)

Congenital coxa vara (decreased abduction associated with decreased femoral neck-shaft angle)

Congenital short femur (limb-length discrepancy)

Fracture of the femur (limited motion associated with pain and swelling)

## ADVERSE OUTCOMES OF THE DISEASE

The longer the hip is dislocated, the less likely that closed reduction will be successful. If left untreated, DDH can lead to premature degenerative joint disease (osteoarthritis), causing pain and limited function.

## TREATMENT

Treatment depends on the magnitude of the problem and the age of the patient. The goal of treatment is to concentrically reduce the femoral head into the socket and maintain the reduction while the acetabulum develops and the hip stabilizes. If DDH is detected within the first 3 months, most hips will reduce and stabilize with a dynamic positioning device, such as a Pavlik harness. The harness holds the hips in flexion and abduction, allowing the femoral head to reduce concentrically into the acetabulum. Consistent, full-time wearing of the splint is necessary for the child with an unstable joint to develop a stable hip joint.

The Pavlik harness is less successful if the DDH is detected in an infant between 3 and 9 months of age. At this age, an orthosis may be tried for 2 to 3 weeks to see if the femoral head will reduce into the acetabulum. If it does not, the harness should be abandoned because the brace will aggravate the deformity if the femoral head remains dislocated. For older infants, an examination under anesthesia, arthrogram, and either closed or open reduction with application of a spica cast are necessary.

## ADVERSE OUTCOMES OF TREATMENT

Failure of reduction of the femoral head into the socket, persistent hip instability, and osteonecrosis of the femoral head are serious complications associated with treatment. Osteonecrosis can interfere with the growth of the proximal femur and the acetabulum, resulting in a deformity.

## REFERRAL DECISIONS/RED FLAGS

An infant who has suspected instability or dislocation requires specialty evaluation.

# DISKITIS

ICD-9 Codes
722.92
    Thoracic diskitis
722.93
    Lumbar diskitis

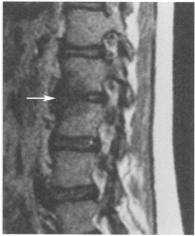

**Figure 1**
T1-weighted MR image showing the characteristic signal changes of diskitis at L2-3.

## DEFINITION

Diskitis is an infection that occurs in or around the intervertebral disk and, in children, is most often a bacterial infection of hematogenous origin. MRI consistently shows inflammation at the anterior corner of one or both adjacent vertebrae (**Figure 1**). These findings, together with the results of microvascular studies, support the concept that diskitis begins as a foci of osteomyelitis in the anterior metaphyseal corner of one vertebra and subsequently spreads to the adjacent disk. Diskitis can occur anywhere in the spine, but it most commonly affects the low thoracic and lumbar regions. Children between ages 2 and 7 years are most commonly affected, and in this age group, diskitis often can be treated with oral antibiotics. Diskitis can develop in young adolescents as well, and in this age group the causative organisms and treatment requirements are similar to those of adults.

## CLINICAL SYMPTOMS

Onset of symptoms is insidious, and delay in diagnosis is usual. Children who are able to communicate may be able to localize the pain to the back, but they also may perceive their pain as abdominal or thigh discomfort. Toddlers are frequently first seen when they refuse to walk. Therefore, the differential diagnosis must include not only spinal disorders, but abdominal, pelvic, and lower extremity processes as well.

## TESTS

### PHYSICAL EXAMINATION

Children rarely appear systemically ill. Fever, if present, may be low grade. Toddlers may refuse to walk or even sit unsupported. Those who will walk often lean forward and place their hands on their thighs for support (psoas sign). Percussion of the spinous processes may help localize the pain. Passive spinal motion is resisted. If both lower extremities are elevated simultaneously, the back and hips are held rigid. The single straight-leg raising test also may be positive.

### DIAGNOSTIC TESTS

White blood cell count is often within normal limits, but the erythrocyte sedimentation rate and C-reactive protein usually are elevated. Blood cultures may be positive.

AP and lateral radiographs of the spine should be obtained as part of the initial assessment. However, irregularity of the vertebral end plates and narrowing of the disk usually are not apparent until 2 or 3 weeks after onset of symptoms.

MRI will confirm the diagnosis and clearly define the extent of the process. A bone scan is usually, but not always, positive early in the disease and may be of value when localization is unclear.

Because of the low yield and necessity for general anesthesia, aspiration of the disk usually is not recommended in young children who have a typical clinical picture.

A tuberculin skin test should be performed, unless done recently.

## DIFFERENTIAL DIAGNOSIS

Epidural abscess (rare, neurologic symptoms)

Herniated disk (teenagers, radicular symptoms)

Pyelonephritis (flank pain, pyuria)

Retrocecal appendicitis (systemic symptoms, pain with hip extension)

Retroperitoneal mass (may require MRI to differentiate)

Septic arthritis of the hip (marked pain on movement of the hip)

Spinal tuberculosis (spares the disk, involves bone, usually thoracolumbar area)

Spine tumor (neurologic abnormalities, may require MRI to differentiate)

## ADVERSE OUTCOMES OF THE DISEASE

Even though persistent disk space narrowing is common and may progress to spontaneous fusion of the adjacent vertebrae, residual problems are rare unless chronic osteomyelitis occurs.

## TREATMENT

Because *Staphylococcus aureus* is the most common organism identified, a penicillinase-resistant antibiotic or cephalosporin usually is used. A common regimen consists of 2 to 4 days of intravenous administration, followed by 4 to 6 weeks of oral antibiotics.

Initial bed rest should be followed by a gradual return to activities, as symptoms permit. With the routine use of antibiotics, immobilization in a body cast or brace is required less frequently but can be quite successful in reducing severe or recalcitrant pain. Physical therapy programs are not recommended.

Surgical debridement is almost never necessary.

## ADVERSE OUTCOMES OF TREATMENT

Antibiotic allergies or secondary gastrointestinal problems can develop.

## REFERRAL DECISIONS/RED FLAGS

Persistent fever, vertebral osteomyelitis and/or collapse, diagnostic dilemma, presence of a psoas abscess, and any neurologic deficit or suspicion of epidural abscess indicate the need for further evaluation.

# EVALUATION OF THE LIMPING CHILD

ICD-9 Code
719.7
   Difficulty in walking

## DEFINITION

Many conditions cause a child to limp. Establishing the correct diagnosis can be challenging because the possibilities are extensive and include various diseases and injuries, as well as various anatomic sites, ranging from the spine to the foot (**Table 1**). In addition, the history is often vague, the complaints nonfocal, and the examination unremarkable despite diagnostic possibilities that carry significant implications.

## CLINICAL SYMPTOMS

### IS THE PROBLEM ACUTE OR CHRONIC?

A recent onset of limping makes infectious or traumatic conditions more likely, although trauma is not as common as might be expected. Young children often fall, and parents tend to attribute one of these episodes as the cause of the limp. Therefore, the history should begin by asking the parents how long they have noticed the limp rather than what caused the child to limp. Unless an infection or other serious process is suspected, problems of short duration may be observed, but chronic problems need further evaluation with laboratory and radiographic studies.

### WHAT TIME OF THE DAY IS THE LIMP WORST?

Most musculoskeletal conditions are exacerbated by activity and relieved by rest. Therefore, parents often report that the pain or limp is worst in the afternoon. However, with transient synovitis of the hip or juvenile rheumatoid arthritis, the limp is more pronounced in the morning. Pain at night suggests leukemia or other neoplasms.

### ARE THERE SYSTEMIC SYMPTOMS?

Questions about malaise, swelling, fever, and loss of endurance are important, even with an acute onset. With chronic symptoms, the review of systems should be more extensive.

## TESTS

### PHYSICAL EXAMINATION

Ask older children to place one finger on "the one spot that hurts the most" to localize the anatomic site and narrow the differential diagnosis. Palpate the spine and lower extremities of younger children to identify areas of tenderness. Inspect the spine and lower extremities for swelling or skin changes. Muscle weakness or atrophy is a sentinel sign of a significant process. In a young child, these findings are best determined by measuring and comparing limb girths at symmetric locations. For example, asymmetry in thigh girth of

## Table 1
### Causes of Limping in Children

| | With trauma | With fever or systemic illness | Without trauma, fever, or systemic illness |
|---|---|---|---|
| Bones | Fracture<br>Child abuse fracture<br>Stress fracture<br>Periostitis | Osteomyelitis<br>Hemoglobinopathy<br>Hand-foot syndrome<br>Sickle cell crises<br>Gaucher crises<br>Neuroblastoma<br>Leukemia<br>Ewing sarcoma | Benign bone tumor<br>    Aneurysmal bone cyst<br>    Unicameral bone cyst<br>    Osteoid osteoma<br>Fibrous dysplasia<br>Langerhans cell histiocytosis<br>Ewing sarcoma<br>Limb-length discrepancy<br>Malignant bone tumor<br>Osteogenic sarcoma<br>Unicameral bone cyst |
| Joints | Sprain<br>Dislocation<br>Hemarthrosis | Septic arthritis<br>Lyme arthritis<br>Systemic juvenile<br>  rheumatoid arthritis<br>Systemic lupus erythematosus<br>Other collagen vascular<br>  disease<br>Reactive arthritis/arthralgia<br>Acute rheumatic fever<br>Sarcoidosis<br>Sickle cell disease<br>Leukemia | Juvenile rheumatoid arthritis<br>    Pauciarticular<br>    Polyarticular<br>Hemophilic arthropathy<br>Pigmented villonodular synovitis |
| Soft tissue | Bursitis<br>Contusion<br>Enthesitis<br>Muscle strain<br>Nerve injury | Abscess<br>Cellulitis<br>Dermatomyositis/poly-<br>  myositis<br>Spider/insect bite<br>Trichinosis<br>Viral myositis | Charcot-Marie-Tooth disease<br>Diastematomyelia<br>Muscular dystrophy<br>Overuse syndrome<br>Rhabdomyosarcoma<br>Spinal cord tumor |
| Spine and pelvis | Avulsion fracture vertebra<br>Disk herniation | Diskitis<br>Osteomyelitis–pelvis<br>Sacroiliac septic arthritis<br>Ankylosing spondylitis | Spondylolysis/spondylolisthesis<br>Disk herniation |
| Hip | Avulsion fracture<br>Anterior superior iliac<br>  spine–sartorius<br>Anterior inferior iliac<br>  spine–rectus femoris<br>Slipped capital femoral<br>  epiphysis, acute | Septic arthritis–hip<br>Osteomyelitis–proximal femur | Developmental dysplasia of the hip<br>Transient synovitis<br>Legg-Calvé-Perthes disease<br>Slipped capital femoral epiphysis,<br>  chronic |

## Table 1 continued
### Causes of Limping in Children

| | With trauma | With fever or systemic illness | Without trauma, fever, or systemic illness |
|---|---|---|---|
| Knee | Avulsion fracture–patella<br>Toddler's fracture of the tibia<br>Referred hip pain | Septic arthritis–knee<br>Osteomyelitis adjacent bone | Popliteal cyst<br>Discoid meniscus<br>Meniscal tear<br>Osgood-Schlatter disease<br>Sinding-Larsen-Johansson disease<br>Osteochondritis dissecans<br>Patella instability |
| Foot and ankle | Toddler's fracture of the tibia<br>Stress fracture–foot<br>Puncture wound–foot | Septic arthritis–ankle<br>Puncture wound<br>Osteomyelitis<br>Foreign body | Accessory navicular<br>Freiberg infraction<br>Köhler disease<br>Sever apophysitis<br>Tarsal coalition |

1 cm or more measured 6 to 8 cm above the patella indicates a significant knee problem that requires additional laboratory and radiographic studies.

## DIAGNOSTIC TESTS

A temperature of 99.5°F (37.5°C) or higher suggests an inflammatory or neoplastic process and the need for additional studies, such as a CBC, erythrocyte sedimentation rate, and appropriate radiographs. AP and lateral radiographs are indicated when a fracture or a chronic process is suspected. Different diagnostic possibilities dictate special views. For example, a tunnel view is indicated to rule out osteochondritis dissecans in an older child who has been limping and had knee pain for several weeks after sports activity. A bone scan often localizes the site of disease in patients with a limp that cannot be diagnosed by routine studies. However, this test is not always positive, even with a chronic process. For example, leukemia may cause increased, decreased, or even normal uptake on bone scans. CT is generally best for benign bony lesions. MRI provides better information on soft-tissue lesions and sarcomas; however, before proceeding to these tests, consult with an appropriate specialist to avoid ordering expensive studies that provide limited information.

# FLATFOOT

## SYNONYMS

Flexible flatfoot
Valgus foot
Pronated foot
Peroneal spastic flatfoot
Pes planus

## DEFINITION

Flatfoot is defined as an abnormally low or absent longitudinal arch. Flexible flatfoot is more common and is considered a normal foot shape in infants and in up to 20% of adults. Rigid flatfoot is an uncommon condition that is discussed in greater detail in the chapter on tarsal coalition.

Flexible flatfoot in children is always bilateral. These patients have a visible arch when they are not standing and have normal mobility of the subtalar joint (inversion and eversion of the hindfoot). Rigid flatfoot may be unilateral or bilateral. These patients have persistent flattening of the longitudinal arch in non–weight-bearing positions and have restricted subtalar motion.

Patients with neuromuscular conditions and underlying hypotonia and patients with pathologic ligamentous laxity (Marfan syndrome, Ehlers-Danlos syndrome, Down syndrome) may have a flatfoot that initially is flexible but with time may progress to a rigid deformity.

## CLINICAL SYMPTOMS

Flexible flatfoot usually is asymptomatic. Occasionally, however, children with flexible flatfeet report activity-related generalized pain and fatigue in the feet, ankles, and legs, as well as aching pain at night. Adolescents with flexible flatfeet often have an associated contracture of the Achilles tendon and may report focal pain and have redness and callosities under the bony prominence beneath the sagging arches.

## TESTS

### PHYSICAL EXAMINATION

The heel is in valgus alignment, which gives the medial malleolus a prominent appearance, and the foot is rotated outward in relation to the leg (**Figure 1**). With severe pes planovalgus, the medial border of the foot is convex, and the lateral border is concave. In addition to noting the longitudinal arch when the child is sitting, the examiner can recreate the arch by passive extension of the toe (jack toe test and by having the patient stand on tiptoes, **Figure 2**). The arch cannot be recreated by any means in a rigid flatfoot.

Contracture of the Achilles tendon with limited ankle dorsiflexion often can accompany a flexible flatfoot in adolescents.

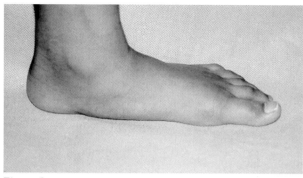

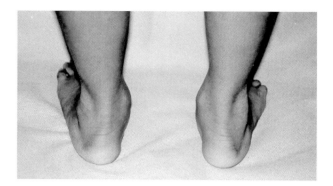

**Figure 1**
Flatfoot, medial and posterior views.

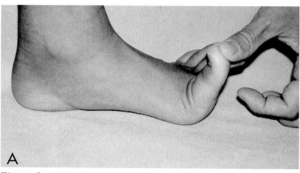

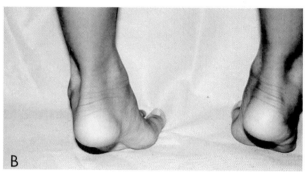

A                                    B

**Figure 2**
Elevation of the arches in flexible flatfeet by (A) jack toe extension test and (B) standing on toes.

### DIAGNOSTIC TESTS

Radiographs are not indicated in children who have symptomatic flexible flatfeet. However, weight-bearing AP, lateral, and oblique radiographs are indicated in the evaluation of a rigid deformity.

### DIFFERENTIAL DIAGNOSIS

The primary decision is whether the child has a flexible or rigid flatfoot.

### ADVERSE OUTCOMES OF THE DISEASE

Flexible flatfoot is a normal variation of the shape of the foot that rarely causes disability or requires treatment. However, leg aches and uneven shoe wear may occur. Pain, disability, and the need for treatment are more common in children who have a contracted Achilles tendon in association with flexible flatfoot.

### TREATMENT

Young children typically are asymptomatic, but the parents are concerned about the appearance of the feet. Parents should be advised that flattening of the longitudinal arch will improve most often and that corrective shoes and orthotics have not been proved effective in the development of arches. Furthermore, it is helpful to remind parents that adults with high arches (cavus feet) are more likely to have pain, whereas most adults with flatfeet are asymptomatic.

Older children and adolescents with medial arch pain related to a contracted Achilles tendon can benefit from daily heel cord stretching exercises. Orthotics, particularly the hard, molded type, will generally increase foot pain, but over-the-counter, inexpensive orthoses worn in regular running shoes can often decrease leg aching and change the pattern of wear to extend the useful life of shoes.

Surgery is rarely indicated for flexible flatfoot. The exception is the older child whose symptoms persist despite a vigorous program of Achilles tendon stretching and shoe modifications. Osteotomy to lengthen the lateral column of the foot, as opposed to arthrodesis, is a recently accepted principle for managing this condition.

## ADVERSE OUTCOMES OF TREATMENT

Surgical procedures to treat flatfeet in young children have been reported but have been mostly abandoned because they are rarely necessary and, furthermore, often do not achieve or maintain correction of the deformity.

## REFERRAL DECISIONS/RED FLAGS

An older child or adolescent with a contracted Achilles tendon and persistent pain with callosities under the sagging arch requires further evaluation. Children with a flexible flatfoot who have persistent pain at any other site in the foot, especially if associated with redness, swelling, or warmth, also require further evaluation.

# FRACTURES IN CHILDREN

Fractures are more common in children than in adults, due in part to their boisterous play and in part to the different characteristics of their bone. The strength of bone gradually increases as a child grows, but it is not until late adolescence that a child's bone is as strong as that of most adults. As a result, bone is the weak link in children, and ligamentous injuries are uncommon until late adolescence.

Fractures are uncommon in children younger than 3 years of age. Infants and young children usually are protected by their restrained activity, even though their bones are weaker. However, intentional abuse as a cause of fracture is significantly higher in young children, as described in the chapter on child abuse. After age 3 years, the incidence of fractures gradually increases until it peaks during adolescence. The incidence is also higher in boys and during the summer months.

Plasticity of bone, or the modulus of elasticity, is greater in children. Therefore, a child's bone can bend or deform without completely breaking. As a result, torus and greenstick fractures are common fracture patterns in children, but these injuries are rarely seen in adults.

Bone healing also is more rapid in children. For example, a fracture of the femur in an adult requires 16 to 20 weeks of immobilization if treated by closed means. By comparison, the same fracture requires only 2 weeks of immobilization in an infant and 4 to 6 weeks of casting in young children. Because of more rapid healing, nonunion is very uncommon in children.

Fractures involving the growth plate or physis are unique to children, accounting for 15% to 20% of all pediatric fractures. These injuries are described in a separate chapter.

Bone remodeling is greater in children, and some deformities will spontaneously correct. The potential for remodeling is greater in younger children, in fractures close to the physis, and in fractures angulated in the plane of motion. For example, a fracture of the distal radius with 35° of volar or dorsal angulation in a 5-year-old child will completely remodel in 1 to 2 years, even if no reduction is performed. In this instance, the primary reason for reduction is to relieve the pressure on adjacent soft tissues. Angular correction in other planes is less predictable, and rotational deformities typically do not correct.

Pediatric fractures present special problems in diagnosis and management. A fracture might not be visible on routine radiographs when it involves only the physis and when the secondary ossification center has not ossified. Young children are also less tolerant of major blood loss, and a child with a displaced femur fracture or multiple trauma needs to be monitored carefully.

The most common management of displaced fractures in children is closed reduction and casting, whereas displaced fractures in adults often require internal or external fixation devices. The thick periosteum in children helps in maintaining the reduction. Pediatric fractures also heal more rapidly, which reduces the duration of and complications associated with immobilization. Furthermore, unlike adults, complications of prolonged bed rest such as pneumonia and thrombophlebitis are very uncommon in children. Thus, body casts can be used to treat complex pediatric fractures involving the spine, pelvis, and lower extremities.

# FRACTURE OF THE GROWTH PLATE

## DEFINITION

Any fracture that involves the epiphyseal growth plate (the physis) is called a physeal fracture. The five-part Salter-Harris classification has been the system most commonly used to describe these injuries. However, there is concern that a Salter-Harris type V fracture does not occur and that this system does not describe all fracture patterns. Recently, a new classification system, the Peterson classification, was proposed that delineates six types and has sound anatomic, epidemiologic, and outcome associations (**Figure 1**). Fracture types progress from lesser to greater seriousness of injury, frequency of occurrence, and level of surgical intervention required.

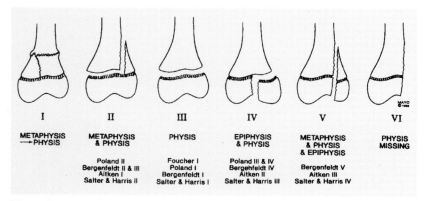

**Figure 1**
Peterson classification of physeal injuries.

*Reproduced with permission from Peterson HA: Physeal Fractures: Part 3. Classification. J Pediatric Orthop 1994:14:439-448.*

## CLINICAL SYMPTOMS

Patients have acute pain, localized tenderness and swelling, and may have deformity and restricted motion of the involved site. There is always a history of trauma.

## TESTS

### PHYSICAL EXAMINATION

Tenderness and swelling are localized and always present with maximum tenderness over the growth plate. Vascular and neurologic compromise are rare, as the fracture does not involve muscle compartments.

### DIAGNOSTIC TESTS

AP and lateral radiographs usually identify the fracture. If not, oblique views will nearly always identify the fracture. Nondisplaced type III fractures only show soft-tissue swelling.

## DIFFERENTIAL DIAGNOSIS

Contusion (swelling and ecchymosis near a joint, negative radiographs)

Dislocation (evident on radiographs)

Fracture of the metaphysis of a long bone (radiographs show no involvement of the physis)

Sprain (swelling, maximum tenderness over the ligament, and negative radiographs)

Osteochondral fracture (involves articular surface but not the physis)

## ADVERSE OUTCOMES OF THE DISEASE

Premature arrest (partial or complete) of growth will result in diminished bone length and angulation deformity. Nonunion and overgrowth are rare.

## TREATMENT

The goal is reduction, maintaining the reduction during the healing process, and avoiding growth arrest. These fractures heal rapidly, usually within 4 to 6 weeks.

Closed reduction and cast immobilization are indicated in fracture types I, II, and III. Some fractures will be minimally displaced and need only immobilization. In adolescents (over age 14 years in boys and 12 years in girls), mild displacement is acceptable because in the event that premature arrest occurs, these patients have little growth remaining in which significant limb-length discrepancy or deformity can develop. Conversely, in these same patients, less angular deformity can be accepted because there is less time for the fracture to remodel before the patient reaches skeletal maturity.

Fracture types IV and V involve the cartilage of both the growth plate and the articular surface. Therefore, anatomic reduction is required to ensure a congruous joint surface and to prevent development of a bone bridge (usually called a physeal bar) between the epiphysis and metaphysis. In most instances, open reduction and internal fixation are necessary to obtain and maintain reduction.

Fracture type VI is by definition always an open fracture; therefore, immediate surgical attention is necessary. Physeal bars always develop after this injury and, if the patient has significant growth remaining, reconstructive surgery will be required.

## ADVERSE OUTCOMES OF TREATMENT

Failure to recognize the fracture and its potential for growth arrest and failure to maintain anatomic reduction are the most common causes of a poor outcome. Physeal bars do not become evident for at least 3 months after fracture, and some not for many months. Follow-up of at least 1 year (unless the patient reaches skeletal maturity earlier) is mandatory. Longer follow-up is needed for physeal fractures of the femur, tibia, and the more complex injuries (types IV, V, and VI).

## REFERRAL DECISIONS/RED FLAGS

Displaced physeal fractures require reduction and maintenance of reduction. All type VI fractures, and many type IV and V fractures, require immediate surgery. All patients require long-term follow-up.

# FRACTURE OF THE CLAVICLE AND PROXIMAL HUMERUS

ICD-9 Codes

810.00
   Clavicle fracture, closed, unspecified part
812.00
   Proximal humerus fracture, closed, unspecified part

## DEFINITION

The clavicle is a common site of fracture in children, with most occurring in the middle third. However, fractures can occur at either end as well. Those close to the sternoclavicular joint can be serious because the great vessels are located just posterior to the joint. Those at the distal third of the clavicle generally heal rapidly in children and typically do not require surgery.

Fractures of the proximal humerus account for about 5% of fractures in children. These fractures can occur in neonates during delivery or in older children as a result of a fall. Metaphyseal fractures typically occur in children between ages 5 and 12 years, while physeal fractures (those involving the growth plate) most commonly occur in children between ages 13 and 16 years. Peterson type III (Salter type II) is the most common pattern of physeal fracture.

## CLINICAL SYMPTOMS

Newborns with a fracture of the clavicle or proximal humerus may refuse to move the arm, a condition called pseudoparalysis. Clavicle fractures in children are characterized by acute pain, tenderness, swelling, and a palpable deformity. Fractures of the proximal humerus are less obvious because of the overlying deltoid muscle.

## TESTS

### PHYSICAL EXAMINATION

Identify the point of maximum tenderness, and check the overlying skin for any tenting or blanching. Assess motor and sensory functions of the axillary, musculocutaneous, median, ulnar, and radial nerves. Radial and ulnar pulses should be checked as well.

### DIAGNOSTIC TESTS

For suspected injury to the clavicle, obtain an AP radiograph of the clavicle. AP and axillary views of the shoulder are necessary for suspected injury of the proximal humerus (**Figure 1**).

## DIFFERENTIAL DIAGNOSIS

Cleidocranial dysostosis (absence of some or all of the clavicle, frontal bossing)

Congenital muscular torticollis (asymmetric neck motion, plagiocephaly)

Congenital pseudarthrosis of the clavicle (atrophic ends of bone at "fracture")

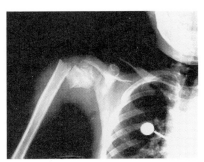

**Figure 1**
Proximal humerus fracture in a 5-year-old boy who fell from a tree.

Obstetric brachial plexus palsy (inability to spontaneously move fingers/wrist/elbow)

Pathologic fracture (injury through a bone cyst or underlying bone disorder)

Septic arthritis/osteomyelitis of the shoulder (no visible fracture, fever, pain with range of motion)

Shoulder dislocation (evident on radiographs)

Soft-tissue injury to shoulder (contusion)

## ADVERSE OUTCOMES OF THE DISEASE
Malunion, physeal bar and growth arrest, neurologic or vascular compromise of the involved extremity, and/or osteomyelitis in an open fracture can occur.

## TREATMENT
### NEWBORNS
These fractures heal without incident and fully remodel. No treatment is needed for fractures of the clavicle. For fractures of the proximal humerus, immobilize the arm for comfort.

### YOUNG CHILDREN
Middle-third clavicle fractures do not require realignment, as they will remodel and straighten with time. Observation and immobilization in a sling or a figure-of-eight strap is satisfactory. Unless posterior displacement with involvement of the great vessels and/or respiratory difficulties are present, fractures of the proximal third also can be treated with a sling. Distal-third clavicle fractures generally heal without reduction or surgery. Fractures of the proximal humerus usually are best treated with a sling. Reduction usually is not needed unless there is more than 40° of angulation.

### ADOLESCENTS
Clavicle fractures in this age group usually require only a sling or figure-of-eight strap unless the fracture is tenting or blanching the overlying skin. Fractures of the proximal humerus can be treated with a sling but may require reduction if there is more than 30° to 40° of angulation or less than 50% apposition of the fragments. Physical therapy rarely is required unless the patient has poor range of motion or atrophy several weeks after the fracture has healed.

## ADVERSE OUTCOMES OF TREATMENT
Recurrence, malunion, growth arrest of the physis, and resulting deformity are possible.

## REFERRAL DECISIONS/RED FLAGS
Neurovascular compromise, difficulty in breathing, skin tenting or blanching over the fracture site, open fractures, displacement of more than 50%, and/or angulation of more than 40° indicate the need for further evaluation.

# FRACTURE OF THE DISTAL FOREARM

ICD-9 Codes

813.42
    Galeazzi fracture
    Greenstick fracture of the distal
    radius
    Metaphyseal fracture of the distal
    radius, complete
    Physeal fracture of the distal radius
    Torus fracture of the distal radius
813.44
    Complete fracture of the distal
    radius and ulna
    Greenstick fractures of the distal
    radius and ulna

## SYNONYMS

Torus fracture

Both-bone fracture of the forearm

Greenstick fracture

Galeazzi fracture

Impaction fracture

## DEFINITION

The distal third of the forearm is the most common location for fractures in children, accounting for 20% to 40% of all pediatric fractures. The different types of fractures, in order of relative severity, are listed in Table 1. Fractures of the distal forearm are uncommon before age 4 years, but torus and greenstick fractures may occur in this younger age group. After age 10, fractures involving the growth plate of the distal radial physis are more common.

Table 1
Types of Distal Radius Fractures in Children

Torus fracture*

Metaphyseal fracture, complete*

Greenstick fracture

Greenstick fractures of the distal radius and ulna

Complete fracture of the distal radius and greenstick
    fracture of the distal ulna

Complete fracture of the distal radius and ulna

Physeal fracture

Galeazzi fracture

* Typically nondisplaced or minimally displaced

A torus fracture is characterized by buckling of the cortex on only one side of the bone and is the least complicated injury. The most common torus fracture involves the dorsal surface of the distal radius. A metaphyseal fracture isolated to the distal radius typically is nondisplaced. In a greenstick fracture, the cortex is disrupted on the tension side but is intact or only buckled on the compression side. A Galeazzi fracture is a displaced fracture of the distal radius with a dislocation of the distal ulna or a fracture of the distal ulnar physis.

## CLINICAL SYMPTOMS

Patients typically report a fall on an outstretched extremity. Acute pain, tenderness, and swelling are noted. With displaced fractures, the deformity is obvious. Symptoms following a torus fracture may not be immediately obvious.

## TESTS

### PHYSICAL EXAMINATION

Evaluate the status of the median, ulnar, and radial nerves distal to the fracture. Assess circulation at the fingertips. Examine the skin carefully, as puncture wounds are indicative of a grade I open fracture.

### DIAGNOSTIC TESTS

AP and lateral radiographs of the forearm should show both the wrist and elbow joints. Comparison views are rarely needed with these injuries.

## DIFFERENTIAL DIAGNOSIS

Child abuse (multiple injuries)

Osteomyelitis of the distal radius or ulna (no history of injury, fever, marked tenderness)

Pathologic fracture through a bone cyst or other tumor (evident on radiographs)

Septic arthritis of the wrist (subacute onset, no history of injury, fever, marked swelling)

Wrist sprain (acute symptoms, but uncommon in children)

## ADVERSE OUTCOMES OF THE DISEASE

Malunion or crossunion (synostosis) with loss of forearm rotation, compartment syndrome (uncommon), and osteomyelitis in open fractures are possible.

## TREATMENT

Most of these fractures heal without incident and can be treated by closed means. Residual angulation typically will remodel completely if 1 to 2 years of growth remain. The considerable remodeling potential of distal forearm fractures is related to the large amount of growth from the distal radial and ulnar physis, which contributes approximately 80% of forearm length.

Torus fractures and nondisplaced fractures of the distal radius are stable but should be immobilized in a short arm cast or splint for comfort and to protect the bone from a second fall that could cause exacerbation of the injury. To ensure compliance and prevent further injury, most children are better treated in a short arm cast. Displaced fractures are treated initially by immobilization in a long arm cast to prevent forearm rotation (**Figure 1**). The duration of immobilization depends on the age of the child and extent of injury.

For displaced fractures of the distal forearm, the degree of angulation that can be accepted depends on the plane of angulation and the amount of

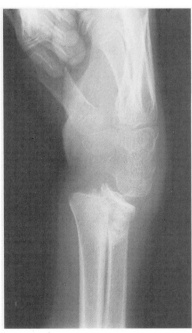

**Figure 1**
Radiograph of an 11-year-old boy who presented late with a significantly displaced fracture of the distal radial physis.

*Reproduced with permission from Waters PM: Forearm and foot fractures, in Richards BS (ed): Orthopaedic Knowledge Update: Pediatrics. Rosemont, IL, American Academy of Orthopaedic Surgeons, 1996, pp 251–257.*

growth remaining. Loss of rotational alignment is the only absolute indication for both reduction and remanipulation. Distal forearm fractures that are angulated in the volar or dorsal plane often remodel in children, even if a reduction was not performed. The principal reason for reduction is to relieve the pressure on adjacent soft tissues; therefore, closed reduction generally is indicated for angulation of 10° to 15° or more.

Unlike adults, most children with Galeazzi injuries can be treated by closed reduction.

Exploration of the fracture under general anesthesia with irrigation and debridement is critical for any open fracture, even if the wound is only a small puncture.

## ADVERSE OUTCOMES OF TREATMENT

Reangulation is fairly common in completely displaced fractures, particularly when reduction is incomplete. The decision to remanipulate the fracture depends on the age of the child, the degree of healing, and the plane of angulation. Significant malunion with loss of functional wrist and forearm motion can occur but is relatively uncommon. Synostosis with loss of forearm pronation and supination is more common with open fractures. Physeal fractures may be complicated by an arrest of growth and resulting deformity at the wrist.

## REFERRAL DECISIONS/RED FLAGS

Inability to extend all fingers, pain not relieved by over-the-counter medications, neurologic dysfunction, dislocation of the distal ulna, and/or angulation of greater than 10° to 15° require further evaluation.

# FRACTURE OF THE PROXIMAL AND MIDDLE FOREARM

## ICD-9 Codes
813.00
Fracture, closed, upper end of forearm, unspecified
813.20
Fracture, middle forearm, closed, unspecified part

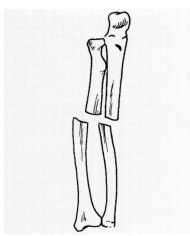

**Figure 1**
Fracture of the middle third of the forearm.

*Adapted with permission from Müller ME, Nazarian S, Koch P, et al (eds): The Comprehensive Classification of Fractures of Long Bones. Berlin, Germany, Springer-Verlag, 1990, pp 96–105.*

## SYNONYMS
Monteggia fracture-dislocation
Both-bone fracture of the forearm

## DEFINITION
In children, fractures of the proximal or midportion of the forearm typically cause disruption of both the radius and the ulna (**Figure 1**). Other injury patterns include a Monteggia fracture-dislocation (radial head dislocation associated with a fracture of the ulna) or isolated fracture of the ulna. An isolated ulna fracture usually occurs secondary to a direct blow as the child places the forearm in front of the face to deflect an oncoming blow.

## CLINICAL SYMPTOMS
Patients have acute pain, tenderness, and swelling, usually in association with a fall on the outstretched arm.

## TESTS
### PHYSICAL EXAMINATION
Assess median, ulnar, and radial nerve function distal to the fracture site. Severe or inordinate pain on passive extension of the fingers should raise concern for possible compartment syndrome.

### DIAGNOSTIC TESTS
Full-length AP and lateral radiographs of the forearm that include the wrist and elbow are indicated. The radial head should align with the capitellum on both views. A Monteggia injury should be excluded if a fracture of the ulna is present. In a Monteggia injury, dislocation of the radial head is usually anterior but could be posterior or lateral.

## DIFFERENTIAL DIAGNOSIS
Child abuse (multiple injuries)

Osteogenesis imperfecta (previous history, thin bony cortices)

Osteomyelitis of the proximal radius or ulna (fever, swelling)

Pathologic fracture through a bone cyst or tumor (evident on radiographs)

Septic arthritis of the elbow (fever, swelling, markedly restricted motion)

## ADVERSE OUTCOMES OF THE DISEASE
If recognized early, a Monteggia fracture-dislocation in children can be treated by closed reduction. However, failure to diagnose the injury in a timely fashion will necessitate open reduction, reconstructive surgery, or acceptance

of the deformity. Proximal forearm fractures are more likely to cause complications such as malunion, compartment syndrome, or loss of forearm rotation.

## TREATMENT

Irrigation and debridement of open fractures are indicated. Both-bone forearm fractures that are angulated more than 15° and all Monteggia fracture-dislocations require closed reduction and immobilization in a long arm cast for 6 to 10 weeks. In adolescents, internal fixation may be required.

## ADVERSE OUTCOMES OF TREATMENT

Recurrence of the deformity, malunion, loss of forearm rotation, and compartment syndrome are possible. Both-bone fractures can develop a synostosis or bony bar connecting the radius and ulna.

## REFERRAL DECISIONS/RED FLAGS

Inability to extend all fingers, pain not relieved by over-the-counter pain medications, and angulation greater than 15° indicate the need for further evaluation.

# FRACTURES ABOUT THE ELBOW

### ICD-9 Codes

812.40
  Fractures of distal humeral physis
812.41
  Supracondylar fracture, distal humerus
812.42
  Lateral condyle fracture; lateral epi-condyle fracture, distal humerus
812.43
  Medial condyle fracture; medial epicondyle fracture, distal humerus
813.01
  Olecranon fracture, proximal forearm
813.06
  Radial neck fracture, proximal forearm

## DEFINITION

Fractures about the elbow are common in children. Injuries involving the distal humerus account for more than 80% of these fractures (Table 1).

### Table 1
### Types of Elbow Fractures in Children

| Distal humerus | Proximal forearm |
| --- | --- |
| Supracondylar | Radial neck |
| Lateral condyle | Olecranon |
| Medial condyle | |
| Lateral epicondyle | |
| Medial epicondyle | |
| Distal humeral physis | |

Supracondylar fractures of the distal humerus are the most common elbow fractures in children, typically affecting children between the ages of 2 and 12 years. This fracture is above the physis. Most are extension fractures with the distal fragment displaced posteriorly (Figure 1).

The next most common injury is a fracture of the lateral condyle of the distal humerus. Fracture of the medial condyle is uncommon; however, whether on the lateral or medial side, condylar fractures are serious because the fracture typically involves the growth plate of the distal humerus and the articular surface of the elbow (Figure 2).

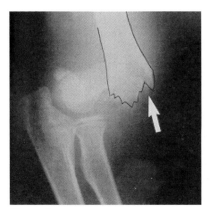

**Figure 1**
Radiograph of a displaced supracondylar fracture.

*Reproduced with permission from Sullivan JA, Anderson SJ (eds) Care of the Young Athlete, Rosemont, IL, American Academy of Orthopaedic Surgeons, 2000, p 317.*

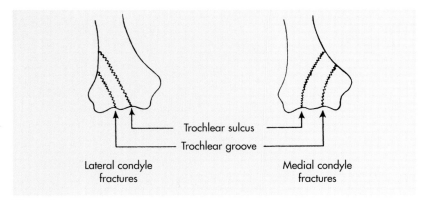

**Figure 2**
Typical fracture patterns of lateral and medial condyles of distal humerus in children.

*Reproduced with permission from Milch H: Fractures and fracture-dislocations of the humeral condyles. J Trauma 1963;3:592–607.*

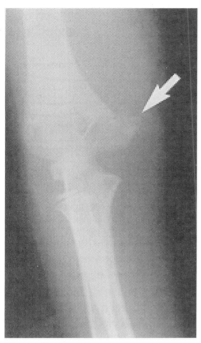

**Figure 3**
Displaced fracture of the medial epicondyle.

*Reproduced with permission from Sullivan JA, Anderson SJ (eds) Care of the Young Athlete, Rosemont, IL, American Academy of Orthopaedic Surgeons, 2000, p 314.*

Fracture of the lateral epicondyle is uncommon. Fracture of the medial epicondyle is the third most common elbow fracture (**Figure 3**). The epicondyles are secondary ossification centers at sites of muscle origin. Fractures of the medial or lateral epicondyle do not involve the articular surface and do not adversely affect growth. Therefore, epicondyle fractures of the distal humerus, even when displaced, have limited consequences unless the elbow joint is concomitantly dislocated and the fragment is incarcerated into the joint.

Fractures across the entire physis of the distal humerus are uncommon. These injuries occur most frequently in infants and small children as a result of child abuse.

In children, the metaphyseal portion of the radial neck is the weak link. Therefore, the valgus force that causes a fracture of the radial head in adults will result in a fracture of the radial neck in children.

Olecranon fractures are uncommon in children. These injuries usually involve the articular surface and, when displaced, require an open or closed reduction.

## CLINICAL SYMPTOMS

Patients have acute pain, tenderness, swelling, and most often a history of falling on an outstretched arm. The child often refuses to use the limb and holds it at the side with the elbow flexed. Swelling can be severe, but with nondisplaced or minimally displaced fractures, swelling may be mild.

## TESTS

### PHYSICAL EXAMINATION

Evaluate the status of the median, ulnar, and radial nerves distal to the injury. Assess distal pulses and capillary filling. With obvious deformity, position or splint the limb in a position of comfort and order radiographs. In other children, attempt to find the site of maximum tenderness and gently evaluate elbow motion.

### DIAGNOSTIC TESTS

AP and lateral radiographs of the elbow are necessary. The fracture may be obvious or subtle. Oblique views and comparison radiographs of the opposite elbow are helpful with subtle injuries. The radial head should be directed toward the distal humerus (capitellum) on both AP and lateral views.

An abnormal posterior fat pad sign is associated with fractures about the elbow, and the presence of this sign is particularly helpful with subtle or occult fractures. In a normal elbow, the anterior fat pad can be seen on a lateral radiograph, but the posterior fat pad is not visualized. Any process that causes an elbow effusion will elevate both anterior and posterior fat pads (**Figure 4**). The posterior fat pad is, therefore, often visible with elbow fractures in children, even when these injuries are not obvious on initial radiographs.

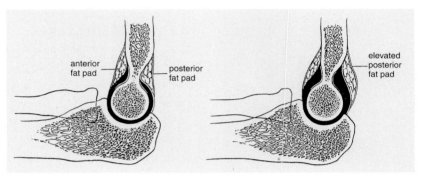

**Figure 4**
Normal anterior and posterior fat pads (left) and anterior and posterior fat pads elevated from an effusion (right).

*Reproduced with permission from Skaggs DL, Mirzayan R: The posterior fat pad sign in association with occult fracture of the elbow in children. J Bone Joint Surg, 1999;81A:1429-1433.*

## DIFFERENTIAL DIAGNOSIS

Dislocation of the elbow (typically posterior, evident on radiographs)

Hemarthrosis of the elbow (swelling, limited motion, no other positive findings)

Monteggia fracture-dislocation (fracture of proximal ulna and dislocation of the radial head)

Sprain (swelling, tenderness over the involved ligament, no evidence of fracture)

Subluxation of the radial head (typical history and age, tenderness over radial head, negative radiographs)

## ADVERSE OUTCOMES OF THE DISEASE

Supracondylar fractures have the highest incidence of neurovascular problems. Median, ulnar, and radial nerve injuries are associated with this fracture. The brachial artery may be injured, and compartment syndrome involving the volar forearm muscles may develop. Failure to recognize this problem in a timely fashion will result in necrosis of forearm muscles and subsequent contractures (Volkmann ischemic contracture). Malunion with loss of the normal carrying angle (cubitus varus) may occur.

Condyle fractures may be missed, particularly in very young children who have limited ossification of the distal humerus. In these children, only a thin wafer of metaphyseal fragment will be apparent, with the rest of the fracture involving the cartilaginous physis and trochlea and, therefore, not visible on plain radiographs. Fractures displaced 2 mm or more are often associated with delayed union, nonunion, or malunion (rotational and/or cubitus valgus). Condyle fractures of the humerus that are initially nondisplaced may become displaced, even when immobilized, by contraction of the forearm muscles attaching at the condyle. These injuries require close follow-up and repeat radiographs.

Medial epicondyle fractures of the distal humerus do not commonly cause residual problems, even when markedly displaced, unless associated with dislocation of the elbow and a fracture fragment that is not recognized as being entrapped in the joint.

Fractures across the entire distal physis of the humerus have complications that are similar but typically less severe than supracondylar fractures. In addition, the potential for child abuse should be recognized and appropriately investigated.

Fractures of the radial neck that are angulated more than 30° may be associated with loss of forearm rotation, premature closure of the growth plate, and osteonecrosis of the radial head.

Fractures of the olecranon that have 2 mm or more disruption of the articular surface need reduction to prevent progressive arthritic changes.

## TREATMENT

Nondisplaced fractures can be treated with splint or cast immobilization. Condyle fractures, in particular, need repeat radiographs in 3 to 5 days. Displaced fractures need reduction and, in most cases, pinning. The exception is medial or lateral epicondyle fractures of the humerus and radial neck fractures with less than 30° of angulation.

## ADVERSE OUTCOMES OF TREATMENT

These are the same as the adverse outcomes of the disease. In addition, postoperative infection can develop.

## REFERRAL DECISIONS/RED FLAGS

Any displacement or angulation, inability to extend all fingers of the affected hand, failure of over-the-counter medications to provide pain relief, and absent or diminished radial pulse are signs that further evaluation is necessary.

# FRACTURES OF THE FEMUR

ICD-9 Codes
820.00
   Femoral neck fracture, closed, unspecified type
820.21
   Intertrochanteric femur fracture, closed
821.00
   Femoral shaft fracture, closed, unspecified part
821.22
   Distal femoral physeal fracture, closed
821.23
   Supracondylar femur fracture, closed

## DEFINITION

Fractures of the femur in children are usually the result of significant trauma, although they can occur after simple falls. Fractures can occur anywhere in the femur (eg, femoral neck, intertrochanteric region, femoral shaft, supra-condylar region, distal femoral physis) and can be transverse, oblique, spiral, or comminuted. Most involve the femoral shaft and heal without incident in 6 to 12 weeks. Traditional closed treatment, such as traction or spica casting, is giving way to surgical fixation in older children and adolescents to enable early mobility and improve outcome.

## CLINICAL SYMPTOMS

Patients have acute pain, swelling, inability to bear weight, deformity, and a history of trauma.

## TESTS

### PHYSICAL EXAMINATION

Pain and disability will be immediate. Tenderness, deformity, or swelling may localize the fracture. Tibial and peroneal nerve function distal to the knee should be evaluated, as should circulation at the ankle.

### DIAGNOSTIC TESTS

AP and lateral radiographs of the femur, including the hip and knee joints, should be obtained. Stress views may be necessary to identify physeal fractures of the distal femur.

## DIFFERENTIAL DIAGNOSIS

Child abuse (metaphyseal corner fractures or multiple fractures in various stages of healing)

Knee injury (especially collateral ligament tears)

Osteogenesis imperfecta (multiple fractures after trivial trauma)

Pathologic fracture through a cyst or bony tumor (evident on radiographs)

Slipped capital femoral epiphysis (common in overweight adolescents)

## ADVERSE OUTCOMES OF THE DISEASE

Malunion, either angular or rotational, along with growth derangement and limb-length discrepancy are possible. Osteonecrosis of the femoral head may occur with a displaced or nondisplaced fracture of the femoral neck. Fractures of the distal femoral physis may be misdiagnosed as a knee sprain.

## TREATMENT

The type of treatment depends on the location of the fracture in the femur, the fracture pattern, and the age of the patient. Immobilization by a spica cast or initial treatment by traction followed by casting are time-honored and effective modalities, especially well suited to young children who tolerate recumbency and heal rapidly.

Nondisplaced femoral neck and intertrochanteric fractures may be treated with cast immobilization. These injuries should be monitored closely with radiographs for evidence of displacement. Displaced fractures should be treated by immediate reduction and fixation to minimize the risk of complications.

Femoral shaft fractures can be treated with immediate spica casting or traction until early callus formation provides enough stability for the fracture to maintain alignment in a spica cast. This treatment is routine for young children up to age 6 years and for children 6 to 10 years of age who do not meet the indications for other types of treatment. Minor angulation will remodel.

Older children may be candidates for fixation of femoral shaft fractures that enables them to get out of bed and return to school earlier. Supracondylar fractures and fractures of the distal femoral physis are difficult to reduce and hold in casts and often will require surgical fixation to maintain the reduction.

## ADVERSE OUTCOMES OF TREATMENT

These are similar to the adverse outcomes of the disease.

## REFERRAL DECISIONS/RED FLAGS

Virtually all femoral fractures require at least a short hospitalization. Open fractures and fractures with vascular compromise require urgent treatment.

# FRACTURES OF THE TIBIA

ICD-9 Code
823.80
Fracture of tibia, unspecified part, closed

## DEFINITION

Diaphyseal and proximal metaphyseal fractures occur more commonly in younger children, but growth plate and intra-articular fractures are more prevalent in older children. The tibia is a common site of fracture in children who are victims of child abuse. A list of various fracture types, age of peak incidence, and potential complications is provided in Table 1.

## Table 1
### Types of Tibial Fractures

| Proximal | Diaphyseal | Distal |
|---|---|---|
| Tibial spine fracture (older child)<br>    Failure to recognize<br>    Chronic laxity of knee | Toddler's fracture (1-3 years)<br>    Failure to recognize<br>    Overdiagnosis | Physeal fracture (older child;<br>    adolescent)<br>    Malunion<br>    Growth arrest |
| Tibial tubercle avulsion (older child;<br>    adolescent)<br>    Growth arrest<br>    Compartment syndrome | Stress fracture (older child;<br>    adolescent)<br>    Failure to recognize<br>    Overdiagnosis | Triplane/Tilleaux fractures*<br>    (adolescent)<br>    Failure to recognize<br>    Degenerative arthritis |
| Metaphyseal fracture (younger child)<br>    Genu valgum | Complete fracture<br>    Varus malunion<br>    Compartment syndrome | *Complex fracture of distal tibia<br>    occurring near end of growth |

## CLINICAL SYMPTOMS

Most patients present with a history of injury causing the acute onset of pain and inability to walk. Toddler's fractures, minimally displaced or incomplete metaphyseal fractures, and stress fractures are characterized by a vague history or insidious onset with minimal swelling or localizing signs and a limp.

## TESTS

### PHYSICAL EXAMINATION

Assess superficial peroneal, deep peroneal, and posterior tibial nerve function. Evaluate dorsalis pedis and posterior tibialis pulses, as well as capillary refill. Assess for possible compartment syndrome, particularly in proximal physeal and midshaft fractures with muscle contusion. Look carefully for any puncture wounds or abrasions that would signify an open fracture.

### DIAGNOSTIC TESTS

AP and lateral radiographs of the tibia that show the knee and ankle are necessary. For injuries thought to involve the knee or ankle, center the radiographs in these areas. Oblique radiographs and CT can be helpful in visualizing complex fractures of the distal tibia, such as triplane or Tilleaux fractures. A bone scan can be helpful in identifying a stress fracture or other occult injuries.

## DIFFERENTIAL DIAGNOSIS

Child abuse (multiple injuries, metaphyseal beak or corner fractures)

Ligament injuries (unusual in prepubertal children)

Osteogenesis imperfecta (previous history, thin bony cortices)

Pathologic fracture through a bone cyst or tumor (evident on radiographs)

Stress fracture (indolent onset)

## ADVERSE OUTCOMES OF THE DISEASE

Early potential problems include compartment syndrome and vascular injuries. These complications are less common but may be more difficult to diagnose in children. Remodeling is unpredictable in deformities of greater than 10°, and malunion with subsequent degenerative arthritis may occur. Growth arrest is common with distal tibial physeal injuries but less likely with proximal injuries.

## TREATMENT

Treatment focuses on minimizing angular deformity, restoring joint congruity, and avoiding or identifying compartment syndrome or vascular injuries. Toddler's fractures, stress fractures, and certain nondisplaced fractures can be managed with immobilization in a short leg walking cast. Displaced shaft fractures often require manipulative reduction and long leg casting. These patients are best managed with hospital admission overnight for observation and elevation. Early splitting of the cast to accommodate swelling may be necessary. The duration of casting depends upon the age of the child and the extent of the fracture.

Displaced intra-articular or physeal fractures need closed or open reduction and limited internal fixation supplemented by cast immobilization. All open fractures require surgical exploration and debridement.

## ADVERSE OUTCOMES OF TREATMENT

These are the same as adverse outcomes of the disease. In addition, infection may develop after open treatment.

## REFERRAL DECISIONS/RED FLAGS

Patients who report pain after immobilization that is not relieved by mild analgesics or over-the-counter medications need further evaluation. Patients who have lacerations or deep abrasions overlying the fracture site should be treated as if they have an open fracture. Inability to correct angular deformities to less than 10° is considered a problem. Proximal or distal tibial fractures that involve the physis or articular surface need further evaluation.

# GENU VALGUM

ICD-9 Code

736.41
    Genu valgum, acquired

## DEFINITION

Genu valgum (knock-knees) is alignment of the knee with the tibia laterally deviated (valgus) in relation to the femur. At birth, the child is bowlegged, with a genu varum of 10° to 15°. The bowing gradually straightens to 0° by 12 to 18 months of age. Continued growth produces maximum genu valgum at age 3 to 4 years that averages 10° to 15°. With subsequent growth, the genu valgum decreases, and normal adult alignment of 5° to 10° genu valgum occurs by early adolescence. Young children have a fairly wide range of normal knee alignment (two standard deviations typically is ± 10°).

## CLINICAL SYMPTOMS

Parental concern is the usual reason for the visit.

## TESTS

### PHYSICAL EXAMINATION

Measure the child's height and then plot it on a height nomogram. Measure the tibiofemoral angle using a goniometer or by measuring the intermalleolar (IM) distance. The IM distance is the distance between the medial malleoli with the medial femoral condyles touching. The IM distance is easy to measure and follow but has the disadvantage of being a relative rather than an absolute measurement because it is dependent on leg length.

### DIAGNOSTIC TESTS

Radiographs usually are not necessary, but should be considered when the valgus is more than 15° to 20°, or if the child is short statured. A weight-bearing AP radiograph on a 36- × 43-cm cassette with the film centered at the knees and the feet pointing straight ahead provides screening for a possible skeletal dysplasia, as well as accurate measurement of the tibiofemoral angle (genu valgum).

## DIFFERENTIAL DIAGNOSIS

Hypophosphatemic rickets (short stature, wide physis, low serum phosphorus)

Multiple epiphyseal dysplasia (short stature, multiple joint involvement)

Pseudoachondroplasia (short stature, early arthritic change)

## ADVERSE OUTCOMES OF THE DISEASE

None

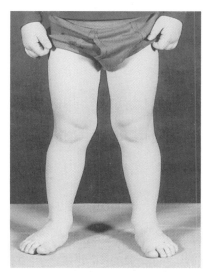

**Figure 1**
Boy referred for evaluation of "knock-knees."

*Reproduced with permission from Greene WB: Genu varum and genu valgum in children, in Schafer M (ed): Instructional Course Lectures 43. Rosemont, IL, American Academy of Orthopaedic Surgeons, 1994, pp 151–159.*

## TREATMENT

Observation is the treatment of choice for an otherwise normal 3- to 4-year-old child with marked genu valgum. Shoe modifications are ineffective, and long leg braces are not indicated because this condition spontaneously corrects more than 99% of the time. The child shown in Figure 1 is a 3-year, 6-month-old boy referred for evaluation of knock-knees. His height is in the 70th percentile, and his development is normal. Genu valgum measured 18° by clinical examination. The patient was considered to be within normal limits, and an explanation was provided to the mother. No radiographs or further follow-up was required.

## ADVERSE OUTCOMES OF TREATMENT

None

## REFERRAL DECISIONS/RED FLAGS

Patients of short stature and those with asymmetric or excessive genu valgum need further evaluation (greater than two standard deviations from normal for age).

SECTION 9 | PEDIATRIC ORTHOPAEDICS

# GENU VARUM

ICD-9 Code
736.42
Genu varum, acquired

## DEFINITION

Genu varum (bow legs) is an angular deformity at the knee with the tibia medially deviated (varus) in relation to the femur. At birth, genu varum of 10° to 15° is normal. The bowing gradually straightens to 0° by age 12 to 18 months. Continued growth then results in progressive valgus with maximum genu valgum of 10° to 15° occurring at age 3 to 4 years. Young children have a fairly wide range of normal knee alignment (two standard deviations is ± 10°).

The most common cause of bow legs in children 18 to 36 months of age is physiologic genu varum, a condition that resolves without treatment (normal variation of growth).

## CLINICAL SYMPTOMS

Parental concern is the usual reason for the visit.

## TESTS

### PHYSICAL EXAMINATION

Measure the child's height and then plot it on a height nomogram. Quantify the genu varum either by using a goniometer to measure the genu varum or by measuring the intercondylar (IC) distance, which is the distance between the medial femoral condyles when the lower extremities are positioned with the medial malleoli touching. The IC distance is easier to measure in small children but is affected by leg length. As a result, the IC distance has the disadvantage of being a relative rather than absolute measurement. Also assess tibial torsion.

### DIAGNOSTIC TESTS

Radiographs are appropriate if the child is under the 25th percentile for height, the varus is relatively severe for the child's age, there is excessive internal tibial torsion, the varus is increasing after age 16 months, or there is significant asymmetry of the two sides. Obtain weight-bearing AP radiographs of the lower extremities on a 36- × 43-cm cassette with the film centered at the knees and the feet pointing straight ahead (**Figure 1**). Assess radiographs for the tibiofemoral angle, the width of the growth plate (widened in rickets and certain skeletal dysplasias), and the slope of the proximal tibia (medial aspect depressed in infantile tibia vara). Infantile tibia vara and physiologic genu varum can be difficult to differentiate in children under age 3 years, but radiographic measurement can help. The right limb shown in Figure 1 has medial depression of the tibial physis and an increased tibial metaphyseal-diaphyseal angle of 20°. This radiographic picture suggests a high probability of infantile tibia vara, and a long leg brace was prescribed.

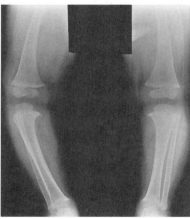

**Figure 1**
1-year, 6-month-old girl with genu varum.

*Reproduced with permission from Greene WB: Infantile tibia vara, in Heckman JD (ed): Instructional Course Lectures 42. Rosemont, IL, American Academy of Orthopaedic Surgeons, 1993, pp 525–538.*

## DIFFERENTIAL DIAGNOSIS

Hypophosphatemic rickets (short stature, widened physis, and low serum phosphorus level)

Infantile tibia vara (obese children who begin walking at an early age; associated internal tibial torsion, depression of the medial aspect of the proximal tibial physis)

Metaphyseal chondrodysplasia (short stature, widened physis, normal serum phosphorus level)

Physiologic genu varum (spontaneous correction by age 2½ to 3 years, normal tibial metaphyseal-diaphyseal angle)

## ADVERSE OUTCOMES OF THE DISEASE

The principal adverse outcome is persistent varus deformity.

## TREATMENT

For young children with infantile tibia vara, bracing can be successful. After age 30 to 36 months, tibial osteotomy may be required.

## ADVERSE OUTCOMES OF TREATMENT

The deformity can recur.

## REFERRAL DECISIONS/RED FLAGS

The presence of disorders other than physiologic genu varum indicates the need for further evaluation.

# INTOEING AND OUTTOEING

**ICD-9 Codes**
736.89
Acquired deformity of lower limb
781.2
Abnormality of gait

## SYNONYMS

### INTOEING
Pigeon-toed
Femoral torsion
Femoral anteversion
Internal tibial torsion

### OUTTOEING
External rotation contracture of infancy
Femoral retroversion
External tibial torsion
External femoral torsion

## DEFINITION

Intoeing means that the foot turns in more than expected during walking and running activities. With outtoeing, the child's foot turns out more than expected.

By age 2 years, children typically walk with the foot turned out relative to the line of progression, a phenomenon that is obvious when observing a child's footprints in the snow or sand. When walking on level ground, the foot typically is turned out at an angle of 10° to 20° to the line of progression.

Intoeing may be secondary to foot deformities or may be due to inward rotation of the femur or tibia, or a combination of the two. Increased internal torsion of the femur (femoral anteversion) is the most common finding. Excessive outtoeing, although not as frequent a concern as intoeing, is similar in that excessive rotation may occur in the femur (femoral retroversion), the tibia (external tibial torsion), or both. In many cases, intoeing and outtoeing are variations of normal development.

Understanding normal development of femoral and tibial torsion, as well as the changes that occur in hip rotation, is critical in evaluating these children. Inward femoral rotation (anteversion) is greatest at birth (approximately 40°) and gradually declines to adult values of 10° to 15° by age 8 years. The tibia normally twists outward between the knee and ankle. Tibial torsion is typically neutral or 0° at birth and gradually increases to 20° to 40° by age 3 to 4 years. Tibial torsion is often asymmetric, with the left side commonly less severe.

Although not an absolute measurement, the easiest way to assess femoral anteversion is by measuring hip rotation. It is important to realize that clinical measurement of hip rotation does not profile the degree of bony femoral torsion until neonatal tightness of the hip joint capsule resolves. Due to intrauterine positioning, a neonate is born with tightness of the hip joint capsule. This creates an external contracture and increased external rotation of the hip even though femoral torsion is maximum at birth. The effect of this capsular contraction on measurement of hip rotation does not completely resolve until the infant is at least age 1 year and sometimes even up to age 2 years.

## CLINICAL SYMPTOMS

Typically, medical attention is sought because parents or grandparents are concerned about how the child is walking. In children, intoeing and outtoeing usually do not cause pain or interfere with development or stability in gait. With severe intoeing, children may stumble or trip more frequently as they catch their toes on the back of the trailing leg.

## TESTS

### PHYSICAL EXAMINATION

The physical examination should include the following steps:

- Measurement of foot progression angle (angle that the foot makes relative to the line of progression as the child walks)

- Measurement of hip rotation (femoral torsion)

- Measurement of tibial torsion (thigh-foot angle)

- Observation of the posture of the foot

- Evaluation for possible neuromuscular disorders

Observe the child walking and estimate the foot progression angle. The foot progression angle does not identify the site of the problem; however, it quantifies the severity of the problem and distinguishes whether there is an intoeing or outtoeing disorder.

Hip rotation approximates femoral torsion. Hip rotation should be measured with the hip in extension. Placing the child in the prone position is the most reliable method to measure hip rotation. Flex the knee to 90° and position the leg in the Zero Starting Position (**Figure 1**). Rotate both legs simultaneously to measure internal rotation. The degree of internal rotation is the angle of the leg from the Zero Starting Position (**Figure 2**). To assess external rotation, place one hand on the buttocks and move the leg into external rotation. The degree of external rotation is the angle of the leg when the pelvis starts to tilt.

The average range of hip rotation for a child older than age 2 years is approximately 50° of internal rotation and 40° of external rotation. An excessive amount of internal rotation (greater than 65°) coupled with a limited degree of external rotation indicates increased femoral anteversion. Likewise, after 2 years of age, an excessive amount of external rotation coupled with limited internal rotation indicates reduced femoral torsion (femoral retroversion).

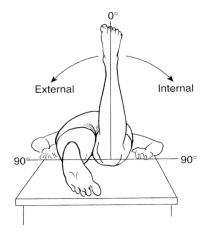

**Figure 1**
Rotation: Zero Starting Position.

*Reproduced with permission from Greene WB, Heckman JD (eds): The Clinical Measurement of Joint Motion. Rosemont, IL, American Academy of Orthopaedic Surgeons, 1994, pp 106-107.*

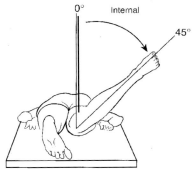

**Figure 2**
Internal rotation.

*Reproduced with permission from Greene WB, Heckman JD (eds): The Clinical Measurement of Joint Motion. Rosemont, IL, American Academy of Orthopaedic Surgeons, 1994, pp 106-107.*

Tibial torsion is most easily assessed by measuring the thigh-foot angle (the axis of the foot relative to the axis of the thigh with the knee flexed to 90° and the hip and foot in a neutral or Zero Starting Position alignment) (**Figure 3**). A neutral or internal thigh-foot angle indicates internal tibial torsion (**Figure 4**).

Foot posture is assessed for metatarsus adductus, a possible cause of intoeing, as well as hindfoot alignment. Increased heel valgus or pes planovalgus may be perceived by the parents as the leg turning out.

Neuromuscular disorders may cause intoeing or outtoeing. Furthermore, these children may be brought to a physician with the parents concerned

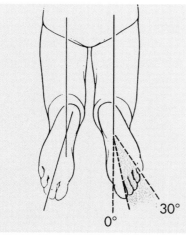

**Figure 3**
Normal range of thigh-foot angle.

*Adapted with permission from Alexander IJ: The Foot: Examination and Diagnosis, ed 1. New York, NY, Churchill Livingstone, 1990, p 115.*

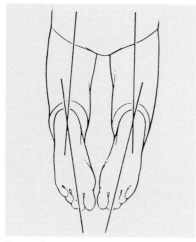

**Figure 4**
Bilateral internal tibial torsion.

*Adapted with permission from Alexander IJ: The Foot: Examination and Diagnosis, ed 1. New York, NY, Churchill Livingstone, 1990, p 115.*

## Table 1
### Gross Motor Developmental Screens During Early Childhood

| Age | Activity |
|---|---|
| 2 years | Stairs, one step at a time |
| 2½ years | Jumps |
| 3 years | Stairs, alternating feet |
| 4 years | Hops on one foot |
| 5 years | Skips |

*Adapted from Paine RS, Oppe TE: Neurological examination of children, Clinics in Developmental Medicine, Nos 20/21. London, England, William Heinemann Medical Books.*

about intoeing or outtoeing before the underlying disorder has been diagnosed. This is particularly common in patients with mild cerebral palsy. Therefore, assess for appropriate motor milestones (**Table 1**) and examine for spasticity, muscle contractures, clonus, and a stiff or imbalanced gait.

External rotation contracture of infancy may persist and cause concern. These children are typically brought to a physician between the ages of 6 to 12 months, a time when they are starting to pull to a stand or are in walkers. The parents are concerned about the posture of the lower extremities. Boys and blacks are more commonly affected. The right leg typically is affected more often. Examination reveals 60° to 70° of external rotation and only 20° to 30° of internal rotation. The hip rotation is usually symmetric, but the right leg typically is more externally rotated because the tibial torsion has advanced to a greater degree on that side. In the absence of neuromuscular disease and muscle imbalance, normal growth will correct this condition without the need for special shoes, braces, or exercise therapy.

## DIAGNOSTIC TESTS
Radiographs are rarely needed unless the child has evidence of short stature.

## DIFFERENTIAL DIAGNOSIS

Cerebral palsy or other neuromuscular disorders (developmental delay, spasticity, muscle weakness)

Femoral anteversion (increased internal rotation of the hip)

Femoral retroversion (increased external rotation of the hip)

Metatarsus adductus (forefoot adducted)

Skeletal dysplasia (short stature)

Tibial torsion (increased internal or external rotation of the tibia)

## ADVERSE OUTCOMES OF THE DISEASE

If intoeing persists, the child may have a cosmetically unpleasant gait pattern and may trip more frequently, but this condition has not been linked to degenerative arthritis in adulthood. If intoeing caused by increased femoral anteversion persists, the tibia may compensate and external tibial torsion may develop. This condition can be associated with patellofemoral disorders during adolescence, but this is rare.

Outtoeing, except in neuromuscular disorders, often improves with age and rarely requires treatment.

## TREATMENT

Shoe modifications, braces, and exercises do not alter developmental changes in femoral or tibial torsion. Casting occasionally is necessary in metatarsus adductus.

Slow correction of femoral anteversion to an acceptable degree is typical. An associated increase in external tibial torsion will diminish the degree of intoeing. In rare cases, children may have persistent tripping or an unsightly gait and surgical correction by rotational osteotomy of the femur may be indicated. The procedure generally is done after age 7 to 8 years to allow for spontaneous resolution.

In children with cerebral palsy and other neuromuscular disorders, both abnormal femoral and tibial torsion persist in a much higher percentage of patients and are more likely to require surgical correction due to their impact on gait.

## ADVERSE OUTCOMES OF TREATMENT

Risks of surgery include failure to heal, infection, over- or undercorrection of the deformity, or postoperative angular deformity. Risks of casting for metatarsus adductus are minimal.

## REFERRAL DECISIONS/RED FLAGS

Physicians who are familiar with the evaluation and examination of this problem can adequately reassure parents regarding the frequent resolution of these deformities. When metatarsus adductus persists in an infant older than age 6 months, or internal tibial torsion or abnormal femoral anteversion persists past age 4 years and the deformity is significant, further evaluation is warranted. Specialty evaluation is sometimes necessary to allay parents' or grandparents' concern.

# JUVENILE RHEUMATOID ARTHRITIS

ICD-9 Codes
714.30
  Polyarticular juvenile rheumatoid arthritis, chronic or unspecified
714.32
  Pauciarticular juvenile rheumatoid arthritis

## SYNONYMS

JRA

Still's disease

## DEFINITION

The American Rheumatic Association lists four criteria for diagnosing juvenile rheumatoid arthritis (JRA): 1) chronic synovial inflammation of unknown cause; 2) onset in children younger than age 16 years; 3) objective evidence of arthritis in one or more joints for 6 consecutive weeks; and 4) exclusion of other diseases. Pauciarticular JRA involves four or fewer joints after 6 months of symptoms, whereas polyarticular JRA involves five or more joints. Systemic JRA is the subgroup characterized by an illness beginning with high spiking fevers—temperatures above 102.7°F (39.3°C). The number of joints involved is not included in the definition of systemic-onset JRA, but most patients in this group have several affected joints.

## CLINICAL SYMPTOMS

Pain, swelling, and stiffness are less severe in JRA than in the adult form.

Pauciarticular JRA is the most common pattern. Age at onset typically is younger than age 4 years, and girls are affected four times more often than boys. The parents will comment that the child is irritable, lethargic, or shows a reluctance to play. The disease commonly begins in a single joint, most frequently the knee, ankle, wrist, or finger joints. Uveitis is most likely to develop in children with this type of JRA and a positive antinuclear antibody (ANA) test.

The polyarticular form is characterized by symmetric involvement of the knees, wrists, fingers, and ankles and is more common in girls. The onset of the seronegative form typically occurs in children between ages 1 and 3 years, and the seropositive form usually begins in adolescence and is virtually indistinguishable from adult rheumatoid arthritis.

Systemic onset commonly occurs in children between the ages of 4 and 9 years and at onset is associated with spiking fevers, polyarthralgias, myalgias, an evanescent maculopapular rash with central clearing, and a high erythrocyte sedimentation rate.

## TESTS

### PHYSICAL EXAMINATION

Evaluate the joints for swelling effusion, warmth, decreased range of motion, and adjacent muscle atrophy.

## DIAGNOSTIC TESTS

The erythrocyte sedimentation rate is often normal. A positive ANA test indicates a tendency for uveitis.

## DIFFERENTIAL DIAGNOSIS

Leukemia (night pain, bone pain more than joint pain or effusion)

Osteomyelitis (fever, more severe pain)

Septic arthritis (fever, single joint involvement, more severe pain and effusion)

## ADVERSE OUTCOMES OF THE DISEASE

Spontaneous remission is common, but end-stage arthritis may occur. Blindness may develop with untreated uveitis.

## TREATMENT

NSAIDs are the mainstay of treatment. Other medications, such as methotrexate, are used if synovitis is persistent. Splinting and orthotics help maintain functional joint alignment. Physical therapy is helpful in maintaining joint motion and strength when the pain has diminished. Regular ophthalmologic slit lamp examinations for uveitis are necessary, with the frequency of this examination dependent on the type of JRA, results on ANA test, and age of the child.

## ADVERSE OUTCOMES OF TREATMENT

NSAIDs can cause gastric, renal, or hepatic complications.

## REFERRAL DECISIONS/RED FLAGS

Failure of NSAIDs, splinting, and therapy to relieve symptoms indicates the need for further evaluation. Persistent active synovitis also is an indication that the patient needs additional evaluation.

# KYPHOSIS

## SYNONYMS

Postural round back

Scheuermann disease

Juvenile kyphosis

## DEFINITION

Kyphosis is a curvature of the sagittal plane of the spinal column. It originates from the Greek word *kyphos* meaning "hump backed" and refers to a curve pointing backward (the apex of the curve is posterior). The normal thoracic spine has a kyphosis of 20° to 40° (Cobb angle measured from T5 to T12). Kyphosis measuring between 40° and 50° is considered borderline normal. Any kyphosis greater than 50° is considered hyperkyphosis. Conditions associated with kyphosis in children are listed in the differential diagnosis.

Postural kyphosis and Scheuermann disease are the most common causes of hyperkyphosis in children. Both conditions present during adolescence. Postural kyphosis is more common in girls, and Scheuermann disease is more common in boys. The kyphosis usually is more severe in Scheuermann disease, but radiographs are necessary to differentiate these disorders. By definition, Scheuermann disease has irregularities of the vertebral end plates, and more than 5° of anterior wedging must be observed in at least three successive vertebra.

## CLINICAL SYMPTOMS

Most patients are seen because of either poor posture or poor posture with back pain. When present, the pain usually is activity related and relieved by rest.

## TESTS

### PHYSICAL EXAMINATION

The Adams forward bend test is the best way to profile the kyphosis. This test is done by viewing the child from the side. Children with Scheuermann disease and other pathologic causes of kyphosis usually have sharp angulation in the spine, while patients with postural kyphosis have a more normal spinal profile (**Figure 1**). Patients with postural kyphosis have normal flexibility (ie, the spine flattens in the supine position).

### DIAGNOSTIC TESTS

Standing AP and lateral radiographs of the spine should be obtained. The x-ray tube should be positioned 6' from the patient, preferably with a 14" × 36" film and a grid. The patient's breasts and gonads should be shielded when possible. Look for bony abnormalities, including congenital abnormalities.

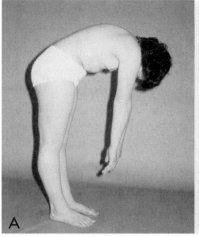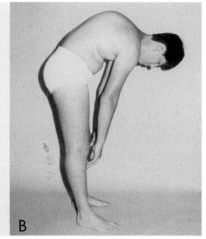

**Figure 1**
Adams forward bend test. A, Normal spine profile. B, Angulated spine profile as in Scheuermann disease.

*Reproduced with permission from Staheli L (ed); Pediatric Orthopaedic Secrets. Hanley&Belfus, Inc. Philadelphia, PA, 1998, p 286.*

Measure curve magnitude on the lateral radiograph using the Cobb method. The upper thoracic vertebrae may not be well visualized; therefore, by definition, kyphosis is measured from T5 to T12. The angle is a line drawn along the superior end plate of T5 and a line drawn on the inferior end plate of T12. Any curvature exceeding 50° is considered abnormal.

## DIFFERENTIAL DIAGNOSIS

Congenital (hemivertebra or anterior failure of segmentation)

Iatrogenic (eg, after laminectomy)

Juvenile rheumatoid arthritis (severe systemic JRA requiring prolonged steroids)

Neurofibromatosis (café au lait spots, subcutaneous neurofibromas, inguinal and/or axillary freckling)

Neuromuscular (cerebral palsy, poliomyelitis)

Pathologic fracture (leukemia, Gaucher disease, thalassemia, osteogenesis imperfecta, juvenile osteoporosis, and any condition requiring prolonged use of steroids)

Tuberculosis (Pott disease)

## ADVERSE OUTCOMES OF THE DISEASE

Scheuermann kyphosis can progress to significant deformities. Respiratory function, however, is not affected until the curve is well over 100°. Congenital kyphosis may cause stretch and dysfunction of the spinal cord.

## TREATMENT

Postural kyphosis can be observed or treated with an exercise program. Scheuermann kyphosis in a skeletally immature patient requires brace treatment and possibly spinal fusion, if the condition is severe. Bracing is not effective in patients with congenital deformities, and progressive deformities often require operative management.

## ADVERSE OUTCOMES OF TREATMENT

Bracing may fail to prevent progression. Operative treatment may be complicated by pseudarthrosis, wound infection, pneumonia, and/or spinal cord injury.

## REFERRAL DECISIONS/RED FLAGS

Patients with Scheuermann kyphosis or any type of congenital kyphotic deformity require further evaluation.

# Legg-Calvé-Perthes Disease

ICD-9 Code

732.1
   Juvenile osteochondrosis of hip and
   pelvis

## Synonyms

Idiopathic osteonecrosis of the femoral head
Avascular necrosis of the femoral head
Aseptic necrosis of the femoral head

## Definition

Legg-Calvé-Perthes disease (LCPD) is idiopathic osteonecrosis of the femoral head in children. LCPD typically affects children between the ages of 4 and 8 years, but the range of onset is 2 to 12 years of age. It is unilateral in 90% of patients, four times more common in boys, and uncommon in blacks. The prognosis is worse in older children and in those who have more severe involvement (ie, greater degree of osteonecrosis).

After the bone dies and loses structural integrity, the articular surface of the femoral head may collapse, leading to deformity and arthritis. However, because bone repair is relatively rapid in children, the prognosis in LCPD is significantly better when compared with adults who develop osteonecrosis of the femoral head.

## Clinical symptoms

Typically, the child has been limping for 3 to 6 weeks at the initial visit. Activity worsens the limp, making symptoms more noticeable at the end of the day. If the child reports pain, it is typically an aching in the groin or proximal thigh.

## Tests

### Physical examination

Examination reveals mild to moderate restriction of hip motion. Abduction, in particular, is limited and typically measures 20° to 30° compared with 60° to 70° on the uninvolved side. However, limited abduction may not be apparent unless movement of the pelvis is recognized. Examine abduction by placing one hand on the opposite pelvis and using the other hand to abduct the hip. The degree of abduction is recorded when the pelvis starts to move or tilt. Another technique is to align the pelvis in neutral and abduct (spread) both extremities.

### Diagnostic tests

AP and frog-lateral radiographs of the pelvis should be obtained. Increased density of the femoral head is an early sign of LCPD. The crescent sign indicates that a shear fracture has occurred in the subchondral bone (**Figure 1**). In the early stage of LCPD, plain radiographs may be normal, and MRI may be necessary to demonstrate the osteonecrosis. In a child with bilateral

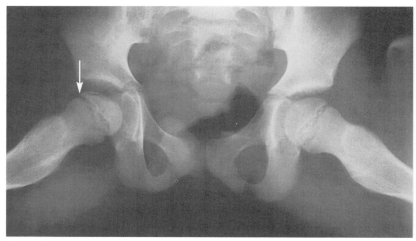

**Figure 1**
A 7-year-old boy with a 2-month history of right hip pain. The subchondral fracture (arrow) is through 75% of the femoral head.

*Reproduced with permission from Beaty JH: Legg-Calvé-Perthes disease: Diagnostic and prognostic techniques, in Barr JS (ed): Instructional Course Lectures 38. Park Ridge, IL, American Academy of Orthopaedic Surgeons, 1989, pp 291–296.*

involvement, screening AP radiographs of the hand and knee are needed to rule out epiphyseal dysplasia or thyroid disease.

## DIFFERENTIAL DIAGNOSIS

Atypical septic arthritis (increasing pain and constitutional symptoms)

Gaucher disease (osteonecrosis secondary to cerebroside and infarcts)

Hypothyroidism (delayed development)

Multiple epiphyseal dysplasia (bilateral, mild short stature, autosomal dominant)

Sickle cell anemia (osteonecrosis secondary to vascular infarcts)

Spondyloepiphyseal dysplasia (bilateral, marked short stature)

Stickler syndrome (bilateral, short stature)

Transient synovitis (pain more noticeable in the morning)

## ADVERSE OUTCOMES OF THE DISEASE

Residual deformity of the femoral head may progress to osteoarthritis of the hip; however, the onset of severe arthritic symptoms varies ranging from adolescence to the geriatric years. The latter is obviously more common and preferred.

## TREATMENT

The physiology of the healing process in LCPD involves revascularization of the femoral head, removal of necrotic bone, and replacement with viable bone that is initially relatively weak (woven bone) and remodeling of woven bone to the normal lamellar bone. While this process occurs more rapidly and with greater consistency in children, it is still a biologic phenomenon that requires many months. Unfortunately, no current interventions accelerate this process.

Furthermore, no treatment modality consistently produces good outcomes or prevents deformity of the femoral head.

Observation may be acceptable for children who are unlikely to develop significant deformity. Therefore, observation is commonly indicated for children younger than age 6 years who do not exhibit significant subluxation and who maintain at least 40° to 45° of abduction. Older children who have no involvement of the lateral portion of the femoral head also may be observed.

The principal reason for treatment with an abduction brace is to contain the femoral head within the acetabulum, thus maintaining the femoral head in as much of a spherical state as possible. An abduction brace that extends only to the distal thigh does not alter the natural history of severe LCPD in children who are ≥ 6 years of age. As a general rule, osteotomy is reserved for older children. Note that none of these treatment modalities completely contains the femoral head during all phases of gait.

Before any treatment is initiated, motion must be regained. A short period of bed rest and traction is commonly required. The abduction brace is generally worn all day and is discontinued when the lateral portion of the femoral head has regenerated, a process that generally takes 12 to 18 months.

## ADVERSE OUTCOMES OF TREATMENT

No improvement in natural history, postoperative infection, and limb-length discrepancy are all possible.

## REFERRAL DECISIONS/RED FLAGS

Children younger than age 6 years who have significant involvement of the femoral head or less than 40° of abduction require further evaluation. Children age 6 years or older require further evaluation.

# METATARSUS ADDUCTUS

ICD-9 Code
754.53
    Metatarsus varus

## SYNONYM
Metatarsus varus

## DEFINITION
Metatarsus adductus is a common congenital deformity characterized by medial deviation (adduction) of the forefoot (**Figure 1**). In one prospective study, the deformity was observed in 13% of full-term infants. Metatarsus adductus often resolves spontaneously, but it may persist.

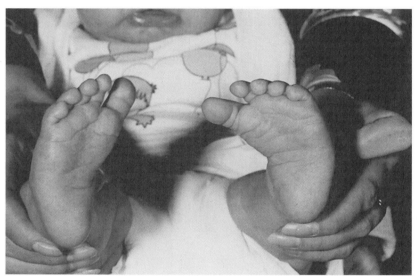

**Figure 1**
Three-month-old infant with obvious metatarsus adductus. The foot appears to be supinated; however, when the foot was placed in a weight-bearing position, the hind-foot alignment was normal.

*Reproduced with permission from Greene WB: Metatarsus adductus and skewfoot, in Schafer M (ed): Instructional Course Lectures 43. Rosemont, IL, American Academy of Orthopaedic Surgeons, 1994, pp 161–177.*

## CLINICAL SYMPTOMS
Symptoms are absent during infancy. Parental concern typically initiates evaluation.

## TESTS
### PHYSICAL EXAMINATION
The most striking feature is convexity of the lateral border of the foot. The hindfoot is in neutral or increased valgus and never demonstrates a varus posture. Normal ankle dorsiflexion is also present. These latter two findings are important because some children with severe metatarsus adductus may, at first inspection, appear to have a clubfoot deformity.

The severity of metatarsus adductus can be assessed using the heel bisector line (**Figure 2**). Normally, a line bisecting the heel crosses the forefoot between the second and third toes. Metatarsus adductus is considered mild when the heel bisector crosses the third toe, moderate when the heel bisector goes between the third and fourth toes, and severe when the heel bisector crosses between the fourth and fifth toes. Flexibility of the forefoot should be assessed, and perhaps the simplest criteria is to define a flexible foot as one in which the second toe can easily be brought in line with the heel bisector.

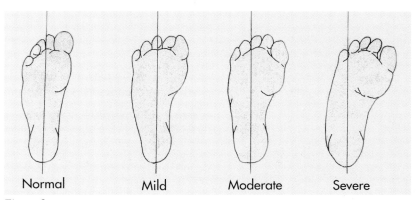

**Figure 2**
Classification of metatarsus adductus as described by Bleck.

*Reproduced with permission from Bleck EE: Metatarsus adductus: Classification and relationship to all kinds of treatment. J Pediatr Orthop 1983;3:2–9.*

## DIAGNOSTIC TESTS

Radiographs are rarely needed, but stress views can be useful in differentiating this condition from an atypical clubfoot. Obtaining serial photocopies of the foot is a low-cost, no-risk method of charting the progression of metatarsus adductus (**Figure 3**).

## DIFFERENTIAL DIAGNOSIS

Cavus foot (high arch, heel in varus)

Clubfoot (heel in varus, ankle in equinus)

Hyperactive abductor hallucis ("monkey toe," lateral border of the foot straight)

Internal tibial torsion (foot rotated in; lateral border of the foot straight)

Skeletal dysplasia (most common in diastrophic dwarfism)

Skewfoot (Z or serpentine foot; valgus hindfoot and midfoot, severe forefoot adduction)

## ADVERSE OUTCOMES OF THE DISEASE

Abnormal shoe wear and subsequent discomfort with prolonged standing are possible. Some children are emotionally stressed when teased about their foot alignment.

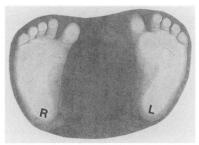

**Figure 3**
Photocopy of feet of a 9-month-old infant with bilateral metatarsus adductus.

*Reproduced with permission from Greene WB: Metatarsus adductus and skewfoot, in Schafer M (ed): Instructional Course Lectures 43. Rosemont, IL, American Academy of Orthopaedic Surgeons, 1994, pp 161–177.*

# Treatment

Most newborns are not treated, although parents are advised to avoid positioning the infant prone with the feet turned in, a position that accentuates metatarsus adductus. Because metatarsus adductus corrects spontaneously in most children, the decision to begin treatment may be delayed until the infant is 6 months old; however, it is reasonable to initiate treatment earlier if the deformity is severe and inflexible.

Stretching exercises done by the parents, and the use of nighttime splints or outflare shoes, have not been proved effective. The reports advocating these modalities have included younger patients whose metatarsus adductus may have resolved spontaneously.

Serial casting is the gold standard of nonoperative management, and if started at age 6 to 9 months, has a high degree of success. Casts are applied for 2-week periods, and usually three or four casts will suffice. Casting can be successful in children ages 1 to 3 years, but at these ages, casting is more difficult and is associated with a higher rate of failure. The cast should be applied in a manner that molds the forefoot into abduction without accentuating heel valgus. A long leg cast is probably more effective.

Operative treatment has limited indications.

# Adverse outcomes of treatment

Recurrent deformity may occur despite serial casting. Exacerbating heel valgus while casting may result in development of a severe flatfoot or skewfoot deformity. Degenerative changes at the tarsometatarsal joints have been noted after a complete tarsometatarsal surgical release. Damage to the physis of the first metatarsal and subsequent shortening of that bone is the unique complication of correcting metatarsus adductus by metatarsal osteotomies.

# Referral decisions/Red flags

Residual metatarsus adductus in an infant age 6 months or a rigid metatarsus adductus in an infant older than age 3 months signals the need for further evaluation.

# NEONATAL BRACHIAL PLEXUS PALSY

### ICD-9 Code
767.6
  Injury to brachial plexus

## SYNONYM
Obstetrical palsy

## DEFINITION
Neonatal brachial plexus palsy, sometimes called obstetrical palsy, is a motor and sensory deficit of the upper extremity that results from a stretch injury to the brachial plexus during labor and delivery. Three patterns of palsy may occur: Erb palsy, Klumpke palsy, and pan plexus palsy. Erb palsy is most common and is defined as a lesion involving the upper portion of the brachial plexus. An Erb palsy primarily affecting C5 and C6 results in weakness of elbow flexion and weakness of shoulder abduction, flexion, and external rotation. If the Erb palsy includes C7, then wrist flexion and elbow extension also are affected. Klumpke palsy is a lesion of the lower plexus that affects primarily the hand and wrist. Pan plexus palsy is involvement of the entire plexus.

The injury can range from a minor stretch of the nerves to a partial or complete rupture of the nerve substance or to an avulsion of the nerve root from the spinal cord. Prognosis for neurologic recovery depends on the severity of the injury. With a mild injury, nerve signal transmission is interrupted temporarily, but the nerve structure itself is not disrupted. Recovery is complete with this type of injury.

The prognosis is poorer with disruption of nerve substance (ie, axon, sheath, or supporting connective tissue), and these infants are likely to have some degree of permanent impairment. Most patients have a "mixed" lesion, with different nerve branches having different degrees of neural disruption.

## CLINICAL SYMPTOMS
Irritability in the supraclavicular triangle may be present during the first few weeks after birth.

## TESTS
### PHYSICAL EXAMINATION
Examination findings vary depending on the pattern of nerve injury and include diminished movement and sensation in the upper extremity. Initially, the upper extremity appears to be flail. The classic appearance of a neonate with Erb palsy is the "head waiter's tip" position (ie, shoulder adducted and internally rotated, elbow extended, forearm pronated, and wrist flexed) (Figure 1). A Horner sign can appear in lower plexus lesions. Phrenic nerve paralysis occurs in approximately 5% of patients.

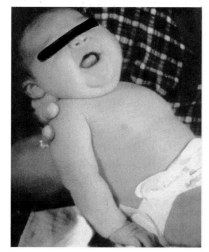

**Figure 1**
Typical posture of child with Erb palsy.

Repeated examinations of muscle and sensory function are needed to correlate the physical findings with an anatomic location of injury and to assess the degree and rate of neurologic recovery. Failure to recover muscle balance results in contractures and limited motion, particularly at the shoulder and elbow.

### DIAGNOSTIC TESTS

Radiographs should be ordered if results of physical examination suggest a fracture of the clavicle or humerus. If the infant does not recover full function, electromyography and nerve conduction velocity studies may help guide decision making for surgical options. These studies are best obtained by the surgeon who can direct specific questions to the electromyographer.

## DIFFERENTIAL DIAGNOSIS

Clavicle fracture (tenderness and deformity on palpation, pain on passive range of motion, possible pseudoparalysis)

Humerus fracture (swelling, deformity, and pain with range of motion of the arm, possible pseudoparalysis)

Proximal humeral osteomyelitis (cessation of normal motion, but infant may not appear toxic)

Septic shoulder joint (cessation of normal motion, but infant may not appear toxic)

## ADVERSE OUTCOMES OF THE DISEASE

The prognosis varies depending on the severity of the neurologic injury. A good prognosis correlates with early spontaneous recovery of function. Joint contractures and limited motion develop if the patient has significant muscle weakness. In children with Erb palsy, muscle imbalance also can result in posterior dislocation of the shoulder and/or radial head instability.

## TREATMENT

Initial treatment consists of a 3-month program designed to rest and then stretch the muscles while awaiting spontaneous recovery. During the first month, management focuses on protecting the injured extremity. Careful examination and documentation of the initial functional deficit allow for an accurate assessment of the amount and timing of later recovery. After the first month, gentle passive range of motion is needed several times a day to stretch the strong muscles and to move the joints through a full range of motion. Special attention to external rotation of the shoulder with the flexed elbow at the side will help prevent posterior subluxation of the shoulder.

During the third month, the infant should be reexamined to document recovery of muscle function. Additional evaluation is appropriate at this time for those infants who do not recover palpable function in all muscle groups.

No single treatment predictably restores full function. Therefore, accurate assessment of the level and severity of injury, prevention of secondary deformity, and a plan to optimize recovery and ultimately the functional outcome for the child are the cornerstones of treatment.

Recent advances in intraoperative electrodiagnostic testing and microsurgical techniques have led to a greater interest in early operative treatment. The dilemma is that some spontaneous recovery will be sacrificed if surgery is done too early, but a longer period of observation may compromise potential results. Furthermore, there is no true repair of these lesions, and the neural reconstruction is a complex process of nerve grafts and nerve transfers. Determining whether an early operation alters the natural history of recovery, and which procedure is best, is difficult to measure and is still being assessed.

Early plexus surgery is an option for certain carefully evaluated infants because it may improve the level of ultimate recovery. An infant who has plateaued in recovery without regaining palpable elbow flexion, shoulder abduction, or external rotation by age 4 to 6 months should be considered for plexus exploration. An infant who has a pan plexus palsy has a poor prognosis for recovery of hand function and should be considered for plexus exploration even earlier than 4 to 6 months.

Children ages 2 to 4 years with significant muscle imbalance about the shoulder, elbow, and hand should undergo appropriate muscle releases and tendon transfers to provide a balanced upper extremity. Earlier procedures may be indicated if shoulder dislocation or significant contracture occurs.

## ADVERSE OUTCOMES OF TREATMENT

Neurologic deficit may not improve after operative treatment. Bony deformities can develop and progress despite tendon transfers. Diminished overall growth potential of the extremity may occur.

## REFERRAL DECISIONS/RED FLAGS

If full recovery does not occur within 3 to 4 months, further evaluation is recommended. Sepsis or skeletal trauma (child abuse) must be suspected if there is sudden loss of function in an extremity that moved well at birth.

# OSGOOD-SCHLATTER DISEASE

ICD-9 Code

732.4
Osgood-Schlatter disease

## SYNONYM

Osteochondritis of the tibial tuberosity

## DEFINITION

Osgood-Schlatter disease (or condition) results from repetitive injury and small avulsion injuries at the bone-tendon junction of the patellar tendon insertion into the secondary ossification center of the tibial tuberosity, which is a weak link to repetitive quadriceps contraction. Onset during early adolescence coincides with development of this secondary ossification center. Overuse explains the fivefold greater incidence in patients who are active in sports and the two to three times greater incidence in boys.

## CLINICAL SYMPTOMS

Patients report pain that is exacerbated by running, jumping, and kneeling activities. Pain also can occur after prolonged sitting with the knees flexed.

## TESTS

### PHYSICAL EXAMINATION

Examination reveals tenderness and swelling at the insertion of the patellar tendon into the tibial tubercle. Osgood-Schlatter disease may be bilateral, but one side is typically more symptomatic. Although knee motion usually is not restricted, kneeling is painful during the acute phase. The knee and patellofemoral joint are stable.

### DIAGNOSTIC TESTS

AP and lateral radiographs of the knee may be normal or show soft-tissue swelling and small spicules of heterotopic ossification anterior to the tibial tuberosity (**Figure 1**). When a patient has bilateral symptoms, radiographs are rarely needed but should be obtained with unilateral involvement to rule out tumors.

## DIFFERENTIAL DIAGNOSIS

Infection (rare, elevated erythrocyte sedimentation rate)

Neoplasm (rare, unilateral)

Sinding-Larsen-Johansson syndrome (similar overuse condition at the inferior pole of the patella, most commonly affects 9- to 11-year-old boys)

## ADVERSE OUTCOMES OF THE DISEASE

The long-term prognosis for patients who undergo nonoperative treatment is good, with minimal adult disability. Some residual prominence of the tibial

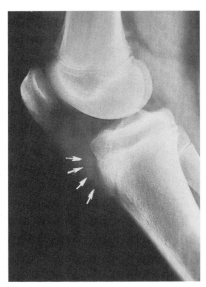

**Figure 1**
Symptomatic tibial tubercle ossicle (arrows) in a 13-year-old boy.

*Reproduced with permission from Stanitski CL: Knee overuse disorders in the pediatric and adolescent athlete, in Heckman JD (ed): Instructional Course Lectures 42. Rosemont, IL, American Academy of Orthopaedic Surgeons, 1993, pp 483–495.*

tubercle is common, particularly in patients who have fragmentation of the epiphysis and heterotopic ossification during the active phase of the disease. In one long-term study, 76% of patients reported no limitation of activity, 18% had tenderness that was similar to but not as painful as the original condition, and the remaining 6% had anterior knee pain but no symptoms referable to the tibial tuberosity. On directed questioning, 60% of patients reported discomfort when kneeling, but this was not typically perceived as a disability.

## TREATMENT

Symptoms are often controlled adequately with intermittent use of ice after sports, coupled with occasional use of NSAIDs, and use of a protective knee pad. Decreasing activity to permit healing of the microscopic avulsion fractures is the key to treating severe symptoms.

Occasionally, immobilization is needed for severe or recalcitrant symptoms. This usually can be accomplished with a prefabricated knee immobilizer that is removed once a day for bathing and range-of-motion exercises.

If the patient is a competitive athlete, the parents and patient will need to understand the duration that sports activities may be affected. In one study of highly competitive athletes affected by Osgood-Schlatter disease, the sport had to be discontinued for an average of 2 to 3 months, and fully effective training was not possible for an average of 6 to 7 months.

Operative treatment is not commonly needed and with rare exceptions should be limited to patients who have persistent symptoms after growth is completed. At that time, excision of heterotopic ossification and the prominence of the tibial tuberosity will usually relieve discomfort and aching after running activities.

## ADVERSE OUTCOMES OF TREATMENT

These are the same as the adverse outcomes of the disease.

## REFERRAL DECISIONS/RED FLAGS

Unilateral pain at rest or pain not directly over the tibial tubercle should raise concerns of a neoplastic or another disorder.

# OSTEOMYELITIS

ICD-9 Codes

730.00
    Acute osteomyelitis, site
    unspecified
731.00
    Chronic osteomyelitis, site
    unspecified

## DEFINITION

Osteomyelitis is an infection in bone that is usually bacterial in origin. In children, osteomyelitis usually develops as a result of hematogenous seeding but can be secondary to direct contamination (eg, open fracture, nail puncture wound).

The metaphysis of long bones is the most common location of osteomyelitis in children. This is because the circulation is sluggish at the metaphyseal-physeal barrier, where small vessels are required to make a "U-turn." Untreated, the infection spreads through the medullary canal and penetrates the metaphyseal cortex causing a subperiosteal abscess. The growth plate usually is not penetrated.

Acute osteomyelitis presents within 2 weeks of disease onset and is the main focus of this chapter.

Subacute osteomyelitis is a more balanced response between host and organism that results in a quasi-contained lesion in the bone and typically presents after 1 month to several months. The diagnosis is often delayed because symptoms are often vague and other findings such as fever and abnormal laboratory studies are not remarkable. There are two types of subacute osteomyelitis. Cavitary subacute osteomyelitis occurs in the epiphysis or metaphysis and is characterized by a small, localized area of radiolucency surrounded by reactive bone. In cavitary osteomyelitis, cultures are often negative and similar to diskitis. Initial treatment may be a 6-week trial of oral antibiotics. The second type of subacute osteomyelitis simulates a neoplastic process and, therefore, mandates a biopsy with or without debridement. These lesions typically are in the diaphysis but also may be metaphyseal. Periosteal elevation and cortical thickening are the early radiographic signs.

Chronic osteomyelitis also is typically of 1 month's to several months' duration and is characterized by necrotic bone harboring bacteria (sequestrum).

## CLINICAL SYMPTOMS

Pain, swelling, tenderness, erythema, increased localized warmth, and generalized malaise are associated with acute osteomyelitis. When the lower extremity, pelvis, or spine is involved, refusal to walk or limping is an early symptom, particularly in a young child. Pseudoparalysis (failure to use a limb despite normal neuromuscular structures) is observed when the upper extremity is affected.

# TESTS

## PHYSICAL EXAMINATION

An elevated temperature of 100.4°F (38°C) or higher is typical but not always present. Tenderness is common in the involved region. Motion of the adjacent joint may be limited, but not to the degree observed in septic arthritis. Other sites of infection such as cellulitis and septic arthritis should be investigated.

## DIAGNOSTIC TESTS

Laboratory studies should include a CBC with differential and erythrocyte sedimentation rate, as these tests confirm an inflammatory process and are parameters in monitoring response to treatment. A C-reactive protein is a better test for monitoring early response to treatment, but whether this study is helpful at diagnosis is unclear. Neonates and children who are seen early in the disease process may not have an abnormal WBC, elevated erythrocyte sedimentation rate, or significant fever. A blood culture should be obtained, as it will identify the infecting organism in 40% to 50% of patients.

AP and lateral radiographs of the suspected area are necessary. Early in the disease process, radiographs are normal or show only soft-tissue swelling, but negative radiographs help in ruling out a fracture or neoplastic process. Seven to 10 days after the onset of symptoms, osseous changes are apparent and include periosteal elevation and/or destruction of bone with areas of radiolucency and no surrounding reactive bone.

Although not often needed in acute osteomyelitis, MRI or a bone scan should be considered in unclear situations. MRI is more definitive but more expensive. Ultrasound may show an area of periosteal elevation and provide direction for aspiration.

Aspiration should be done if the area of potential bone involvement is identified, the site is accessible, and a neoplastic process has been ruled out. A 20-gauge or larger bore needle and syringe should be used to obtain the specimen. Positive results can confirm the diagnosis, and the specimen can help guide antibiotic therapy through evaluation of a Gram stain and the subsequent results of culture.

# DIFFERENTIAL DIAGNOSIS

Acute leukemia (indolent onset, diffuse tenderness, night pain)

Acute rheumatic fever (migratory arthralgia)

Cellulitis (erythema and swelling of subcutaneous tissues)

Langerhan cell histiocytosis (pain, "hole in a bone" appearance)

Malignant bone tumors (Ewing sarcoma most often simulates osteomyelitis)

Septic arthritis (joint swelling and severe restriction of motion)

# ADVERSE OUTCOMES OF THE DISEASE

Growth disturbance and limb-length discrepancy, chronic osteomyelitis, destruction of adjacent joints, pathologic fracture, and bone defects leading to limb dysfunction are possible.

# TREATMENT

Intravenous antibiotic should be started immediately after obtaining initial diagnostic tests and cultures. *Staphylococcus aureus* is the most common pathogen, and antibiotic selection should cover that possibility in all age groups. Group B streptococci and enteric rod organisms also should be covered in neonates. In children ages 6 months to 4 years, *Haemophilus influenzae* is also covered if vaccination is incomplete.

Surgical drainage is needed more often when the patient is seen approximately 4 to 7 days after onset, or when symptoms and fever persist despite antibiotic therapy. Surgery for acute osteomyelitis consists primarily of drainage of the subperiosteal abscess. In chronic osteomyelitis, resection of necrotic and avascular tissue is required.

The typical course of antibiotics is 6 weeks but may be longer depending on clinical response and laboratory values. The indication and time to switch from intravenous to oral antibiotics is controversial at present, but an early change to oral medication (after up to 7 days of intravenous therapy) is feasible in many patients, particularly those who present early.

Immobilization of the affected bone decreases pain and should continue for 3 weeks or more to assist the healing process and protect against pathologic fracture. The bone is weaker not only from osseous destruction, but the woven bone that is initially formed in the healing process does not have the same strength as lamellar bone.

Osteomyelitis secondary to nail puncture wounds usually is caused by *Pseudomonas aeruginosa*. This infection requires operative debridement and antibiotic therapy for 2 to 3 weeks. Failure to debride this infection adequately can lead to chronic osteomyelitis that is difficult to eradicate. A shorter course of antibiotics may be acceptable if the contaminated area is small and can be aggressively debrided.

## ADVERSE OUTCOMES OF TREATMENT

These are the same as the adverse outcomes of the disease.

## REFERRAL DECISIONS/RED FLAGS

A team approach provides the best management of osteomyelitis.

# Pediatric Sport Participation

Sports participation during childhood offers a number of potential benefits that lead to lifelong habits of fitness. Children develop specific skills, learn the importance of teamwork, acquire leadership skills, and develop confidence. All of these attributes result in improved self-esteem. Physical activity also provides an appropriate outlet for releasing stress.

Organized sports also are associated with some potential disadvantages, such as an overemphasis on winning, burnout, and injuries. Adults who lead children's sports activities sometimes forget that sports should be for the child and should be fun.

Children are more heat sensitive than adults and tend to be inadequately hydrated. Therefore, practices should be scheduled during the cooler hours of the day, and adequate amounts of fluids that children like to drink should be readily available and encouraged.

## Readiness for sports participation

Overall readiness must be based on the individual child and his or her eagerness to participate, not the parents' desire. A variety of sport activities should be offered and the child allowed to choose.

The attrition rate for youth sport participation is 35% annually. Many athletes drop out because of burnout, not being able to participate, or because they are not matched to their level of skill.

Motor development in infants and toddlers is limited, but aquatic programs for infants and toddlers are popular. A recent policy statement developed by the American Academy of Pediatrics noted that children generally are not developmentally ready for swimming lessons until after their fourth birthday and that aquatic programs for infants and toddlers have not been shown to decrease the risk of drowning.

Children 3 to 5 years of age have developed the fundamental skills of crawling, walking, jumping, and running. Vision, however, is relatively imprecise. Children at this age have difficulty tracking moving objects. Therefore, "keeping their eye on the ball" will be difficult. Furthermore, children in this age group have very short attention spans and are egocentric in their learning. Appropriate activities for this age include running, tumbling, throwing, and swimming, but team and competitive sports are inappropriate.

Children between the ages of 6 and 10 years begin transitional skill development. Prior to this age they could throw, but now they are ready to work on accuracy. Some children at this age are very proficient; others are not. At about age 7 to 8 years, children begin to communicate and cooperate as a group effort; however, their attention span is still limited. Team sports in this group should be modified to ensure that practices are short and fun and that skills instruction is limited to 10 to 20 minutes. Include egocentric activities to practice the material taught. Modify the rules to stress high scoring and full participation.

Adolescents can develop complex sport skills that require execution of complex motor skills coupled with rapid decision making. Certainly for some children, waiting until adolescence to become involved in competitive sports that require complex skills and interactions, such as football, wrestling, hockey, and basketball, prevents the burnout that occurs when these sports are pushed on the child at an earlier age. Older children also have good learning skills and attention spans. Chalk talks and the like can be used with this group.

A comprehensive discussion of the many issues affecting the young athlete is beyond the scope of this text. The reader is referred to *Care of the Young Athlete*, a comprehensive text published jointly by the American Academy of Orthopaedic Surgeons and the American Academy of Pediatrics.

# Preparticipation Physical Evaluation

## Definition

Although it is not intended to substitute for a routine annual physical examination, the preparticipation physical evaluation (PPE) is often the only contact an older child or adolescent has with a physician. Therefore, this examination should be as comprehensive as possible.

The PPE has a number of goals, as listed below:

1. Identify conditions that would predispose children to serious injury or death.

2. Identify current medical or psychological conditions that could be worsened by exercise.

3. Diagnose previously undetected conditions.

4. Assess general health and risk-taking behaviors.

5. Satisfy school, state, and insurance requirements.

6. Assess fitness level and performance parameters (optional).

## Types of evaluations

One of two types of PPE is appropriate. The first is an examination by the athlete's personal physician. This is perhaps the preferred method; however, it is not always feasible because of lack of access, cost considerations, or time constraints. The second is the "station" method in which athletes move through several stations for different parts of the evaluation. This approach allows for large numbers of athletes to be evaluated in a short time at relatively little cost. Specialists are often available to expedite consultations, and coaches and athletic trainers usually are involved to help maintain order and facilitate communication.

A standard form can be used with either of these methods (**Figures 1** and **2**).

## Components of the PPE

### Timing and interval

Optimal timing for the PPE is 6 weeks prior to the beginning of the athletic season. This allows adequate time for further consultation, diagnostic testing, or rehabilitation of identified problems. Comprehensive evaluations should be performed at every new level of school (elementary school, middle school, high school), with either interval or comprehensive evaluations repeated annually.

## HISTORY

Most clinically relevant conditions should be uncovered during the medical history. Often the history given by adolescents is inaccurate or incomplete; therefore, parental input is desirable. Questions should emphasize symptoms related to the cardiovascular system, such as dizziness or syncope with exercise, chest pain, shortness of breath, palpitations, and fatigability. Use of a questionnaire often helps to ensure completeness and reminds athletes or parents of previous injuries and illnesses. Because many important cardiovascular conditions have a hereditary component, obtaining a family history also is critical. The family history should include details about any sudden death in a close relative prior to the age of 50 years, Marfan syndrome, long QT syndrome, or other significant cardiovascular conditions.

## PHYSICAL EXAMINATION

The examination component begins with a thorough general examination, including inspection for any of the physical signs of Marfan syndrome. Because evaluation of the cardiovascular system is key, heart rate and blood pressure measurements should be obtained and femoral pulses palpated. Precordial auscultation should be done with the athlete in both supine and standing positions in an effort to elucidate the murmur of hypertrophic cardiomyopathy. The physical examination also should include a musculoskeletal screening examination (**Figure 3**).

## DIAGNOSTIC TESTS

Routine screening radiographs and laboratory tests are not indicated. These tests should be ordered based on information solicited during the history and physical examination.

## REFERRAL DECISIONS/RED FLAGS

Any history of the following physical findings indicates the need for further evaluation and possible specialty consultation.

1. Early fatigue, dizziness, syncope, chest pain, shortness of breath, or palpitations with exercise

2. Family history of sudden death or significant cardiovascular condition

3. Physical signs of Marfan syndrome

4. Significant head or spinal injury

5. Best-corrected vision of less than 20/40 in either eye

6. Previous heat illness

7. Significant musculoskeletal problem or injury

Once the PPE has been completed, recommendations for unrestricted clearance, clearance after further evaluation or treatment, limited participation, or total restriction can be made. Often these decisions will be made together with the athlete, parents, and consultants. Guidelines for conditions referable to the cardiovascular system can be found in the 26th Bethesda Conference published in the *Journal of the American College of Cardiology*.

# Preparticipation Physical Evaluation

**HISTORY**

DATE OF EXAM _____

Name _____ Sex _____ Age _____ Date of birth _____

Grade ____ School _____ Sport(s) _____

Address _____ Phone _____

Personal physician _____

*In case of emergency, contact*

Name _____ Relationship _____ Phone (H) _____ (W) _____

---

**Explain "Yes" answers below.**
**Circle questions you don't know the answers to.**

| | Yes | No |
|---|---|---|
| 1. Have you had a medical illness or injury since your last check up or sports physical? | ☐ | ☐ |
| Do you have an ongoing or chronic illness? | ☐ | ☐ |
| 2. Have you ever been hospitalized overnight? | ☐ | ☐ |
| Have you ever had surgery? | ☐ | ☐ |
| 3. Are you currently taking any prescription or nonprescription (over-the-counter) medications or pills or using an inhaler? | ☐ | ☐ |
| Have you ever taken any supplements or vitamins to help you gain or lose weight or improve your performance? | ☐ | ☐ |
| 4. Do you have any allergies (for example, to pollen, medicine, food, or stinging insects)? | ☐ | ☐ |
| Have you ever had a rash or hives develop during or after exercise? | ☐ | ☐ |
| 5. Have you ever passed out during or after exercise? | ☐ | ☐ |
| Have you ever been dizzy during or after exercise? | ☐ | ☐ |
| Have you ever had chest pain during or after exercise? | ☐ | ☐ |
| Do you get tired more quickly than your friends do during exercise? | ☐ | ☐ |
| Have you ever had racing of your heart or skipped heartbeats? | ☐ | ☐ |
| Have you had high blood pressure or high cholesterol? | ☐ | ☐ |
| Have you ever been told you have a heart murmur? | ☐ | ☐ |
| Has any family member or relative died of heart problems or of sudden death before age 50? | ☐ | ☐ |
| Have you had a severe viral infection (for example, myocarditis or mononucleosis) within the last month? | ☐ | ☐ |
| Has a physician ever denied or restricted your participation in sports for any heart problems? | ☐ | ☐ |
| 6. Do you have any current skin problems (for example, itching, rashes, acne, warts, fungus, or blisters)? | ☐ | ☐ |
| 7. Have you ever had a head injury or concussion? | ☐ | ☐ |
| Have you ever been knocked out, become unconscious, or lost your memory? | ☐ | ☐ |
| Have you ever had a seizure? | ☐ | ☐ |
| Do you have frequent or severe headaches? | ☐ | ☐ |
| Have you ever had numbness or tingling in your arms, hands, legs, or feet? | ☐ | ☐ |
| Have you ever had a stinger, burner, or pinched nerve? | ☐ | ☐ |
| 8. Have you ever become ill from exercising in the heat? | ☐ | ☐ |
| 9. Do you cough, wheeze, or have trouble breathing during or after activity? | ☐ | ☐ |
| Do you have asthma? | ☐ | ☐ |
| Do you have seasonal allergies that require medical treatment? | ☐ | ☐ |

| | Yes | No |
|---|---|---|
| 10. Do you use any special protective or corrective equipment or devices that aren't usually used for your sport or position (for example, knee brace, special neck roll, foot orthotics, retainer on your teeth, hearing aid)? | ☐ | ☐ |
| 11. Have you had any problems with your eyes or vision? | ☐ | ☐ |
| Do you wear glasses, contacts, or protective eyewear? | ☐ | ☐ |
| 12. Have you ever had a sprain, strain, or swelling after injury? | ☐ | ☐ |
| Have you broken or fractured any bones or dislocated any joints? | ☐ | ☐ |
| Have you had any other problems with pain or swelling in muscles, tendons, bones, or joints? | ☐ | ☐ |

*If yes, check appropriate box and explain below.*

☐ Head    ☐ Elbow    ☐ Hip
☐ Neck    ☐ Forearm    ☐ Thigh
☐ Back    ☐ Wrist    ☐ Knee
☐ Chest    ☐ Hand    ☐ Shin/calf
☐ Shoulder    ☐ Finger    ☐ Ankle
☐ Upper arm    ☐ Foot

| | Yes | No |
|---|---|---|
| 13. Do you want to weigh more or less than you do now? | ☐ | ☐ |
| Do you lose weight regularly to meet weight requirements for your sport? | ☐ | ☐ |
| 14. Do you feel stressed out? | ☐ | ☐ |

15. Record the dates of your most recent immunizations (shots) for:

Tetanus _____  Measles _____
Hepatitis B _____  Chickenpox _____

**FEMALES ONLY**

16. When was your first menstrual period? _____
When was your most recent menstrual period? _____
How much time do you usually have from the start of one period to the start of another? _____
How many periods have you had in the last year? _____
What was the longest time between periods in the last year? _____

**Explain "Yes" answers here:** _____
_____
_____
_____
_____
_____
_____
_____
_____
_____
_____
_____

---

**I hereby state that, to the best of my knowledge, my answers to the above questions are complete and correct.**

Signature of athlete _____ Signature of parent/guardian _____ Date _____

© 1997 *American Academy of Family Physicians, American Academy of Pediatrics, American Medical Society for Sports Medicine, American Orthopaedic Society for Sports Medicine, and American Osteopathic Academy of Sports Medicine.*

**Figure 1**
Preparticipation physical evaluation form: history questionnaire.

# Preparticipation Physical Evaluation

PHYSICAL EXAMINATION

Name _____ Date of birth _____

Height _____ Weight _____ % Body fat (optional) _____ Pulse _____ BP___/____ (___/___ , ___/___)

Vision R 20/ _____ L 20/ _____    Corrected: Y  N    Pupils: Equal _____ Unequal _____

|  | NORMAL | ABNORMAL FINDINGS | INITIALS* |
|---|---|---|---|
| **MEDICAL** | | | |
| Appearance | | | |
| Eyes/Ears/Nose/Throat | | | |
| Lymph Nodes | | | |
| Heart | | | |
| Pulses | | | |
| Lungs | | | |
| Abdomen | | | |
| Genitalia (males only) | | | |
| Skin | | | |
| **MUSCULOSKELETAL** | | | |
| Neck | | | |
| Back | | | |
| Shoulder/arm | | | |
| Elbow/forearm | | | |
| Wrist/hand | | | |
| Hip/thigh | | | |
| Knee | | | |
| Leg/ankle | | | |
| Foot | | | |

* Station-based examination only

CLEARANCE

❑ **Cleared**

❑ **Cleared after completing evaluation/rehabilitation for:** _____

_____

_____

_____

❑ **Not cleared for:** _____ **Reason:** _____

**Recommendations:** _____

_____

_____

_____

**Name of physician (print/type)** _____ **Date** _____

**Address** _____ **Phone** _____

**Signature of physician** _____ **, MD or DO**

© 1997 *American Academy of Family Physicians, American Academy of Pediatrics, American Medical Society for Sports Medicine, American Orthopaedic Society for Sports Medicine, and American Osteopathic Academy of Sports Medicine.*

Figure 2
Preparticipation physical evaluation form: physical examination record.

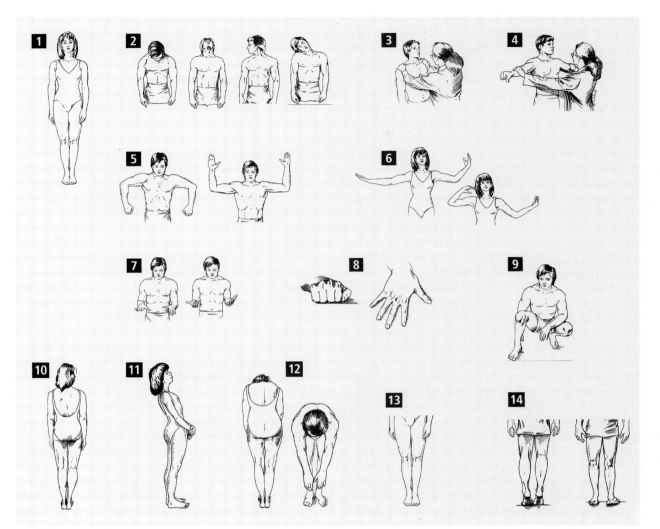

**Figure 3**

1. Inspection, athlete standing, facing toward examiner (symmetry of trunk, upper extremities);

2. Forward flexion, extension, rotation, lateral flexion of neck (range of motion, cervical spine);

3. Resisted shoulder shrug (strength, trapezius);

4. Resisted shoulder abduction (strength, deltoid);

5. Internal and external rotation of shoulder (range of motion, gleno-humeral joint);

6. Extension and flexion of elbow (range of motion, elbow);

7. Pronation and supination of elbow (range of motion, elbow and wrist);

8. Clench fist, then spread fingers (range of motion, hand and fingers);

9. "Duck walk" four steps (motion of hip, knee, and ankle; strength; balance);

10. Inspection, athlete facing away from examiner (symmetry of trunk, upper extremities);

11. Back extension, knees straight (spondylolysis/ spondylolisthesis);

12. Back flexion with knees straight, facing toward and away from examiner (range of motion, thoracic and lumbosacral spine; spine curvature; hamstring flexibility);

13. Inspection of lower extremeties, contraction of quadriceps muscles (alignment, symmetry);

14. Standing on toes, then on heels (symmetry, calf; strength; balance).

*Figures 2.1-2.9 and 2.11-2.14 © Rebekah Dodson; Figure 2.10 © Terry Boles.*

Guidelines for most other conditions are presented in the *Preparticipation Physical Evaluation* monograph published by the Physician and Sports Medicine, 4530 W. 77th Street, Minneapolis, MN 55435. To obtain a copy of this monograph, contact AAP Publications, 1-800-433-9016.

# SCOLIOSIS

## DEFINITION

Scoliosis is a lateral curvature of the spine of greater than 10°. The curve(s) can occur in the thoracic or lumbar spine (occasionally in both) and are associated with rotation of the vertebrae and sometimes with excessive kyphosis or lordosis. Idiopathic scoliosis is most common, but it can develop secondary to other problems (Table 1).

Table 1
### Etiologic Classification of Structural Scoliosis

| Type | Possible cause |
|---|---|
| Idiopathic | |
| Congenital | Failure of formation—hemivertebra <br> Failure of segmentation—bony bar joining one side of two or more adjacent vertebrae |
| Neuromuscular | Cerebral palsy <br> Muscular dystrophy <br> Myelomeningocele <br> Spinal muscular atrophy <br> Friedreich ataxia (spinocerebellar degeneration) |
| Vertebral disease | Tumor <br> Infection <br> Metabolic bone disease |
| Spinal cord disease or anomaly | Tumor <br> Syringomyelia |
| Disease associated | Neurofibromatosis <br> Marfan syndrome <br> Connective tissue disorders |

Idiopathic scoliosis usually develops in early adolescence. The male-to-female ratio is nearly equal in patients with curves of less than 20°. However, girls are seven times more likely than boys to have a significant, progressive curvature that requires treatment. Progression typically occurs in girls between the ages of 10 and 16 years.

## CLINICAL SYMPTOMS

Parents may notice that the child's clothes do not hang correctly. More commonly, the curvature is identified during a school screening program or routine examination. Pain is not characteristic in adolescents with idiopathic scoliosis. The presence of significant pain suggests another condition and requires further evaluation.

# TESTS

## PHYSICAL EXAMINATION

Mild degrees of scoliosis may not be apparent when the patient is standing. Findings such as uneven shoulder height or pelvic asymmetry are inaccurate in detecting mild degrees of scoliosis; such findings are often present in the absence of spinal curvature.

The forward bending test is the most sensitive clinical method of documenting the problem; this test accentuates the vertebral and rib rotational deformities that are part of the abnormality (**Figure 1**). Observe the back from behind as the patient bends forward with the feet together, knees straight, and the arms hanging free. Elevation of the rib cage and/or prominence of the lumbar paravertebral muscle mass on one side is a positive finding. The deformity can be quantified in degrees using an inclinometer such as the scoliometer. Inclinations of greater than 5° to 7° should be evaluated further.

The examination should include evaluation for other conditions associated with scoliosis. Assess the trunk and lower extremities for skin lesions, cavus feet, limb-length discrepancy, abnormal joint laxity, and, most importantly, neuromuscular abnormalities. Left-sided thoracic curvatures have a significant association with spinal cord abnormalities, and these patients require detailed evaluation and further diagnostic testing.

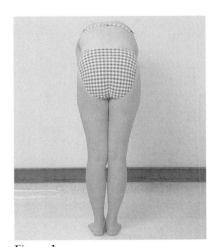

**Figure 1**
Forward bending test.

## DIAGNOSTIC TESTS

Posteroanterior and lateral full-length radiographs with the patient standing and the knees straight should be obtained. The x-ray tube should be positioned 6' from the cassette, a 14" × 36" grid. Positioning patients with their backs to the x-ray source and using modern image-enhancing equipment minimizes exposure of the breasts and gonads.

The Cobb angle is the standard method of quantifying the degree of curvature and is determined by measuring the intersecting angle of perpendiculars (congruent angle) to the upper end plate of the most superior and the lower end plate of the most inferior vertebrae in the curve (**Figure 2**). By convention, radiographs of the spine are viewed, measured, and described as if the patient were being examined from behind.

# DIFFERENTIAL DIAGNOSIS

See Table 1 for a list of differential diagnoses.

# ADVERSE OUTCOMES OF THE DISEASE

Progression of the curve is possible. If the curve is less than 50° at skeletal maturity, progression usually ceases. When an idiopathic thoracic curve is greater than 60°, progression in adulthood is common and can compromise respiratory function, although significant reduction in pulmonary function is unusual with a curve of less than 90° in an otherwise healthy individual. Back pain can occur in adulthood. In most patients, the back pain is not a major disability, but disabling pain is more likely to develop in patients who have decompensated lumbar or thoracolumbar curvatures.

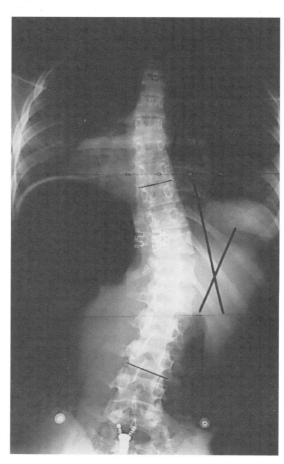

**Figure 2**
Posteroanterior radiograph of the entire spine on a long cassette demonstrating a scoliotic deformity and the Cobb method of measuring its magnitude.

## TREATMENT

Many idiopathic curves never progress to a degree that requires brace or operative treatment. Regular observation during adolescence is appropriate. The frequency of observation depends on the degree of curve and the amount of growth remaining (Table 2).

## Table 2
### Guidelines for Observation

|  | Premenarche | Postmenarche |
|---|---|---|
| Scoliometer < 5° | Recheck 3 months | Recheck 5 to 6 months |
| > 5° | Radiographs | Radiographs |
| Curve magnitude | Risser 0-2* | Risser 3-5* |
| < 20° | Recheck 3 months | Recheck 6 to 12 months |
| 20°–30° | Brace or recheck 3 months | Repeat radiograph 3 months |
| 30°–45° | Brace | Brace or repeat radiograph 3 months |

*Risser sign is progression of ossification of the iliac apophysis

Exercise therapy does not influence progression of scoliosis.

Brace treatment is reserved for patients with progressive curves in the range of 20° to 45°. The goal of bracing is to arrest progression; therefore, bracing is not necessary for curves that are unlikely to progress or when limited growth remains. Bracing also is ineffective for large curves even when several years of growth remain. Bracing is not always effective, even with a well-made orthosis and good patient compliance.

Surgery consisting of a spinal fusion is appropriate for idiopathic curves of greater than 50° or for curves of 40° to 50° that are likely to progress. Scoliosis of other etiologies is more likely to progress, and bracing and/or surgery may be advisable prior to reaching the guidelines for adolescent idiopathic scoliosis.

## ADVERSE OUTCOMES OF TREATMENT

The spinal curve may progress despite brace treatment, requiring operative intervention. Operative results can be adversely affected by infection, neurologic injury, or failure of the fusion mass to become solid. Regardless of the technique or instrumentation used, a solid bony fusion is the goal of any operative procedure.

## REFERRAL DECISIONS/RED FLAGS

Patients with an obvious curvature or mild scoliosis with more than 5° of inclination should be evaluated radiographically to document the degree of scoliosis and estimate the likelihood of progression. Patients with unusual findings—convex left thoracic curves, pain, abnormal neurologic findings, bowel or bladder dysfunction, or deformities of the feet—require further evaluation for other than an idiopathic etiology.

# SEPTIC ARTHRITIS

ICD-9 Code

711.0
Pyogenic arthritis

## SYNONYMS

Pyarthrosis

Infected joint

## DEFINITION

Joint infections are more common in children and develop as a result of either hematogenous seeding from sources such as respiratory infection or impetigo or by direct extension from penetrating wounds or an adjacent osteomyelitis. The latter occurs mostly in the hip. Septic arthritis typically affects the large joints of the lower extremities and occasionally the sacroiliac joint. As a result of the release of proteolytic enzymes from the bacteria, neutrophils, and other inflammatory cells, microscopic articular cartilage damage can be detected within 48 to 72 hours of inoculation.

## CLINICAL SYMPTOMS

Patients typically have an acute onset of guarding of the involved joint. The pain is often poorly localized initially. Children will frequently limp or stop walking or refuse to move the upper extremity (pseudoparalysis). Malaise, elevated temperature, and loss of appetite soon develop.

## TESTS

### PHYSICAL EXAMINATION

The patient typically appears ill at presentation. For comfort, the joint is held in a position that accommodates distention. The child is apprehensive and resists attempts to examine the affected extremity. An affected hip will be positioned in flexion, abduction, and external rotation, while an involved knee or elbow is positioned in slight flexion.

### DIAGNOSTIC TESTS

Any suspicion of joint infection requires immediate aspiration and analysis of the joint fluid. The results are corroborated with the findings on physical examination and results of other laboratory tests (Table 1).

Plain radiographs typically are not helpful in confirming an early diagnosis but are useful in excluding other disorders. Initial radiographs appear normal. Joint space widening, fat pad signs, and soft-tissue swelling develop later. Ultrasound can be useful, particularly in the hip, in the early screening for a joint effusion; however, this imaging study has a variety of technical limitations. Furthermore, the absence of joint effusion on ultrasound does not rule out a septic process.

## Table 1
### Typical Laboratory Results Associated with Septic Arthritis

| Condition | Erythrocyte sedimentation rate | Blood culture | Joint culture | Blood WBC | Joint WBC |
|---|---|---|---|---|---|
| Septic joint | 30 mm/h in most patients; gradual decrease unpredictable in neonates | Positive 30% to 40% | Positive 60% to 70% | 15,000/mm$^3$ (variable) often not elevated early | 20 to 250,000/mm$^3$ |
| Transient synovitis | < 20 mm/h (average 18) | Negative | Negative | Normal | Normal |
| Juvenile rheumatoid arthritis | Normal to 40 mm/h (average 25) | Negative | Negative | Normal | Variable |

## DIFFERENTIAL DIAGNOSIS

Acute leukemia (bone pain more common, less swelling of the joint)

Acute osteomyelitis (no significant joint effusion)

Juvenile rheumatoid arthritis (more gradual onset, less "sick" appearance)

Lyme disease (indolent onset)

Reactive arthritis (less severe pain and effusion)

Rheumatic fever (arthralgia, less effusion)

Transient synovitis (hip only, less "sick" appearance)

Traumatic hemarthrosis (history of trauma)

## ADVERSE OUTCOMES OF THE DISEASE

If untreated, septic arthritis invariably causes articular cartilage erosions, capsular scarring, and subsequent painful arthritis. Delay in treatment may result in secondary joint arthrosis developing later in life with associated joint stiffness and pain. Delay in treating septic arthritis of the hip joint in a young child can result in subluxation, dislocation, and/or osteonecrosis of the femoral head.

## TREATMENT

Prompt intravenous antibiotic administration and joint drainage is the treatment of choice. The selection of the initial antibiotic is based on the most likely infecting organism(s) (**Table 2**). Changes in treatment are based on results of culture studies (**Table 3**). If the infection is diagnosed early and is not severe, and if the joint can be decompressed by aspiration, then treatment by antibiotics alone may be satisfactory. Otherwise, surgical decompression is indicated. To minimize the risk of osteonecrosis, a septic hip joint requires prompt surgical drainage.

## Table 2
### Causative Organisms and Preferred Antibiotics for Septic Arthritis

| Organism | Typical age | Antibiotic |
|---|---|---|
| *Staphylococcus aureus* | All ages | Oxacillin |
| Group B streptococci | Neonate to 3 months | Ampicillin |
| Group A streptococci | 3 months to adolescence | Oxacillin |
| *Kingella kingae* | Neonate to 6 years | Cefotaxime |
| *Haemophilus influenzae* | Neonate to 3 months | Cefotaxime |
| Gram-negative coliforms | Neonate to 3 months | Ceftriaxone |
| Gonococcus | Adolescence | Ceftriaxone |

## Table 3
### Preferred Antibiotics Pending Culture Results

| Patient age | Antibiotic |
|---|---|
| Neonate | Oxacillin plus cefotaxime or gentamicin |
| Younger than 6 years old | Oxacillin plus cefotaxime |
| 6 years to adolescence | Oxacillin |
| Adolescence | Oxacillin plus ceftriaxone |

## ADVERSE OUTCOMES OF TREATMENT

The adverse outcomes of treatment have more to do with failure to diagnose and/or properly treat a septic joint. Surgical decompression must be done promptly and thoroughly. Failure to adequately debride the joint may prolong the duration of infection and/or increase the risk for recurrence. To be predictably effective, antibiotics must be selected based on culture reports or historic guidelines. Antibiotics must be delivered in therapeutic doses for an appropriate period of time (usually 2 to 3 weeks).

## REFERRAL DECISIONS/RED FLAGS

A team approach provides best management of septic arthritis in children. Joint aspiration and fluid analysis are essential in confirming the diagnosis.

# SERONEGATIVE SPONDYLOARTHROPATHIES

## SYNONYMS

Reiter syndrome

Ankylosing spondylitis

Psoriatic arthritis

## DEFINITION

The seronegative spondyloarthropathies have the following characteristics in common: 1) inflammation of tendon, fascia, or joint capsule insertions (enthesitis); 2) pauciarticular arthritis, usually involving the lower extremity; 3) extra-articular inflammation involving the eye, skin, mucous membranes, heart, and bowel; and 4) association with the HLA-B27 antigen.

## CLINICAL SYMPTOMS

Unlike that in adults, the onset of ankylosing spondylitis in children is more likely to affect the joints of the lower extremities. Asymmetric pauciarticular arthritis involving the lower extremity in children age 9 years or older, particularly in boys, should suggest the possibility of ankylosing spondylitis. The family history is often positive.

Reiter syndrome, with its triad of conjunctivitis, enthesitis, and urethritis, may be triggered in young children by infectious diarrhea caused by *Yersinia*, *Campylobacter*, *Salmonella*, or *Shigella*. In adolescents, nongonococcal urethritis secondary to *Chlamydia* or trachoma may cause Reiter syndrome. All three components of the disorder are not necessarily present in every patient, nor are they always present at the same time. The Achilles tendinitis or plantar fasciitis associated with Reiter syndrome can be extremely painful.

Psoriatic arthritis is considered uncommon in children, but approximately one third have the onset of this disorder before age 15 years, especially girls. Arthritis frequently antedates skin problems when this disorder occurs in childhood. A family history of psoriasis is a helpful clue when joint symptoms occur first.

Arthritis of inflammatory bowel disease, either ulcerative colitis or Crohn disease, typically causes symptoms before age 21 years, but only 15% of patients are diagnosed before age 15 years. Arthralgia without joint effusion is twice as common as arthritis with joint effusion.

## TESTS

### PHYSICAL EXAMINATION

A purplish discoloration may occur around the joint and is one of the distinguishing features of a juvenile spondyloarthropathy. Likewise, a child with ankylosing spondylitis may have an enthesitis, such as patellar tendinitis,

Achilles tendinitis, or plantar fasciitis. Although children with ankylosing spondylitis may not have back pain, limited mobility of the spine can be present.

Mild conjunctivitis or an acute anterior uveitis causing painful red eyes and photophobia also are associated with Reiter syndrome.

In psoriatic arthritis, monoarticular involvement of the knee is the most common presentation. Progression to other joints proceeds in an asymmetric fashion. Compared with other spondyloarthropathies, upper extremity involvement and tenosynovitis involving the digits and nail pits is more common in psoriatic arthritis.

Pauciarticular arthritis of the lower extremity in inflammatory bowel disease typically is of short duration and either resolves spontaneously or with treatment of the bowel lesion. However, progressive ankylosing spondylitis may develop in some patients.

## DIAGNOSTIC TESTS

The presence of the HLA-B27 antigen and a positive family history for spondyloarthropathy support the diagnosis of ankylosing spondylitis. Sterile pyuria supports the diagnosis of Reiter syndrome.

## DIFFERENTIAL DIAGNOSIS

Juvenile rheumatoid arthritis (often younger age at onset, upper extremity joint commonly affected, synovitis more impressive)

Various overuse syndromes (localized and more often unilateral)

## ADVERSE OUTCOMES OF THE DISEASE

Many lower extremity problems associated with the childhood spondyloarthropathies resolve spontaneously, but persistent erosive arthritis may develop. Ultimately, changes in the sacroiliac joint develop in children with ankylosing spondylitis.

## TREATMENT

NSAIDs, muscle strengthening, orthotics for the painful joint, and counseling about activity modifications are indicated.

## ADVERSE OUTCOMES OF TREATMENT

NSAIDs can cause gastric, renal, or hepatic complications.

## REFERRAL DECISIONS/RED FLAGS

Loss of function or inability to control pain indicates the need for further evaluation.

# SHOES FOR CHILDREN

A child's shoes were once considered an indicator of the family's economic status. A barefooted child suggested poverty and deprivation. Later the child's shoe became a focus of medical treatment. Many physicians thought that by modifying the child's shoes, lower limb deformity could be corrected and disability in later life prevented. During the past several decades, clinical studies have clarified the role shoes play in a child's life. The accumulated data are now sufficiently large to establish recommendations for children's footwear.

## NORMAL FOOT DEVELOPMENT

Clinical studies have consistently shown that the bare human foot has the following attributes: 1) excellent mobility; 2) thickening of the plantar skin to as much as 1 cm; 3) alignment of the phalanges with the metatarsals, causing the toes to spread; 4) variable arch height; and 5) an absence of most common foot deformities. These findings show that satisfactory foot development occurs in the barefoot environment.

Arch development has been documented in several studies. The arch develops spontaneously during a child's first 6 to 8 years, and the range of normal is very broad. About 15% of adults have flexible flatfeet, which are considered a variation of normal and typically are not associated with disability.

## EFFECTS OF SHOES ON THE FOOT

The primary role of shoes is to protect the foot. Indeed, if shoes are not fitted properly, toe deformities are likely to develop.

Wearing shoes does not affect how soon a child will begin to walk. Infants do well in stockings around the house. At this age, soft shoes may be used for appearance or to protect the foot when outside. Soft, flexible shoes are best for the toddler. If the toddler's foot is chubby, a high-top shoe can be helpful to keep the shoe on the foot, but this type of shoe does not affect the growth or development of the foot. High-top shoes also may be necessary in children with conditions that cause ligamentous laxity or hypotonia.

## CHARACTERISTICS OF A GOOD SHOE

For children, the features of a good shoe include the following:

Flexible. The shoe should allow as much free motion as possible. As a test, make certain that the shoe can be easily flexed in your hand.

Flat. Avoid high heels that force the foot forward, cramping the toes.

Foot-shaped. Avoid pointed toes or other shapes that are different from the normal foot.

Fitted generously. Better too large than too short. Allow about a finger-breadth of room for growth.

Friction like skin. The sole should have about the same friction as skin. Soles that are slippery or adherent can cause the child to fall.

## THE "CORRECTIVE" SHOE

The concept that shoes could be therapeutic appears to be based on the once widely accepted assumption that the growing foot needs support and could be molded by a corrective shoe. The assumption that external forces could correct deformity led to the development of various orthotic inserts and heel modifications. Although uncontrolled studies reported improvements with such devices, two controlled prospective studies on the effect of shoe modifications and arch development published in 1989 showed no difference between treated and untreated feet. In essence, shoe inserts do not modify or alter intoeing, outtoeing, or flexible flatfeet. In fact, shoe inserts can be harmful. Adults who wore shoe modifications as children often remember the experience as negative and, in one study, were shown to have lower self-esteem than control subjects.

Some shoe modifications are useful. These are not corrective but produce some immediately desirable effect: Shoe lifts for the short leg equalize limb length and improve walking. Shoe inserts for older children or adolescents with rigid foot deformities can redistribute weight-bearing forces and reduce discomfort or skin breakdown if sensation is impaired. Shock-absorbing footwear with cushioned soles can help in the management of overuse syndromes.

## CURRENT PROBLEMS

The design of shoes has improved over the past decade. Currently, the major problems in shoes affect girls. The prevalence of constrictive and deforming shoes for girls, including heel elevations, pointed toes, and tight fit, causes deformity (bunions) and instability, both of which increase the risk of ankle injuries.

## RECOMMENDATIONS

1. Shoes should be regarded as a form of clothing, designed to simulate the barefoot state.

2. Walking and playing barefooted in a safe environment is an acceptable alternative to wearing shoes for infants and children.

3. For most children, shoes should be flexible, flat, shaped like the foot, and have soles that provide friction similar to skin.

4. Cushioning of the sole can reduce the risk of overuse conditions around the foot.

5. Shoe modifications are not "corrective." Inserts are useful only for load redistribution and do not change the shape of the foot.

6. Physicians should promote public education about healthy footwear for children.

7. Prescribing unnecessary shoe inserts and modifications is expensive for the family and society. More importantly, these can be uncomfortable and embarrassing for the child.

# SLIPPED CAPITAL FEMORAL EPIPHYSIS

ICD-9 Code

732.2
Nontraumatic slipped upper
femoral epiphysis

## SYNONYM
Slipped epiphysis

## DEFINITION
Slipped capital femoral epiphysis (SCFE) is displacement of the femoral head through the physis that typically occurs during the adolescent growth spurt.

During adolescence, the orientation of the physis of the proximal femur changes from horizontal to oblique. That, coupled with the patient's increased body size, may cause intolerable shear at the relatively weak physis. The result is microscopic fractures and gradual slippage of the femoral head posteriorly and usually also medially. Occasionally, an acute event causes sudden displacement of the femoral head—in essence, a fracture or unstable slip.

Obesity, male gender, and greater involvement with sports activities are predisposing factors. Increased femoral retroversion also is a risk factor and probably explains the greater incidence of SCFE among blacks.

A small percentage of patients with SCFE have an endocrine disorder that alters the strength or growth of the physis. Hypothyroidism and growth hormone deficiency are most common, but SCFE also has been observed in panhypopituitarism, hyperthyroidism, and multiple endocrine neoplasia. Growth hormone deficiency usually is diagnosed before SCFE develops, but in children with hypothyroidism, SCFE often occurs before the endocrine disorder has been diagnosed.

The mean age at presentation is 12 years for girls (typical range: 10 to 14 years) and 13 years for boys (typical range: 11 to 16 years). Onset before or after the typical age range is associated with some type of endocrinopathy.

Bilateral involvement is more common than originally understood and is seen in 40% to 50% of patients who are followed to closure of the growth plate.

## CLINICAL SYMPTOMS
Pain exacerbated by activity is the most common presenting symptom. Pain usually is localized to the anterior proximal thigh, but in one third of patients it is referred to the distal thigh and, on rare occasions, at the ankle. The clinical examination is easy and almost pathognomonic. Therefore, it is worthwhile to perform a screening examination for SCFE on all adolescents who present with lower extremity pain.

# TESTS

## PHYSICAL EXAMINATION

Loss of hip internal rotation is the most sensitive and specific finding and is readily apparent, even with minimal displacement of the femoral head. SCFE is the only pediatric disorder that causes greater loss of internal rotation when the hip is moved into a flexed position. Assessing internal rotation with the hip flexed to 90° is an effective screening maneuver and is easily done on all adolescents who have lower extremity pain.

Abduction and extension also are decreased. The affected extremity is between 1 and 3 cm shorter than the unaffected extremity, depending on the severity of the slip. In addition, patients typically walk with the affected extremity externally rotated.

## DIAGNOSTIC TESTS

AP and frog-lateral radiographs of the pelvis confirm the diagnosis (**Figure 1**). On rare occasions, the femoral head is displaced only in a posterior direction. In these situations, the AP radiograph will appear normal or will show slight valgus malalignment of the femoral head. No displacement is evident in a few patients, but in this preslip phase, the physis is widened.

The severity of displacement is classified as mild, moderate, or severe as measured by the degree of posterior displacement. Most authors rate a mild SCFE as less than 30°, moderate as 30° to 50°, and severe as greater than 50°.

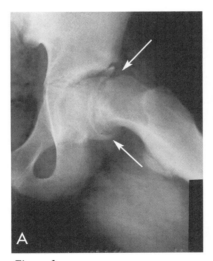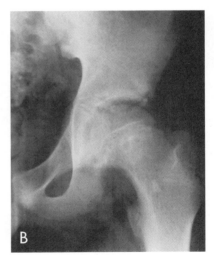

**Figure 1**
AP and frog-lateral radiographs of the pelvis showing mild SCFE of the right hip. A, Posterior displacement of the femoral head (arrows) is profiled on the lateral radiograph. B, On the AP radiograph, mild degrees of medial displacement can be recognized by drawing a line on the lateral aspect of the femoral neck. In this situation, the line on the involved hip will either miss or transect less of the femoral head.

## DIFFERENTIAL DIAGNOSIS

Endocrinopathy (atypical age, constitutional symptoms)

Legg-Calvé-Perthes disease (in younger age range)

Meralgia paresthetica (lateral femoral cutaneous nerve entrapment)

Neoplasm (night pain, no restriction of hip internal rotation in flexion)

## ADVERSE OUTCOMES OF THE DISEASE

Progressive arthritis, chondrolysis, and osteonecrosis may occur. Individuals vary, but on average, the degree of displacement correlates with the duration of symptoms. Severe SCFE predisposes the hip to symptomatic degenerative changes by the time the patient is a young or middle-aged adult, but stabilization of a mild or moderately displaced SCFE provides good long-term function, with symptomatic arthritis either not occurring or not developing until the older adult years. Therefore, making the diagnosis as early as possible is important.

## TREATMENT

The goals of treatment for adolescents with SCFE are to prevent further slippage of the femoral head, promote closure of the physis, and avoid osteonecrosis and chondrolysis. Treatment is based on the duration of symptoms and the degree of displacement. Most patients are treated by in situ stabilization. Patients with severe deformity may require a realignment osteotomy. With an unstable SCFE, patients have severe pain after a fall, are unable to walk, and have radiographic evidence of severe displacement. These patients require emergent reduction and stabilization.

## ADVERSE OUTCOMES OF TREATMENT

Patients are at risk for recurrent slippage until the physis closes. After stabilization, this problem is not common because the typical patient with SCFE is nearing completion of growth. Furthermore, insertion of the screw promotes closure of the growth plate. Chondrolysis and osteonecrosis also may occur.

## REFERRAL DECISIONS/RED FLAGS

Further evaluation for operative treatment should occur immediately upon diagnosis.

# SPONDYLOLISTHESIS

## ICD-9 Codes

738.4
   Spondylolisthesis, traumatic or acquired
756.11
   Spondylolysis, lumbar, congenital
756.12
   Spondylolisthesis, lumbar, congenital

## DEFINITION

Spondylolisthesis occurs when one vertebral body slips forward in relation to the vertebral body below. In children, spondylolisthesis occurs most frequently between L5 and S1 when a defect develops at the junction of the lamina with the pedicle (pars intra-articularis) (**Figure 1**). The resultant spondylolysis means that the posterior elements (lamina and spinous process) have only a fibrous tissue connection to the anterior elements (pedicle and vertebral body). As a consequence, the vertebral body may slide forward, producing the "slip" or spondylolisthesis. Most likely this condition is a fatigue or stress fracture that occurred in the preadolescent years and failed to heal. Children who participate at a high level in activities that place hyperextension stresses on this area, such as gymnastics and football, have a higher incidence of this condition.

## CLINICAL SYMPTOMS

Back pain that radiates posteriorly to or below the knees and that is worse with standing may develop (**Figure 2**). Symptoms are more common with more than 50% slippage. Spasms in the hamstring muscles, manifested by the inability to bend forward, accompanied by limited straight leg raising test are frequently found in symptomatic patients. True nerve root compression symptoms (radiculopathy), however, are infrequent in children.

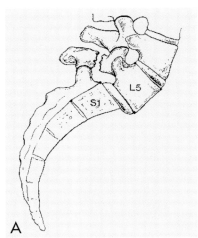

**Figure 1**
A, Lateral drawing of a grade I L5-S1 spondylolisthesis. B, Determination of slip percentage.

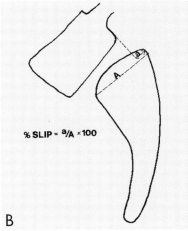

% SLIP = ᵃ/A ×100

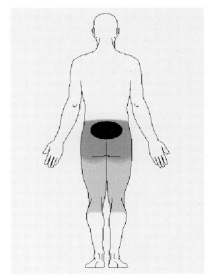

**Figure 2**
Typical pain diagram for a patient with adolescent spondylolisthesis.

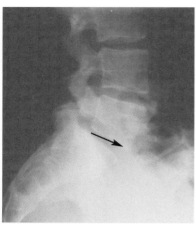

**Figure 3**
Lateral radiograph of a grade I L5-S1 spondylolisthesis.

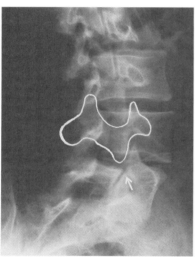

**Figure 4**
Oblique radiograph shows a normal "Scotty dog" appearance (outlined area). In the vertebra below, the neck of a Scotty dog is broken (arrow) and is the site of the pars interarticularis defect of spondylolisthesis.

## TESTS

### PHYSICAL EXAMINATION

Typical posture includes flexion of the hips and knees, backward tilting of the pelvis, and flattening of the normal lumbar lordosis. With marked slippage, a step-off can be palpated, with the spinous process of the slipped vertebra more prominent than the one above.

Hamstring spasm is manifested by marked limitation in forward bending and a limited passive straight leg raising test. Motor and sensory function of the lumbosacral nerve roots should be assessed, although objective neurologic deficits are uncommon.

### DIAGNOSTIC TESTS

With spondylolisthesis, lateral radiographs demonstrate forward translation of L5 relative to S1 (expressed as percentage of the anterior-posterior width of the vertebral body) (**Figure 3**). If only spondylolysis has occurred, there is no forward translation of L5, but a defect in the pars interarticularis is evident on the oblique views (an absent neck in the Scotty dog) (**Figure 4**).

## DIFFERENTIAL DIAGNOSIS

Intervertebral disk injury or herniation (no step-off or slip, and no defect seen on plain radiographs, radiculopathy occasionally present)

Intervertebral diskitis (elevated erythrocyte sedimentation rate and fever, disk space narrowing on radiographs)

Osteoid osteoma (night pain, abnormal bone scan, pain relieved by aspirin)

Spinal cord tumor (sensory findings, upper motor neuron signs)

Ankylosing spondylitis (HLA antigen, sacroiliac joint changes)

## ADVERSE OUTCOMES OF THE DISEASE

Progressive or complete slip of the vertebral body, chronic back pain and disability, weakness or paralysis of the lower lumbar nerve roots, or bowel and bladder involvement (cauda equina syndrome) are possible.

## TREATMENT

Observation to evaluate the possibility of increasing slippage is indicated until growth is completed. The frequency of evaluation depends on the amount of growth remaining, the degree of slippage, and whether a patient is symptomatic. A standing spot lateral radiograph is usually adequate for follow-up. In symptomatic patients, activities that aggravate the condition should be discontinued. An exercise problem that targets strengthening of the abdominal and paraspinal muscles, stretching of the hamstring muscles, and postural adaptations may be helpful. A custom-fitted thoracolumbar orthosis may control pain in patients who remain symptomatic despite activity modifications. Spinal fusion is indicated in children who have a documented progression and a slip of greater than 50% and significant growth remaining. Patients whose symptoms cannot be relieved through nonoperative treatment also should be considered for surgery.

## Adverse outcomes of treatment

Despite treatment, the slip may progress. Spinal fusions may be complicated by pseudarthrosis and continued pain.

## Referral decisions/Red flags

Patients with significant pain and/or a confirmed spondylolisthesis need further evaluation.

# TARSAL COALITION

## SYNONYMS

Calcaneal bar
Talocalcaneal bar
Peroneal spastic flatfoot
Rigid flatfoot

## DEFINITION

Tarsal coalition is an abnormal connection between any two tarsal bones. Initially, the coalition may be fibrous or cartilaginous, but it often ossifies during early adolescence and restricts hindfoot motion. The two most common locations for a tarsal coalition are between the calcaneus and navicular (calcaneonavicular coalition) and between the talus and calcaneus (talocalcaneal coalition). The condition is bilateral in approximately 50% of patients and may be found in other family members who are asymptomatic but have no hindfoot motion.

## CLINICAL SYMPTOMS

If symptoms develop, they usually occur during adolescence, when ossification of the bar starts to occur. Calcaneonavicular coalitions generally become symptomatic in children between the ages of 9 and 13 years, while symptoms from a talocalcaneal coalition generally develop later, between the ages of 13 and 16 years.

The onset of pain usually is insidious but can be associated with an injury or change in activity. Parents may observe a limp and the foot turning out. Pain from a talocalcaneal coalition usually is vague and located deep within the hindfoot, while a calcaneonavicular coalition usually causes pain laterally over the area of the coalition.

## TESTS

### PHYSICAL EXAMINATION

Hindfoot motion (inversion and eversion) is markedly restricted. Spasm of the peroneal muscles is frequent and can be demonstrated by quickly inverting the foot. Peroneal spasm holds the foot in a stiff, everted flatfoot posture; however, regardless of whether peroneal spasm is present, patients with tarsal coalition typically have a rigid flatfoot; the longitudinal arch is absent whether in a weight-bearing position or not.

## DIAGNOSTIC TESTS

AP, lateral, and oblique radiographs of the foot will delineate a calcaneonavic-ular coalition (**Figure 1**). Talocalcaneal bars are difficult to see on routine radiographs, even with special views; therefore, CT is necessary to confirm the diagnosis.

## DIFFERENTIAL DIAGNOSIS

Accessory navicular (medial prominence and pain over the navicular)

Congenital vertical talus (rigid flatfoot deformity noted in the neonate)

Flexible flatfoot (no restriction of subtalar motion, usually without pain)

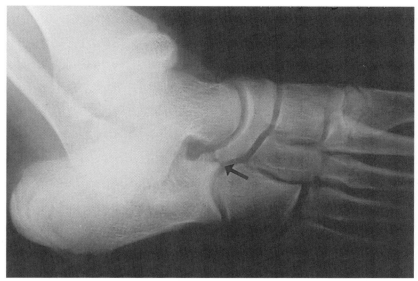

**Figure 1**
Oblique radiograph of a foot with a cartilaginous calcaneonavicular coalition (arrow).

## ADVERSE OUTCOMES OF THE DISEASE

Pain, restricted inversion and eversion of the foot, and limited walking and running are possible consequences.

## TREATMENT

Treatment options include observation, short leg cast immobilization, resec-tion of the coalition, and arthrodesis. Observation or activity modifications are appropriate for children who are asymptomatic or who have minimal symp-toms. For more severe symptoms or if milder symptoms persist, a 4- to 6-week trial in a short leg walking cast may be of benefit. For patients with per-sistent symptoms that do not respond to nonoperative treatment, resection of the coalition is the preferred treatment. Resection reduces pain in most patients, but this procedure is more reliable for calcaneonavicular coalitions. Hindfoot arthrodesis (joint fusion) is reserved for patients who have not responded to resection procedures or patients who are not candidates for coalition resection (the coalition is too large or arthritic changes are already present).

## ADVERSE OUTCOMES OF TREATMENT

Complications include cast sores, postoperative infection, failure of fusion, recurrence of a resected coalition, inadequate pain relief, and arthritic changes.

## REFERRAL DECISIONS/RED FLAGS

Significant pain following nonoperative treatment indicates the need for further evaluation.

# TOE WALKING

ICD-9 Code
781.2
  Abnormality of gait

## DEFINITION

Toe walking can be a normal variation of gait in children as they begin to walk; however, when it persists in children who are older than 18 months and who are otherwise normal and have no underlying neurologic deficit, it is known as idiopathic toe walking. This condition involves both legs and also is referred to as habitual toe walking.

## CLINICAL SYMPTOMS

Children with idiopathic toe walking generally are active, asymptomatic, and have no functional difficulties or other medical problems. Parental concern or a history of a sibling with toe walking usually is the impetus for seeking medical attention.

## TESTS

### PHYSICAL EXAMINATION

The diagnosis of idiopathic toe walking is one of exclusion; therefore, pathologic causes must be ruled out. Obtaining a thorough history is critical, particularly a detailed birth history. Cerebral palsy is suggested by a history of prematurity, anoxia, hypoxia, or perinatal infection. Muscular dystrophy is suggested by a positive family history and proximal muscle weakness. The time of onset also is important. In children with idiopathic toe walking, the onset of walking is normal, and toe walking begins with the onset of gait. Children with cerebral palsy usually have delayed gross motor milestones. Children with Duchenne muscular dystrophy initially walk with a heel-toe gait but develop toe walking at a later age.

Toe walking varies in severity (**Figure 1**), but children with idiopathic toe walking generally can stand with their feet flat on the floor and can walk heel-toe if reminded. Some will have decreased ankle dorsiflexion, while others do not.

### DIAGNOSTIC TESTS

Diagnostic tests should be ordered only if the history is unclear or if the examination reveals some abnormality suggestive of another disorder.

## DIFFERENTIAL DIAGNOSIS

Cerebral palsy (delayed developmental milestones, spasticity of gastrocnemius-soleus complex)

Intraspinal abnormality (cavus feet, unilateral or asymmetric involvement)

Muscular dystrophy (proximal muscular weakness, positive family history)

Occult hydrocephalus (upper motor neuron signs)

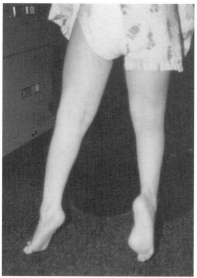

**Figure 1**
Example of a child with idiopathic toe walking.

## ADVERSE OUTCOMES OF THE DISEASE

The prevalence of long-term sequelae has not been documented; however, in some patients, persistent callosities and pain in the forefoot develop during late adolescence.

## TREATMENT

Treatment depends on the age of the child and the severity of the problem. In the toddler who has just begun to walk, the condition often resolves spontaneously after 3 to 6 months. Observation is appropriate for older toddlers who only occasionally walk on their toes. Stretching exercises may be tried for young children with mild contractures; however, children at this age typically do not tolerate extensive therapy. Serial casting for 6 to 8 weeks is often successful in children 3 to 8 years of age who have persistent toe walking and a persistent equinus. A short leg cast is applied with the ankle in near maximal dorsiflexion, and the casts are changed at 2- to 3-week intervals, with the amount of dorsiflexion increased at each cast change. After casting, many of these children will walk heel-toe, but some will revert to their previous gait pattern. Physical therapy that focuses on heel cord stretching or use of an ankle-foot orthosis may be helpful in preventing recurrence.

Operative treatment also is an option and typically is indicated for an older child with a fixed heel cord contracture when nonoperative treatment is ineffective or poorly tolerated. Heel cord lengthening is a relatively simple outpatient procedure that requires approximately 6 weeks of cast immobilization.

## ADVERSE OUTCOMES OF TREATMENT

Observation and stretching exercises are complicated only by failure or recurrence. Recurrence and skin problems can occur with casting or with heel cord lengthening.

## REFERRAL DECISIONS\RED FLAGS

Any child with persistent toe walking despite stretching and physical therapy or with evidence of a neuromuscular impairment requires further evaluation. Unilateral toe walking is never normal. In these instances, thorough examination is required to identify the underlying pathologic process. The most common causes of unilateral toe walking are limb-length discrepancy, cerebral palsy, and intraspinal abnormality.

# TORTICOLLIS

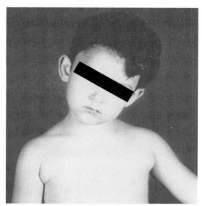

**Figure 1**
Congenital muscular torticollis. The chin is rotated to the right and the head inclined to the left.

## SYNONYM
Wry neck

## DEFINITION
Torticollis is a head position characterized by rotation of the chin toward one shoulder combined with tilting of the head to the opposite shoulder. Torticollis is a finding, not a diagnosis. Congenital muscular torticollis and atlanto-axial rotary subluxation are the most common causes.

Congenital muscular torticollis is a unilateral contracture of the sternocleidomastoid (SCM) muscle. Scar tissue in the muscle impedes growth of the SCM muscle. As a result, the involved muscle develops a contracture that causes the head to tilt toward the affected side and rotate toward the unaffected side (**Figure 1**). Facial asymmetry also develops.

Atlanto-axial rotary subluxation (AARS) is a rotational displacement of C1 on C2. Approximately 50% of neck rotation occurs between C1 and C2. Children between 2 and 12 years are most commonly affected. Greater ligamentous laxity in children probably explains its increased incidence in this population. AARS may be associated with minor trauma or develop after an upper respiratory infection (Grisel syndrome).

## CLINICAL SYMPTOMS
Parental concern about the head posture is the usual reason for the visit for both conditions. For congenital muscular torticollis, the parents also may note a lump or swelling in the muscle at 4 to 6 weeks of age. If present, this mass disappears in a few weeks. Children with AARS may report neck pain, but the discomfort typically is minimal.

## TESTS

### PHYSICAL EXAMINATION
Infants with congenital muscular torticollis hold the head in a "cock robin" position. Contracture of the left SCM muscle directs the chin to the right shoulder and tilts the left ear to the left shoulder and limits neck rotation to the left and lateral tilt to the right. The opposite deformity is seen with contracture of the right SCM muscle. Flattening of the face is noted on the side of the contracted SCM muscle.

Patients with AARS hold the head in a similar position. SCM muscle spasm, however, may be noted on the "chin" side. This spasm differs from that of congenital muscular torticollis in which the SCM muscle on the "ear" side is tight.

The examination also should include assessment for ocular or neurologic disorders. Congenital muscular torticollis can be associated with developmental hip dysplasia, and that possibility should be investigated.

### DIAGNOSTIC TESTS

AP and lateral radiographs of the cervical spine should be obtained in patients with congenital muscular torticollis to rule out underlying congenital bony anomalies. Patients with AARS also should have open mouth views of the odontoid; however, good views are difficult to obtain in this condition. CT with the head maximally rotated to the right and then maximally rotated to the left may be required to document AARS. Before CT, obtain flexion-extension lateral views to rule out upper cervical instability. Despite possible limitation by muscle spasm, these views should be obtained only with active, never passive, motion.

## DIFFERENTIAL DIAGNOSIS

### CONGENITAL MUSCULAR TORTICOLLIS

Benign paroxysmal torticollis (intermittent torticollis)

Congenital anomalies of the base of the skull (rare, evident on radiographs)

Klippel-Feil syndrome (congenital cervical spine anomalies, short neck, low hair line)

Ocular disorders (torticollis may improve when eyes are closed or vision blocked)

### ATLANTO-AXIAL ROTARY SUBLUXATION

Fractures of the upper cervical spine (history of trauma, evident on radiographs)

Neoplasms of the cervical spine (indolent onset, pain, evident on radiographs)

Osteomyelitis of the cervical spine (evident on radiographs, laboratory studies)

Posterior fossa or spinal cord tumor (neurologic examination, gentle passive motion may not be as limited, MRI)

## ADVERSE OUTCOMES OF THE DISEASE

Facial asymmetry and persistent limited motion are possible with congenital muscular torticollis. With AARS, persistent limited motion also is possible. Upper cervical instability may be present, which could increase the risk of neurologic injury.

## TREATMENT

Nonoperative treatment of congenital muscular torticollis consists of frequent stretching exercises that tilt and rotate the head. Supervision by a physical therapist is helpful, but parents must actually do the stretching exercises several times a day. The infant's bed and changing table can be positioned to encourage the infant to look away from the limited side. If the problem persists after 12 to 18 months, surgical release/lengthening of the SCM should be considered.

Initial management of AARS is immobilization in a soft cervical collar and analgesics for pain. Range-of-motion exercises are not helpful. If reduction does not occur in approximately 1 week, cervical traction with a head halter and better pain management should be attempted. Conditions that persist for several months may require upper cervical fusion for relief of symptoms.

## ADVERSE OUTCOMES OF TREATMENT

For patients with congenital muscular torticollis, failure of stretching programs and a persistent deformity are possible. Even with operative treatment, the contracture may recur with growth.

For patients with AARS, persistent deformity is possible. Recurrence is rare in patients diagnosed and treated promptly. Upper cervical arthrodesis permanently limits neck motion.

## REFERRAL DECISIONS/RED FLAGS

For infants with congenital torticollis, failure to improve following 2 to 3 months of nonoperative treatment, the presence of anomalies of the skull or cervical spine, or abnormal results of neurologic or eye examination indicate the need for further evaluation.

Children with acquired torticollis who have an abnormal neurologic examination or evidence of instability on lateral radiographs need urgent specialty evaluation. Acquired torticollis that persists for more than 2 or 3 weeks or situations in which initial treatment has failed usually need further evaluation as well.

# TRANSIENT SYNOVITIS OF THE HIP

ICD-9 Code

719.05
Effusion of joint, pelvic region and thigh

## SYNONYMS

Observation hip

Toxic synovitis

## DEFINITION

Transient synovitis of the hip is a sterile effusion of the joint that resolves without therapy or sequelae. Children 2 to 5 years of age are most commonly affected, and boys are affected two to three times more often than girls. The etiology is unknown, but mild trauma at an age when the socket or acetabulum is not fully developed seems to be the best explanation. This theory fits the demographics. Another theory proposes an infectious etiology, but numerous studies have not demonstrated a bacterial or viral agent. Therefore, the term "toxic synovitis" should not be used to describe this disorder.

## CLINICAL SYMPTOMS

Typically, the child awakens with a limp or refuses to walk. Children who can communicate, typically localize their pain to the groin or proximal thigh. After "loosening up," the limp may improve but will worsen toward the end of the day.

## TESTS

### PHYSICAL EXAMINATION

Examination reveals a limp and mild restriction of hip motion, particularly abduction. Most children are afebrile.

### DIAGNOSTIC TESTS

Because transient synovitis is a diagnosis of exclusion, the extent of the evaluation process depends on the degree and duration of symptoms. If a child is seen 1 to 3 days after onset, is afebrile, does not appear ill, has only mildly restricted abduction (movement of at least 25° to 30°), and does not guard when the hip is moved in other directions, then radiographs and laboratory studies are not necessary. However, if the symptoms have been present for several days but the child is afebrile and has only mildly restricted motion, then AP and frog-lateral radiographs of the pelvis are appropriate to rule out a latent osteomyelitis or other chronic process. Diagnostic studies, such as a CBC, erythrocyte sedimentation rate, blood cultures, and radiographs, are indicated if the patient has very limited motion or a temperature that is higher than 99.5°F (37.5°C).

Radiographs usually are normal; however, they may show widening of the joint space. Ultrasound and bone scan often demonstrate changes but are rarely necessary. A joint effusion will be seen on ultrasound, and a bone scan can demonstrate mild uptake.

Aspirate the joint if there are findings compatible with septic arthritis.

## DIFFERENTIAL DIAGNOSIS

Juvenile rheumatoid arthritis (multiple joints, persistent symptoms, systemic symptoms)

Legg-Calvé-Perthes disease (limp worse at the end of the day, present after 2 to 6 weeks of symptoms, abnormal radiographs)

Rheumatic fever (arthralgias progress in a migratory fashion to other joints, systemic symptoms)

Septic arthritis of the hip (primary disorder to exclude: temperature above 99.5°F [37.5°C], an erythrocyte sedimentation rate greater than 20 mm/h)

## ADVERSE OUTCOMES OF THE DISEASE

The symptoms and associated limp typically resolve within 3 to 14 days. Recurrence is possible but uncommon. No sequelae have been associated with transient synovitis. Legg-Calvé-Perthes disease subsequently develops in 1% to 3% of patients, but whether the disorders have any association is unclear. A delay in diagnosing septic arthritis also is possible.

## TREATMENT

Most children can be treated by bed rest at home, with the parents periodically checking the temperature. When the diagnosis is equivocal or if the patient is uncomfortable, hospitalization for observation and traction are indicated.

## ADVERSE OUTCOMES OF TREATMENT

None

## REFERRAL DECISIONS/RED FLAGS

A temperature higher than 99.5°F (37.5°C) or an erythrocyte sedimentation rate greater than 20 mm/h suggests septic arthritis, in which case patients need further evaluation. Also, patients need additional evaluation if radiographs suggest Legg-Calvé-Perthes disease.

# GLOSSARY OF ICD-9 CODES

## SECTION 1: GENERAL ORTHOPAEDICS

088.81 Lyme disease
238.0 Neoplasm of uncertain behavior of other and unspecified sites and tissues, bone and articular cartilage
238.1 Neoplasm of uncertain behavior of other and unspecified sites and tissues, connective and other soft tissue
274.0 Gouty arthropathy
337.21 Reflex sympathetic dystrophy of the upper limb
337.22 Reflex sympathetic dystrophy of the lower limb
355.8 Mononeuritis of lower limb, unspecified (Chronic compartment syndrome)
451.1 Phlebitis and thrombophlebitis, of deep vessels of lower extremities
696.0 Psoriatic arthropathy
711.0 Pyogenic arthritis
711.1 Arthropathy associated with Reiter disease and nonspecific urethritis
712.2 Chondrocalcinosis due to pyrophosphate crystals
712.3 Chondrocalcinosis, unspecified
713.1 Arthropathy associated with gastrointestinal conditions other than infections
714.0 Rheumatoid arthritis
715.0 Osteoarthrosis, generalized
715.1 Osteoarthrosis, localized, primary
715.2 Osteoarthrosis, localized, secondary
715.3 Osteoarthrosis, localized, not specified whether primary or secondary
716.1 Traumatic arthropathy
720.0 Ankylosing spondylitis
721.6 Ankylosing vertebral hyperostosis
729.1 Myalgia and myositis, unspecified
729.5 Pain in limb

730 Osteomyelitis, periostitis and other infections involving bone
733.00 Osteoporosis, unspecified
840 Sprains and strains of shoulder and upper arm
841 Sprains and strains of elbow and forearm
842 Sprains and strains of hand and wrist
843 Sprains and strains of hip and thigh
844 Sprains and strains of knee and leg
845 Sprains and strains of ankle and foot
846 Sprains and strains of sacroiliac region
847 Sprains and strains of other and unspecified parts of back
958.8 Other early complications of trauma (Acute compartment syndrome)
997.60 Amputation stump complication, unspecified

## SECTION 2: SHOULDER

353.0 Brachial plexus lesions
714.0 Rheumatoid arthritis
715.11 Osteoarthrosis, localized, primary, shoulder
715.21 Osteoarthrosis, localized, secondary, shoulder
716.11 Traumatic arthropathy, shoulder
716.91 Arthropathy, unspecified, shoulder
718.81 Instability of shoulder joint, NOS
723.4 Brachial neuritis or radiculitis NOS
726.0 Adhesive capsulitis of shoulder
726.10 Rotator cuff syndrome NOS
727.61 Rupture of tendon, nontraumatic, complete rupture of rotator cuff
810.00 Fracture of clavicle, closed, unspecified part
811.00 Fracture of scapula, unspecified part, closed

812.00 Fracture of humerus, upper end, closed, unspecified part
812.21 Fracture of humerus, closed, shaft of humerus
831.00 Dislocation of shoulder, closed, unspecified
831.04 Dislocation of shoulder, closed, acromioclavicular (joint)
840.4 Sprains and strains of shoulder and upper arm, rotator cuff
840.8 Sprains and strains of shoulder and upper arm, unspecified site

## SECTION 3: ELBOW AND FOREARM

354.2 Mononeuritis of upper limb and mononeuritis multiplex, lesion of ulnar nerve
384.3 Posterior interosseous nerve syndrome
714.12 Rheumatoid arthritis of the elbow
715.12.1 Osteoarthritis, primary, of the elbow
715.22 Osteoarthritis, secondary, of the elbow
716.12 Traumatic arthritis of the elbow
726.31 Medial epicondylitis
726.32 Lateral epicondylitis
726.33 Olecranon bursitis
812.40 Fracture of the distal humerus, unspecified
813.01 Fracture of radius and ulna, olecranon process of ulna
813.05 Fracture radial head
813.06 Fracture radial neck
832.0 Dislocation of elbow, unspecified
841.9 Sprains and strains of elbow and forearm, unspecified site

## SECTION 4: HAND AND WRIST

054.6 Herpetic whitlow
195.4 Malignant neoplasm, upper limb

213.5    Benign neoplasms of short bones of upper limb

229.8    Benign neoplasms of other and unspecified sites

354.0    Carpal tunnel syndrome

354.2    Lesion of ulnar nerve

681.01   Felon

681.02   Paronychia of finger

712.23   Pseudogout of the wrist

714.0    Rheumatoid arthritis

715.13   Osteoarthritis of the wrist, primary

715.14   Osteoarthritis, primary, localized to the hand

715.23   Osteoarthrosis of the wrist, secondary

715.24   Osteoarthritis, secondary, localized to the hand

715.93   Osteoarthritis of the wrist, unspecified

715.94   Osteoarthritis, unspecified, localized to the hand

716.13   Traumatic arthropathy of the hand

716.14   Traumatic arthropathy of the hand

716.94   Arthropathy, unspecified, hand

727.03   Trigger finger

727.04   de Quervain tenosynovitis

727.41   Ganglion of joint

727.42   Ganglion of tendon sheath

727.64   Rupture of flexor tendons of hand and wrist, nontraumatic

727.89   Abscess of bursa or tendon

728.6    Dupuytren contracture

732.3    Kienböck disease

736.1    Mallet finger

736.21   Boutonnière deformity

813.41   Colles fracture, Smith fracture

813.42   Other fractures of distal end of radius (alone)

814.01   Fracture of carpal bone, closed-navicular (scaphoid) of wrist

815.00   Fracture of metacarpal bone(s), site unspecified, closed

816.00   Fracture of one or more phalanges of hand, site unspecified, closed

834.00   Dislocation of finger or thumb, closed, unspecified site

842.1    Tendon injuries of the wrist and hand, unspecified site

842.10   Sprains and strains of hand, unspecified site

882.0    Open wound of hand, except fingers, without mention of complication

883.0    Open wound of finger(s) without mention of complication

885.0    Traumatic amputation of thumb without mention of complication

886.0    Traumatic amputation of fingers without mention of complication

927.3    Crushing injury of finger(s)

E906.0   Dog bite

E906.3   Cat bite

# SECTION 5: HIP AND THIGH

355.1    Meralgia paresthetica

710.05   Systemic lupus erythematosus

714.05   Rheumatoid arthritis

715.15   Primary (idiopathic) osteoarthritis of the hip

715.25   Secondary osteoarthritis of the hip (eg, Legg-Calvé-Perthes disease)

716.15   Traumatic arthritis of the hip

719.65   Snapping hip

720.05   Ankylosing spondylitis

726.5    Enthesopathy of hip region

733.09   Osteoporosis not elsewhere classified or drug-induced

733.42   Aseptic necrosis of femoral head and neck

808.0    Fracture of the acetabulum

808.2    Fracture of the pubis

808.41   Fracture of the ilium

808.42   Fracture of the ischium

808.43   Multiple fractures pelvis (unstable pelvic ring fracture)

820.00   Femoral neck (transcervical) fracture

820.21   Intertrochanteric femur fracture

821.01   Fracture of the femoral shaft, closed

835.01   Posterior dislocation

835.02   Anterior dislocation

843.9    Sprains and strains of hip and thigh, unspecified site

# SECTION 6: KNEE AND LEG

274.0    Gouty arthropathy

440.4    Vascular claudication

682.6    Other cellulitis and abscess, leg, except foot

710.05   Systemic lupus erythematosus

712.96   Unspecified crystal arthropathy, lower leg

714.06   Rheumatoid arthritis, lower leg

715.16   Osteoarthrosis, localized, primary, lower leg

715.26   Osteoarthrosis, localized, secondary, lower leg

716.16   Traumatic arthropathy, lower leg

717.3    Old tear of medial meniscus, unspecified

717.40   Old tear of lateral meniscus, unspecified

717.7    Chondromalacia of patella

717.81   Old disruption of lateral collateral ligament

717.82   Old disruption of medial collateral ligament

717.83   Chronic disruption of anterior cruciate ligament

717.84   Old disruption of posterior cruciate ligament

717.9    Unspecified internal derangement of knee

718.36   Recurrent dislocation of joint, lower leg

719.46   Pain in joint, knee

721.42   Thoracic or lumbar spondylosis with myelopathy

724.02   Lumbar spinal stenosis

726.60   Enthesopathy of knee, unspecified

726.61   Pes anserinus tendinitis or bursitis

726.64   Patellar tendinitis

726.65   Prepatellar bursitis

726.8    Shin-splints

727.00   Synovitis and tenosynovitis, unspecified

727.51   Popliteal cyst

729.5    Pain in limb

732.4    Juvenile osteochondrosis of lower extremity, excluding foot

732.7    Osteochondritis dissecans

733.16   Stress fracture, tibia or fibula

733.43   Aseptic necrosis of bone, medial femoral condyle

755.64   Congenital deformity of knee joint

821.2    Fracture of other and unspecified parts of femur, lower end, closed

822.0    Fracture of patella

823.0    Fracture of tibia and fibula, upper end, closed

836.0    Acute tear of medial meniscus of knee

836.1    Acute tear of lateral meniscus of knee

836.3    Dislocation of patella, closed

844.0   Acute lateral collateral ligament sprain

844.1   Acute medial collateral ligament sprain

844.2   Acute posterior cruciate ligament tear

844.8   Sprains and strains of knee and leg, other specified sites

844.9   Medial gastrocnemius tear

924.10   Contusion of lower limb

958.8   Compartment syndrome

959.7   Injury, other and unspecified, knee, leg, ankle, and foot

## SECTION 7: FOOT AND ANKLE

078.19   Viral warts, unspecified; other specified viral warts

110.1   Dermatophytosis, of nail

355.5   Tarsal tunnel syndrome

355.6   Mononeuritis of lower limb; lesion of plantar nerve

700   Corns and calluses

703.0   Diseases of nail; ingrowing nail

713.5   Arthropathy associated with neurologic disorders

714.0   Rheumatoid arthritis

715.17   Osteoarthritis, localized, primary; ankle and foot

715.27   Osteoarthritis, localized, secondary; ankle and foot

716.17   Traumatic arthritis

718.87   Ankle/foot instability

719.47   Pain in joint, foot and ankle

726.70   Enthesopathy of ankle and tarsus, unspecified

726.71   Achilles bursitis or tendinitis

726.72   Posterior tibial tendinitis

726.79   Peroneal tenosynovitis

727.06   Tenosynovitis and synovitis of foot and ankle

727.1   Bunion

727.43   Ganglion and cyst of synovium, tendon, and bursa, unspecified

728.71   Plantar fascial fibromatosis

733.99   Sesamoiditis

734.8   Claw toe (acquired)

735.0   Hallux valgus (acquired)

735.2   Hallux rigidus

735.4   Hammer toe (acquired)

735.8   Other acquired deformities of toe

780.8   Hyperhidrosis

824   Fracture of ankle

824.8   Fracture of ankle; unspecified, closed

825.0   Fracture of calcaneus, closed

825.2   Fracture of tarsal and metatarsal bones

825.25   Fracture of other tarsal and metatarsal bones, closed; metatarsal bones(s)

826.0   Fracture of one or more phalanges of foot; closed

838.03   Closed dislocation tarsometatarsal joint

845.00   Sprains and strains of the ankle and foot

845.09   Sprains and strains of ankle and foot; Achilles tendon

845.12   Sprains and strains of ankle and foot; metatarsophalangeal (joint)

## SECTION 8: SPINE

198.5   Secondary malignant neoplasm of other specified site, bone and bone marrow

344.60   Cauda equina syndrome, without mention of neurogenic bladder

721.0   Cervical spondylosis without myelopathy

721.1   Cervical spondylosis with myelopathy

722.0   Displacement of cervical intervertebral disk without myelopathy

722.10   Displacement of thoracic or lumbar intervertebral disk without myelopathy

722.52   Degeneration of thoracic or lumbar intervertebral disk, lumbar, or lumbosacral disk

723.0   Spinal stenosis in cervical region

723.4   Other disorders of cervical region, brachial neuritis or radiculitis

724.02   Spinal stenosis other than cervical, lumbar region

724.2   Low back pain

724.4   Thoracic or lumbosacral neuritis or radiculitis, unspecified (Radicular syndrome of lower limb)

733.13   Pathologic fracture, vertebrae

737.30   Scoliosis (and kyphoscoliosis), idiopathic

737.43   Curvature of spine associated with other conditions, scoliosis

738.4   Acquired spondylolisthesis

805.0   Fracture of vertebral column without mention of spinal cord injury, cervical, closed

805.2   Fracture of the vertebral column without mention of spinal cord injury, dorsal (thoracic), closed

805.4   Fracture of the vertebral column without mention of spinal cord injury, lumbar, closed

847.0   Sprains and strains of other and unspecified parts of back, neck

847.1   Sprains and strains of other and unspecified parts of back, thoracic

847.2   Sprains and strains of other and unspecified parts of the back, lumbar

## SECTION 9: PEDIATRIC ORTHOPAEDICS

682.7   Abscess, foot

696.0   Psoriatic arthritis

711.0   Pyogenic arthritis

711.1   Reiter syndrome

713.1   Arthritis of inflammatory bowel disease

714.30   Polyarticular juvenile rheumatoid arthritis, chronic or unspecified

714.32   Pauciarticular juvenile rheumatoid arthritis

717.9   Pathologic plica

719.05   Effusion of joint, pelvic region and thigh

719.42   Pain in joint, upper arm

719.7   Difficulty in walking

720.0   Ankylosing spondylitis

722.92   Thoracic diskitis

722.93   Lumbar diskitis

723.5   Torticollis, unspecified

724.1   Pain in thoracic spine

724.2   Low back pain

729.5   Pain in limb

730.00   Acute osteomyelitis, site unspecified

731.00   Chronic osteomyelitis, site unspecified

732.0   Scheuermann disease

732.1   Juvenile osteochondrosis of hip and pelvis

732.2   Nontraumatic slipped upper femoral epiphysis

732.4   Sinding-Larsen-Johannson syndrome

        Osgood-Schlatter disease

732.5 Juvenile osteochondrosis of foot
    Calcaneal apophysitis
    Accessory navicular
    Freiberg infraction
    Osteochondral lesion of talus
    Os trigonum
732.7 Osteochondritis dissecans
733.49 Osteonecrosis of navicular
734.0 Pes planus (acquired)
736.41 Genu valgum, acquired
736.42 Genu varum, acquired
736.6 Patellofemoral dysfunction
736.6 Bipartite patella
736.75 Cavovarus deformity of foot, acquired
736.89 Acquired deformity of lower limb
737.0 Postural kyphosis
737.30 Idiopathic scoliosis
737.39 Unspecified curvature of the spine
738.4 Spondylolisthesis, traumatic or acquired
754.1 Congenital sternomastoid torticollis
754.30 Congenital dislocation of the hip, unilateral
754.31 Congenital dislocation of the hip, bilateral
754.41 Congenital dislocation of the knee
754.43 Anterolateral bowing of the tibia
    Posteromedial bowing of the tibia
754.44 Congenital dislocation of the patella
754.51 Talipes equinovarus
754.53 Metatarsus varus
754.59 Varus deformities of feet, other (Talipes cavovarus)
754.61 Congenital vertical talus
    Congenital pes planus
    Tarsal coalition
754.62 Calcaneovalgus foot
755.01 Polydactyly of fingers
755.02 Polydactyly of toes
755.11 Syndactyly of fingers without fusion of bone
755.21 Transverse deficiency of the forearm
755.26 Radial hemimelia
755.27 Ulnar hemimelia
755.29 Hypoplasia of the thumb
755.34 Proximal femoral focal deficiency

755.36 Tibial hemimelia
755.37 Fibular hemimelia
755.38 Congenital short first metatarsal
755.50 Congenital dislocation of the radial head
755.53 Congenital radial-ulnar synostosis
755.60 Congenital deformities of the lower extremity
755.62 Coxa vara
755.66 Hallux valgus
755.67 Anomalies of the foot, not elsewhere classified
756.11 Spondylolysis, lumbar, congenital
756.12 Spondylolisthesis, lumbar, congenital
767.6 Injury to brachial plexus
781.2 Abnormality of gait
810.00 Clavicle fracture, closed, unspecified part
812.00 Proximal humerus fracture, closed, unspecified part
812.40 Fracture of distal humeral physis
812.41 Supracondylar fracture, distal humerus
812.42 Lateral condyle fracture; lateral epicondyle fracture, distal humerus
812.43 Medial condyle fracture; medial epicondyle fracture, distal humerus
813.00 Fracture, closed, upper end of forearm, unspecified
813.01 Olecranon fracture, proximal forearm
813.06 Radial neck fracture, proximal forearm
813.20 Fracture, middle forearm, closed, unspecified part
813.42 Torus fracture of the distal radius
    Metaphyseal fracture of the distal radius, complete
    Greenstick fracture of the distal radius
    Physeal fractures of the distal radius
    Galeazzi fracture
813.44 Greenstick fractures of the distal radius and ulna
    Complete fracture of the distal radius and ulna
820.00 Femoral neck fracture, closed, unspecified type

820.21 Intertrochanteric femur fracture, closed
821.00 Femoral shaft fracture, closed, unspecified part
821.22 Distal femoral physeal fracture, closed
821.23 Supracondylar femur fracture, closed
823.80 Fracture of tibia, unspecified part, closed
995.50 Child abuse, unspecified
E920.9 Nail puncture wound

ICD-9 CODES

# INDEX

Page numbers with *f* indicate figures;
Page numbers with *t* indicate tables.

Antibiotics
    for animal bites, 211
    for diskitis, 635
    for fingertip infections, 238
    for human bites, 268
    for Lyme disease, 44
    for nail fungus infection, 483
    for nail injuries, 274
    for osteomyelitis, 688
    for prepatellar bursitis, 402–403
    for septic arthritis, 75, 76t, 701,
        702, 702t
    for septic olecranon bursitis, 190
    for septic tenosynovitis, 211, 248
Antinuclear antibody test
    for inflammatory arthritis, 315
    for juvenile rheumatoid arthritis,
        670–671, 672
Apprehension sign
    for anterior talofibular ligament,
        114, 114f
    for patellar instability, 350, 350f,
        391
    for shoulder instability, 148
Arch fracture. See Metatarsals, fractures
        of
Arterial circulation to the hand, Allen
        test for, 209, 209f
Arthritis, 2–3. See also Fibromyalgia
        syndrome; Inflammatory
        arthritis; Juvenile rheumatoid
        arthritis (JRA); Posttraumatic
        arthritis; Radiocarpal arthritis;
        Rheumatoid arthritis (RA);
        Septic arthritis
    of the anterior cruciate joint, 117
    clinical symptoms, 118–119, 119f
    corticosteroid injections for, 120,
        218, 220–221, 220f, 223,
        224, 365, 370, 428,
        429–430, 429f
    of the elbow, 165–172, 170f
    of the foot and ankle, 409,
        426–428, 426f, 427f
    glenohumeral, 118
    gout and, 24
    of the hand, 213–215, 213f
    inflammatory bowel disease and, 78
    of the knee, 363–365, 364f
    midfoot, 427
    NSAIDs for, 48, 120, 175, 365, 428
    postinjection infectious, 23
    psoriatic, 77–78
    of the shoulder, 118–120, 118f,
        119f
    subtalar, 427
    talocalcaneal, 427
    talonavicular, 426, 427
    of the thumb carpometacarpal joint,
        217–219, 217f, 218f
    traumatic, 294
    variables in pediatric, 581
    of the wrist, 222–223, 222f
Arthrocentesis for pain relief, 377

Arthrodesis
    for cavus foot deformity, 608
    for osteoarthritis, 52
    for rheumatoid arthritis, 73
    for tarsal coalition, 715–716
Arthrofibrosis, 362
Arthrography, 41
    for shoulder instability, 148
Arthrogryposis, 613
Arthrotomy for septic arthritis, 75
Aseptic necrosis. See Legg-Calvé-Perthes
        disease; Osteonecrosis
Aspiration
    in crystalline deposition disease, 26
    of ganglia, 265, 265f
    in hand/wrist arthritis, 224
    in meniscal tears, 380
    of olecranon bursitis, 191–192,
        191f
    of popliteal cysts, 398
    of prepatellar bursitis, 402
Atlanto-axial rotary subluxation
        (AARS), 719, 720, 721
Atraumatic or voluntary instability
        (AMBRI), 148, 149
Autonomic nervous system dysfunc-
        tion, 66
Avascular necrosis. See Legg-Calvé-
        Perthes disease; Osteonecrosis
Aviator's fracture. See Talus, fractures of
Axial loading test, 45, 533, 533f
Axial rotation, 45

# B

Babinski sign, 534, 534f
    for back pain, 543, 550, 589
Back pain. See also Low back pain
    in children, 589–591, 590t
        adverse outcomes, 591
        clinical symptoms, 589
        definition, 589
        differential diagnosis, 590–591,
            590t
        referral decisions, 591
        synonyms, 589
        tests, 589–590
        treatment, 591
            adverse outcomes, 591
Bacteroides in bite wounds, 210
Baker cyst, 100. See also Popliteal cyst
Balanitis circinata, 77
Bankart lesions, 147
Barlow sign, in developmental dysplasia
        of the hip, 583, 583f, 630,
        630f
Barton fracture, 249, 249f
Baseball finger. See Mallet finger
Bell palsy, 43
Below-knee amputation, 12
Bennett fracture, 259, 259f, 260
Biceps, testing of, 530, 530f
Biceps femoris, 330

Biceps tendon
    inspection/palpation of, 110, 110f
    rupture of, 144–146
        adverse outcomes, 146
        clinical symptoms, 144
        definition, 144
        differential diagnosis, 145
        distal
            adverse outcomes, 194
            clinical symptoms, 193
            definition, 193
            differential diagnosis,
                193–194
            referral decisions, 194
            treatment, 194
                adverse outcomes, 194
        referral decisions, 146
        tests, 144–145, 145f
        treatment, 146
            adverse outcomes, 146
Bilateral crutches for inflammatory
        arthritis, 317
Bimalleolar injuries, 448
Biofeedback for complex regional pain
        syndromes, 68
Biopsy
    for bone tumors, 96
    for soft-tissue tumors, 98
Bipartite patella, 343, 366–367, 366f
    adverse outcomes, 366
    in children, 586–587, 586f
    clinical symptoms, 366
    definition, 366, 366f
    differential diagnosis, 366
    referral decisions, 367
    tests, 366
    treatment, 367
        adverse outcomes, 367
Bites
    animal, 210–212, 212t
    human, 266–268, 266f, 268t
Black tea, soaking malodorous feet in,
        473
Bleomycin for plantar warts, 496
Blood culture
    for septic arthritis, 700, 701t
    for transient synovitis of the hip,
        722
Board-lasting technique, 504
Bone cancer. See under Tumors
Bone lesion. See under Tumors
Bone marrow edema syndrome. See
        Transient osteoporosis of the
        hip
Bone mineral density (BMP)
    calcium supplement and, 60
    for osteoporosis, 58
Bone-on-bone crepitus, 119
Bone scans, 42
    for complex regional pain syn-
        dromes, 66–67
    for diabetic foot, 443
    for diskitis, 635
    for foot and ankle pain in children,
        597

for fracture of the growth plate, 645
for fractures about the elbow, 657
for metatarsal fractures, 454
for metatarsus adductus, 670, 680
for osteonecrosis of the navicular, 598
for proximal and middle forearm fractures, 653
for scaphoid fractures, 253–254
for stress fractures, 509
for tarsal coalition, 715
for tibial fractures, 661
for toe walking, 718
Cauda equina, 537
Cauda equina syndrome, 520, 525, 537–538, 537f, 562, 565
adverse outcomes of, 538
clinical symptoms, 537, 537f
definition, 537
differential diagnosis, 538
referral decisions, 538
tests, 537–538
treatment, 538
adverse outcomes of, 538
Causalgia. *See* Complex regional pain syndromes; Reflex sympathetic dystrophy (RSD)
Cavitary subacute osteomyelitis, 686
Cavovarus, 606
Cavus foot deformity, 412, 412f
in children, 606–608, 607f
adverse outcomes, 607
clinical symptoms, 606
definition, 606
differential diagnosis, 607
orthotic devices for, 486f
referral decisions, 608
synonyms, 606
tests, 606–607, 607f
treatment, 607–608
adverse outcomes, 608
Cellulitis, 24, 100
Central slip extensor tendon injury. *See* Boutonnière deformity
Cerebral hemorrhage, frozen shoulder and, 124
Cerebral palsy, 581, 717
femoral and tibial torsion in, 670
Cervical arthritis. *See* Cervical spondylosis
Cervical collars for cervical spinal fractures, 549
Cervical disk herniation, frozen shoulder and, 124
Cervical lordosis, 539
Cervical myelopathy, 28, 539, 542
Cervical radiculopathy, 539–541, 542
adverse outcomes, 541
clinical symptoms, 539, 540f
definition, 539
differential diagnosis, 541
referral decisions, 541
tests, 539–540, 540ft
treatment, 541
adverse outcomes, 541

Cervical spine disorders
diffuse idiopathic skeletal hyperostosis and, 28
fractures of, 548–549
adverse outcomes, 549
clinical symptoms, 548
definition, 548
differential diagnosis, 549
referral decisions, 549
tests, 548–549
treatment, 549
radiographs of, in diagnosing metastatic disease, 567
Cervical spondylosis, 542–544, 542f, 543f
adverse outcomes, 544
clinical symptoms, 542–543, 542f
definition, 542
differential diagnosis, 544
referral decisions, 544
synonyms, 542
tests, 543, 543f
treatment, 544
adverse outcomes of, 544
Cervical sprain, 545–547, 545f
adverse outcomes, 546
clinical symptoms, 545, 545f
definition, 545
differential diagnosis, 546
referral decisions, 547
synonym, 545
tests, 545–546
treatment, 546–547
adverse outcomes, 547
Charcot arthropathy, 24, 442, 443. *See also* Diabetic foot
distinguishing from osteomyelitis, 443
treatment for, 444
Charcot joint, initial stage of, 444
Charcot-Marie-Tooth disease, 412, 412f, 513
Chauffeur's fracture, 249, 249f
Chemotherapy
for bone tumors, 97
for metastatic disease, 568
for soft-tissue tumors, 99
Child abuse, 609–612, 610f, 611f
definition, 609
distal humerus fractures in, 655
final diagnosis, 612
investigative interview, 609–610
reporting, 612
synonyms, 609
tests, 610–611, 610f
Chondrocalcinosis, 24, 25
Chondroitin sulfate
for arthritis, 120
for osteoarthritis, 53–54
Chondromalacia, 390. *See also* Patellofemoral pain of the patella, 585
Chondrosarcomas, 287, 343
Chronic ankle/subtalar instability, 435
Chronic arthropathy, 24

Chronic lateral ankle pain, 434–436
clinical symptoms, 434
definition, 434
differential diagnosis, 435–436
tests, 434
Chronic low back pain. *See* Lumbar degenerative disk disease
Chronic osteomyelitis, 686
Chronic pain syndrome, 14
Chronic pyrophosphate arthropathy, 25
Chronic synovitis, 499
Claudication, 358–359
comparison of vascular to neurogenic, 563t
neurogenic, 29, 358, 359
vascular, 358, 359
Clavicle
fracture of, 127–128
adverse outcomes, 128
in children, 647–648, 647f
adverse outcomes, 648
clinical symptoms, 647
definition, 647
differential diagnosis, 647–648
referral decisions, 648
tests, 647, 647f
treatment, 648
adverse outcomes, 648
clinical symptoms, 127
definition, 127
differential diagnosis, 128
referral decisions, 128
synonym, 127
tests, 127–128
treatment, 128
adverse outcomes, 128
separation of, 115
Clavus. *See* Calluses; Corns
Claw toes, 412, 412f, 437, 475, 499, 513
orthotic devices for, 486f
Clenched fist injury. *See* Human bites
Clonus, 543
Clubfoot, 613–615, 613f
adverse outcomes, 614
clinical symptoms, 613
definition, 613, 613f
differential diagnosis, 614
gender and, 580
referral decisions, 615
synonyms, 613
tests, 613–614
treatment, 614–615
adverse outcomes, 615
Coaptation splint, 130, 130f
Cobb angle for scoliosis, 398f, 697
Cobb method in measuring curve magnitude on radiograph, 673
Colchicine for gouty arthritis, 26
Cold sensitivity, 242
Cold stress tests for reflex sympathetic dystrophy and complex regional pain syndromes, 67

for soft-tissue masses of foot and
ankle, 507
for trigger finger, 283, 285–286,
285f
for trochanteric bursitis, 336,
337–338, 337f
Cortisol suppression, transient serum,
23
Cortisone injections for arthritis, 214,
215
Cosmesis, 620
COX-1, 48
COX-2, 48
COX-2 inhibitors, 48, 50
Coxa vara, 616–617, 616f
acquired, 616–617
congenital, 616, 616f
developmental, 617
Craniofacial abnormalities, 628
C-reactive protein
for diskitis, 634
for inflammatory arthritis, 315
for osteomyelitis, 687
Crohn disease, 78, 703
Cross-body adduction, 113, 113f
Cruciate ligament. See Anterior cruciate
ligament (ACL)
Crutches, 15–16
gait patterns used with, 16, 16t
Cryotherapy, 70t
for plantar warts, 496
Crystal-induced arthritis, corticosteroids for, 21
Crystalline deposition diseases, 2–3,
24–27, 164
adverse outcomes, 26
clinical symptoms, 24–25
definition, 24
differential diagnosis, 26
referral decisions, 27
synonyms, 24
tests, 25
treatment, 26
adverse outcomes, 26
Cubital tunnel syndrome, 195. See also
under Ulnar nerve
Cubitus valgus, 195
Cumulative trauma disorders, 3. See
also Overuse syndromes
Curettage for plantar warts, 496
Cyclobenzaprine
for fibromyalgia syndrome, 35
tachyphylaxis as side effect of, 35
Cyclooxygenase (COX), 48
Cysts
epidermal inclusion, 287, 288t
flexor tendon, 261–262
ganglion, 287, 288t, 506
mucous, 261-263
in osteoarthritis, 320, 320f
popliteal, 397–398, 398f
rupture of popliteal, 355

# D

Dancer's toe. See Sesamoiditis
Debridement
for animal bites, 211
for ankle fractures, 450
for elbow arthritis, 171–172
for human bites, 267
for meniscal tears, 380–381
for osteochondritis dissecans, 383
for osteomyelitis, 444
Decompression
for cauda equina syndrome, 537,
538
for cervical spondylosis, 543
for metastatic disease, 568
for radial tunnel syndrome, 178
for septic arthritis, 75, 702
for septic olecranon bursitis, 190
for subungual hematomas, 274
for ulnar nerve compression, 197
Deep space infection, 211
Deep venous thrombosis (DVT), 100
Degenerative arthritis, 108. See also
Arthritis; Osteoarthritis (OA)
of the glenohumeral joint, 106
Degenerative disk disease of the cervical
spine. See Cervical spondylosis
Degenerative joint disease, 2. See also
Arthritis; Osteoarthritis (OA)
Degenerative spondylolisthesis, 569
Deltoid, testing of, 111, 111f, 530, 530f
de Quervain tenosynovitis, 21, 201,
203, 232–233, 232f
adverse outcomes, 233
clinical symptoms, 232
definition, 232
differential diagnosis, 232
Finkelstein test for, 208, 208f
injection for, 233, 234, 234f
referral decisions, 233
synonym, 232
tests, 232, 232f
treatment, 233
adverse outcomes, 233
trigger finger and, 282
Dermatophytic onychomycosis. See
under Nails
Destructive synovitis, 3
Developmental coxa vara, 617
Developmental dysplasia, 294,
630–633, 631f, 632f
adverse outcomes, 632
clinical symptoms, 630
definition, 630
differential diagnosis, 632
referral decisions, 633
risk for osteoarthritis and, 320, 321
synonyms, 630
tests, 630–632, 631f, 632f
treatment, 632–633
adverse outcomes of, 633
Diabetes mellitus, 442
corticosteroid injections and, 23
frozen shoulder and, 124
trigger finger and, 282, 283

Diabetic foot, 442–444, 442f, 443f
adverse outcomes, 444
care of, 445–447
clinical symptoms, 442, 442f
definition, 442
differential diagnosis, 443
referral decisions, 444
synonyms, 442
tests, 443, 443f
treatment, 444
adverse outcomes of, 444
Diabetic ulcers, 443
treatment of, 444
Die-punch fracture, 249, 249f
Diffuse idiopathic skeletal hyperostosis
(DISH), 28–29, 28f, 522, 525
adverse outcomes, 29
clinical symptoms, 28, 28f
definition, 28
differential diagnosis, 29
referral decisions, 29
synonyms, 28
tests, 28, 28f
treatment, 29
adverse outcomes, 29
Digital anesthetic block
for foot, 461–462, 461f
for hand, 240, 240f, 274, 280, 281
Direct load transfer, 13f
DISH. See Diffuse idiopathic skeletal
hyperostosis (DISH)
Disk herniation, 122, 295, 537. See also
Lumbar herniated disk
Diskitis, 634–635, 634f
adverse outcomes, 635
clinical symptoms, 634
definition, 634, 634f
differential diagnosis, 635
referral decisions, 635
tests, 634–635
treatment, 635
adverse outcomes, 635
Dislocations
of distal interphalangeal joint, 281
of elbow, 173–175, 173f, 174f, 594
of glenohumeral joint, 107
of hip, 303–305, 303f, 304f
of knee, 617, 617f
Lisfranc, 426
of metacarpophalangeal joint, 278,
279, 280, 280f
of metatarsophalangeal joint, 499
of midfoot, 456–458, 456f, 457f
of patella, 342, 617
of radial head, 622, 622f
of shoulder, 135, 151–152, 151f
of wrist, 278–281, 278f, 279f, 280f
Distal interphalangeal (DIP) joint
boutonnière deformity and, 226
closed reduction of, 280
ganglion cyst and, 287
mallet finger and, 271–272, 271f,
272f
mucous cysts in, 261, 262
Dog bite wounds. See also Animal bites
bacteria isolated in, 210

Estrogen deficiency, trabecular bone
loss and, 57
Etodolac (Lodine), 50
Ewing sarcoma, 95, 599
Exercise programs
for ankle sprains, 424
for arthritis of the knee, 365
for biceps tendon rupture, 146
for brachial plexus injuries, 123
for bursitis, 370
for cervical sprains, 546
for complex regional pain syndromes, 67
for degenerative spondylolisthesis,
574
for fibromyalgia syndrome, 35
for flatfoot, 641
for frozen shoulder, 125
for impingement syndrome, 138
for inflammatory arthritis, 317
for isthmic spondylolisthesis, 576
for low back sprain, 555
for lumbar degenerative disk disease, 557
for lumbar spinal stenosis, 565
for osteoarthritis, 52
for plantar fasciitis, 489
for radial tunnel syndrome, 178
for rotator cuff tears, 143
for shoulder rehabilitation,
153–154, 153f, 154f, 155f,
156
for toe walking, 718
for torticollis, 720–721
Exertional compartment syndromes,
62, 63, 357–358
Extensor hallucis longus, testing, 416,
416f, 532, 532f
Extensor mechanism tendinitis. See
Patellar tendinitis; Quadriceps
tendinitis
Extensor tendon injury. See Mallet finger
External femoral torsion. See Outtoeing
External rotation contracture of infancy.
See Outtoeing
External rotation test in diagnosing
injury to the syndesmosis, 423
External tibial torsion. See Outtoeing

# F

FABER test, 78, 302, 302f
Facet joint arthritis, 295
Falls and musculoskeletal injuries in
elderly patient
adverse outcomes, 31
clinical symptoms, 31
definition, 30
referral decisions, 32
tests, 31
treatment, 31–32
adverse outcomes, 32
Fanconi anemia, 627

Fasciotomy. See also Surgery
for compartment syndrome, 18–19
Fat embolism, femoral shaft fractures
and, 308
Fat pad sign
as sign of distal humeral fracture,
183, 183f
as sign of elbow fractures, 655, 656f
as sign of occult fractures, 593, 593f
Feet. See Foot and ankle disorders;
Lower extremities
Felons, 237, 237f. See also under
Fingertips
Femoral anteversion, 388, 390–391,
666. See also Intoeing
correction of, 669
Femoral condyle, osteonecrosis of,
385–386
adverse outcomes, 386
clinical symptoms, 385
definition, 385
referral decisions, 386
synonym, 385
tests, 385
treatment, 386
adverse outcomes, 386
Femoral retroversion, 666, 667. See also
Outtoeing
Femoral torsion, 667. See also Intoeing
Femur
distal fracture of, 376–377, 376f
fracture of, 306-308, 307f
adverse outcomes, 308
in children, 658–659
adverse outcomes, 658
clinical symptoms, 658
definition, 658
differential diagnosis, 658
referral decisions, 659
tests, 658
treatment, 659
adverse outcomes, 659
clinical symptoms, 306
definition, 306
differential diagnosis, 306, 308
referral decisions, 308
tests, 306, 307f
treatment, 308
adverse outcomes, 308
Legg-Calvé-Perthes disease,
675–677, 676f
adverse outcomes, 676
clinical symptoms, 675
definition, 675
differential diagnosis, 676
gender and, 580
referral decisions, 677
synonyms, 675
tests, 675–676, 676f
treatment, 676–677
adverse outcomes, 677
proximal fracture of, 312–314,
312f, 313f
adverse outcomes, 313
clinical symptoms, 312

definition, 312
differential diagnosis, 312
referral decisions, 314
tests, 312, 312f, 313f
treatment, 313–314
adverse outcomes, 314
shaft fractures, 659
slipped capital femoral epiphysis,
708–710, 709f
adverse outcomes, 710
assessment of hip rotation in,
585
clinical symptoms, 708
definition, 708
differential diagnosis, 710
referral decisions, 710
synonyms, 708
tests, 709, 709f
treatment, 710
adverse outcomes, 710
Fibroma, 98
Fibromatosis. See Soft-tissue masses of
the foot and ankle
Fibromyalgia syndrome, 3, 33–35, 33f
adverse outcomes, 35
clinical symptoms, 33–34, 33f
definition, 33
differential diagnosis, 34–35
referral decisions, 35
tests, 34
treatment, 35
adverse outcomes, 35
Fibula
congenital absence of, 623–624,
624f
fracture of distal, 448
stress fractures of, 356–357, 357f
Fibular hemimelia, 623–624, 624f
Fight bite. See Human bites
Fighter's fracture. See Metacarpals, fractures of; Phalangeal fractures
Fingertips. See also Nails
infections of, 237–239, 238f, 239f
adverse outcomes, 238
clinical symptoms, 237
definition, 237
differential diagnosis, 238
referral decisions, 239
synonyms, 237
tests, 237–238
treatment, 238–239, 238f, 239f
adverse outcomes, 239f
injuries/amputations of, 241–243
adverse outcomes, 242
clinical symptoms, 241
definition, 241
differential diagnosis, 242
referral decisions, 243
tests, 241
treatment, 242–243
adverse outcomes, 243
Finkelstein test, 203
for de Quervain tenosynovitis, 208,
208f, 232, 232f
First metatarsophalangeal joint sprain.
See Turf toe

INDEX

INDEX

INDEX

Olecranon bursa, 189
    aspiration of, 189, 191–192, 191*f*
Olecranon bursitis, 164, 165, 189–190,
    189*f*
    adverse outcomes, 190
    clinical symptoms, 189
    definition, 189, 189*f*
    differential diagnosis, 190
    referral decisions, 190
    septic, 190
    tests, 189–190
    treatment, 190
        adverse outcomes, 190
Olecranon fractures, 655
Oligoarticular peripheral joint arthritis,
    2
Onychocryptosis. *See* Ingrown toenail
Onychomycosis, 482
Opponens strength, 207, 207*f*
Oral hypoglycemic agents, 50
Orthotics, 484–486
    application of, 486, 486*f*
    for bunionettes, 431–432
    cervical
        halo brace, 571
        Philadelphia collar, 571
        rigid cervical orthotics, 571
        soft cervical collar, 571
    definition, 484
    for flatfoot, 641
    foot types and functions, 484, 484*f*
    for hallux rigidus, 427
    for isthmic spondylolisthesis, 576
    for juvenile rheumatoid arthritis,
        672
    lumbar
        elastic belts, 572
        lumbosacral corset, 572
        rigid orthotics, 572
    for metatarsal fractures, 454
    for midfoot arthritis, 428
    for plantar fasciitis, 489
    for posterior tibial tendon dysfunc-
        tion, 498
    for rheumatoid foot and ankle, 500
    for seronegative spondylo-
        arthropathies, 704
    for spondyloisthesis, 713
    for tarsal tunnel syndrome, 512
    thoracic
        Jewett or other similar three-
            point orthosis, 572
        thoracolumbosacral corset, 571
        total-contact thoracolumbar
            orthosis, 572
    for turf toe, 517
    types of, 484–485
Ortolani maneuver, 630–631, 631*f*
Ortolani sign, dislocated hip and, 584,
    584*f*, 631, 631*f*
Os acromiale, 135
Osgood-Schlatter disease, 581, 588,
    588*f*, 684–685, 684*f*
    adverse outcomes, 684–685
    clinical symptoms, 684

definition, 684
differential diagnosis, 684
referral decisions, 685
synonyms, 684
tests, 684, 684*f*
treatment, 685
    adverse outcomes, 685
Osteoarthritis (OA), 2, 24, 50, 51–52.
    *See also* Arthritis
    adverse outcomes, 52
    alternative therapies for, 53–54
        chondroitin sulfate, 53–54
        glucosamine, 53–54
        S-adenosyl-L-methionine, 54
        viscosupplements, 54
    clinical symptoms, 51
    corticosteroids for, 21
    definition, 51
    differential diagnosis, 51
    in elbow, 170
    of the hip, 320–321, 320*f*
        adverse outcomes, 321
        clinical symptoms, 320
        definition, 320
        differential diagnosis, 321
        referral decisions, 321
        synonyms, 320
        tests, 320, 320*f*
        treatment, 321
            adverse outcomes, 321
    midfoot, 426
    primary, 2, 213
    referral decisions, 52
    secondary, 2, 213
    of shoulder, 118–119, 118*f*
    synonyms, 51
    tests, 51
    treatment, 52
        adverse outcomes, 52
Osteoarthrosis. *See* Osteoarthritis (OA)
Osteochondral lesion, 409
    of the talus, 597
Osteochondral loose body, 595
Osteochondritis dissecans, 382–384,
    382*f*
    adverse outcomes, 383
    in children, 587–588, 587*f*, 595,
        595*f*
    clinical symptoms, 382
    definition, 382, 382*f*
    differential diagnosis, 384
    referral decisions, 384
    tests, 384
    treatment, 383
        adverse outcomes, 384
Osteochondritis of the tibial tuberosity.
    *See* Osgood-Schlatter disease
Osteogenesis imperfecta, 57
    pediatric, 611
Osteoid osteoma, 599
Osteomalacia, 57
Osteomyelitis, 37, 55–56, 211
    acute, 686
    adverse outcomes, 56
    cavitary subacute, 686

in children, 686–688
    adverse outcomes, 687
    clinical symptoms, 686
    definition, 686
    differential diagnosis, 687
    referral decisions, 688
    tests, 686–687
    treatment, 688
        adverse outcomes, 688
chronic, 686
clinical symptoms, 55
definition, 55
differential diagnosis, 56
distinguishing from Charcot
    arthropathy, 443
referral decisions, 56
subacute, 686
synonym, 55
tests, 55–56
treatment, 56, 444
    adverse outcomes, 56
Osteonecrosis. *See also* Kienböck dis-
    ease
    arthritis and, 315
    of the capitellum, 595
    of the femoral condyle, 385–386
        adverse outcomes, 386
        clinical symptoms, 385
        definition, 385
        referral decisions, 386
        synonym, 385
        tests, 385
        treatment, 386
            adverse outcomes, 386
    of the femoral head, 304, 317, 658
    of the hip, 322–324, 322*ft*, 323*f*
        adverse outcomes, 324
        clinical symptoms, 322
        definition, 322, 322*t*
        differential diagnosis, 323
        referral decisions, 324
        synonyms, 322
        tests, 322–323, 322*f*, 323*f*
        treatment, 324
            adverse outcomes, 324
    of the navicular, 598, 598*f*
    risk of, 304, 322*t*
    scaphoid fractures and, 252
    of the shoulder, 118
    of the talus, 452
Osteopenia, pediatric, 611
Osteophytes, 2, 51
    in osteoarthritis, 320, 320*f*
Osteoporosis, 3, 57–61
    adverse outcomes, 59
    clinical symptoms, 57
    definition, 57
    differential diagnosis, 58
    fracture management and, 31
    of the hip
        fractures and, 312
        transient, 333–334
            adverse outcomes, 334
            clinical symptoms, 333
            definition, 333

INDEX

Radiation
    for metastatic disease, 568
    for plantar warts, 496
    for soft-tissue tumors, 99
Radicular arm pain, 522, 523f
Radicular leg pain, 522, 524–525, 525f
Radiculopathy, 541, 559–560
Radiocapitellar joint, 164
Radiocarpal arthritis, 202
Radiographs, 25, 40–41, 40t
    of accessory navicular, 602, 602f
    of acromioclavicular injuries, 116,
        361
    of animal bites, 211
    of ankle fractures, 448–449, 448f,
        449f
    of ankle sprains, 423
    of anterior knee pain in children,
        585
    of arthritis, 119, 119f, 170f, 171,
        174, 213f, 214, 217, 217f,
        218f, 222, 222f, 364, 364f,
        427, 427f
    of back pain, 589–590
    of bipartite patella, 366
    of bone tumors, 95, 95f
    of boutonnière deformity, 225, 225f
    of brachial plexus injuries, 122
    of bursitis of the knee, 369
    of calcaneal apophysitis, 604–605,
        604f
    of calcaneus and tallus fractures,
        451
    of carpal tunnel syndrome, 228
    of cauda equina syndrome, 538
    of cavus foot deformity, 606, 607f
    of cervical radiculopathy, 540
    of cervical spinal fractures, 548–549
    of cervical spondylosis, 543, 543f
    of cervical sprains, 545–546
    of child abuse, 610–611, 610f, 611f
    of chronic lateral ankle pain, 434
    of clavicle fractures, 127f, 128, 647
    of collateral ligament tears, 374
    of complex regional pain syn-
        dromes, 66
    of congenital deformities, 616, 616f,
        617f, 618f, 622f, 624f
    of degenerative spondylolisthesis,
        573, 573f
    of de Quervain tenosynovitis, 232
    of developmental dysplasia of the
        hip, 631
    of diabetic foot, 443, 443f
    of diffuse idiopathic skeletal hyper-
        ostosis, 28, 28f
    of diskitis, 634
    of dislocations, 278–279, 279f
    of distal biceps tendon rupture, 193
    of distal forearm fractures, 650,
        650f
    of distal humeral fractures, 182f,
        183, 183f
    of distal radius fractures, 250
    of elbow dislocation, 173f, 174

    of elbow fractures, 655
    of elbow pain, 593
    of epicondylitis, 178
    of femoral shaft fractures, 306, 307f
    of femur fractures, 658
    of fingertip injuries, 241
    of flexor tendon injuries, 246
    of foot and ankle pain in children,
        596–597
    of fracture-dislocation of the mid-
        foot, 456–457, 457f
    of fracture of the growth plate, 644
    of fractures, 36
    of frozen shoulder, 125
    of ganglia, 263
    of genu valgum, 662
    of genu varum, 664, 664f
    of hallux rigidus, 464, 464f
    of hip dislocations, 303, 304f
    of hip strains, 328
    of human bites, 267
    of humeral shaft fractures, 129,
        129f
    of impingement syndrome, 136f,
        137
    of ingrown toenails, 468
    of isthmic spondylolisthesis, 575,
        576f
    of Kienböck disease, 269, 269f, 270
    of knee fractures, 377
    of kyphosis, 672–673
    of lateral femoral cutaneous nerve
        syndrome, 318
    of Legg-Calvé-Perthes disease,
        675–676, 676f
    of limping children, 638
    of low back sprain, 554
    of lumbar degenerative disk disease,
        556–557, 557f
    of lumbar herniated disk, 561
    of lumbar spinal fractures,
        550–551, 550f, 551f
    of lumbar spinal stenosis, 564
    of mallet finger, 271
    of meniscal tears, 380
    of metastatic disease, 567
    of metatarsal fractures, 453, 454f
    of metatarsalgia, 475
    of Morton neuroma, 478
    of nail injuries, 273, 274
    of neonatal brachial plexus palsy,
        682
    of olecranon fracture, 186
    of Osgood-Schlatter disease, 684,
        684f
    of osteoarthritis, 51, 171, 320, 320f
    of osteochondritis dissecans, 383
    of osteomyelitis, 55, 687
    of osteonecrosis, 322–323, 322f,
        385
    of osteoporosis, 333
    of overuse syndromes, 63
    of patellar/quadriceps tendinitis,
        393
    of patellofemoral instability and
        malalignment, 388, 388f

    of patellofemoral pain, 391, 391f
    of pelvic fractures, 309f, 310
    of phalangeal fractures, 459
    of plantar fasciitis, 487–488, 488f
    of plica syndrome, 395
    of posterior cruciate ligament
        sprain, 400
    of posterior heel pain, 494, 494f
    of posterior tibial tendon dysfunc-
        tion, 498
    of prepatellar bursitis, 402
    of proximal and middle forearm
        fractures, 652
    of proximal femur fractures, 312,
        312f
    of proximal humerus fractures, 132,
        132f, 133f, 647, 647f
    of quadriceps and patellar tendon
        rupture, 405
    of rheumatoid arthritis, 72
    of rotator cuff tears, 142, 142f
    of scaphoid fractures, 252–253,
        253f
    of scapular fractures, 134, 135f
    of scoliosis, 569
    of septic arthritis, 74–75
    of seronegative spondylo-
        arthropathies, 78, 79f
    of sesamoiditis, 502
    of shoulder instability, 148, 149f
    of shoulder problems, 108
    of slipped capital femoral epiphysis,
        709, 709f
    of snapping hip, 325
    of soft-tissue masses of foot and
        ankle, 506
    of spondylolisthesis, 712, 712f
    of sprains, 92, 278–279, 279f
    of stress fractures, 508, 508f, 509f
    of tarsal coalition, 715, 715f
    of tarsal tunnel syndrome, 512
    of thigh strains, 330
    of thoracic outlet syndrome, 158
    of thoracic spinal fractures,
        550–551, 550f, 551f
    of tibial fractures, 660–661
    of toe deformities, 514
    of torticollis, 720
    of transient synovitis of the hip,
        722–723
    of trochanteric bursitis, 335
    of tumors of hand and wrist, 288,
        289
    of turf toe, 516
Radiohumeral synostosis, 628
Radioulnar joint, proximal, 164
Radius
    congenital dislocation of head, 622,
        622f
    congenital radial-ulnar synostosis
        and, 621, 622f
    distal fractures of, 65, 249–251,
        249f, 251f
        adverse outcomes, 250
        clinical symptoms, 250

definition, 249, 249f
differential diagnosis, 250
referral decisions, 251
synonyms, 249
tests, 250
treatment, 250–251, 251f
adverse outcomes, 251
fractures of head, 178, 187-188,
187f
clinical symptoms, 187
definition, 187, 187f
differential diagnosis, 187–188
referral decisions, 188
tests, 187
treatment, 188
Range of motion, 7
arthritis and, 119
for cervical spine, 527–528, 527f,
528f
for elbow and forearm, 167–168,
167f, 168f
for foot and ankle, 414–415, 414f,
415f
for hand and wrist, 205–206, 206f
for hip and thigh, 298–300, 298f,
299f, 300f
for knee and lower leg, 350, 350f
for lumbar spine, 528–529, 528f,
529f
musculoskeletal problems and, 6
in pediatric orthopaedics, 583, 583f
for shoulder, 107, 110–111,
110–111f
Range-of-motion brace for anterior cruciate ligament tear, 362
Range-of-motion exercises
for anterior cruciate ligament tear,
362
for bipartite patella, 367
Raynaud phenomenon, 242
Rectus femoris, strain of, 328
Recurrent dislocation. See under
Shoulder disorders
Recurrent paronychia infections, 288
Reflex sympathetic dystrophy (RSD),
65–68, 66f
adverse outcomes, 67
clinical symptoms, 65–66, 66f
definition, 65
differential diagnosis, 67
referral decisions, 68
synonyms, 65
tests, 66–67
treatment, 67–68
adverse outcomes, 68
Rehabilitation, 69
for collateral ligament tears, 374
definition, 69
for fractures, 38
for hip strains, 329, 329t
referral decisions, 69
for shoulder, 153–156, 153f, 154f,
155f
for thigh strains, 331
treatment, 69, 70t
adverse outcomes, 69

Reiter disease, 77, 79. See also
Seronegative spondylo-
arthropathies
Reiter syndrome, 704. See also
Seronegative spondylo-
arthropathies
Renal transplantation, osteonecrosis of
the femoral condyle and, 385
Repetitive strain injury. See Overuse
syndromes
Residual limb pain, 14
Residual limb ulcers or infection, 13
Resisted pronation, 168, 168f
Resisted supination, 168, 168f
Resisted wrist extension, 169, 169f
Resisted wrist flexion, 169, 169f
Rest, ice, compression, and elevation
(RICE), 89
for collateral ligament tears, 374
for meniscal tears, 381
for sprains and strains, 93
for turf toe, 517
Retrocalcaneal bursitis, 493
Retrolisthesis, 573
Retropatellar pain, 387–388
Retroperitoneal lesions, 525
Reverse straight-leg raising test, 535,
535f, 560
Reversible hepatotoxicity, 49
Rheumatoid arthritis (RA), 2–3, 71–73.
See also Arthritis; Juvenile
rheumatoid arthritis (JRA)
adverse outcomes, 72
clinical symptoms, 71–72, 119
corticosteroids for, 21
crystalline deposition disease and,
24
definition, 71
differential diagnosis, 72
in the elbow, 164, 170, 171
in the hands, 214
in the hip, 294
medical management of, 171
nonsteroidal anti-inflammatory
drugs for, 48, 50
popliteal cysts and, 397
referral decisions, 73
in the shoulder, 118, 119
tests, 72
in the toe, 513
treatment, 72–73
adverse outcomes, 73
trigger finger and, 282, 283
Rheumatoid factor
for arthritis, 222
for inflammatory arthritis, 315
for rheumatoid foot and ankle, 499
Rheumatoid foot and ankle, 499–500,
499f, 500f
adverse outcomes, 500
clinical symptoms, 499, 499f
definition, 499
differential diagnosis, 499
referral decisions, 500
tests, 499, 500f

treatment, 500
adverse outcomes, 500
Rheumatoid synovitis, 213
Rhomboid, muscle testing of, 113
Rib fractures, 134
in child abuse, 610–611
Rickets, 581
Rigid cervical orthotics, 571
Rigid flatfoot. See Tarsal coalition
Rigid orthotics, 572
Rolando fracture, 259
Rotator cuff, 136
deficiency, 119
muscles of, 141, 141f
pathology, 106
strengthening program for, 138
tears of, 106, 107, 108, 119, 119f,
141–143, 141f
adverse outcomes, 143
arthropathy of, 118, 119, 119f
clinical symptoms, 142
definition, 141, 141f
differential diagnosis, 142–143
referral decisions, 143
synonyms, 141
treatment, 143
adverse outcomes, 143
tendinitis, 137 (See also
Impingement syndrome)
RSD. See Reflex sympathetic dystrophy
Run-around abscess, 237
Runner's painful knee, orthotic devices
for, 486f
Ruptured popliteal cyst, 100

## S

Sacroiliac joint, 294
Sacroilitis, 2, 77
Sacrum, 294
S-adenosyl-L-methionine (SAM), for
osteoarthritis, 54
Salsalate (Disalcid), 50
Salter-Harris fracture classification, 644
Saphenous nerve, compression of, 369
Sarcomas, 98
Ewing, 599
synovial cell, 599
Scaphoid, fracture of, 252–254
adverse outcomes, 253, 254
clinical symptoms, 252
definition, 252
differential diagnosis, 253
referral decisions, 254
tests, 252–253
treatment, 253–254
adverse outcomes, 254
Scapholunate joint, ganglion over, 262
Scapular fractures, 134–135, 135f
adverse outcomes, 135
clinical symptoms, 134
definition, 134
differential diagnosis, 134–135
referral decisions, 135

INDEX

INDEX

Synovial cell sarcoma, 599
Synovial cyst. *See* Ganglia; Popliteal cyst
Synovial inflammation, detection of, 315
Synovitis. *See also* Arthritis
  chronic, 499
  destructive, 3
  of the hip (*See* Inflammatory arthritis)
  metatarsophalangeal, 499
  rheumatoid, 213
  subtalar, 409
Synovium, hypertrophy of, 74
Syringomyelia, 591
Systemic lupus erythematosus
  arthritis and, 315
  and osteonecrosis of the femoral condyle, 385

## T

Tachyphylaxis as side effect of amitriptyline and/or cyclobenzaprine, 35
Tailor's bunion. *See* Bunionettes
Talipes equinovarus, 624. *See also* Clubfoot
Talocalcaneal arthritis, 427
Talocalcaneal bars. *See also* Tarsal coalition
  distinguishing on radiographs, 597
Talocalcaneal coalition, 714
Talonavicular arthritis, 426, 427, 428
Talonavicular joint, amputations at, 12
Talus, fractures of, 451–452, 452*f*
  adverse outcomes, 452
  clinical symptoms, 451
  definition, 451
  differential diagnosis, 451
  referral decisions, 452
  synonyms, 451
  tests, 451, 452*f*
  treatment, 452
    adverse outcomes, 452
Tardy ulnar palsy. *See* Ulnar nerve, compression of
Tarsal coalition in children, 596, 597, 714–716, 715*f*
  adverse outcomes, 715
  clinical symptoms, 714
  definition, 714
  differential diagnosis, 715
  referral decisions, 716
  synonyms, 714
  tests, 714–715, 715*f*
  treatment, 715–716
    adverse outcomes, 716
Tarsal navicular bone, accessory navicular and, 602–603
  adverse outcomes, 602
  clinical symptoms, 602
  definition, 602
  differential diagnosis, 602
  referral decisions, 603

tests, 602, 602*f*
  treatment, 603
    adverse outcomes, 603
Tarsal tunnel syndrome, 409, 452, 511–512, 511*f*, 512*f*
  adverse outcomes, 512
  clinical symptoms, 511
  definition, 511, 511*f*
  differential diagnosis, 512
  referral decisions, 512
  synonyms, 511
  tests, 511–512, 512*f*
  treatment, 512
    adverse outcomes, 512
Tarsometatarsal dislocation, 426
TAR syndrome (thrombocytopenia), 628
Tendinitis, 3
  Achilles, 598, 703, 704
  flexor, 62
  NSAIDs in treating, 48
  patellar, 62, 393–394, 393*f*, 703
  quadriceps, 393–394, 393*f*, 586
  rotator cuff, 137
  tibial, 62
Tendoachilles rupture. *See* Achilles tendon, rupture of
Tendon rupture, 23. *See also* Flexor tendon injuries
Tennis elbow, 62. *See also* Epicondylitis
  injection for, 178, 180–181, 180*f*
Tenosynovitis, 3, 436. *See also* de Quervain tenosynovitis
  corticosteroids for, 21
  flexor, 21, 62
  septic flexor, 247, 247*f*
Teres minor muscle testing, 112, 112*f*
Testosterone deficiency, trabecular bone loss and, 57
Tetanus immunization status, 242
Tetanus prophylaxis in wound management, 212*t*, 268*t*, 277
Tethered spinal cord, 591
Tetracycline
  for human bites, 268
  for seronegative spondyloarthropathies, 78
Thenar atrophy, 227, 227*f*
Thermotherapy, 70*t*
Thigh, strains of, 330–332, 331*f*, 332*f*
  adverse outcomes, 331
  clinical symptoms, 330
  definition, 330
  differential diagnosis, 331
  referral decisions, 332
  tests, 330, 331*f*
  treatment, 331, 332*f*
    adverse outcomes, 332
Thomas test in diagnosing hip flexion contracture, 299, 299*f*
Thompson test in diagnosing Achilles tendon rupture, 420
Thoracic kyphosis, 57

Thoracic outlet syndrome, 157–160, 159*f*, 203
  adverse outcomes, 159
  clinical symptoms, 157–158
  definition, 157
  differential diagnosis, 158
  referral decisions, 160
  tests, 158
  treatment, 159–160, 159*f*
    adverse outcomes, 160
Thoracic spine, fractures of, 550–552, 550*f*, 551*f*
  adverse outcomes, 551
  clinical symptoms, 550
  definition, 550
  differential diagnosis, 551
  referral decisions, 552
  tests, 550–551, 550*f*, 551*f*
  treatment, 551
    adverse outcomes, 551
Thoracolumbar corset, 551
Thoracolumbosacral corset, 571
Three-point orthosis, 572
Thrombophlebitis, 324
Thumb
  absence of, 627
  arthritis of carpometacarpal joint, 217–219, 217*f*
    injection for, 220–221, 220*f*
  flexion/extension of, 206, 206*f*
  fracture of base, 259–260, 259*f*
    adverse outcomes, 260
    clinical symptoms, 259
    definition, 259, 259*f*
    differential diagnosis, 260
    referral decisions, 260
    synonyms, 259
    tests, 260
    treatment, 260
      adverse outcomes, 260
  gamekeeper's, 278
  range of motion testing for, 206, 206*f*
  skier's, 278
  Watson stress test for carpometacarpal arthritis of, 209, 209*f*
Thumb sign for posterior cruciate ligament, 352, 352*f*, 400, 400*f*
Thumb spica cast, 279
Thyroid function tests to rule out hyperthyroidism or hyperparathyroidism, 58
Tibia
  anterolateral bowing of, 618, 618*f*
  congenital absence of, 624–625, 625*f*
  fractures of the, in children, 660–661, 660*t*
    adverse outcomes, 661
    clinical symptoms, 660
    definition, 660, 660*t*
    differential diagnosis, 661
    referral decisions, 661
    tests, 660–661

treatment, 661
    adverse outcomes, 661
    posteromedial bowing of, 617*f*, 618
    stress fractures of, 356–357, 357*f*
Tibial hemimelia, 624–625, 625*f*
Tibialis, testing for, 532, 532*f*
Tibial nerve entrapment, 512
Tibial plateau fractures, 376, 376*f*
Tibial tendinitis, 62
Tibial torsion, 388, 666, 668
Tibiofemoral instability, 344–345
Tilleaux fractures, 661
Tinea ungulum. *See* Nails, fungus infection in
Tinel test
    for carpal tunnel syndrome, 228, 228*f*
    for chronic ankle/subtalar instability, 435
    for tarsal tunnel syndrome, 512
    for thoracic outlet syndrome, 203
    for ulnar nerve compression, 195
    for ulnar nerve entrapment, 290–291
Toddler's fracture, 611
Toes. *See also* Turf toe
    amputation of, 11
    congenital curly, 619
    deformities of, 513–515, 513*f*
        adverse outcomes, 514
        clinical symptoms, 513–514
        definition, 513, 513*f*
        differential diagnosis, 514
        referral decisions, 515
        tests, 514
        treatment, 514, 514*f*
            adverse outcomes, 515
Toe walking in children, 717–718, 717*f*
    adverse outcomes, 718
    clinical symptoms, 717
    definition, 717
    differential diagnosis, 717
    referral decisions, 718
    tests, 717, 717*f*
    treatment, 718
        adverse outcomes, 718
Too many toes sign, 411, 411*f*, 497, 497*f*
Tophi, 25, 189
Torn cartilage. *See* Meniscal tears
Torn cruciate. *See under* Anterior cruciate ligament (ACL)
Torticollis in children, 719–721, 719*f*
    adverse outcomes, 720
    clinical symptoms, 719
    definition, 719, 719*f*
    developmental dysplasia and, 630
    differential diagnosis, 720
    referral decisions, 721
    synonyms, 719
    tests, 719–720
    treatment, 720–721
        adverse outcomes, 721
Torus fracture, 649
Total-contact thoracolumbar orthosis, 572

Toxic synovitis. *See* Transient synovitis of the hip in children
Trabecular bone loss, 57
Traction for femoral shaft fractures, 308
Transcutaneous electrical nerve stimulation (TENS)
    for complex regional pain syndromes, 68
    for reflex sympathetic dystrophy, 68
    for thoracic outlet syndrome, 160
Transfemoral amputation, 12
Transient hyperglycemia, 23
Transient osteoporosis of the hip, 333–334
    adverse outcomes, 334
    clinical symptoms, 333
    definition, 333
    differential diagnosis, 333
    referral decisions, 334
    synonym, 333
    tests, 333
    treatment, 334
        adverse outcomes, 334
Transient serum cortisol suppression, 23
Transient synovitis of the hip in children, 722–723
    adverse outcomes, 723
    clinical symptoms, 722
    definition, 722
    differential diagnosis, 723
    referral decisions, 723
    synonyms, 722
    tests, 722–723
    treatment, 723
        adverse outcomes, 723
Transmetatarsal amputation, 11–12
Transtibial amputation, 12
Transverse deficiency of the forearm, 628–629, 628*f*
Trauma, 3
    lower extremity amputations and, 11
    repetitive, as cause of ulnar nerve entrapment, 290
    spinal, 525
Traumatic arthritis, 294
    in foot and ankle, 426
Traumatic compartment syndrome, 3
Trendelenburg test, 302, 302*f*
Triceps, testing of, 530, 530*f*
*Trichophyton mentagrophytes* in nail fungus infection, 482
*Trichophyton rubrum* in nail fungus infection, 482
Tricyclic antidepressants
    for complex regional pain syndromes, 68
    for fibromyalgia syndrome, 35
Trigger finger, 282–284, 282*f*, 285*f*
    adverse outcomes, 283
    clinical symptoms, 282–283
    definition, 282, 282*f*
    differential diagnosis, 283
    injection for, 285–286, 285*f*

referral decisions, 284
synonyms, 282
tests, 283
treatment, 283
    adverse outcomes, 283
Trimalleolar injuries, 448
Triplane fracture, 661
Trochanteric bursitis, 325, 335–336, 335*f*, 524
    adverse outcomes, 336
    clinical symptoms, 335
    definition, 335, 335*f*
    differential diagnosis, 335–336
    injection, 337–338, 337*f*
    referral decisions, 336
    synonym, 335
    tests, 335, 335*f*
    treatment, 336
        adverse outcomes, 336
Tumors. *See also* Metastatic disease
    about the elbow, 595
    bone, 94–97, 94*t*, 95*f*
        adverse outcomes, 97
        clinical symptoms, 95
        definition, 94, 94*t*
        differential diagnosis, 96–97
        referral decisions, 97
        synonyms, 94
        tests, 95–96, 95*f*
        treatment, 97
            adverse outcomes, 97
    frozen shoulder and, 124
    of the hand and wrist, 287–289, 288*t*, 289*f*
        adverse outcomes, 289
        clinical symptoms, 287
        definition, 287
        differential diagnosis, 288, 288*t*, 289*f*
        referral decisions, 289
        tests, 287–288
        treatment, 289
            adverse outcomes, 289
    pediatric foot, 599
    soft tissue, 98–99
        adverse outcomes, 99
        clinical symptoms, 98
        definition, 98
        differential diagnosis, 99
        referral decisions, 99
        tests, 98
        treatment, 99
            adverse outcomes, 99
Turf toe, 89, 516–517
    adverse outcomes, 516
    clinical symptoms, 516
    definition, 516
    differential diagnosis, 516
    referral decisions, 517
    synonyms, 516
    tests, 516
    treatment, 517
        adverse outcomes, 517
Type II osteoporosis, 57
Type I osteoporosis, 57

INDEX

# COMMON ORTHOPAEDIC TERMS

**Abduction** The movement of a body part away from the midline.

**Adduction** The movement of a body part towards the midline.

**Ankylosis** Marked stiffness of a joint typically observed with end stage arthritis, following a complex intra-articular fracture, delayed treatment of septic arthritis, or severe rheumatoid arthritis.

**Arthrodesis** The surgical fusion of a joint. The procedure removes any remaining articular cartilage and positions the adjacent bones to promote bone growth across a joint. A successful fusion eliminates the joint and stops motion. The usual purpose is pain relief or stabilization of an undependable joint.

**Arthroplasty** A procedure to replace or mobilize a joint, typically performed by removing the arthritic surfaces and replacing them with an implant. Total joint arthroplasty is replacement of both sides of the joint. Hemiarthroplasty replaces only one side of a joint.

**Capsule** A collagenous structure that surrounds a joint like a sleeve. The capsule allows motion of joints and protects the articular cartilage. The capsule, along with ligaments, tendons, and bony structure, provides stability of the joint.

**Cavus** Excessive height of the longitudinal arch of the foot.

**Closed fracture** A fracture that does not disrupt the integrity of the surrounding skin.

**Closed reduction** A procedure to restore normal alignment of a fractured bone or dislocated joint; no incision is needed, the fractured bones are simply manipulated.

**Comminuted** A fracture that has more than two fragments.

**Condyle** A rounded process at the end of a long bone.

**Cox-, Coxa** Hip. Coxa vara is a varus (or adduction) deformity of the hip. Coxa valgus is aligned in the opposite direction.

**Cubitus** Elbow. Cubitus varus is a bowing (or adduction) deformity of the elbow. Cubitus valgus is aligned in the opposite direction.

**Delayed union** A delay in normal fracture healing; not necessarily a pathologic process.

**Diaphysis** The shaft of a long bone.

**Dislocation** Complete disruption in the normal relationship of two bones forming a joint (ie, no contact of the articular surfaces). The direction of the dislocation is described by the position of the distal bone (ie, with an anterior dislocation of the shoulder, the humerus is displaced anterior to the scapula).

**Equinus** Plantar flexed position of the ankle.

**Epiphysis** The end of a long bone in a child that is formed from one or more secondary ossification centers.

**External fixation** Stabilization of a fracture or unstable joint by inserting pins into bone proximal and distal to the injury that are then attached to an external frame.

**Fracture** A disruption in the integrity of a bone.

**Fracture-dislocation** A fracture of bone associated with a dislocation of its adjacent joint.

**Genu** Knee. Genu valgum is knock-knee deformity; genu varum is a bowleg deformity.

**Greenstick** A fracture that disrupts only one side of the bone. This fracture pattern is seen in children because of the greater plasticity of their bones.

**Hallux** The great toe.

**Impacted** A fracture pattern in which the fragments are pushed together; therefore, imparting some stability.

**Internal fixation** Surgical insertion of a device that stops motion across a fracture or joint to encourage bony healing or fusion.

**Kyphosis** Curvature of the spine that is convex posteriorly.

**Ligament** A collagenous tissue that spans two bones to stabilize a joint. Some ligaments are mere thickenings of the joint capsule while other ligaments are distinct structures.

**Lordosis** Curvature of the spine that is convex anteriorly.

**Malunion** Healing of a fracture in an unacceptable position.